OPHTHALMOLOGY

PRINCIPLES AND CONCEPTS

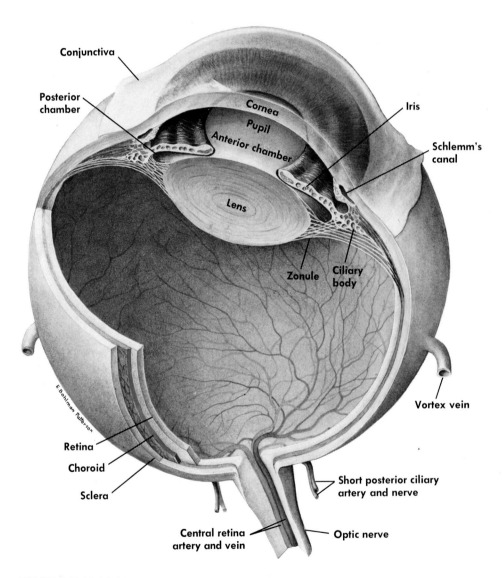

Conjunctiva

Posterior
chamber

Cornea

Pupil

Anterior chamber

Iris

Schlemm's
canal

Lens

Zonule

Ciliary
body

E. Bohlman Patterson

Vortex vein

Retina

Choroid

Sclera

Short posterior ciliary
artery and nerve

Central retina
artery and vein

Optic nerve

THE HUMAN EYE

OPHTHALMOLOGY
PRINCIPLES AND CONCEPTS

FRANK W. NEWELL, M.D., M.SC. (Ophth.)

The James N. and Anna Louise Raymond Professor,
and Chairman, Department of Ophthalmology,
The University of Chicago;
Profesor Extraordinario de Oftalmólogia,
Universidad Autónoma de Barcelona

FOURTH EDITION

with 448 illustrations

THE C. V. MOSBY COMPANY

Saint Louis   1978

FOURTH EDITION

Copyright © 1978 by The C. V. Mosby Company

All rights reserved. No part of this book may be reproduced
in any manner without written permission of the publisher.

Previous editions copyrighted 1965, 1969, 1974

Printed in the United States of America

The C. V. Mosby Company
11830 Westline Industrial Drive, St. Louis, Missouri 63141

Library of Congress Cataloging in Publication Data

Newell, Frank W.
  Ophthalmology.

  Bibliography: p.
  Includes index.
  1. Ophthalmology. I. Title.
RE46.N57   1978   617'.7   78-6733
ISBN 0-8016-3640-X

CB/CB/B 9 8 7 6 5 4 3 2 1

To
Marian, Frank, Mary Susan,
Elizabeth Ann, *and* David Andrew

PREFACE

This text is an introduction to ophthalmology intended for the undergraduate and graduate student. As with earlier editions, its purpose is to integrate knowledge of the basic disciplines with understanding of ocular disorders and ocular manifestations of systemic disease. To meet the needs of nonophthalmologists, diseases of the eye are discussed without emphasis on refraction, optics, biomicroscopy, and related areas. Discussion of systemic disorders emphasizes the basic abnormality of the primary disease process rather than involvement of a particular portion of the eye. The text has been organized so that the student may intelligently interpret the symptoms arising from various abnormalities in order to carry out a meaningful examination.

The general format of the previous three editions has been retained, but nearly all sections have been revised to reflect the surge of information in the last few years: phagocytosis and renewal photoreceptor outer segment disks, the aldose-reductase pathway of galactose cataract formation, improved cytologic methods, photocoagulation, microsurgery, intraocular lenses, vitrectomy, enzyme assay of fibroblast cell culture, tear film abnormalities, computed tomography, ultrasonography, corneal endothelial function, visual evoked potential, glaucoma management, mechanisms of amblyopia, soft contact lenses, and new antibiotics. These and other changes have made ophthalmology far different from what it was a generation ago.

Many individuals took time from busy schedules to review various sections: Karl J. Fritz, Ronald N. Gaster, Walter M. Jay, Herbert E. Kaufman, Irving H. Leopold, Steven M. Podos, Joel M. Pokorny, David J. Schanzlin, Vivianne C. Smith, Daniel Snydacker, H. Stanley Thompson, Brenda J. Tripathi, Ramesh C. Tripathi, and Gunter K. von Noorden. They have my warm appreciation for their instruction and clarification of ambiguities of expression.

Professor Ramesh C. Tripathi and Mr. Ernest H. Heath, of the University of Chicago Department of Ophthalmology, and Charles S. Wellek, of the University of Chicago Audiovisual Department, provided numerous new illustrations. Lee Allen, of Iowa City, provided several new drawings.

As in the past, Mrs. Karin Cassel provided exceptional organizational and clerical skills and was generally indispensable in the completion of the text.

FRANK W. NEWELL

CONTENTS

ix

PART ONE
Basic mechanisms

Chapter 1

ANATOMY AND EMBRYOLOGY

ANATOMY

To an unusual extent, the understanding of ocular functions and their modification in disease depends on an appreciation of the anatomy of the eye, the surrounding structures, and the central vascular and nervous connections. Dissection of a fresh animal eye readily reveals the interrelationship of the intraocular tissues and the organization of the eye as a multichambered, nearly spherical structure. The surface anatomy is easily studied in a living subject by direct inspection with a small penlight for illumination and a +20 diopter lens for magnification.

THE EYE

The eye (frontispiece) rests in the front half of the cavity of the orbit upon a fascial hammock surrounded by fat and connective tissue; only its anterior aspect is exposed, and it is protected by the bony orbital rim. Attached to the eye are four recti and two oblique muscles. These are innervated by the oculomotor (N III), trochlear (N IV, superior oblique muscle), and abducent (N VI, lateral rectus muscle) cranial nerves, which enter the orbit through the superior orbital fissure in the posterior orbit. The optic nerve connects the eye with the brain and leaves the orbit through the optic foramen, which also transmits the ophthalmic artery and the sympathetic innervation of the eye. The ophthalmic branch of the trigeminal nerve (N V) that transmits sensory fibers from the upper face and the eye also enters the cranial cavity through the superior orbital fissure. The exposed anterior one third of the eye consists of a central transparent portion, the cornea, and a surrounding opaque portion, the sclera. The sclera is covered with the bulbar conjunctiva, which is continuous with the palpebral conjunctiva lining the inner surface of the protective tissue curtains, the eyelids. Located in the upper outer portion of the bony orbit is the lacrimal gland.

The anterior pole of the eye is the center of curvature of the cornea. The posterior pole marks the center of the posterior curvature of the globe, and it is located to the temporal side of the optic nerve. The geometric axis is a line connecting these two poles. The equator encircles the eye midway between the two poles (Fig. 1-1).

The anteroposterior diameter of the normal eye, measured by roentgen ray or ultrasonic methods, is about 22 to 27 mm. The circumference is between 69 and 85 mm. In the average eye (24 mm in diameter), the equator is on the surface of the sclera 16 mm posterior to the corneoscleral limbus. The posterior pole is 32 mm behind the corneoscleral limbus.

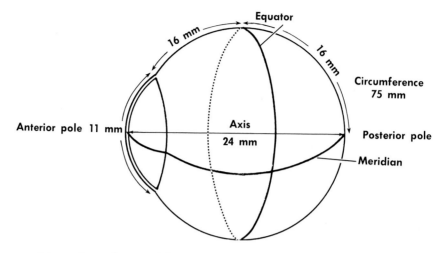

Fig. 1-1. Principal coordinates of the eye. The geometric axis connecting the anterior and posterior poles does not correspond exactly with the visual axis, which is a line connecting an object in space with the fovea centralis. The sizes given are average; the normal eye may vary in length from 22 to 27 mm.

The anterior termination of the sensory retina, the ora serrata, is approximately 8 mm posterior to the corneoscleral limbus.

The globe has three main layers, each of which is further divided. The outer supporting coat is composed of the transparent cornea, the opaque sclera, and their junction, the corneoscleral sulcus or limbus. The middle vascular layer, or the uvea, consists of the choroid, the ciliary body, and the iris, which contains a central opening, the pupil. The inner layer consists of the retina, which is composed of two parts, a sensory portion and a layer of pigment epithelium.

The lens is a transparent structure located immediately behind the iris and supported in position by a series of fine fibers, the zonule. These are attached to the ciliary body and the capsule of the lens.

The eye encloses three chambers: (1) the vitreous cavity, (2) the posterior chamber, and (3) the anterior chamber. The *vitreous cavity*, by far the largest, is located behind the lens and zonule and is adjacent to the retina throughout. The *posterior chamber* is minute in size and is bounded by the lens and zonule behind and the iris in front. The *anterior chamber* is located between the iris and the posterior surface of the cornea and communicates with the posterior chamber through the pupil. Aqueous humor is secreted by the ciliary processes into the posterior chamber and passes through the pupil into the anterior chamber. The trabecular meshwork opens into the canal of Schlemm, an endothelium-lined channel that encircles the anterior chamber.

Outer coat

The outer coat of the eye consists of relatively tough fibrous tissues shaped as segments of two spheres: the sclera, with a radius of curvature of about 13 mm, and the cornea, with a radius of curvature of about 7.5 mm. The white, opaque sclera constitutes the posterior five sixths of the globe, and the transparent cornea provides the anterior one sixth of the globe. The junction of the cornea and the sclera, the corneoscleral limbus, contains the trabecular meshwork and the aqueous

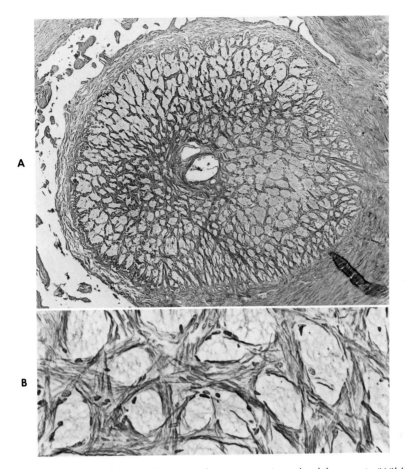

Fig. 1-2. A, Flat section of human lamina cribrosa (posterior scleral foramen). (Wilder stain; ×45.) **B,** The fibers are continuous with the scleral fibers but are lined with microglia. (Wilder stain; ×400.) (Courtesy Ramesh C. Tripathi.)

humor drainage system, the canal of Schlemm, which is an important functional and anatomic area.

The sclera. The sclera is a dense, fibrous, almost entirely collagenous structure that comprises the posterior five sixths of the eye. Anteriorly, it forms the "white" of the eye and is covered with a richly vascular episclera, the fascia bulbi (Tenon capsule), and the conjunctiva. The fine blood vessels of the Tenon capsule are visible anteriorly through the nearly transparent conjunctiva. Posteriorly, the sclera is connected by loose, fine collagen fibers to the dense fascia bulbi (Tenon capsule, p. 47).

The sclera has two large openings, the anterior and posterior scleral foramina, and numerous smaller openings through which nerves and blood vessels pass. The sclera is perforated 3 mm medial to the posterior pole by the posterior scleral foramen, the canal through which the optic nerve passes from the eye. The canal is cone-shaped and measures 1.5 to 2.0 mm in diameter on the inner surface of the sclera and 3.0 to 3.5 mm on the outer surface. The scleral foramen is bridged by a sievelike structure, the lamina cribrosa (Fig. 1-2), the most posterior portion of which is formed by scleral fibers. The anterior portion, derived from the choroid and Bruch membrane, is rich in elastic tissue. As a result of prolonged high intraocular pressure in glaucoma, the lamina cribrosa bulges outward to form a glaucomatous cup.

The anterior scleral foramen is a transitional area between the cornea and sclera. On its inner surface is the scleral spur to which the longitudinal portion of the ciliary muscle (N III) is attached. Slightly anterior to this is the canal of Schlemm (p. 13). The sclera is thickest (1.0 mm) in the region surrounding the optic nerve, where the meningeal coverings of the nerve blend into the sclera. It is thinnest (0.3 mm) immediately posterior to the insertions of the recti muscles. About 4 mm posterior to the equator in the region between the recti muscles are the openings for the four vortex veins that are the collecting channels for choroidal veins. In the area surrounding the optic

nerve, the sclera is perforated by the long and short ciliary nerves. About 4 mm posterior to the corneoscleral limbus and just anterior to the rectus muscle insertions, the anterior ciliary arteries pierce the sclera at a site sometimes marked with a dot of uveal pigment. Occasionally, a loop of a long ciliary nerve extends through the sclera, returns to the ciliary body, and appears as a small pigmented dot 2 to 4 mm from the corneoscleral limbus.

Structure. The sclera (Fig. 1-3) has three parts: (1) the episclera, (2) the scleral stroma, and (3) the lamina fusca.

The *episclera* is the outermost layer. It is a moderately dense, vascularized con-

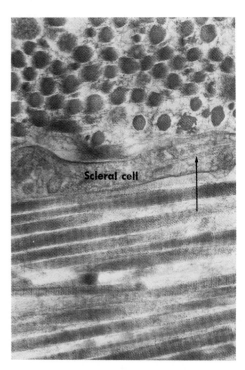

Fig. 1-4. Electron micrograph of the sclera in cross section showing collagen bundles of the sclera. The collagen fibrils in lamellae are of irregular diameter and much more irregularly arranged than those of the cornea. Part of a scleral fibroblast is seen in the interlamellar space *(arrow).* (×40,000.) (Courtesy Ramesh C. Tripathi.)

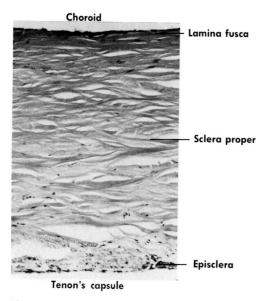

Fig. 1-3. Transverse section of sclera. (Masson trichrome stain; ×160.)

nective tissue that merges with the scleral stroma and sends connective tissue bundles into the fascia bulbi (Tenon capsule). The episclera becomes progressively thinner toward the back of the eye. Both the fascia bulbi and the episclera are attenuated behind the equator; this accounts for the relative avascularity of the posterior sclera.

The dense *scleral stroma* consists mainly of bundles of typical collagen fibers (Fig. 1-4) that vary in diameter from 10μ to 16μ and in length from 30μ to 140μ. Fibers are oriented parallel to the corneoscleral limbus to form an interlacing basket weave in that region. In the region of the insertion of the extraocular muscles, they become more meridional, apparently in response to mechanical stresses. The white appearance of the sclera arises because its stroma contains different mucopolysaccharides in lower concentrations than in the cornea and because of the variable size and less regular arrangement of the collagen fibers. When the water content of the sclera (usually between 65% and 70%) is reduced to less than 40% or increased to more than 80%, the sclera becomes transparent.

The *lamina fusca* is the innermost layer of the sclera; it is located adjacent to the choroid, which provides many melanocytes that give it a brown color. Fine collagen fibers blend with the choroid and form delicate connections between the choroid and the sclera.

Blood supply. The scleral stroma derives its nutrition from the episcleral and choroidal vascular network. Anterior to the insertion of the rectus muscle, the anterior ciliary arteries form a dense episcleral plexus. These vessels become congested in "ciliary injection" (p. 173). Small branches of the posterior ciliary arteries supply the scleral stroma posterior to the recti muscles.

Nerve supply. The posterior sclera has branches of the short ciliary nerves, which enter the sclera close to the optic nerve. The long ciliary nerves provide sensory innervation anteriorly. Because of the rich supply of nerves, inflammations of the sclera are unusually painful.

The cornea. The cornea is the transparent tissue at the anterior one sixth of the eye. Its anterior peripheral portion is covered with conjunctiva, whereas its posterior margin terminates at the trabecular meshwork. Anteriorly, it measures about 10.6 mm vertically and about 11.7 mm horizontally; posteriorly, it is circular with a diameter of 11.7 mm. The central portion is 0.52 mm thick with almost parallel anterior and posterior surfaces. It thickens to about 0.7 mm at the periphery. Its growth is complete in humans at about 6 years of age. The radius of curvature of the anterior surface is 7.8 mm, and the radius of curvature of the concave posterior surface is 6.2 to 6.8 mm. The cornea separates air with an index of refraction of 1.00 and aqueous humor with an index of refraction of 1.34; thus, it is the main refracting structure of the eye. Variations in the radius of curvature in different corneal meridians cause astigmatism.

Structure. The cornea (Fig. 1-5) has three layers: (1) the epithelium, with its basement membrane; (2) the substantia propria (stroma), with its anterior condensation, Bowman zone; and (3) the endothelium, with its basement membrane (Descemet membrane) that separates it from the stroma.

The *epithelium* is 50μ to 90μ thick and covers the stroma anteriorly. It is continuous with the epithelium of the conjunctiva. The epithelium is stratified, 5 to 6 cell layers thick. It has an outermost layer that is some 2 to 3 cell layers thick, a midzone layer formed by 2 or 3 layers of polyhedral cells (wing cells), and a single layer of tall, columnar germinal cells that rest upon a delicate basement membrane. These cells form in the basal

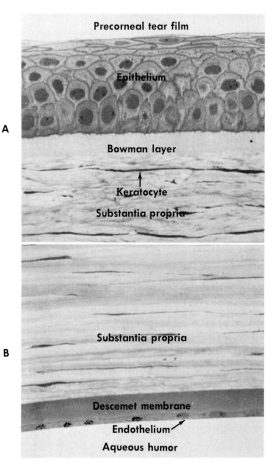

A

B

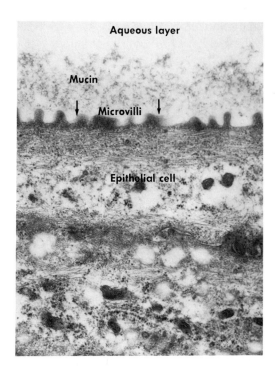

Fig. 1-6. The anterior surface of the corneal epithelium shows a degenerating epithelial cell with its microvilli covered with mucin. (×25,000.) (Courtesy Ramesh C. Tripathi.)

Fig. 1-5. Cross section of the axial area of the cornea. The substantia propria constitutes some 90% of the thickness. **A,** The epithelium rests upon a basement membrane, the Bowman layer, which is adjacent to the anterior condensation of the substantia propria. **B,** The lamellae of the posterior substantia propria are much more regularly arranged than those of the anterior substantia propria. (×500.) (Courtesy Ramesh C. Tripathi.)

layer, become progressively flatter, and are shed from the superficial layer some 7 days later. The superficial squamous cells (Fig. 1-6) have many microvilli and microplicae. These cells are flat, have horizontal nuclei, and are joined to each other with zonula occludens, an important factor in corneal drug penetration. With age, they lose their interdigitation

and disintegrate or are swept away by the eyelids in blinking. Cells in the midzone are polyhedral with a convex anterior surface, paralleling the surface of the cornea, and a concave posterior surface. Those immediately adjacent to the columnar epithelium have round nuclei that become successively flatter as the cells approach the surface. The cells are joined together by desmosomes and macula occludens. The basal cells are tall and columnar in shape. They have a flattened base that rests on the basement membrane and is attached to it by hemidesmosomes. The interdigitating adjacent cell borders are joined by desmosomes. Cells often show mitosis. The basement membrane is PAS-positive and is firmly attached to the underlying anterior condensation of the substantia propria (Bow-

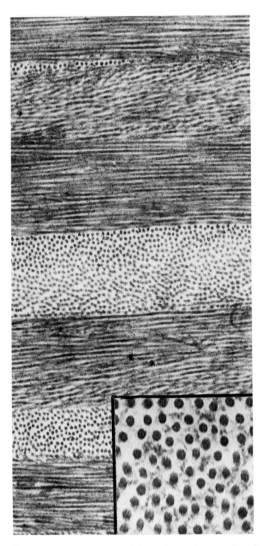

Fig. 1-7. Cross section of the substantia propria of the cornea. The collagen fibers are in bundles of approximately 200 lamellae that are arranged tangentially and at right angles to each other. Collagen fibrils are embedded in a mucopolysaccharide matrix and are separated by a distance of about 200 nm (one-half the wavelength of blue light, so that the cornea is transparent). The collagen fibrils (*inset,* ×90,000) generally are of uniform size; interspersed among them is a microfibrillar structure that may be a precursor of collagen. (×32,500.) (Courtesy Ramesh C. Tripathi.)

man zone) by irregular filaments. After injury, this attachment may take up to 6 weeks to reestablish itself, and it generally constitutes a barrier, separating superficial processes in the cornea from the underlying substantia propria.

The *substantia propria* (Fig. 1-7), or stroma, constitutes some 90% of the corneal thickness. Its anterior portion, the Bowman zone (Bowman membrane to the light microscopist), is an acellular region made up of randomly oriented collagen fibers that form a feltlike area resistant to deformation, trauma, and the passage of foreign bodies or infecting organisms. Once destroyed, its typical architecture is not restored, and scarring results. The stroma is composed of bundles of collagen fibers (lamellae) of uniform diameter that extend the entire width of the cornea. In the posterior cornea, the lamellae are of almost equal width; they become more irregular in the anterior portion. The bundles of lamellae cross mainly at almost right angles to each other, but a transitional zone exists between adjacent lamellae in which the fibers are tangential. The lamellae are enmeshed in a ground substance consisting predominantly of mucoproteins and glycoproteins. Scattered throughout are fixed, long, flattened, and pressed cells known as keratocytes or corneal corpuscles that correspond to fibroblasts in other tissues. There are a few wandering cells (leukocytes and macrophages).

The posterior surface of the stroma is lined with a PAS-positive glassy membrane, the Descemet membrane. This is formed of atypical collagen fibers together with amorphous material and fine fibrils arranged in a hexagonal pattern. The Descemet membrane is the basement membrane of endothelial cells.

The *endothelium* of the cornea is a single layer of endothelial cells (Fig. 1-8) with centrally located large oval nuclei. These cells are rich in intracellular orga-

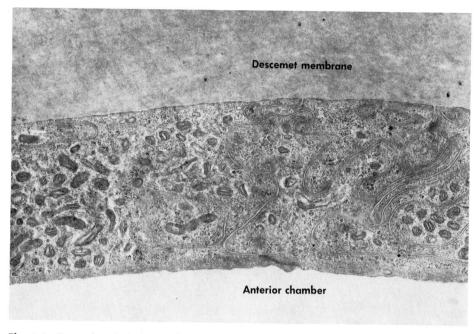

Fig. 1-8. Corneal endothelium. The cells are rich in organelles; adjacent cell borders are markedly convoluted but parallel and are attached by zonulae occludens on the anterior chamber aspect. (×24,000.) (Courtesy Ramesh C. Tripathi.)

nelles. The posterior border is in direct contact with the aqueous humor and has occasional microvilli. The cells are tightly bound together with macula occludens; near the apical zone a terminal bar is constantly present. The endothelium is responsible for the relative dehydration of the corneal stroma. Injury to the endothelium (or epithelium) causes edema of the overlying corneal stroma (p. 254).

At the corneal periphery, the Bowman membrane and the Descemet membrane stop abruptly. A line connecting these terminations constitutes the anterior margin of the corneoscleral limbus.

Nerve supply. The corneal nerves are branches of the ophthalmic division of trigeminal nerve and are entirely sensory. Within the cornea the nerves are nonmyelinated, but they gain a myelin sheath at the corneoscleral limbus. Most

are concentrated in the anterior stroma beneath the Bowman zone and send branches forward into the epithelium with either beadlike thickening or bare fibers. The Descemet membrane and the endothelium are not innervated. The axons pass in the long ciliary nerves through the ciliary ganglion to the semilunar ganglion.

Blood supply. The central cornea is avascular, but the corneoscleral limbus is generously supplied by the anterior conjunctival branches of the anterior ciliary arteries. These run circumferentially around the corneoscleral limbus, giving off small radial branches that end either as a deep corneal plexus or as a superficial corneal plexus with recurrent branches that anastomose with posterior conjunctival arteries (p. 55).

Corneoscleral limbus. The corneoscleral limbus or junction (Fig. 1-9) is a transi-

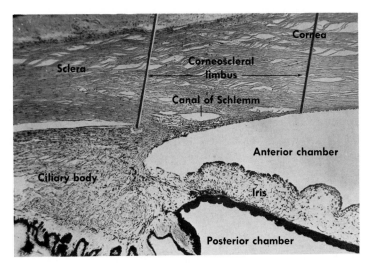

Fig. 1-9. Corneoscleral limbus. The central margin of the corneoscleral limbus is a line drawn between the termination of the Bowman membrane and the point where the Descemet membrane becomes discontinuous. The posterior margin is a line drawn parallel to the central margin and passing through the scleral spur. (Hematoxylin and eosin stain; ×105.)

tional zone 1 to 2 mm wide between the cornea, sclera, and conjunctiva. In this region, the corneal epithelium loses its regular structure and becomes continuous with the conjunctival epithelium that contains goblet cells and lymphatic channels. The regularity of the stromal collagen is lost, and the collagen fibers have variable diameters, some characteristic of the central cornea and others characteristic of the sclera. Blood vessels, nerves, and mast cells, which are absent from the cornea, are more frequent here than elsewhere in the sclera. The Bowman zone of the stroma ends abruptly in a loose arrangement of collagen fibers, fine filaments, and amorphous material. A thin layer of episcleral fibrous tissue adheres closely to the underlying sclera. The Descemet membrane loses its membranous character and splits into narrow bands that cover the inner trabecular sheets of the anterior chamber angle. The endothelium loses its regular character and continues as the endothelial lining of the trabecular meshwork.

The anterior margin of the corneoscleral limbus is usually a line drawn between the termination of the Bowman membrane and the end of the nonfenestrated portion of the Descemet membrane. The distal margin is less distinct; it is generally considered to be a plane drawn perpendicular to the scleral spur parallel to the anterior margin. Enmeshed in the corneoscleral limbus is the trabecular meshwork with its canal of Schlemm, which forms the drainage system of the anterior chamber. Clinically, the area is viewed with a gonioscope (p. 398).

Trabecular meshwork. Encircling the circumference of the anterior chamber is the trabecular meshwork, the conventional drainage route that is a porelike structure through which aqueous humor passes to the canal of Schlemm (Fig. 1-10). In cross section, the trabecular meshwork forms an obtuse triangle with a short base and two long sides. The base of the triangle is in contact with the scleral spur, the anterior face of the ciliary body,

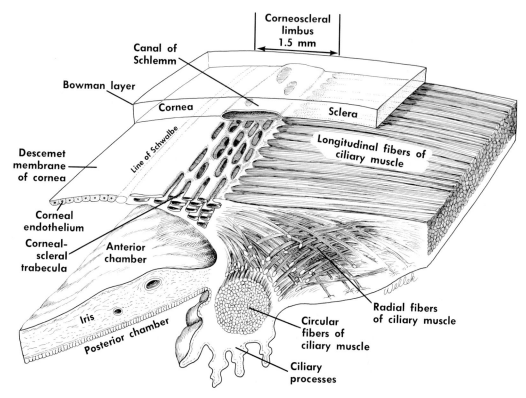

Fig. 1-10. Schematic construction of the ciliary body and angle recess in humans. Anteriorly the area is covered by the cornea and posteriorly by the sclera, which contains the canal of Schlemm. The termination of the corneal endothelium is marked by the line of Schwalbe. The ciliary muscle consists of longitudinal fibers, which are mainly parallel to the sclera; radial fibers, which are intermediate; and a circular muscle, which is most internal. The corneoscleral trabecula provides a filtering area between the anterior chamber angle and the canal of Schlemm. (Redrawn from Rohen, J. W.: Das Auge und seine Hilfsorgane. In Von Mollendorf, W., and Bargmann, W., editors: Handbuch der mikroskopischen Anatomie des Menschen, Berlin, 1964, Springer-Verlag.)

and the iris root. The apex terminates in the deep corneal lamellae and the termination of the continuous Descemet membrane. The inner side, the corneo-scleral portion, is in contact with the cornea and the sclera and opens into the canal of Schlemm. The opposite side, the uveal portion, faces into the anterior chamber. The meshwork is composed of a number of superimposed beamlike (L. *trabecula,* beam) fibrocellular cords that enclose oval, circular, or rhomboidal spaces (Fig. 1-11). A mucinous substance coats the anterior surface. The anterior

termination of the trabecular meshwork at the Descemet membrane forms the border line of Schwalbe surrounding the corneal circumference.

The trabecular meshwork is innervated by a plexus of delicate axons that terminate without specialized endings within the endothelium of the canal of Schlemm. The nerves arise from both divisions of the autonomic nervous system and from the trigeminal nerve. Fibers of the longitudinal portion of the ciliary muscle terminate in the region adjacent to the canal of Schlemm.

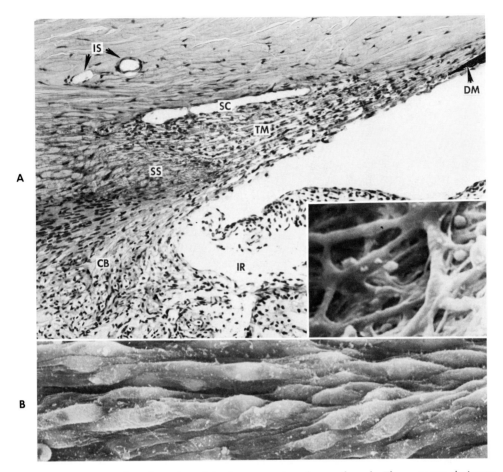

Fig. 1-11. A, Meridional section of the human trabecular meshwork. The aqueous drainage pathway consists of the trabecular meshwork *(TM),* Schlemm canal *(SC),* and intrascleral collector channels *(IS).* The trabecular meshwork, located in the inner corneoscleral limbus, extends from the scleral spur *(SS),* anterior face of the ciliary body *(CB),* and iris root *(IR)* to the deeper corneal lamellae and peripheral termination of the Descemet membrane *(DM).* (×138.) The inset shows the rounded trabeculae from the anterior chamber aspect. **B,** Scanning electron microphotograph of the endothelial lining of the trabecular wall of the Schlemm canal viewed from the anterior chamber aspect. Note the crypts between the cells, their spindle shape, and the central bulges that correspond to the location of nuclear and microvascular structures. The long axes of the cells usually parallel the canal circumference. (With permission from Tripathi, R. C.: Exp. Eye Res. **25:**65, 1977. Copyright by Academic Press Inc. [London] Ltd.)

Canal of Schlemm. The canal of Schlemm is a channel, approximately oval in cross section, that surrounds the entire circumference of the anterior chamber. It is lined with a single layer of mesothelial cells (endothelium) that contain giant vacuoles. On its inner surface, it communicates with the anterior chamber through the trabecular meshwork. Its outer wall is buried in the stroma of the corneoscleral sulcus. The canal of Schlemm connects with the venous

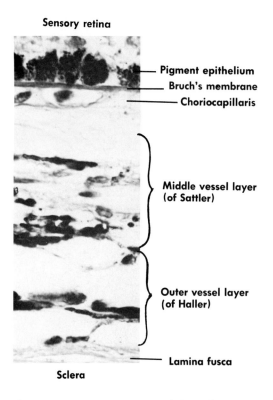

Sensory retina

— Pigment epithelium
— Bruch's membrane
— Choriocapillaris

Middle vessel layer
(of Sattler)

Outer vessel layer
(of Haller)

— Lamina fusca

Sclera

Fig. 1-12. Transverse section of choroid. (Hematoxylin and eosin stain; ×625.)

system through a system of 25 to 35 collector channels that anastomose to form a deep scleral plexus. This scleral plexus drains aqueous humor from the canal of Schlemm into anterior ciliary veins and episcleral veins. The anterior ciliary veins may appear subconjunctivally as minute vessels containing clear aqueous, the aqueous veins.

Middle coat

The middle, or uveal, coat of the eye (L. *uva*, grape) consists of the choroid, the ciliary body, and the iris. The choroid is a vascular layer that provides the blood supply to the retinal pigment epithelium and the outer half of the sensory retina adjacent to it. The ciliary body secretes aqueous humor and contains the smooth muscle responsible for the change in shape of the lens, causing accommodation (p. 105). The iris surrounds a central opening, the pupil, that controls the amount of light entering the eye.

The choroid is of mesodermal origin, whereas the epithelium of the ciliary

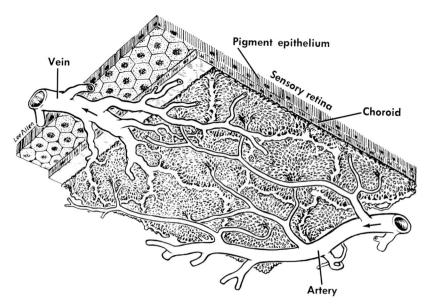

Vein

Pigment epithelium

Sensory retina

Choroid

Artery

Fig. 1-13. Lobular structure of the choroidal circulation viewed from the underside. The short posterior arteries divide soon after their entry into the eye and send branches to the center of each lobule, which drains into peripheral veins. (Courtesy Lee Allen.)

body and the pigment layer of the iris are the anterior extremities of the primitive secondary optic vesicle. The dilatator and sphincter muscles of the iris arise from neural ectoderm, and the ciliary muscles arise from mesoderm.

The choroid. The choroid (Fig. 1-12) is the vascular sheet that provides the blood supply for the retinal pigment epithelium and the outer half of the sensory retina adjacent to it. It is composed of an inner layer of fenestrated, large-diameter capillaries (21μ), the choriocapillaris, and successively larger collecting veins approximately arranged in layers. The choroid extends from the optic nerve posteriorly to the ciliary body anteriorly. Possibly reflecting a variation in nutritional requirements of the different parts of the retina, it is thickest (0.25 mm) at the posterior pole and gradually thins anteriorly to 0.10 mm. It is attached firmly to the sclera in the region of the optic nerve where the posterior ciliary arteries enter the eye and at the points of exit of the four vortex veins.

Structure. The three layers of blood vessels of the choroid have supporting structures on either side: the suprachoroid (lamina fusca) on the outer side and the basal lamina (Bruch membrane) on the inner side.

The outermost layer, the *suprachoroid (lamina fusca)*, is made up of delicate lamellae composed of elastic and collagenous fibers to form a syncytium that is dense posteriorly and becomes looser anteriorly. Melanocytes (fibroblasts that contain pigment) are abundant in this layer and decrease in number in the vascular layers. Smooth muscle fibers, fibroblasts, endothelial cells, long and short posterior ciliary arteries, and nerves are found in this layer. The short posterior ciliary arteries have but a short course in the suprachoroid and extend directly to the choriocapillaris layer.

The blood vessel layer has three components: (1) the outer (nearest the sclera)

vessel layer (of Haller), which consists of large veins that lead to the vortex veins and have no valves; (2) the middle vessel layer (of Sattler), which consists of medium-sized veins and some arterioles and which contains a loose, collagenous stroma with numerous elastic fibers, fibroblasts, and melanocytes; and (3) the choriocapillaris, which consists of large fenestrated capillaries that form a dense, flat network extending from the optic disk to the ora serrata. The choriocapillaris (Fig. 1-13) has a distinct lobular structure with a feeding arteriole in the center and draining venules at the lobular periphery.

The *lamina basalis choroideae (Bruch membrane)* (Fig. 1-14) is about 7μ thick and separates the choriocapillaris from the retinal pigment epithelium. It arises

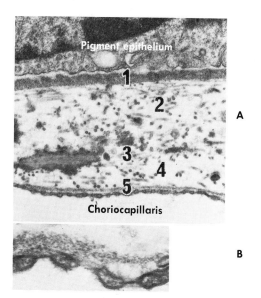

Fig. 1-14. Electron microscopy of the Bruch layer, which separates the choriocapillaris from the pigment epithelium. **A** (1) The basement membrane of the pigment epithelium; (2) inner collagen layer; (3) elastic layer; (4) outer collagen layer; (5) basement membrane of the choriocapillaris. **B,** View of the choriocapillaris showing its fenestrations bridged by membranous diaphragms. (**A,** ×21,000; **B,** ×77,000.) (Courtesy Ramesh C. Tripathi.)

from both the choroid and the retinal pigment epithelium. The outer layer, nearest the choroid, is composed of the basement membrane of the endothelial cells of the choriocapillaris. Adjacent to this is a delicate layer of collagen fibers. Centrally, a layer of elastic tissue fibers extends outward to form the supporting structure of the choriocapillaris. The inner (cuticular) layer originates from the retinal pigment epithelium and is composed of collagen fibers surrounded by acid mucopolysaccharides. Resting upon this is the delicate basement membrane of the retinal pigment epithelium. At the optic nerve, the Bruch membrane stops abruptly as does the pigment epithelium.

Blood supply. The blood supply of the choroid is derived from the short posterior ciliary arteries, the two long posterior ciliary arteries, and the seven anterior ciliary arteries (Fig. 1-15). The short posterior ciliary arteries usually arise as two or three branches of the opthalmic artery. These branches subdivide into 10 to 20 branches that perforate the sclera at the central retina and at the circumference of the optic nerve. The majority pass at once into the choroid and communicate directly with the choriocapillaris layer. The two long posterior ciliary arteries perforate the sclera on either side of the optic nerve and extend anteriorly in the suprachoroidal space on

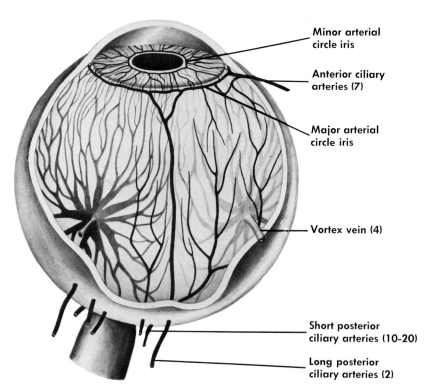

Minor arterial circle iris

Anterior ciliary arteries (7)

Major arterial circle iris

Vortex vein (4)

Short posterior ciliary arteries (10-20)

Long posterior ciliary arteries (2)

Fig. 1-15. Blood supply of the uveal tract. The two long posterior arteries mainly supply the iris. The anterior ciliary arteries supply the ciliary body, whereas the short posterior ciliary arteries supply the choroid. Note that there are no corresponding veins; rather, the blood is collected into four vortex veins that empty into the superior and inferior ophthalmic veins, which drain into the cavernous sinus.

the medial and lateral sides of the globe to the ciliary body. There each divides into two branches that extend circumferentially to form the major arterial circle of the iris, located in the ciliary body. Branches extend anteriorly to the iris. Recurrent choroidal branches extend posteriorly to the choriocapillaris.

The anterior ciliary arteries are the terminal branches of the two muscular arteries of each rectus muscle (except the lateral rectus muscle, which has but one muscular artery). The anterior ciliary arteries bifurcate into vessels that penetrate the sclera and nonpenetrating vessels that extend toward the cornea. The penetrating vessels provide the blood supply to the ciliary body and send branches to the anterior extremity of the choriocapillaris of the choroid and the major arterial circle of the iris. The nonpenetrating vessels extend forward in the episclera as anterior conjunctival arteries, anastomose with posterior conjunctival arteries, and terminate in the superficial (conjunctival) and deep (episcleral) pericorneal plexus (p. 56).

Venous blood is collected from the choroid, ciliary body, and iris by a series of veins of increasingly larger diameter. These lead to four large vortex veins located behind the equator of the globe. Additionally, the vortex veins contain blood from the iris and from the ciliary body. The vortex veins empty into the superior and inferior ophthalmic veins, each of which drains into the cavernous sinus.

Nerve supply. The choroid is innervated mainly by sympathetic nerves that pass through the ciliary ganglion without synapse and are distributed by the short ciliary nerves. As they enter the suprachoroid, they branch repeatedly to form plexuses of increasing delicacy. Numerous adrenergic vesicles are present in close association with arterioles.

The ciliary body. The ciliary body (Fig. 1-16) is a ring of tissue about 6 mm wide located between the root of the iris and the choroid.

In cross section, the ciliary body forms an approximate right triangle. The right angle is attached to the scleral spur. The base faces the anterior and posterior chambers and is divided by the insertion of the iris. The hypotenuse faces the vitreous cavity and posterior chamber; the adjacent side is apposed to the sclera.

Structure. The ciliary body is divided into uveal and epithelial portions. The uveal portion is adjacent to the sclera and

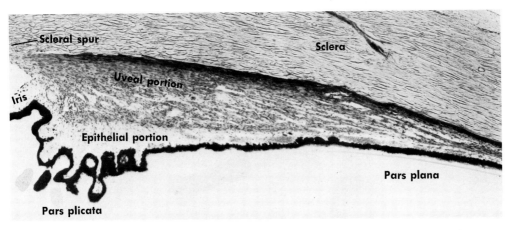

Fig. 1-16. Ciliary body, which encircles the eye. (×60.) (Courtesy Ramesh C. Tripathi.)

includes the ciliary muscle, the supra-choroid (lamina fusca), the vessel layer, the lamina basalis choroideae (lamina vitrea), and connective tissue. The epithelial portion (the tissues forming the hypotenuse) is adjacent to the posterior chamber and includes the pars plana (orbiculus ciliaris) and the pars plicata (corona ciliaris).

UVEAL PORTION. The ciliary muscle is the most prominent structure in the uveal portion of the ciliary body. It is composed of three groups of smooth muscle: (1) the longitudinal fibers (Brücke muscle), which are the outermost, parallel the surface of the overlying sclera and constitute the main bulk of the muscle; (2) the radial fibers arise from the anterior portion of the longitudinal fibers and run obliquely to become continuous with circular fibers; and (3) the circular fibers (Müller muscle) are the innermost portion of the ciliary muscle and parallel the lens equator.

Contraction of the longitudinal portion may place traction on the scleral spur and open the canal of Schlemm. Contraction of the circular fibers may relax the lens zonule, permitting a more convex shape of the lens (accommodation, p. 105). The motor innervation is from short ciliary branches of the inferior division of the oculomotor nerve (N III). These fibers arise in the Edinger-Westphal nucleus and synapse with postganglionic fibers in the ciliary ganglion.

The scleral surface of the ciliary body is the suprachoroid (lamina fusca), which is comparable to that of the choroid but contains fewer lamellae. The vessel layer is composed mainly of the major arterial circle of the iris, its tributaries, and veins. There is no choriocapillaris. The lamina basalis choroideae (Bruch membrane) is

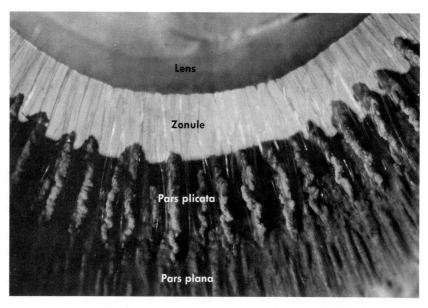

Lens

Zonule

Pars plicata

Pars plana

Fig. 1-17. Posterior view of the epithelial portion of the ciliary body. The suspensory ligament (zonule) extends from the equator of the lens to insert into the valleys between the ciliary processes of the pars plicata ciliaris. (Courtesy Patricia N. Farnsworth, Ph.D., Physiology and Ophthalmology Department, College of Medicine and Dentistry of New Jersey.)

split by connective tissue at the anterior termination of the choroid. The elastic layer derived from the choroid diminishes and disappears, but the cuticular layer, which arises from the retinal pigment epithelium, continues forward to the root of the iris as the basement membrane of the pigmented epithelium of the ciliary body.

EPITHELIAL PORTION. The epithelial portion of the ciliary body forms the hypotenuse of the triangular ciliary body and faces the vitreous cavity and the posterior chamber. It is divided into (1) the pars plana (orbiculus ciliaris), about 4 mm wide and closest to the choroid, and (2) the pars plicata (corona ciliaris), the anterior 2 mm. The pars plicata is thrown into some 60 to 70 folds, the ciliary processes, each of which is 0.8 mm high and 1 mm wide. The junction of the pars plana portion of the ciliary body with the retina has a toothed or scalloped margin, the ora serrata (Fig. 1-17). Each tooth corresponds with the valley of a ciliary

process, and narrow striae extend to them from the ora serrata. In this region the sensory retina abruptly changes into a single layer of elongated, columnar, nonpigmented ciliary epithelium.

Each ciliary process consists of a delicate finger of tissue with a covering of nonpigmented epithelium over a layer of pigmented epithelium surrounding a vascular core (Fig. 1-18). Each process has an arteriole extending to the apex, where it breaks into a rich capillary system.

The covering epithelium of the ciliary body consists of a single layer of nonpigmented epithelium constituting the anterior continuation of the sensory retina and a single layer of pigment epithelium constituting the anterior continuation of the retinal pigment epithelium. Each layer has a basement membrane at the base of the cells. That of the nonpigmented epithelium is continuous with the internal limiting membrane of the retina and is located on the vitreous side of the cell (its base). The

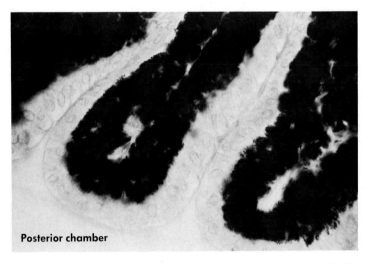

Posterior chamber

Fig. 1-18. Cross section of the ciliary processes. The nonpigmented epithelium is on the surface; its base faces the posterior chamber, and the cell apex faces the pigment epithelium. The nonpigmented epithelium is a forward extension of the sensory retina, whereas the pigmented epithelium is continuous with the retinal pigment epithelium. (Periodic acid–Schiff stain; ×63.)

basement membrane of the pigmented epithelium is the cuticular portion of the Bruch membrane and is on the side of the cell nearest the sclera. The apices of these cells are thus in apposition, and secretion of aqueous humor and hyaluronic acid by the nonpigmented epithelium is through the apex of the cell. Aqueous humor thus must pass in intercellular spaces between the cells. The nonpigmented epithelium of the ciliary processes has prominent Golgi complexes, and the structure is comparable to other secreting glandular cells.

Blood supply. The blood supply is mainly from the major arterial circle of the iris formed by the two long ciliary arteries and the seven anterior ciliary arteries.

Nerve supply. The motor nerve supply to the ciliary muscle is from the oculomotor nerve by postganglionic parasympathetic fibers that synapse in the ciliary ganglion and are distributed by the short ciliary nerves. These nerves also carry the sympathetic nerve supply of the uveal blood vessels.

The iris and pupil. The iris is a delicate diaphragm lying in front of the lens and the ciliary body and separating the anterior and posterior chambers. Located slightly to its nasal side is a circular aperture, the pupil, which reflexly controls the amount of light admitted to the eye (p. 110). The iris inserts into the base of the ciliary body and sends processes anteriorly to insert into the trabecular meshwork. It rests upon the lens, and

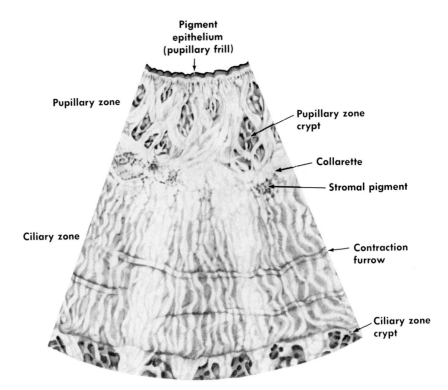

Fig. 1-19. Surface pattern of the iris. The collarette divides the pupillary zone from the ciliary zone and marks the position of the minor vascular circle of the iris, from which the pupillary membrane rises in fetal life.

without this support the iris is tremulous (iridodonesis).

The anterior iris surface (Fig. 1-19) is divided into a central pupillary zone and a peripheral ciliary zone. Their junction is a circular ridge that marks the earlier location of the minor vascular circle of the iris from which the embryonic pupillary membrane originates. Atrophy of the membrane begins in the seventh gestational month and is usually completed by 8½ months, sometimes leaving behind a few delicate strands that extend from the collarette to the anterior lens capsule.

The pupillary zone of the iris is relatively flat, and its width varies with the amount of atrophy of the anterior leaf of the pupillary membrane and the degree of pupillary dilation. The ciliary zone of the iris is marked by many radial interlacing ridges, giving a gossamerlike appearance. In lightly pigmented eyes, concentric contraction furrows may be seen.

Structure. The iris consists of two layers: (1) stroma, located anteriorly and arising from mesoderm, and (2) pigmented epithelium, located posteriorly and arising from neural ectoderm (Fig. 1-20).

The *stroma* may be divided into an anterior and a posterior leaf. The anterior stroma contains numerous vessels radiating at different levels from the major arterial circle of the iris and crossing each other at different angles. There are fine collagen fibers in which chromatophores that vary in pigment content are enmeshed. The anterior limiting membrane of the iris is a condensation of the anterior stroma, producing a dense matting. The anterior leaf is most highly developed about the seventh month of fetal life. Thereafter, atrophy occurs in the pupillary zone of the iris and in irregular areas in the ciliary zone to form crypts. The posterior leaf is similar to the anterior leaf but contains more elastic fibers, fewer chromatophores, and blood vessels that are less likely to atrophy. It is visible in the pupillary zone and at the depth of iris crypts.

The color of the iris depends on the amount of melanin in the stroma. If slight,

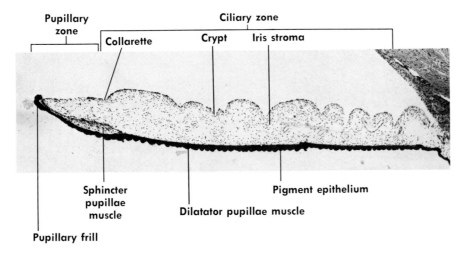

Fig. 1-20. Transverse section of the iris. The stroma is derived from mesoderm, whereas the pigmented epithelium constitutes a fusion of the two layers of the primitive optic vesicle and is a forward extension of both the sensory retina and retinal pigment epithelium. (Hematoxylin and eosin stain; ×43.)

reflection from the pigment of the pigmented epithelium causes scattering and thus a blue color. If marked, the color of the iris is hazel, and if more marked, the color of the iris is brown.

The *pigmented epithelium* consists of two layers of cells densely packed with melanin that constitute a fusion of the two layers of the primitive optic vesicle. The anterior layer of pigment cells is closely identified with the dilatator pupillae muscle and is absent in the region of the sphincter muscle. The posterior layer of epithelium is covered on its lenticular surface with an internal limiting membrane continuous with that of the retina and the ciliary body. Often the pupillary margin has a pigment frill continuous with the ectodermal pigmented epi-

thelium that constitutes the anterior extremity of the secondary optic vesicle.

The sphincter pupillae muscle is located in the pupillary zone of the posterior stroma. It is a smooth muscle about 1 mm wide that forms a sphincter around the pupillary margin. The dilatator muscle is a thin sheet of smooth muscle (myoepithelium) located between the stroma and the posterior layer of the pigmented epithelium. It extends from the iris root at the ciliary body as far as the sphincter pupillae muscle. Both muscles are derived from neural ectoderm from the outer layer of the optic cup.

Blood supply. The iris blood supply is provided by radial vessels in the stromal layer that extend from the major arterial circle of the iris (circulus arteriosus iridis

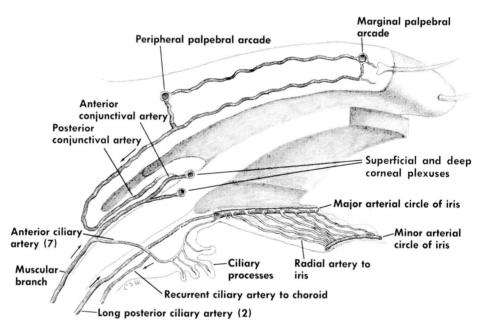

Fig. 1-21. Blood supply of the anterior ocular segment. Two anterior ciliary arteries arise from the muscular branches of each rectus muscle except for the lateral rectus muscle, which contributes only one. Two long posterior ciliary arteries enter the globe on the nasal and temporal sides of the optic nerve and extend forward in the suprachoroidal space to the ciliary body. The vascular arcades of the eyelid are derived from the lateral palpebral branches of the lacrimal artery and the medial palpebral branches of the dorsonasal artery. They have generous anastomoses with branches of the external carotid artery distributed to the face.

major) located in the ciliary body (Fig. 1-21). This is formed by the two long posterior ciliary arteries and the seven anterior ciliary arteries. The iris blood vessels pass radially in a corkscrew pattern toward the pupillary margin, giving rise to the meridional striations of the ciliary portion of the iris. At the collarette they anastomose to form an incomplete minor vascular circle of the iris. The vessels have an unusually thick collagen adventitia but a thin muscularis layer. The endothelia of the veins have a perivascular sheath. They drain into the vortex veins. The endothelial cells lining blood vessels of the iris have tight junctions that prevent the passage of large molecules; together with the epithelium of the ciliary body processes this forms the blood-aqueous barrier. The ciliary body vessels, like those of the choroid, are fenestrated.

Nerve supply. The iris is richly supplied with nerves from the short ciliary and long ciliary nerves that carry sensory, motor, and sympathetic fibers. The nerves are partially medullated and have a thick neurilemma. The motor innervation of the dilatator pupillae muscle arises from sympathetic nerves accompanying the long ciliary nerves. Additionally, the long ciliary nerves transmit sensory fibers from the iris. The sphincter pupillae muscle is innervated by parasympathetic nerves from the oculomotor nerve that synapse in the ciliary ganglion (p. 63) and are distributed with short ciliary nerves. The sympathetic nerve supply of iris arteries is carried by the short ciliary nerves.

Inner coat

The retina. The retina develops from invagination of the optic vesicle (see discussion on embryology, p. 73) to form an outer layer, the retinal pigment epithelium, and an inner layer, the sensory retina. The inner layer is stratified into

many layers, but the pigment epithelium is only one layer thick. The layers of the retina nearest the choroid are designated as the outer layers, and those nearest the vitreous humor as the inner layers. The

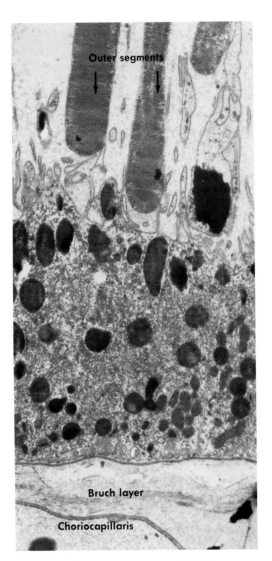

Fig. 1-22. Electron microscopy of the human retinal pigment epithelium. Microvilli at the apex of the pigment epithelial cell closely surround the outer segments of the photoreceptors. The pigment epithelium rests upon the Bruch layer and separates it from the choriocapillaris. (×8,250.) (Courtesy Ramesh C. Tripathi.)

retina extends from the optic nerve posteriorly to the scalloped margin (the ora serrata) anteriorly, where it continues as the epithelium of the ciliary body.

Retinal pigment epithelium. The retinal pigment epithelium (Fig. 1-22) is a single layer of cells that extends to the optic nerve margin posteriorly and to the ora serrata anteriorly, where it fuses with the anterior continuation of the sensory retina and continues forward as the pigmented ciliary epithelium. The cells of the pigment epithelium contain varying amounts of melanin, which, on ophthalmoscopic examination, give a granular appearance to the fundus. In the region underlying the central retina, the cells are slender and tall, but they are more cuboidal and irregular in the periphery. Their basement membrane is firmly attached to the cuticular portion of the Bruch membrane, but the villous projections of the apices surround the outer segments of rods and cones in a mucoid medium without specialized attachments.

In flat section, individual pigment epithelium cells have four to eight sides but are usually hexagonal. They are fitted together like cobblestones in a regular arrangement. In cross section, the pigment epithelium cells are divided into thirds, consisting of a base, a body, and an apex.

The base, which contains little or no pigment but much mitochondria, has prominent infoldings of basal plasma membrane and is in intimate contact with the cuticular portion of the Bruch membrane. The cell body contains the nucleus and, when present, granules of lipofuscin. The apex is topped with microvilli that surround the periphery of the outer segments of rods and cones. Ovoid pigment granules occur in the microvilli, whereas spherical granules occur in the apical cytoplasm. The apices of adjacent cells, but not the microvilli, are tightly bound together by terminal bars containing both zonula occludens and zonula adherens portions. Lipofuscin is particularly prominent in the pigment epithelium underlying the central retina. In fluorescein angiography it obscures the fluorescence from the underlying choroid.

Sensory retina. The sensory retina (pars optica retinae) develops from differentiation of the inner wall of the secondary optic vesicle. It consists of a layer of photoreceptor cells whose axons synapse with cells that modulate their response. These cells in turn synapse with cells that transmit spike discharges to the brain (Table 1-1). The rods and cones, the light-sensitive cells of the retina, correspond to the sensory endings elsewhere in the nervous system. The skeletal support of the retina is derived from the glial system of Müller cells.

PHOTORECEPTOR CELL. The photoreceptor cell (Fig. 1-23) may be divided into: (1) an outer segment intimately related to the pigment epithelium; (2) a cilium, a tubelike structure that connects the outer and inner segments; (3) an inner segment composed of an ellipsoid and a myoid; (4) the outer rod (or cone) fiber connecting the inner segment to the cell body; (5) the cell body that contains the nucleus; and (6) the inner rod (or cone) fiber that terminates in a specialized synaptic ending.

The *outer segment* consists of a dense vertical stack of some 700 flattened sacs or disks that originate from infoldings of a double layer of plasma lamellae. The space within each sac is occupied by the visual pigments. Most (111 to 130 million) outer segments in humans consist of cylindrical disks (rods) containing rhodopsin, whereas other outer segments (6.3 to 6.8 million) have a conical shape (cones) with the apex pointing outward. The outer tip of the rod is surrounded by the microvilli of the retinal pigment epithelium and the extracellular space containing mucopolysaccharides. Outside of

Table 1-1. Coats of the eye

_____

I. Outer coat
  A. Cornea
    1. Epithelium
      a. Precorneal tear film
        (1) Oily layer (from meibomian glands)
        (2) Aqueous layer (from lacrimal glands)
        (3) Mucoid layer (from goblet cells)
    2. Stroma
      a. Anterior condensation (Bowman zone)
    3. Mesothelium (endothelium)
      a. Descemet membrane (basement membrane) separates endothelium from stroma
  B. Sclera
    1. Episclera
    2. Sclera proper
    3. Lamina fusca
II. Middle coat
  A. Choroid
    1. Lamina fusca
    2. Layer of large veins (of Haller)
    3. Layer of smaller veins (of Sattler)
    4. Choriocapillaris (blood supply of the outer retina)
  B. Ciliary body
    1. Uveal portion
      a. Lamina fusca
      b. Vessel layer
      c. Ciliary muscle
        (1) Longitudinal
        (2) Radial
        (3) Circular
    2. Epithelial portion
      a. Pigmented epithelium
      b. Nonpigmented epithelium
  C. Iris
    1. Anterior border layer (fibroblasts and melanocytes, absent in pupillary zone)
    2. Stroma (connective tissue, blood vessels, sphincter pupillae muscle [N III])
    3. Epithelium
      a. Anterior (myoepithelium: dilatator pupillae muscle [sympathetics])
      b. Posterior pigmented layer
III. Transitional coat (lamina basalis choroideae, Bruch membrane, lamina vitrea [obsolete])
  A. Basement membrane of choriocapillaris endothelium
  B. Outer collagen layer
  C. Elastic layer
  D. Inner collagen layer
  E. Basement membrane of pigment epithelium
IV. Inner coat
  A. Retinal pigment coat (outer layer optic vesicle)
    1. Base (plasma membrane, mitochondria)
    2. Body (nucleus, endoplasmic reticulum, lipofuscin)
    3. Apex (pigment, ingested outer segment [phagosomes])
      a. Microvilli
      b. Terminal bars
  B. Sensory retina (inner layer optic vesicle)
    1. Photoreceptor cells
      a. Outer segment (rods and cones)
      b. Cilium

_____

Continued.

Table 1-1. Coats of the eye—cont'd

---

      c. Inner segment
        (1) Ellipsoid
        (2) Myoid
        (3) Outer fiber (surrounded by terminal bars of Müller cells, the external limiting membrane)
        (4) Cell body (nucleus)
        (5) Inner fiber*
        (6) Synaptic vesicle*
   2. Modulator cells (nuclei form inner nuclear layer)
      a. Bipolar*†
        (1) Midget
      b. Horizontal*
      c. Amacrine†
   3. Transmitter cells
      a. Ganglion†
        (1) Nerve fiber layer (axons of ganglion cells)
        (2) Internal limiting membrane (retinal basement membrane from Müller cells)
   4. Skeletal support
      a. Müller cells (nuclei form inner nuclear layer)
      b. Astroglia nerve fiber layer

---

*The axons of photoreceptor cells and horizontal cells and the dendrites of bipolar cells and horizontal cells form the outer plexiform layer of the retina (outer molecular layer).
†The axons of bipolar cells and processes of amacrine cells and the dendrites of ganglion cells form the inner plexiform layer (inner molecular layer).

the fovea the tapered portion of the cone does not reach the retinal pigment epithelium, and the microvilli are lengthened to reach the cone outer segment. In the foveal region cones are more slender and resemble the cylindrical structure of rods.

The outer segment is connected to the inner segment by the *cilium*. The connecting cilium contains nine pairs of microtubules but lacks the central pair seen in mobile cilia. This structure transmits cellular components from the inner segment and cell body to the disks and supporting structures.

The *inner segment* is divided into a refractile outer portion, or ellipsoid, and a nonrefractile, basophilic inner portion, or myoid. The ellipsoid is filled with mitochondria grouped around the base of the cilium. The myoid portion (contractile in some amphibia) of the inner segment contains free and membrane-bound ribosomes, Golgi complexes, and a variety of

vesicles and vacuoles. The division into ellipsoid and myoid portions is more distinct than in cells connected to rods.

The inner segment is connected to the cell body, which contains the nucleus, by a delicate *outer rod* (or cone) fiber, which may be long or short depending on the distance between the myoid and the cell body. Mainly, the inner fibers of cones are shorter than those of rods. The outer fiber is surrounded by the terminal bars of Müller fibers that constitute the outer limiting membrane of the retina in light microscopy. These bars provide vertical orientation for the photoreceptors.

The *cell body*, located in the outer nuclear layer, consists almost entirely of nucleus.

An *inner rod* (or cone) fiber passes in the outer plexiform layer and terminates in a synaptic expansion, the rod spherule, or in a cone pedicle, the cone-foot, that synapses in the outer plexiform layer with cells whose nuclei are in the inner

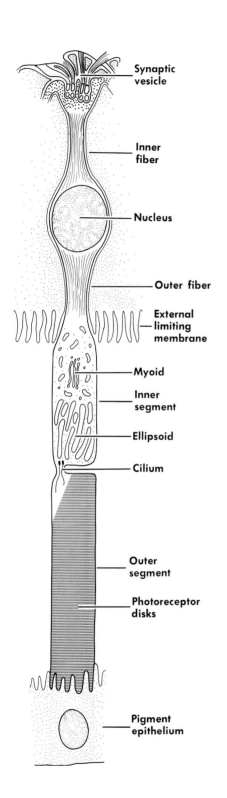

Synaptic
vesicle

Inner
fiber

Nucleus

Outer fiber

External
limiting
membrane

Myoid

Inner
segment

Ellipsoid

Cilium

Outer
segment

Photoreceptor
disks

Pigment
epithelium

nuclear layer. There are several different types of synaptic endings, and it is possible at this level that there are both inhibition and integration of the nervous impulse. At this level chemical intermediates are secreted that are involved in the synaptic transmission of impulses.

Mature visual cells do not replicate, and their DNA is stable. In contrast, ribosomal RNA, transfer RNA, and messenger RNA are constantly renewed by the cell nucleus and passed to the myoid. The ribosomes in the myoid are continually synthesizing acid mucopolysaccharides that surround outer segments and new proteins, particularly opsin, the visual pigment protein (p. 94). These proteins reach the outer segment through the connecting cilium (Fig. 1-24). The phospholipids that combine with proteins to form the disks of the outer segments are synthesized in the myoid portion of the cell. The new protein transported to the outer segment becomes associated with the outer membrane that envelops the stack of disks, and the disks are assembled near the cilium. The rod's oldest disks, which are surrounded by the retinal pigment microvilli, are detached in small groups from the tip of the cell; they are phagocytized and destroyed by the pigment epithelium.

MODULATOR CELLS. The signal initiated by stimulation of the outer segments is modulated and transmitted by three different cell types: (1) bipolar cells, (2)

Fig. 1-23. Diagram of the vertebrate visual cell. Photoreceptor disks of the outer segment are constantly renewed and have a half-life of about 7 days. The youngest disks are adjacent to the inner segment, where they are formed. The older disks are phagocytized by the pigment epithelium. The cell body does not undergo mitosis but constantly creates new photoreceptors. (Redrawn from Young, R. W.: Invest. Ophthalmol. **15**:700, 1976.)

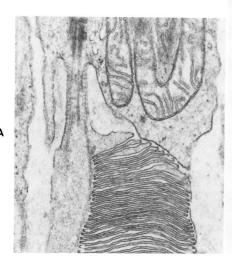
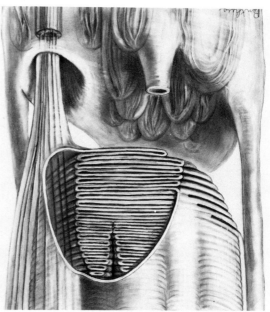

Fig. 1-24. A, Electron micrograph showing the junction of the outer and inner segments of the retinal rod of the rhesus monkey. The membranous disks form by inward folding of the outer cell membrane adjacent to the inner segment. As the disks mature they are displaced away from the base by newer disks and lose their attachment to the outer membrane and to each other. **B,** Drawing of this region reconstructed from electron micrographs to illustrate the process of disk formation. (From Young, R. W.: Invest. Ophthalmol. **15:**700, 1976.)

horizontal cells, and (3) amacrine cells. Horizontal and amacrine cells are called association cells. Their nuclei are located in the inner nuclear layer.

Bipolar cells consist of a cell body located in the inner nuclear layer, an outer dendritic portion, and an inner axon. The outer dendritic portion synapses with the synaptic vesicle of rods or cones in the outer plexiform layer and with horizontal cell processes. The axon synapses with dendrites of ganglion cells in the inner plexiform layer.

In primates there are three varieties of bipolar cells: (1) midget, (2) flat midget, and (3) diffuse bipolars. Their dendrites attach to photoreceptor synaptic vesicles with desmosomelike attachments. Synapse with horizontal cells is by desmosomes and gap junctions. A dense basketlike weave of the dendrites in the outer plexiform layers forms a dense membranelike structure that divides the retina into an outer portion dependent on choroidal circulation and an inner portion nurtured by the sensory retinal vasculature.

All cones synapse with at least one midget bipolar cell and commonly with other bipolar cells, but midget bipolar cells generally synapse with but a single cone. Traditionally, those that synapse with a single cone, the midget bipolars, synapse with but one ganglion cell and characterize the cells transmitting the impulse from the cones in the fovea centralis to the brain. Physiologically, this one-to-one representation of the fovea centralis cones is an oversimplification. Bipolar cells synapse with more than one foveal photoreceptor and ganglion cell but with fewer cells than elsewhere in the retina.

Bipolar axons have branches that terminate in synaptic vesicles comparable to those of photoreceptors. In the inner plexiform layer, they synapse with the dendrites of ganglion cells and the processes of amacrine cells.

The nuclei of *horizontal cells* are located in the outer portion of the inner nuclear layer, and both their axons and dendrites are located in the outer plexiform layer. Horizontal cell dendrites synapse with several closely adjoining photoreceptors, and their axon synapses with several photoreceptors in a distant part of the retina. Other axons synapse with bipolar cells. Possibly, they act as condensers, as in an electric circuit, and collect impulses from a group of photoreceptors and, with discharge, trigger a visual impulse.

Amacrine cells are oriented in the wrong direction to be explained in terms of the transmission of the light impulse. The amacrine cell processes synapse with ganglion cells and bipolar cells. Their cell bodies lie at the inner portion of the inner nuclear layer, and their processes are directed inward toward the ganglion cell layer. Some contain large vesicles in their nuclei and cell processes that may contain dopamine. They may have an inhibitional function in the integration of the visual impulse.

TRANSMITTER CELLS. Ganglion cells transmit spike discharges through their axons to the midbrain. Their nuclei are located in the innermost cellular layer of the retina. In the region surrounding the fovea centralis, the ganglion cell layer is five to seven layers thick. In the retinal periphery, the ganglion cell layer is but a single cell thick. Transmitter cells may be classified anatomically on the basis of their dendrites: nonstratified, multistratified, diffuse, small, or large. Ganglion cell

dendrites synapse with the axons of bipolar cells and the processes of amacrine cells in the inner plexiform layer. Physiologically, they may be divided into those subserving vision and those transmitting afferent impulses for pupillary constriction. X-ganglion cells are small ganglion cells that serve cones and have small fibers extending to the lateral geniculate body. Y-cells, or large ganglion cells, have thick axons that serve rods. W-cells have axons that do not synapse in the lateral geniculate body. They may serve pupillary reactions and have spatial orientation functions.

The axons of ganglion cells form the nerve fiber layer and are arranged with the fiber approximately radial to the optic nerve. The layer is sometimes visible in red-free light and may often be seen ophthalmoscopically in black persons. The nerve fibers arising from ganglion cells in the fovea centralis extend directly medially to the optic nerve almost in a straight line. Other fibers from the temporal retina arch above and below these fibers but do not cross the horizontal raphe of the retina, which extends temporally from the fovea centralis to the ora serrata. The fibers to the nasal side of the optic disk have an approximately straight radial course. The distribution is important in the configuration of field defects in glaucoma. The major branches of the central retinal artery and vein are located in the nerve fiber layer.

THE SUPPORTING ASTROGLIA. Müller cells provide the skeletal support for the retina partially aided by smaller astrocytes and oligodendrocyticlike cells in the nerve fiber layer. The nuclei of Müller cells are located in the middle portion of the inner nuclear layer of the retina. The cell sends delicate processes toward the photoreceptors and sturdy processes inward that enclose neurons and prevent short circuits in the retina. Its outer fibers provide a delicate honeycomb around photoreceptor nuclei and send out villi that form the terminal bars of the external limiting membrane at the level of the inner segments of the rods and cones.

The inner processes envelop the inner retina, sheath the blood vessels, and terminate in the internal limiting membrane of the retina; they constitute the basement membrane of the retina (the internal limiting membrane). Müller cells furnish glucose to nerve cells, synthesize and store glycogen, and contain considerable lactic dehydrogenase activity.

Regions of the retina. The retina has been divided into regions that differ histologically and functionally. The histologic divisions include: (1) the ora serrata, the scalloped anterior termination of the sensory retina; (2) the central retina, which surrounds the fovea centralis; and (3) the extracentral, or peripheral, retina, which includes the other portions of the retina.

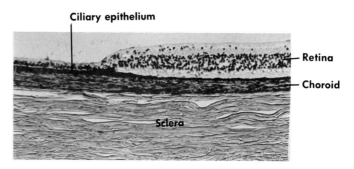

Fig. 1-25. Abrupt termination of the retina to form the ora serrata and the forward continuation as the ciliary epithelium. (Hematoxylin and eosin stain; ×43.)

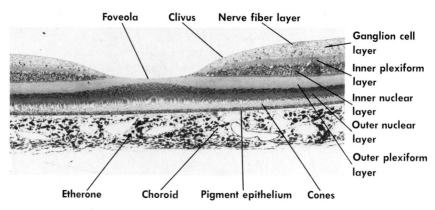

Fig. 1-26. Human central retina. The fovea centralis is a depression with sloping walls, the clivus. The floor of the fovea centralis, the foveola, is flat, although the long, thin cones give this layer a convexity. The fibers of the outer plexiform layer are tangential to the surface of the retina. The inner layers of the retina are absent, so that light falls directly upon the cones. The floor of the fovea centralis corresponds closely to the capillary-free region of the retina, and this area is nurtured solely by the choriocapillaris. (×105.) (Courtesy Ramesh C. Tripathi.)

ORA SERRATA. The ora serrata is the anterior termination of the retina; it consists of scalloped fringe paralleling the ciliary processes (Fig. 1-25). It is located about 8 mm from the corneoscleral limbus. In this area the sensory retina abruptly loses its laminated structure, and the two layers of the primitive optic vesicle fuse and continue forward as the ciliary epithelium.

CENTRAL RETINA. This specialized region is about 6 mm in diameter. (The optic disk is 1.5 mm in diameter and is customarily used as a reference point in the measurement of retinal lesions.) It extends from the fovea centralis nasally almost to the optic disk, about the same distance temporally, and a similar distance above and below. The retinal layers of the central retina from the outer nuclear layer inward have a yellow carotenoid pigment, the macula lutea (yellow spot), which may be seen in red-green light and in eyes opened within 15 minutes after cessation of circula-

tion. Additionally, the ganglion cell layer has more than one layer of cell bodies.

The fovea centralis (Fig. 1-26) is a depressed area located in the central retina about 3 mm temporal to the optic disk and 0.8 mm below the horizontal meridian. It measures 1.5 mm in diameter. The sides of the depression form the clivus; its center is the foveola (Fig. 1-27), measuring about 0.4 mm in diameter. The photoreceptors in the fovea centralis are exclusively cones. The outer segments of cones in the foveola are densely packed, thin, long, and attenuated. Their outer fibers sweep tangentially to their cell bodies, and the inner fibers continue a tangential course to synapse in the outer plexiform layer. The foveola is nurtured solely by the choriocapillaris of the choroid and does not contain the capillaries of the sensory retina located in the inner layers of the retina. All cell layers are displaced peripherally so that light falls directly on the cones' outer segments with-

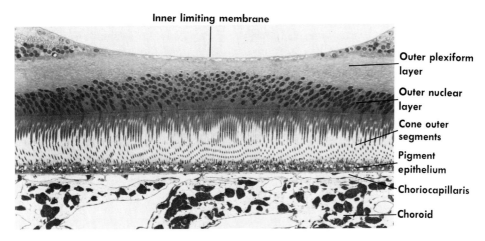

Fig. 1-27. Human foveola. This is the capillary-free zone of the retina, and cones are the sole photoreceptors present. The cell bodies of the cones are seen together with the outer plexiform layer and the inner limiting membrane of the retina. The outer segments have been cut slightly obliquely and do not appear continuous. The choriocapillaris in this region is well demonstrated. The lumina of the blood vessels are far larger than in other capillaries and permit about three erythrocytes to pass through simultaneously. (×350.) (Courtesy Ramesh C. Tripathi.)

out passing through the inner layers of the retina.

PERIPHERAL RETINA. In the peripheral retina the photoreceptors are mainly rods, and the cones present are thicker than those in the central retina. The outer plexiform layer is vertically arranged, and the inner nuclear layer has a regular orientation. The ganglion cells are larger than those in the central retina, and their cell bodies are arranged singly.

Retinal layers. The sensory retina is divided into three layers of nuclei and three layers of fibers. Conventionally, the layers closest to the sclera are the outer layers, and the layers closest to the vitreous are the inner layers.

The three nuclear layers are: (1) the outer nuclear layer, which contains the nuclei of photoreceptors (rods and cones); (2) the inner nuclear layer, which contains the nuclei of bipolar, horizontal, amacrine, and Müller cells; and (3) the ganglion cell layer, which contains the nuclei of ganglion cells. The three nerve layers are: (1) the outer plexiform layer, where there is synapse between cells whose nuclei are located in the outer nuclear layer and cells whose nuclei are located in the inner nuclear layer; (2) the inner plexiform layer, where there is synapse between cells whose nuclei are in the inner nuclear layer and the ganglion cell layer; and (3) the nerve fiber layer composed of axons of ganglion cells.

Functionally, the retina is divided into temporal and nasal portions by a line drawn vertically through the center of the fovea. Nerve fibers originating from cells temporal to this line pass to the lateral geniculate body on the same side. Nerve fibers originating from ganglion cells nasal to this line cross in the optic nerve to the opposite side of the brain.

Ophthalmoscopically, the clinician uses the optic nerve as a hub to divide the retina into superior and inferior temporal portions, superior and inferior nasal portions, and a central area. The different quadrants are further divided into the regions posterior and anterior to the equator.

Blood supply. The retina is nurtured from two sources: (1) the outer portion is nurtured by the choriocapillaris of the choroid (p. 15), and (2) the inner portion is nurtured by the central retinal artery and its branches. This does not provide a double blood supply—both must be intact to maintain active retinal metabolism.

The central retinal artery, the first branch of the ophthalmic artery, enters the inferior medial side of the optic nerve about 12 mm posterior to the globe. It extends forward to the optic disk, where it bifurcates into superior and inferior papillary branches. As the vessel passes through the lamina cribrosa, its wall is reduced to about one-half its previous thickness, the internal elastic lamella is lost, and the medial muscle coat becomes incomplete. Thus, within the eye its primary branches are arterioles.

The superior and inferior papillary branches of the central retinal artery bifurcate on the surface of the disk to form nasal and temporal branches. The nasal branches follow a relatively direct course to the periphery. The temporal vessels arch above and below the fovea centralis and pass to the periphery.

CAPILLARIES. Retinal capillaries have multiple arteriolar connections so that closure of a single feeder vessel will not cause loss of flow in its capillary bed. The capillaries are distributed in a superficial network at the level of the nerve fiber layer and in an intraretinal network at the level of the inner nuclear layer (Fig. 1-28). The intraretinal capillaries receive blood from the capillaries in the nerve fiber layer. Arterial abnormalities (such as vascular hypertension) tend to involve the nerve fiber plexus, whereas venous

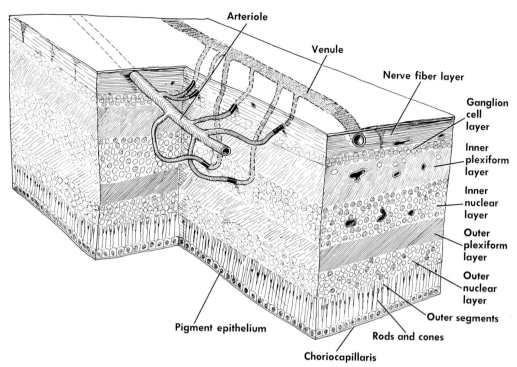

Fig. 1-28. Retinal arterioles provide two major capillary layers in the retina: one in the nerve fiber layer and one in the inner nuclear layer. In general, diseases affecting primarily the arteries, such as vascular hypertension, involve the capillary network in the nerve fiber layer, whereas predominantly venous diseases, such as diabetes mellitus, involve the layer of capillaries in the inner nuclear layer. The outer receptors together with their cell bodies in the outer nuclear layer and a portion of the outer plexiform layer are nurtured by the choriocapillaris of the choroid. Both systems are necessary to the function of the retina.

abnormalities (such as diabetes mellitus) tend to involve the inner nuclear plexus. The arteries have a large capillary-free zone surrounding them.

The endothelial cells line the retinal capillaries and are regularly arranged with their nuclei parallel to the direction of the vessel. The vessel wall contains pericytes (mural cells) that are separated from the endothelium by their basement membrane. The endothelial cells are joined by terminal bars, and the blood-retina barrier is thought to be at this level.

VEINS. The veins in the retina essentially follow the distribution of the arteries. They consist of an endothelial coat supported by a small amount of connective tissue. At points in the retina where arteries cross veins, the vessels are bound together with a common adventitial sheath. Arterioles usually cross a venule on the vitreal side. The central retinal vein emerges from the optic nerve at about the same point where the central retinal artery enters 12 mm behind the globe. As the central retinal vein passes through the meninges surrounding the optic nerve, it is considered vulnerable to increases in intracranial pressure, a factor important in the production of papilledema.

The optic nerve. The optic nerve is a

portion of a white fiber track of the central nervous system that consists of axons of retinal ganglion cells together with nerve fibers extending from the brain to the eye. The optic nerve extends from the optic disk at a level with the retina within the eye to the optic chiasm, where, in normal humans, one half of the fibers decussate to the opposite side of the brain in the optic chiasm (p. 42). Thereafter, crossed nasal fibers and uncrossed temporal fibers constitute the optic tract (p. 42).

The optic nerve is divided into four portions: (1) intraocular, 1 mm; (2) orbital, 30 mm; (3) intracanalicular, 4 to 10 mm; and (4) intracranial, 10 mm.

The *intraocular portion* of the optic nerve includes the optic disk and the portion of the optic nerve within the posterior scleral foramen. The optic disk (Fig. 1-29) is about 3 mm nasal to and about 0.8 mm above the foveola. It is composed of axons of ganglion cells that leave the eye through the sievelike lamina cribrosa (Fig. 1-2). The choroid and all layers of the retina, except the nerve fiber layer, terminate at the disk margin. Inasmuch as the photosensitive rods and cones are absent, this area is blind and gives rise to the blind spot of Mariotte in visual field testing (p. 161).

The central retinal artery and vein are visible on the nerve surface. A central physiologic cup is commonly present and is formed by atrophy of the vascular elements emerging from the central portion of the optic disk during fetal life.

The optic nerve passes from the eye through the scleral foramen bridged with the lamina cribrosa (p. 6) that is formed by fibrous tissue from the sclera, elastic tissue of the sclera, and astroglia derived from the septal system of the nerve. Posterior to the optic disk the nerve fibers are myelinated, whereas anterior to the disk they are normally not myelinated. The

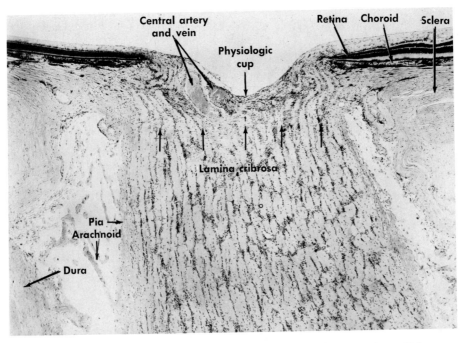

Fig. 1-29. Optic disk and optic nerve. (Hematoxylin and eosin stain; ×43.)

portion of the optic nerve visible within the eye measures about 1.5 mm in diameter.

The *orbital portion* of the optic nerve has an S-shaped curve to permit movements of the eye. It is covered with a dense dural sheath, an arachnoid sheath, and a pia mater. These extend from the optic foramen to the globe, where the dura mater and arachnoid sheaths blend into the sclera. Near the globe the long and short ciliary arteries and nerves are arranged about its circumference. The central retinal artery and vein penetrate the optic nerve 12 mm behind the globe. At the apex of the orbit the optic nerve is surrounded by the tendinous origin of the rectus muscle, the ligament of Zinn.

In its *intracanalicular portion* the optic nerve passes through the optic foramen together with the ophthalmic artery and the sympathetic nerves accompanying this vessel. At the anterior portion of the optic foramen the dural sheath covering the nerve divides so that one portion continues as the periosteum of the orbit and the other continues within the dural sheath of the optic nerve. In the optic foramen the dural sheath is adherent to bone, arachnoid, and pia mater so that the nerve is firmly fixed in this portion.

The *intracranial portion* passes medially to form the chiasm.

Structure. The optic nerve contains between 1.1 and 1.3 million fibers classified as afferent axons of ganglion cells subserving vision and the pupillary reflex, efferent fibers of unknown function, autonomic fibers, and photostatic fibers to the superior colliculi.

The nerve is composed of bundles of nerve fibers separated by septa that are continuous with the pial sheath and carry minute blood vessels to the nerve (Fig. 1-30). As in the brain, nerve fibers are supported by astroglia and oligodendrog-

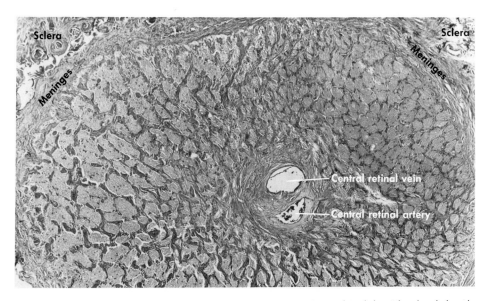

Fig. 1-30. Cross section of the human optic nerve just posterior to the globe. The dural sheath contribution to the sclera is shown. The central artery and vein share a common adventitial sheath, as they do at points of crossings. In the nerve the myelinated nerve fibers are divided into septa by delicate, collagenous fibers from the pia. The nerve fiber bundles are separated from the septal system by a layer of astrocytes. (×70.) (Courtesy Ramesh C. Tripathi.)

lia derived from the neural ectoderm and by mesenchymal microglia that have a phagocytic function. Myelinization of the optic nerve begins at the chiasm at about the twenty-fourth week of fetal life and, at birth, has reached a point just behind the lamina cribrosa. Oligodendrocytes are associated with the synthesis and metabolism of myelin; these cells are more numerous behind the lamina cribrosa. Inasmuch as the optic nerve loses its myelin sheath within the lamina cribrosa, astrocytes are more common in this area. They provide a framework on the intraocular surface of the optic nerve and are probably important in providing mechanical support for nerve fibers that make a right angle turn from the retina.

Blood supply. The blood supply of the optic nerve is derived from several sources. The intraocular portion is supplied by the short posterior ciliary arteries that, as they penetrate the sclera, give off branches to form the anastomotic partial circle of Haller-Zinn. The central retinal artery does not furnish branches to the optic nerve in this region. Much attention has been focused on the blood supply to this area because of involvement of the optic disk in glaucoma.

The intraorbital portion of the nerve has a peripheral and possibly an axial system. The peripheral vessels arise from the pia mater and are derived from the neighboring blood vessels. The axial vessels are derived from the central retinal artery, a branch of the ophthalmic artery. The axial vascular system nurtures the central retinal fibers.

The intracanalicular and intracranial portions of the optic nerve are nurtured by the pial fibrovascular meshwork from branches of the internal carotid artery.

Chambers of the eye. The eye contains three chambers: the anterior chamber, the posterior chamber, and the vitreous cavity.

Anterior chamber. The anterior chamber (frontispiece) is bounded anteriorly by the cornea, posteriorly by the front surface of the iris and lens, and peripherally by the angle recess. The anterior chamber is deepest in its central portion (3 mm) and shallowest at the peripheral insertion of the iris. It has a volume of approximately 0.20 ml in humans.

Posterior chamber. The posterior chamber (frontispiece) is bounded anteriorly by the iris, laterally by the ciliary processes, medially by the equator of the lens, and posteriorly by the anterior face of the vitreous. Its volume in adults is about 0.06 ml. The aqueous humor secreted by ciliary processes flows from the posterior chamber through the pupil into the anterior chamber.

Vitreous cavity. The vitreous cavity is the largest cavity of the eye. It is bounded anteriorly by the lens zonule and ciliary body and posteriorly by the retina and optic nerve. It has a volume of 4.5 ml.

The vitreous body. The vitreous body is a transparent, gel-like structure composed of a network of collagen fibers (Fig. 2-4) suspended in a liquid containing hyaluronic acid. It is sphere-shaped with a segment removed anteriorly to provide a saucer-shaped depression for the lens (lenticular fossa). In the region of this depression the vitreous body is condensed and described clinically as the anterior hyaloid membrane, although it is not a membrane. The vitreous body adheres firmly to the ciliary epithelium in the region of the ora serrata and to the margin of the optic disk. Sometimes the hyaloid surface is loosely attached to the posterior capsule of the lens (Weigert hyaloideocapsular ligament).

In the healthy eye the vitreous body is in contact with the entire retina and is attached to the basement membrane of the retina by scattered collagenous filaments. These attachments are sometimes firm in the region of the central retina and the equator, and they may be a cause of retinal holes (p. 349). The central portion of the vitreous is less fibrillar than elsewhere; this gives the appearance of a hyaloid canal (the canal of Cloquet).

The vitreous may be divided into two portions: a cortical portion, which is adjacent to the retina, and the lens, which circumscribes the entire vitreous body. In the region of the ora serrata, which is the vitreous base, numerous fibrils attach the vitreous to the ora serrata. At the edge of the optic disk, fibrils extend between

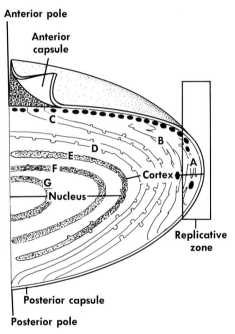

Fig. 1-31. Diagram to show distribution of cells in the human lens. New lens fibers replicate at the lens equator, and their nuclei migrate to the anterior subcapsular area in the nuclear bow (not shown). Young lens cells *(A, B, C)* occupy a thin layer, contain nuclei, and attach to their basement membrane, the capsule. Matured lens fibers *(D, E, F, G)* without nuclei occupy the majority of the lens and form the zones of discontinuity seen clinically with the biomicroscope. Lens fibers are joined together by socket and fine ridge joints. (Redrawn with permission from Kuwabara, T.: Exp. Eye Res. **20:**427, 1975. Copyright by Academic Press Inc. [London] Ltd.)

the vitreous and the basement membrane of Müller cells. Embryologically (p. 77), the vitreous is divided into primary (mesenchymal), secondary (most of the vitreous), and tertiary (the zonule) sections.

The central vitreous has a less dense structure with less fibrils than the vitreous cortex. The vitreous cortex contains a few cells called "hyalocytes," which are believed to be phagocytes, connective tissue cells of the macrophage type.

The lens. The crystalline lens (Fig. 1-31) is a transparent, biconvex structure located immediately posterior to the iris and pupil and anterior to a shallow depression in the anterior viterous face, the lenticular fossa. It is held in position by the zonular fibers. It is approximately 10 mm in diameter and 4 mm thick. The anterior surface has a radius of curvature of approximately 10 mm. The posterior surface has a radius of curvature of about 6 mm. The equator is 0.5 mm distant from the ciliary processes. The zonular fibers insert into the anterior and posterior lens capsule and extend further over the anterior surface than the posterior surface.

One cell type comprises the entire lens. The capsule of the lens is a thickened basement membrane of this ectodermal cell. Nucleated lens cells are found in a single layer beneath the anterior lens capsule only. Embryologically, the posterior lens fibers of the posterior lens cells grow rapidly, fill the lens vesicle, and lose their nuclei. Thereafter, the posterior lens capsule is supported by cells that have their nuclei beneath the anterior capsule.

The cells beneath the anterior capsule continue to form lens fibers throughout life. The replicative activity is near the equator of the lens, where the amino acids required for protein composition pass from the ciliary body through the lens capsule. Old fibers become compressed centrally and form heavier and less elastic lens fibers. Grossly, the lens seems brilliantly transparent; but as revealed by biomicroscopic examination, it has well-defined zones formed at various stages of life by the compression of lens fibers. The anterior lens cell (lens epithelium) attaches to the lens at its apical surface. The basement membrane covers the outer surface. The lateral cell membranes are markedly infolded but have sparse junctions except near the equator, where gap junctions are well formed.

The lens substance consists of elongated lens fibers, which have their cell body at the equator, and mature lens fibers, which have lost their nuclei and form the greatest portion of the substance of the lens, packed into an increasingly dense, central nucleus. The young cells migrate toward the center of the lens to form a bow zone. The posterior portion of the cells attaches to the basement membrane. Their apical ends join at the an-

terior center area and maintain junctions with cells extending from corresponding cells of the opposite side to form the upright, anterior Y-suture of the lens. When cells lose their nuclei, the posterior fibers are detached from the basement membrane and are pushed deeper into the central zone to form the inverted Y-shaped posterior suture. Lens fibers are curved, bandlike, exogenous cylinders that have numerous ridges and knob and socket invaginations, especially in their lateral edges. The apical ends of these cells are flat with lobulated edges. The cells form anterior suture lines with cells extending from the opposite side.

The lens capsule is a smooth, homogenous, acellular structure. The anterior capsule is thicker than the posterior capsule, but both consist of a homogenous structure composed of fine filamentary lamellae embedded in a cementlike substance. The nuclei of the supporting cells of the posterior capsule are located only

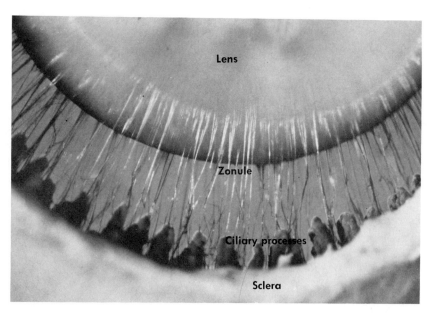

Fig. 1-32. Insertion of the zonules into the anterior portion of the lens capsule at the lens equator. (Courtesy Patricia N. Farnsworth, Ph.D., Physiology and Ophthalmology Department, College of Medicine and Dentistry of New Jersey.)

in the bow zone. The capsule is thickest in its equatorial area, just central to the insertion of the zonular fibers. The superficial zonule is a thin, zonular region composed of acid mucopolysaccharides, which constitute the attachment of the zonule to the lens.

The zonule. The lens zonule (zonule of Zinn, or suspensory ligament of the lens, Fig. 1-32) supports the lens in position. It is composed of a series of fine fibrils modified from the collagenous tissue on the outer surface of the lens capsule. The

zonules arise from the nonpigmented epithelium of the ciliary body and attach to the lamellar portion of the lens capsule on either side of the equator. The zonular fibers attach to the internal limiting membrane covering the ciliary epithelium. They attach to the basement membrane of the ciliary epithelium in the valleys between the ciliary processes and not at their apices. The ciliary attachment is broad, and fibers may extend to the pars plana of the ciliary body. Other fibers attach to the anterior vitreous face. The in-

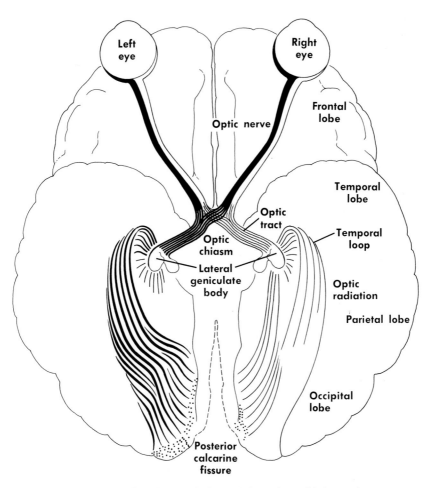

Fig. 1-33. Optic pathways. All of the nasal fibers of the right and left eye decussate (cross) at the optic chiasm.

sertion is to the equator of the lens in a zone that extends about 2 mm in front and 1 mm behind it.

Optic pathways

The retina, as discussed previously, is divided into a central portion (mainly cones), used in central vision and color vision, and a peripheral portion (mainly rods), used in dark adaptation and in the detection of movement. In the distribution of nerve impulses in the visual pathways, the retina is divided into four quadrants by horizontal and vertical lines

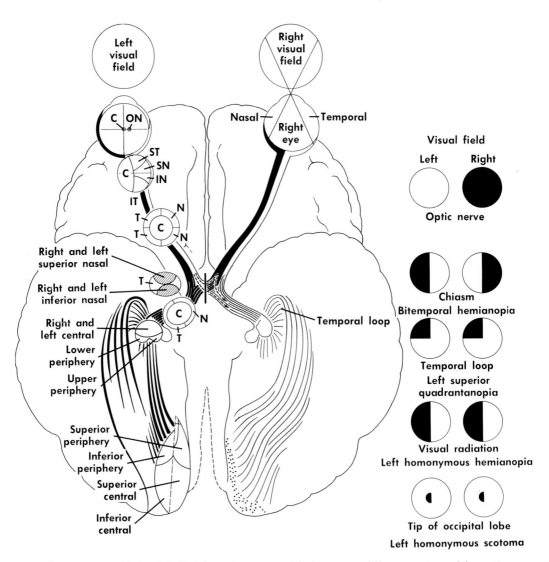

Fig. 1-34. Typical visual field defects that occur with damage to different regions of the optic pathways. Visual fields are diagrammed to reflect the source of the light that stimulates the retina. Light from the temporal side stimulates the nasal portion of the retina, light from above stimulates the lower portion, and so on. Thus, the visual field defect caused by a lesion affecting fibers arising from the nasal half of the retina is diagrammed as a temporal field defect.

ent but are modified by the occurrence of numerous granule (stellate) cells that form a grossly visible band of Gennari.

THE ORBIT

The eyes rest in the anterior portion of two bony cavities, the orbits, located on either side of the nose. Although the orbit appears to be positioned directly forward, only the medial walls are parallel, whereas the lateral walls diverge at an angle of about 45°. The posterior openings of each orbit, the optic foramen, and the superior orbital fissure are thus located medial to the eye, so that the optic nerve, blood vessels, and ocular muscles that originate in the annulus of Zinn near the orbital apex must pass laterally, an important factor in ocular motility.

The anterior two thirds of the orbit are roughly the shape of a truncated quadrilateral pyramid with a base of about 35 to

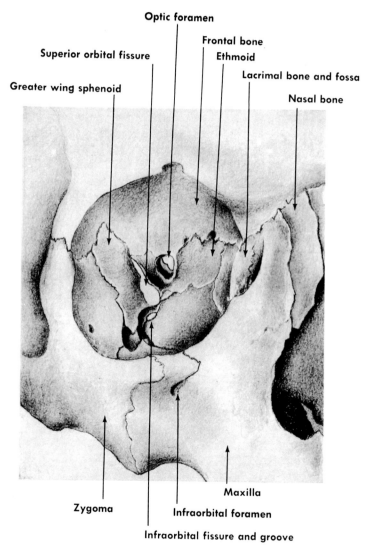

Fig. 1-35. The bony orbit.

40 mm. The floor of the orbit disappears at the posterior third as it narrows to the shape of a triangular pyramid. The orbit is usually considered to be approximately 40 mm in height, width, and depth, and its volume is about 29 ml.

Portions of six bones form the orbit (Fig. 1-35): the maxilla, the palatine, the frontal, the sphenoid, the zygoma, and the ethmoid and lacrimal, which belongs exclusively to the orbit.

Structure

The anterior margin of the orbit narrows so that its greatest width is about 10 mm within the front surface. The anterior margin is thickened and provides protection for the eye. The zygomatic bone and the zygomatic process of the frontal bone form the sturdy lateral margin. The superior margin is formed entirely by the frontal bone. The medial angular process of the frontal bone and the frontal process of the maxilla form the medial margin, which is poorly defined because of the fossa for the lacrimal sac. The inferior margin is formed by the zygoma and the body of the maxilla. Each wall of the orbit, except the medial, is approximately triangular with the base directed forward.

Two bones form the lateral wall: the zygoma anteriorly and the greater wing of the sphenoid posteriorly. The zygomatic portion of the lateral wall is composed of dense bone that separates the orbit from the fossa of the temporalis muscle. The lateral orbital tubercle is situated on the anterior margin of the lateral wall. To it is attached the aponeurosis of the levator palpebrae superioris muscle, the suspensory ligament of the lateral rectus muscle. The greater wing of the sphenoid bone forms the posterior two thirds of the lateral wall. This posterior portion is extremely thin, and it separates the orbit from the temporal lobe of the brain.

The roof of the orbit is formed mainly by the thin orbital plate of the frontal bone. In its lateral portion, the orbital roof is adjacent to the zygoma anteriorly and to the greater wing of the sphenoid posteriorly. Medially, it forms a suture with the lacrimal bone anteriorly and the ethmoid bone posteriorly. The fossa for the lacrimal gland is located in its anterior lateral portion. Medially, near the anterior margin, is the trochlea, a fibrous tissue that forms a pulley for the tendon of the superior oblique muscle. Immediately above the orbital roof is the frontal sinus anteriorly and the frontal lobe of the brain posteriorly.

The orbital floor does not extend to the apex; thus the posterior orbit is triangular or rounded. The floor is formed mainly by the orbital plate of the maxilla. The orbital surface of the zygoma extends laterally, and the orbital process of the palatine bone medially. Posteriorly, the infraorbital sulcus (Fig. 1-36) extends across the floor of the orbit from the infraorbital fissure and contains the infraorbital artery and maxillary nerve. At about its midpoint, this becomes a canal that opens into the infraorbital foramen through which the artery and nerve emerge on the face.

The medial wall is quadrilateral. It is formed mainly by the orbital plate of the ethmoid bone, but it has sutures anteriorly with the lacrimal bone and posteriorly with the body of the sphenoid bone. Because the ethmoid bone is extremely thin (lamina papyracea), this sinus may rupture into the orbit when inflamed, or the bone may fracture and thus permit air to enter the orbit. In the anterior portion of the orbit, the fossa of the lacrimal crest is located between the anterior lacrimal crest of the frontal process of the maxilla and the posterior lacrimal crest of the lacrimal bone. The lacrimal sac occupies this fossa and extends downward through the nasal lacrimal duct into the nose. The medial canthal ligament divides into two leaves

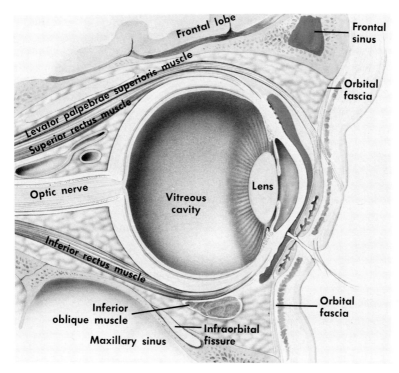

Fig. 1-36. Sagittal section of the orbit. The infraorbital fissure is the weakest area of the orbit and is involved in blow-out fractures.

that insert into the anterior and posterior lacrimal crest. The posterior portion of the medial wall of the orbit formed by the body of the sphenoid bone contains the optic foramen.

Optic foramen and orbital fissures

The optic foramen is located at the posterior medial portion of the orbit in the body of the sphenoid bone. The optic canal measures 4 to 10 mm in length. Through it passes the optic nerve, the ophthalmic artery, and sympathetic nerves from the carotid plexus. Just lateral to the optic foramen is a superior orbital fissure that separates the greater and lesser wings of the sphenoid bone. The fissure is divided into lateral and medial portions by the fibrous annulus of Zinn, from which the ocular muscles

arise. Passing through the superior orbital fissure within the annulus of Zinn are the oculomotor nerve (N III), trochlear nerve (N IV), and all branches of the ophthalmic division of the trigeminal nerve (N V) except the lacrimal and frontal branch. These, together with the trochlear nerve (N IV), emerge from the lateral portion of the superior orbital fissure outside the annulus of Zinn and the muscle cone.

The inferior orbital fissure (sphenomaxillary) is formed at the junction of the orbital plate of the greater wing of the sphenoid bone and the lateral margin of the orbital process of the maxillary bone. It transmits the second branch (maxillary) of the trigeminal nerve and provides anastomosis between the inferior ophthalmic vein and the pterygoid plexus. The fissure is covered by smooth muscle of Müller, which has a doubtful function in humans and is the analogue of the retractor bulbi muscle of lower animals.

The annulus of Zinn encircles the optic foramen and the medial portion of the superior orbital fissure. The dural sheaths accompanying the optic nerve split into two layers at the orbital apex. One portion lines the orbit as the periosteum; the other continues forward as the dural sheath of the optic nerve. The annulus is inserted medially into the cleft formed by this splitting; laterally, it is attached at the spina recti lateralis at the tip of the greater wing of the sphenoid. Each of the recti muscles originates at the annulus of Zinn. The lateral rectus muscle is divided into an upper and lower head by the superior orbital fissure.

Orbital fascia

The orbital contents are bound together and supported by connective tissues that, although connected, divide the

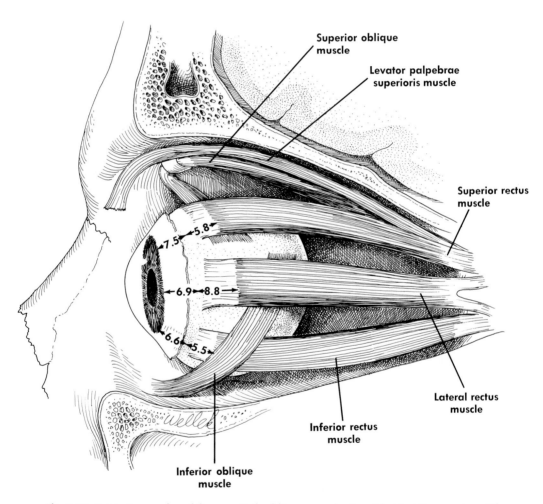

Fig. 1-37. Extrinsic muscles of the eye. Both oblique muscles insert behind the equator of the globe. The inferior oblique muscle passes over the body of the inferior rectus muscle but beneath the lateral rectus muscle. The numbers indicate the distance of the insertion from the corneoscleral limbus and the length of the muscle tendon.

orbit into spaces of clinical importance in limiting the spread of hemorrhage and inflammation. The main orbital fasciae are (1) the periorbital (periosteum of the orbit), (2) the orbital septum (palpebral fascia), (3) the bulbar fascia (Tenon capsule), and (4) the muscular fascia.

The *periorbita (periosteum of the orbit)* is the periosteal lining of the orbit. It is derived from the dura mater, which splits at the optic foramen into two layers, one contributing to the periosteum and the other continuing as the dural sheath of the optic nerve.

The *orbital septum (palpebral fascia)* stretches from the bony margins of the orbit to the lid in close relationship with the posterior surface of the palpebral portion of the orbicularis oculi muscle (p. 52). The septum prevents orbital fat from entering the eyelids and limits the spread of inflammation.

The *bulbar fascia (Tenon capsule)* separates the globe from orbital fat and constitutes the socket in which the eye moves. It extends forward to the insertion of the deeper layers of the conjunctiva at the corneoscleral limbus. Its lower portion is thickened to form a sling (the ligament of Lockwood), upon which the globe rests. Posteriorly, the fascia is thin and perforated by the structures passing to or from the globe.

The *muscular fascia* surrounds the ocular muscles, particularly their anterior portions, like the sleeve of a coat surrounds an arm. The portion that covers the medial and lateral recti muscles sends expansions to the orbital margins as check ligaments. Other fibers extend to the conjunctiva and hold it taut in ocular rotation.

EXTRINSIC MUSCLES

The extrinsic muscles of the eye (Fig. 1-37) are the four recti and the two oblique muscles. (The ciliary muscle and the sphincter and dilatator muscles of the pupil are the intrinsic muscles.)

Origin

The four recti muscles originate at the apex of the orbit from the ligament of Zinn (annulus tendineus communis), which encircles the optic foramen and the medial portion of the superior orbital fissure. The superior oblique muscle originates at the apex of the orbit from the periosteum of the body of the sphenoid bone medial to and above the optic foramen. The inferior oblique muscle arises from the floor of the orbit from the periosteum covering the anteromedial portion of the maxilla. The four recti muscles insert into the sclera anterior to the equator of the globe. The two oblique muscles insert into the sclera posterior to the equator.

The extraocular muscles appear to be the most highly organized of all striated muscles. They contain slow fibers capable of a graded contracture on their exterior surface near the orbit and fast fibers responsible for rapid movements in the central mass of the muscle. The slow fibers correspond to red muscle fibers, which contain a high content of mitochondria and oxidative enzymes. The fast fibers correspond to white muscle fibers and contain greater amounts of glycogen and glycolytic enzymes and less oxidative enzymes than do the slow fibers.

Recti muscles

The recti muscles are (1) the medial rectus muscle, (2) the lateral rectus muscle, (3) the superior rectus muscle, and (4) the inferior rectus muscle. They originate from the ligament of Zinn and pass forward in the orbit, gradually diverging to form the ocular muscle cone. Each muscle is about 40 mm long and 9.5 to 10.5 mm wide at its point of insertion into the sclera. By means of a tendon, the muscles insert into the sclera between 5 and 7 mm from the corneoscleral limbus.

The *medial rectus muscle* arises from the medial portion of the ligament of Zinn in close contact with the optic nerve. It is innervated by the inferior division of the third cranial nerve, which enters on the bulbar side. It functions in adduction (medial rotation) of the globe.

The *lateral rectus muscle* arises by two heads from the upper and lower portions of the ligament of Zinn, where it bridges the superior orbital fissure. It passes forward, over the insertion of the inferior oblique muscle, to insert into the sclera. It is innervated by the abducent nerve (N VI), which enters on its bulbar surface at about the middle. The function of this muscle is abduction (turning out) of the eye (p. 107).

The *superior rectus muscle* arises from the superior portion of the ligament of Zinn in close contact with the meningeal sheaths surrounding the optic nerve.* The muscle passes forward and laterally from the apex, forming an angle of 23° with the sagittal diameter of the globe. Superiorly, it is in close contact with the levator palpebrae superioris muscle throughout its course. The superior rectus muscle is innervated by the superior division of the third cranial nerve, which enters its bulbar surface at the junction of the anterior one third with the posterior two thirds. The muscle functions mainly as an elevator, with elevation becoming more efficient as the eye is turned laterally and becoming entirely absent as the eye is turned medially. When the eye is turned medially, the muscle aids in adduction. The muscle intorts (rotates inward) the superior meridian of the cornea (p. 106).

The *inferior rectus muscle* arises from the inferior portion of the ligament of Zinn and passes forward and laterally, forming an angle of 23° (as does the superior rectus muscle) with the sagittal diameter of the globe. It is innervated by

---

*On movement of the eye in retrobulbar neuritis (p. 367) pain occurs because of the close association of the superior and medial recti muscles with the optic nerve.

the inferior division of the third cranial nerve, which enters on its superior edge at the junction of the anterior one third with the posterior two thirds. The muscle functions mainly as a depressor, with depression becoming more efficient as the eye is turned laterally and becoming entirely absent as the eye is turned medially. In medial rotation, the muscle aids in adduction. The muscle extorts (rotates outward) the superior meridian of the cornea (p. 107).

Oblique muscles

There are two oblique muscles, the superior oblique and the inferior oblique.

The *superior oblique muscle* originates from the periosteal covering of the body of the sphenoid bone above and medial to the optic foramen. It consists of two parts: a direct portion extending from its origin to the trochlea and a reflected portion, composed entirely of tendon, from the trochlea to its insertion on the globe beneath the superior rectus muscle.

The direct portion passes forward in the angle between the roof and the medial wall of the orbit to the trochlea. The trochlear nerve (N IV) enters its upper surface at 8 to 13 mm from its origin. The trochlea is a V-shaped fibrocartilage attached to the trochlear spine of the medial aspect of the frontal bone a few millimeters behind the orbital margin. The tendon of the superior oblique muscle begins about 10 mm behind the trochlea. It is encased in a synovial sheath through the trochlea. From the trochlea the tendon passes downward, laterally, and posteriorly beneath the superior rectus muscle to be inserted on the upper outer quadrant of the eye behind the equator. The tendon is shaped as a fibrous cord about 1 by 2 mm in size, but it becomes flat and wide as it approaches the medial margin of the superior rectus muscle. The main function of the muscle is intorsion (inward rotation) of the 12 o'clock meridian of the cornea; this action is absent when the eye is rotated medially. In medial rotation the muscle depresses the eye, and in the straight ahead position the muscle aids in abduction.

The *inferior oblique muscle* arises from the periosteum covering the orbital plate of the maxilla a few millimeters behind the orbital margin and near the orifice of the nasolacrimal duct. It passes laterally and posteriorly between the inferior rectus muscle and the floor of the orbit, and then it curves upward around the globe to insert into the posterior sclera on the inferior lateral surface of the globe. It has no tendon. The muscle is innervated by the inferior division of the oculomotor nerve (N III), which enters the bulbar surface just after the muscle has passed to the lateral side of the inferior rectus muscle. The main function of the inferior

oblique muscle is elevation, which increases as the eye is rotated medially and is absent in abduction. In lateral rotation the muscle aids in abduction. The muscle extorts (rotates outward) the 12 o'clock meridian of the cornea.

EYELIDS

The eyelids are thin curtains of skin, muscle, fibrous tissue, and mucous membrane that protect the eye from external irritation, interrupt and limit the amount of light entering the eye, and distribute tears over the surface of the globe. The upper eyelid is limited above by the eyebrow; the lower eyelid merges with the cheek. Each eyelid is divided by a horizontal furrow into an orbital and a tarsal portion. The upper furrow is formed by skin insertions of the levator palpebrae superioris muscle (Fig. 1-38). The lower

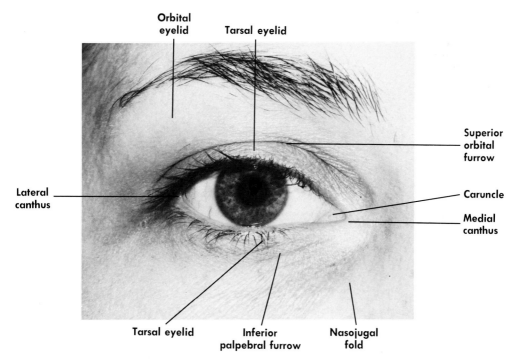

Fig. 1-38. Eyelids and palpebral folds. The superior and inferior palpebral folds divide the eyelids into tarsal and orbital portions.

furrow is poorly defined and is formed by a few cutaneous connections from the orbicularis oculi muscle. The corneoscleral limbus is covered above and below by the eyelids.

When the eyes are open, the eyelids form an elliptic opening, the palpebral fissure, which measures about 12 by 30 mm. Laterally, this fissure forms a 60° angle. The apex of the angle is about 2 mm higher than the medial portion in whites and blacks. In Mongolians and Orientals, the outer canthus may be 4 to 5 mm higher, but the almond shape of the palpebral fissure arises from its asymmetry so that the inner half is wider than the outer half. Medially, the palpebral fissure is rounded. In Mongolians it is obscured by a characteristic vertical skin fold (epicanthus) which, when present in whites, may cause the eyes to appear to be turned in (pseudostrabismus).

Located on the free margin of each eyelid are the opening of the lacrimal canaliculi (the puncta), the eyelashes or cilia, and the openings of glands (Fig. 1-39). Each eyelid margin is 2 mm thick and 30 mm long. At a point 5 mm from the medial angle is a small eminence, the papilla lacrimalis, which contains the minute central opening of the lacrimal canaliculus, the punctum. The medial one sixth of the eyelid, or the lacrimal portion, has no cilia or gland openings, and the eyelid margins are rounded. The lateral five sixths of the eyelid margin has square edges.

The intramarginal sulcus, or gray line, divides the eyelid margin into anterior and posterior leaves. The eyelashes originate anterior to the gray line, and the orifices of the tarsal glands are posterior to it. The junction of the conjunctiva and the stratified epithelium of the skin is at the level of the orifices of the tarsal glands.

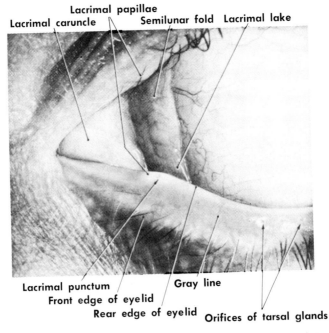

Fig. 1-39. Lacrimal portion of the eyelid margin. (From Gibson, H. L.: Med. Radiogr. Photogr. **28:**126, 1952.)

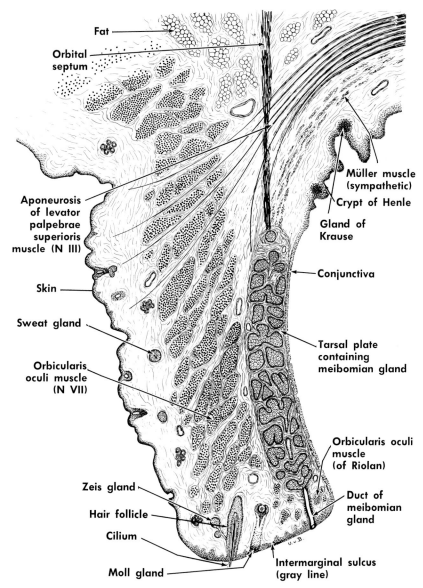

Fat

Orbital septum

Aponeurosis of levator palpebrae superioris muscle (N III)

Skin

Sweat gland

Orbicularis oculi muscle (N VII)

Zeis gland

Hair follicle

Cilium

Moll gland

Müller muscle (sympathetic)

Crypt of Henle

Gland of Krause

Conjunctiva

Tarsal plate containing meibomian gland

Orbicularis oculi muscle (of Riolan)

Duct of meibomian gland

Intermarginal sulcus (gray line)

Fig. 1-40. Eyelid in cross section. The orbital septum separates the intraorbital contents from the eyelid. The intermarginal sulcus provides a line of surgical dissection separating the anterior structures of the eyelid from the tarsus and tarsal conjunctiva.

The eyelashes on the upper eyelid margin curve upward and are more numerous than those on the lower eyelid margin, which curve downward. Opening into the follicle of each cilium are the ducts of the sebaceous glands of Zeis. Large sweat glands (of Moll) open into these follicles or directly onto the eyelid margin between the cilia.

Structure. The eyelids contain the following parts (Fig. 1-40):

Skin
Muscles
    Orbicularis oculi (N VII)
        Orbital portion
        Palpebral portion
    Levator palpebrae superioris (N III)
    Palpebral smooth muscles of Müller (sympathetic nerves)
Fibrous tissue
    Palpebrum fascia or septum orbitale
    Tarsal plates
    Medial and lateral palpebral ligaments

The *skin* of the eyelids is the thinnest in the body. It contains no fat in the subcutaneous areolar area and is thrown into numerous folds. The skin may be markedly distended by blood or fluid and, because of its thinness, underlying blood vessels may appear as dark blue channels.

The *muscles* of the eyelids are the orbicularis oculi (N VII), the levator palpebrae superioris (N III), and the palpebral smooth muscles of Müller (sympathetic nerves).

The orbicularis oculi muscle (N VII) is a thin, oval sheet of striated muscle composed of concentric fibers arranged approximately parallel to the palpebral fissure. There are two main portions: a peripheral orbital part involved in forcible closure of the eyelids and a central palpebral part involved in involuntary blinking. Both portions of the orbicularis oculi muscle originate from the anterior and posterior leaves of the medial palpebral ligament attached to the anterior and posterior lacrimal crests. The muscle inserts into the lateral palpebral ligament attached to the lateral orbital tubercle.

The levator palpebrae superioris muscle (N III) is closely related to the superior rectus muscle in its origin and course. It arises from the periosteal covering of the lesser wings of the sphenoid bone, and its origin blends with that of the superior rectus muscle below and the superior oblique muscle medially. It runs forward beneath the roof of the orbit to a point about 1 cm behind the septum orbitale, where it expands to the aponeurosis, which passes through the septum to find wide insertion. The aponeurosis inserts into the skin of the eyelid to form the superior palpebral furrow, into the anterior surface of the tarsal plate, and into the medial and lateral palpebral ligaments. The nerve supply is from the superior division of the oculomotor nerve (N III), which passes through the underlying superior rectus muscle to reach the levator muscle.

The superior and inferior palpebral smooth muscles of Müller (sympathetics) are small sheets of smooth muscle located immediately beneath the orbital portion of the palpebral conjunctiva. The superior palpebral muscle arises from the undersurface of the levator palpebrae superioris muscle. The inferior palpebral muscle has an indefinite origin from the muscular fascia covering the inferior rectus muscle. Each of the palpebral muscles inserts into the tarsal plate. They function in providing "tone" to the eyelids.

The *fibrous tissue* of the eyelids consists of a peripheral layer, the palpebral fascia or septum orbitale (p. 47), and a thickened central portion, the tarsal plates.

The tarsal plates consist of firm connective tissue (not cartilage) that gives form and density to the free margin of the eyelids. Each tarsal plate is about 1 mm thick and 25 to 30 mm long. They extend from the lacrimal puncta medially to the lateral canthus. The upper tarsus is about 11 mm wide, and the lower tarsus is about 5 mm wide.

The free edge of the tarsal plate extends the length of the ciliary portion of the eyelid margin. The posterior surface of the tarsus is firmly attached to the tarsal conjunctiva and conforms to the curvature of the globe. The anterior surface of the tarsus is separated from the orbicularis oculi muscle by loose areolar tissue, so that the muscle moves freely over its surface. The deep margin of the tarsus gradually merges into the orbital septum. Medially and laterally, the tarsal plates attach to palpebral ligaments.

Each tarsus contains sebaceous (meibomian) glands, the ducts of which open onto the eyelid margin. These glands are arranged in a single row in the tarsal plate, and each consists of 10 to 15 acini placed irregularly around a central canal opening onto the eyelid margin. The sebaceous secretion prevents the overflow of tears, makes possible an airtight closure of the eyelids, provides the superficial layer of the precorneal tear film (p. 84), and prevents the rapid evaporation of tears.

Blood supply. The blood supply to the eyelid is derived from marginal and peripheral vascular arcades (Fig. 1-21). These are formed by the lateral palpebral branches of the lacrimal artery and the medial palpebral branches of the dorsonasal artery, both of which are derived from the internal carotid artery through the ophthalmic artery (p. 58). There is a wide anastomotic circulation provided by branches of the external carotid artery through the facial, superficial temporal, and infraorbital arteries.

Nerve supply. The ophthalmic (first) division of the trigeminal nerve (N V)

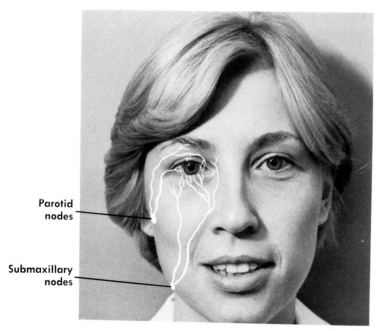

Parotid nodes

Submaxillary nodes

Fig. 1-41. Lymphatic drainage of the eyelids and conjunctiva. The orbit and the globe and its contents have no lymphatics.

provides the sensory innervation to the upper eyelid and to a small lateral portion of the lower eyelid. Innervation of the remaining portion of the lower eyelid is by the maxillary (second) division of the trigeminal nerve through the infraorbital nerve. The facial nerve (N VII) innervates the orbicularis oculi muscle, and the oculomotor nerve (N III) supplies the levator palpebrae superioris muscle. Postganglionic sympathetic fibers from the superior cervical ganglion innervate the palpebral muscles of Müller.

Lymphatic supply. The eyelids are drained by two groups (Fig. 1-41) of lymphatic vessels: (1) a medial group drains the medial two thirds of the lower eyelid and the medial one third of the upper eyelid and ends in the maxillary lymph nodes; and (2) a lateral group drains the remaining portion of the eyelids and ends in the parotid (preauricular) nodes.

THE CONJUNCTIVA

The conjunctiva is a thin, transparent mucous membrane (Fig. 1-42) lining the inner surface of the eyelids and covering the anterior portion of the sclera. Its epithelium is continuous with that of the cornea and the lacrimal drainage system through the puncta. The conjunctiva is divided into three areas: (1) the palpebral conjunctiva, (2) the conjunctiva of the

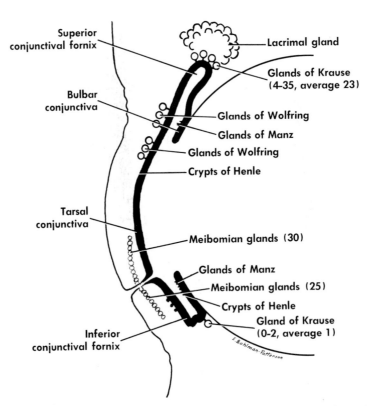

Fig. 1-42. Sagittal section through the eye to show the conjunctival sac and the position of the glands. The glands of Wolfring and Manz secrete the mucinous portion of tears; the lacrimal gland and the glands of Krause secrete the aqueous portion of tears; and the meibomian glands secrete the oily interior layer of the tear surface.

superior and inferior fornices, and (3) the bulbar conjunctiva.

The *palpebral conjunctiva* is divided into marginal, tarsal, and orbital portions. That portion on the margin of the eyelid contributes to the mucocutaneous junction at the gray line. The tarsal portion is closely adherent to the tarsal plate, from which it can be removed only with difficulty. The orbital portion is thrown into folds.

The *conjunctiva of the superior and inferior fornices* forms transitional areas between the palpebral and bulbar conjunctivae. It is but loosely applied to the underlying tissue and may become markedly swollen.

The *bulbar conjunctiva* is closely adherent to the sclera, which can be seen as the "white" of the eye through the transparent conjunctival tissue.

At the medial angle of each eye are two specialized structures formed in part by the conjunctiva: the semilunar fold and the lacrimal caruncle (Fig. 1-39). The semilunar fold (plica semilunaris) consists of a delicate vertical crescent of conjunctiva, the free edge of which is concave and concentric with the corneal margin. It is separated from the bulbar conjunctiva by a cul-de-sac 2 mm deep. The lacrimal caruncle is a minute piece of modified skin located in the lacus lacrimalis medial to the semilunar fold. It is covered by stratified epithelium that is not keratinized. It consists of large sebaceous glands similar to meibomian glands and has fine hairs with sebaceous glands similar to the glands of Zeis. The caruncle is conspicuous when the eye is rotated laterally.

Structure. Like other mucous membranes, the conjuncitva is composed of two layers: (1) stratified columnar epithelium and (2) a lamina propria composed of an adenoid and a fibrous layer.

The *stratified columnar epithelium* varies in thickness from two cell layers in its upper tarsal portion to five to seven layers at the corneoscleral junction. It is never keratinized in healthy individuals.

The *lamina propria* is composed of connective tissue containing blood vessels, nerves, and conjunctival glands. After the age of 3 months, the development of the adenoid layer makes the surface of the conjunctiva moderately irregular. Goblet cells secreting mucin are numerous in the conjunctival fornices and occur less frequently in the bulbar portion. They secrete the innermost layer of the precorneal tear film (p. 84) responsible for wetting the corneal epithelium. The bulbar and fornix conjunctiva and the orbital portion of the palpebral conjunctiva contain the adenoid layer with numerous lymphocytes enmeshed in a fine reticular network. True lymphatic follicles are not present. The fibrous layer of the conjunctiva is continuous with the attached margin of the tarsal plates and contains the smooth palpebral muscle of Müller (sympathetics).

Blood supply. The blood supply of the palpebral conjunctiva arises from the peripheral and marginal arterial arcades of the eyelid. The marginal arcade nourishes the margin and a portion of the tarsal part of the palpebral conjunctiva. The bulbar and fornix conjunctiva is nourished by the peripheral arcade (Fig. 1-21).

The posterior conjunctival branches of the peripheral arterial arcade provide the blood supply of the peripheral bulbar conjunctiva. These vessels are superficial, nearly invisible, and extend within 4 mm of the corneoscleal junction. In this area, anterior conjunctival branches of the seven anterior ciliary arteries pass toward the cornea to form a superficial (conjunctival) and a deep (episcleral) pericorneal plexus. The anterior and posterior conjunctival vessels anastomose.

The posterior conjunctival vessels are dilated in inflammations of the bulbar conjunctiva (p. 217). Because of their superficial position, they appear bright red and move with the conjunctiva. They are most evident in the fornices and fade toward the limbus. Because they are superficial, they may be constricted with the instillation of 1:1,000 epinephrine. The superficial (conjunctival) pericorneal plexus, which is derived from the anterior ciliary arteries, is injected in inflammations of the cornea. The deep (episcleral) pericorneal plexus is injected in inflammations of the iris and the ciliary body and in angle-closure glaucoma. Because of their deep position, these vessels appear dull red to purple and do not move with the conjunctiva. They are not affected by topical epinephrine. These vessels are most evident near the corneoscleral limbus and fade toward the fornices. Because of the generous anastomoses between the anterior and posterior conjunctival arteries, severe inflammations always cause injection of both ciliary and conjunctival vessels.

Nerve supply. The bulbar conjunctiva is innervated by ciliary nerves and by sympathetic nerves accompanying blood vessels. Sensory innervation of the superior palpebral conjunctiva is by the frontal nerve medially and lacrimal nerve laterally. Sensory innervation of the inferior palpebral conjunctiva is by the lateral palpebral branch of the lacrimal nerve laterally (ophthalmic division, N V) and the infraorbital nerve (maxillary division, N V).

Lymphatic supply. The lymphatics of the conjunctiva parallel those of the eyelid (p. 54).

Glands. The conjunctival epithelium, unlike that of the cornea, contains numerous unicellular mucous glands (goblet cells) that secrete the mucoid layer of the precorneal tear film. The glands are most numerous in the bulbar conjunctiva and fornices and are absent at the eyelid margins and corneoscleral limbus (Fig. 1-42). Located deep in the substantia propria in the superior and inferior fornices, particularly laterally, are the accessory lacrimal glands of Krause, which have the histologic structure of the lacrimal gland proper. The accessory lacrimal glands of Wolfring are situated near the upper margin of the superior tarsal plate.

LACRIMAL APPARATUS

The lacrimal apparatus consists of a secretory and a collecting portion. The secretory portion (Fig. 1-42) is composed of the lacrimal gland and the accessory lacrimal glands of Krause and Wolfring. The collecting portion consists of the canaliculi with their orifices (the puncta), the lacrimal sac, and the lacrimal duct, which has its opening in the inferior nasal meatus.

Secretory portion

Lacrimal gland. The lacrimal gland is located in the anterior lateral portion of the roof of the orbit in the lacrimal fossa. It is divided into a large orbital portion and a small palpebral portion by the lateral part of the aponeurosis of the levator palpebrae superioris muscle. The lacrimal gland is of the tubuloalveolar type and has numerous acini composed of a double layer of cells surrounding a central canal. The canals open into the larger ducts that in turn open into excretory ducts. Three to five ducts drain the orbital portion of the gland, and five to seven ducts drain the palpebral portion. The ducts of the orbital portion pass through the palpebral lobe, and each of the ducts opens separately onto the superior temporal fornix.

Secretory innervation to the lacrimal gland arises in the lacrimal (salivary) nucleus in the floor of the fourth ventricle and runs through the facial nerve to the geniculate ganglion. The fibers do not synapse here but leave the facial pathway via the greater superficial patrosal nerve to reach the sphenopalatine (Meckel) ganglion. From here, postganglionic fibers are distributed to the lacrimal gland, passing either directly or with the zygomatic branch of the maxillary branch of the trigeminal nerve (N V). Postganglionic sympathetic fibers from the superior cervical ganglion pass by way of the deep petrosal nerve to the sphenopalatine ganglion, where they are distributed with fibers destined for the lacrimal gland. The sympathetic innervation is mainly to blood vessels of the gland and has no direct effect on secretion.

The lacrimal gland is drained by the lymphatic vessels ending in the preauricular lymph nodes.

Accessory lacrimal glands of Krause and Wolfring. The accessory lacrimal glands of Krause and Wolfring are isolated accumulations of lacrimal tissue distributed throughout the upper and lower cul-de-sac. More of these glands are located in the lateral one third of the conjunctiva than elsewhere. There are 5 to 10 large glands, which may be multilobulated, and 10 to 30 small glands.

Collecting portion

The collecting portion of the lacrimal apparatus (Fig. 1-43) is composed of the puncta, the canaliculi, the lacrimal sac, and the nasolacrimal duct.

Puncta. The puncta are slightly elevated openings that are round or slightly ovoid, about 3 mm in size, and located on the upper and lower eyelid margins about

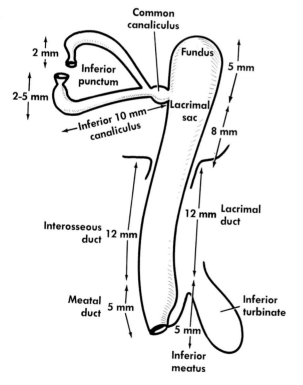

Fig. 1-43. Collecting portion of the lacrimal apparatus. Tears enter the canaliculi through the puncta and then pass through the lacrimal sac and nasal lacrimal duct to the inferior nasal meatus.

6 mm from the medial canthus. The opening is surrounded by relatively dense, avascular connective tissue.

Canaliculi. The upper and lower canaliculi each consist of a vertical portion 2.0 to 3.5 mm in length and a horizontal portion directed medially for about 8 mm where they join to form the common canaliculus. The canaliculi are about 0.5 mm in diameter, lined by stratified squamous epithelium, and surrounding by elastic tissue. Each punctum, the opening of the lacrimal canaliculi, is inverted into the lacrimal lake when the eyelids are closed. The dense surrounding of connective tissue prevents their collapse.

Lacrimal sac. The lacrimal sac is located in the medial portion of the orbit in the lacrimal fossa. The medial palpebral ligament lies anterior to it. The sac inserts in the lacrimal crest and reflects a portion of the ligament to the posterior lacrimal crest. The fundus of the sac rises 3 to 5 mm above the palpebral ligament, and immediately posterior to the ligament the sac receives the canaliculi. Inferiorly, the sac is continuous with the nasolacrimal duct.

Nasolacrimal duct. The nasolacrimal duct is a downward extension of the sac that opens into the inferior nasal meatus. The duct is surrounded by the bone of the nasolacrimal canal, and it opens in the inferior nasal meatus at the anterior portion of the lateral wall. The duct may pass for several millimeters in the nasal mucous membrane before the opening. A variety of constrictions and folds in the sac of the nasolacrimal duct are described as "valves."

BLOOD SUPPLY
Arteries

The eye and the orbital contents receive their main blood supply from the ophthalmic artery. The eyelids and conjunctiva have a generous anastomotic supply from branches of both the external carotid and the ophthalmic arteries. There are numerous variations in the pattern of vasculature.

Ophthalmic artery. The ophthalmic artery is the first intracranial branch of the internal carotid artery that begins just as the artery exits from the cavernous sinus. The ophthalmic artery enters the orbit through the optic foramen below and lateral to the optic nerve, turns forward and upward, and passes over the optic nerve to its medial side. It ascends to the medial wall of the orbit, passes forward with the nasociliary nerve between the medial recti and the superior oblique muscles, and terminates by dividing into dorso-nasal and supratrochlear branches (Fig. 1-44).

The majority of branches of the ophthalmic artery are given off while the vessel is lateral to the optic nerve. These branches include the following arteries.

1. The central retinal artery sends nutrient vessels to the optic nerve. It then divides into superior and inferior optic disk branches, which in turn divide into nasal and temporal branches providing blood to the inner layers of the retina.

2. The medial and lateral posterior ciliary arteries give rise to 6 to 20 branches. The short posterior ciliary artery branches enter the globe around the optic nerve and are distributed to the intraocular portion of the optic nerve and the choriocapillaris. The long posterior ciliary arteries anastomose with the anterior ciliary arteries to form the circulus arteriosus iridis major.

3. The lacrimal artery gives off a large, recurrent meningeal artery that anastomoses with the middle meningeal branch of the maxillary artery. The lacrimal artery terminates in temporal and zygomatic branches that anastomose with the anterior deep temporal and transverse facial arteries. These form lateral palpebral branches that anastomose with

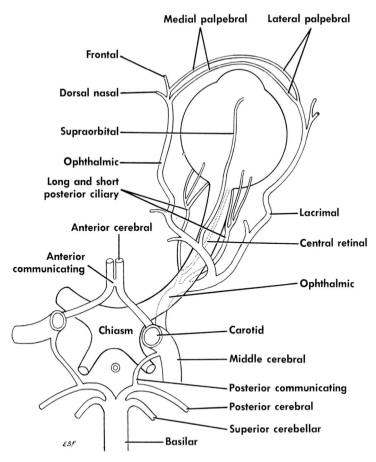

Fig. 1-44. Arteries that supply blood to the orbit and the ocular adnexa. There are many variations.

medial palpebral arterial arcades of the eyelid. Branches of the peripheral arterial arcade are distributed to the conjunctiva as the posterior conjunctival arteries.

4. A variable number of recurrent arteries anastomose with branches of the internal carotid artery. These may replace major blood vessels, even the ophthalmic artery itself.

5. Muscular branches are distributed to each of the extrinsic muscles in the orbit and have many anastomoses. The anterior ciliary arteries (Fig. 1-21) are forward continuations of the muscular arteries of the recti muscles. Each rectus

muscle has two muscular arteries except the lateral rectus muscle, which has one. The anterior ciliary vessels extend to the corneoscleral limbus as the anterior conjunctival arteries and form the pericorneal arcade. The superficial conjunctival arteries anastomose with the posterior conjunctival arteries derived from the palpebral arcade. About 4 mm from the corneoscleral limbus, branches of the anterior ciliary arteries penetrate the sclera to contribute, together with long posterior ciliary arteries, to the circulus arteriosus iridis major and to provide blood vessels to the ciliary processes.

When superior to the optic nerve, the ophthalmic artery gives off the supraorbital artery, which extends anteriorly to anastomose with the superficial temporal and supratrochlear arteries in the scalp.

When medial to the optic nerve, the ophthalmic artery gives off posterior and anterior ethmoidal arteries. The anterior ethmoidal artery has an anterior meningeal branch. Superior and inferior palpebral branches anastomose through the tarsal and peripheral palpebral arcades with the corresponding branches of the lacrimal artery. The ophthalmic artery terminates in two branches: (1) the dorsonasal artery, which is distributed to the skin of the nose and to the lacrimal sac and anastomoses with angular and nasal branches of the facial artery, and (2) the supratrochlear artery.

External carotid artery. The blood supply to the eye and eyelids from branches of the external carotid artery arises from (1) the external maxillary (facial) artery, (2) the superficial temporal artery, and (3) the internal maxillary artery.

The *external maxillary (facial) artery* gives off a number of branches to the face. Its terminal branch is the angular artery, which anastomoses at the medial canthus with the dorsonasal branch of the ophthalmic artery to provide blood for the inferior arterial arcades of the eyelids. It also anastomoses with the infraorbital artery, a branch of the internal maxillary artery.

The *superficial temporal artery* is the smaller terminal branch of the external carotid artery. The transverse facial artery, the largest branch of the superficial temporal artery, anastomoses with the infraorbital and angular arteries. The zygomatico-orbital artery anastomoses with the lacrimal artery and its palpebral branches to participate in the arterial arcade of the eyelids. The frontal artery anastomoses with the supraorbital and frontal branches of the ophthalmic artery

and with the corresponding artery from the opposite side.

The *internal maxillary artery* is the larger of the terminal branches of the external carotid artery. Its largest branch is the middle meningeal artery, which supplies the bone and dura mater at the base of the skull. The internal maxillary artery sends an orbital branch through the superior orbital fissure and anastomoses with a recurrent branch of the ophthalmic artery. The infraorbital artery originates in the pterygopalatine (sphenomaxillary) fossa; it enters the orbit through the infraorbital fissure, runs in the infraorbital sulcus and canal in the orbital plate of the maxilla, and passes forward to emerge on the face from the infraorbital foramen. The infraorbital branch anastomoses with the angular branch of the external maxillary (facial) artery, the transverse facial branch of the superficial temporal artery, and the lacrimal and dorsonasal branches of the ophthalmic artery.

These vessels provide a generous anastomosis for nutrition of the eyelids and the globe. The many anastomoses make it particularly difficult to correct aneurysms involving the circle of Willis.

Veins

Venous drainage of the orbit is mainly through the superior and inferior orbital veins. These are markedly tortuous, have no valves, and empty into the cavernous sinus. The superior orbital vein communicates with the angular vein, which is continuous with the facial vein. The inferior ophthalmic vein communicates with the pterygoid plexus through the inferior orbital fissure. The inferior ophthalmic vein may either communicate directly with the cavernous sinus or may empty into the superior ophthalmic vein. The two superior vortex veins empty into the superior orbital vein, and the two inferior vortex veins join the inferior orbital vein. The central retinal vein usually exits from the optic nerve close to the entrance of the artery. It enters the cavernous sinus separately or empties into the superior ophthalmic vein.

The cavernous sinus (Fig. 1-45) is an irregular-shaped, endothelium-lined venous space situated between the meningeal and periosteal layers of the dura mater on either side of the body of the sphenoid bone. It extends from the medial end of the superior orbital fissure to the apex of the petrous bone behind.

In front, it receives the superior orbital vein, with which it is almost continuous. Medially, it communicates with the opposite sinus, and behind, with the superior and inferior petrosal sinuses. The internal carotid artery passes through the cavernous sinus on its medial wall; the abducent nerve (N VI) is just lateral to the artery. The oculomotor nerve (N III) and trochlear nerve (N IV) are in its medial wall on its superior aspect, whereas the ophthalmic and maxillary branches of

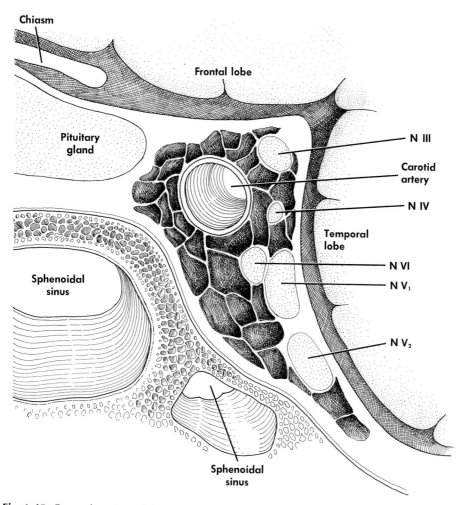

Fig. 1-45. Coronal section of the cavernous sinus posterior to the orbit. It is almost continuous with the superior orbital vein.

the trigeminal nerve (N V) are located lateral to and below the artery. One or a combination of these nerves may be affected by diseases of the cavernous sinus, such as thrombosis (p. 247) and rupture or aneurysm of the internal carotid artery (p. 529).

NERVES TO THE EYES
Cranial nerves

The distribution and function of the cranial nerves to the eyes are as follows:

Motor
  Oculomotor (N III)
    Superior division to superior recti and levator palpebrae superioris muscles
    Inferior division to medial and inferior recti and inferior oblique muscles and motor (short) root to ciliary ganglion (ciliary and sphincter pupillae muscles)
  Trochlear (N IV) to superior oblique muscle
  Abducent (N VI) to lateral rectus muscle
Mixed
  Facial (N VII)
    Motor to face
    Secretory to submaxillary, sublingual, and lacrimal glands
    Taste from anterior two thirds of tongue
  Trigeminal (N V)
    Motor to muscles of mastication
    Sensory from face and eye
    Proprioceptive from muscles of mastication (mesencephalic nucleus and perhaps ocular muscles)

Oculomotor (third cranial) nerve. The oculomotor (third cranial) nerve supplies the superior, medial, and inferior recti

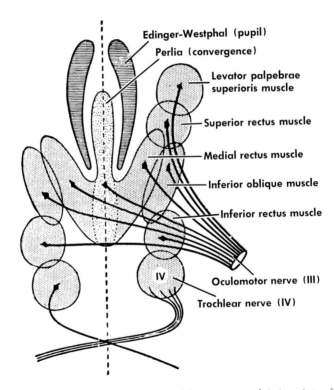

Fig. 1-46. Ventral view of the oculomotor and trochlear nerve nuclei. A variety of arrangements has been suggested. This is Brouwer's modification of Bernheimer's scheme. (From Warwick, R.: Oculomotor organization. In Bender, M. B., editor: The oculomotor system, New York, 1964, Harper & Row, Publishers, Inc.)

muscles and the levator palpebrae superioris muscle. Its visceral efferent fibers innervate the ciliary muscle and the sphincter pupillae muscle after synapse in the ciliary ganglion.

Nucleus. The nucleus of the oculomotor nerve is an elongated mass of cells located beneath the cerebral aqueduct of Sylvius, which connects the third and fourth ventricles. Many different arrangements of its component parts have been described (Fig. 1-46). The nucleus is frequently stated to be composed of two parts: lateral cells that are paired, located posteriorly, and are nearly continuous with the nuclear cells of the trochlear nerve; and medial cells that are unpaired, located at the anterior extremity of the nucleus, and related to convergence. The latter group of cells is the nucleus of Perlia.

The lateral paired cells send fibers to all of the extrinsic muscles of the eye except the superior oblique (N IV) and the lateral recti (N VI) muscles. At their anterior termination on each side is the Edinger-Westphal nucleus, which innervates the sphincter pupillae and ciliary muscles.

The medial (posterior) longitudinal fasciculus connects the lateral motor cells of the oculomotor nerve to each other and to the nuclei of the fourth and sixth cranial nerves, the vestibular nuclei, and the sensory nucleus of the trigeminal nerve. This fiber tract transmits stimuli that coordinate conjugate movements of the eyes (eyes right, eyes left, eyes up, or eyes down). Anterior lesions in this tract produce an internuclear ophthalmoplegia (p. 524) in which convergence is normal but, on attempts to turn the eyes laterally, the adducting eye does not pass beyond the midline and there is a coarse nystagmus of the abducting eye.

Intracerebral course. From the third cranial nerve nucleus, efferent fibers run through the tegmentum, red nucleus, and substantia nigra and leave the midbrain in the interpeduncular fossa between the cerebral peduncles.

Intracranial course. In their intracranial course, the oculomotor nerves are closely associated with the posterior cerebral arteries above and the superior cerebellar arteries below. From the midbrain they pass down forward, outward, and downward to pierce the dura mater and enter the roof and lateral wall of the cavernous sinus about midway between the anterior and posterior clinoid processes. In the cavernous sinus each nerve is close to the trochlear and ophthalmic division of the trigeminal nerve.

Orbital distribution. The oculomotor nerve leaves the cavernous sinus near the lesser wing of the sphenoid bone and enters the orbit through the superior orbital fissure (Fig. 1-47). Here it divides into a small superior and larger inferior division. The superior division is distributed to the superior rectus muscle on its bulbar surface and passes through this muscle to terminate in the levator palpebrae superioris muscle. The inferior division is distributed to the medial and inferior recti muscles. Its terminal portion ends in the posterior border of the inferior oblique muscles. The terminal branch to the inferior oblique muscle sends the short, or motor, root branch to the ciliary ganglion.

Ciliary ganglion. The ciliary ganglion is located between the lateral rectus muscle and the optic nerve near the apex of the orbit.

It has three roots: parasympathetic, sympathetic, and sensory.

Parasympathetic root (N III)
 Ciliary muscle
 Sphincter pupillae muscle
Sympathetic root
 Uveal blood vessels
Sensory root (N V)
 Globe

The *parasympathetic root* consists of visceral motor fibers (Edinger-Westphal

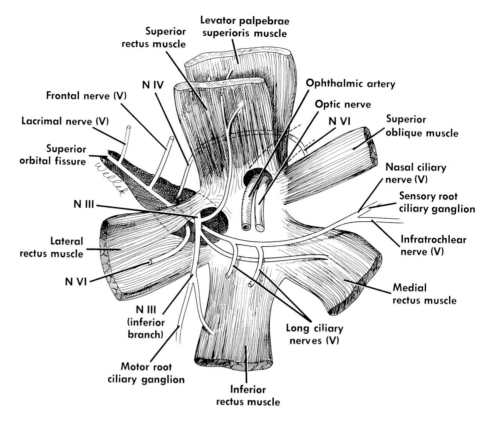

Fig. 1-47. Apex of the right orbit. The optic nerve, ophthalmic artery, and sympathetic nerves are transmitted through the optic foramen. The optic foramen and the medial portion of the superior orbital fissure are encircled by the annulus of Zinn. The lacrimal and frontal branches of the ophthalmic division of the fifth nerve and the trochlear nerve (N IV) enter the orbit in the lateral portion of the superior orbital fissure outside of the annulus. The other branches of the ophthalmic division of the fifth nerve and the oculomotor (N III) and abducent (N VI) nerves enter the orbit more medially with the annulus. The maxillary, or second, division of the trigeminal nerve enters the orbit through the inferior orbital fissure and emerges on the face at the intraorbital foramen. The lateral rectus muscle is divided into upper and lower origin by the annulus of Zinn as it bridges the superior orbital foramen. The superior oblique muscle is exceptional in receiving the motor nerve, the trochlear (N IV), on its orbital surface. All the other muscles are innervated on the side closest to the globe.

nucleus) given off by the terminal branch of the inferior division of the oculomotor nerve, which ends in the inferior oblique muscle. After synapse in the ciliary ganglion, emerging fibers are distributed as postganglionic cholinergic fibers to the ciliary muscle (accommodation) and the sphincter pupillae muscle (pupillary constriction).

The *sympathetic root* consists of fibers derived from the cavernous and internal carotid plexuses. The sympathetic nerves are postganglionic fibers that synapse in the superior cervical ganglion and thus pass through the ciliary ganglion without synapse. These fibers mainly provide vasoconstrictor fibers to uveal blood vessels.

The *sensory root* is derived from the nasal ciliary branch of the ophthalmic division of the trigeminal nerve, and these fibers do not synapse. The sensory root also contains sympathetic fibers that may entirely replace the separate sympathetic root.

The branches of the ciliary ganglion are 6 to 20 short ciliary nerves that branch and pierce the sclera about the optic nerve. They are distributed to the uveal tract and to the ciliary and sphincter pupillae muscles.

Trochlear (fourth cranial) nerve. The trochlear (fourth cranial) nerve innervates the superior oblique muscle only. Its fibers decussate in the brain, and it is the only cranial nerve to emerge from the dorsal surface of the brain.

Nucleus. The nucleus of the trochlear nerve is a small group of cells located at the posterior end of the lateral (paired) portions of the oculomotor nerve. It is located beneath the cerebral aqueduct of Sylvius, near its connection with the fourth ventricle, at about the level of the inferior colliculus (Fig. 1-46). The cells are connected by the medial longitudinal fasciculus to other motor nuclei of the eye, the vestibular nuclei, and the trigeminal sensory nucleus.

Course in the brain stem. The trochlear is the sole cranial nerve to decussate dorsally. The axons pass laterally and then curve around the aqueduct of Sylvius, progressing caudally and passing over the aqueduct, at which point they leave the brain stem.

Intracranial course. After emerging from the brain stem on its dorsal surface, the trochlear nerve passes as a slender filament around the cerebral peduncle to reach the ventral surface of the brain just posterior to the oculomotor nerve. It enters the dura mater posterior to the entrance of the oculomotor nerve at about the level of the posterior clinoid process. It is located in the lateral wall of the cavernous sinus somewhat below the oculomotor nerve. The trochlear nerve emerges from the cavernous sinus and enters the lateral portion of the superior orbital fissure outside the ligament of Zinn. In the orbit it passes anteriorly and medially, crossing above the oculomotor nerve, the levator palpebrae superioris muscle, and the superior rectus muscle. It enters the superior oblique muscle on its orbital surface. This is the only ocular muscle that does not receive its innervation on its bulbar aspect.

Abducent (sixth cranial) nerve. The abducent (sixth cranial) nerve has the longest intracranial course of any of the motor nerves of the eye. It makes a sharp turn over the petrous ridge, which makes it vulnerable to trauma and increased intracranial pressure.

Nucleus. The nucleus of the abducent nerve is located in the gray matter in the floor of the fourth ventricle lateral to the medial longitudinal fasciculus. The genu of the facial nerve curves over the dorsal and lateral surfaces of the abducent nucleus.

Course in the brain stem. The axons of the abducent nerve cells pass anteriorly and ventrally through the pons and between the medially located superior olivary nucleus and the laterally located pyramidal tract. The fibers emerge on the ventral surface of the brain stem in a deep groove between the pons anteriorly and the medulla posteriorly.

Intracranial course. The fibers of the sixth cranial nerve pass anteriorly on the surface of the pons, to which they are bound by the anterior inferior cerebellar artery, the first branch of the basilar artery. The nerve then pierces the dura mater and passes vertically over the posterior part of the petrous portion of the temporal bone to enter the cavernous sinus. Just before entering this sinus, the nerve passes under the petrosphenoid ligament. In the cavernous sinus it is located just below the carotid artery and is the most inferiorly located of the motor nerves to the eye. The nerve enters the orbit through the superior orbital fissure between the two heads of the lateral rectus muscle. It passes forward and laterally in the orbit to innervate the lateral rectus muscle from its bulbar surface.

Facial (seventh cranial) nerve. The facial nerve supplies derivatives of the second branchial arch. It is mainly motor to the muscles of the face and scalp, but it has a small sensory component carrying sensations of taste from the anterior two thirds of the tongue. Additionally, it provides motor fibers to the submaxillary, sublingual, and lacrimal glands.

Nuclei. The motor nucleus of the facial nerve is located in the pons medial to the spinal trigeminal tract and lateral to the fibers of the abducent nerve. The gustatory (taste) nucleus receives fibers from cranial nerves VII, IX, and X. The cell bodies are located in the geniculate ganglion, and the axons extend centrally to the gustatory nucleus in the medulla. Fibers that stimulate salivary and lacrimal secretion originate in the salivary nucleus.

Course in the brain stem. The motor axons pass medially and posteriorly to the floor of the fourth ventricle to form a compact genu around the abducent nucleus. The fibers pass laterally to emerge from the ventral surface of the brain stem at the inferior border of the pons, considerably lateral to the abducent nerve.

Intracranial course. On emerging from the brain stem, the motor fibers of the facial nerve pass in the posterior cranial fossa anterior and lateral to the internal auditory meatus, which they enter in company with the acoustic and vestibular nerves and the intermediate nerve of Wrisberg. The facial nerve makes a sharp backward bend in the temporal bone to enter the facial canal, which curves over the superior and dorsal as-

pects of the middle ear. It emerges from the temporal bone at its lower portion through the stylomastoid foramen.

The nerve then immediately turns anteriorly around the base of the styloid process to enter the parotid gland, where it divides into its terminal divisions, the upper temporofacial and the lower cervicofacial. The temporofacial division gives off temporal and zygomatic branches supplying the orbicularis oculi, the frontalis, the corrugator supercilii, and the anterior and superior auricularis muscles. The cervicofacial division supplies the lower face. These upper and lower branches of the facial nerve have separate areas of origin in the facial nucleus. The upper branches have cortical connections with each hemisphere, but the lower branch has connections only with the opposite motor cortex. Thus, in a unilateral supranuclear lesion, structures innervated by the upper portion of the facial nerve are not affected, but those innervated by the lower portion (opposite side) are affected. The structures are similarly affected in infranuclear lesions.

The taste fibers have a complicated course. Those from the anterior tongue join the chorda tympani nerve, which runs across the middle ear cavity to join the facial nerve. Then the fibers pass with the facial nerve to a point where the internal acoustic meatus joins the facial canal. It is here that the geniculate ganglion is located. Other taste fibers are located in the petrous ganglion (glossopharyngeal nerve) and in the nodose ganglion (vagus nerve).

Motor fibers to the salivary and lacrimal glands are contained in the intermediate nerve of Wrisberg, which passes with the facial nerve into the internal auditory meatus. As the facial nerve turns to enter the facial canal, most of the visceral efferent fibers leave at the apex of the angle as the greater superficial petrosal nerve, which runs forward through the petrous bone to reach the intracranial cavity. The greater superficial petrosal nerve then runs under the semilunar ganglion to emerge from the cranial cavity through the foramen lacerum—it passes through the pterygoid canal to join the spheno-palatine ganglion. Motor fibers to the lacrimal gland join the maxillary branch of the trigeminal nerve, which joins the zygomatic branch to enter the lacrimal gland.

Fibers to the maxillary gland pass with the chorda tympani nerve to emerge from the skull by a fissure between the tympanic and petrous portions of the temporal bone. Fibers join the lingual branch of the mandibular nerve and then synapse with the submaxillary ganglion; postganglionic fibers are distributed almost immediately to the maxillary and sublingual glands. The parotid gland receives its innervation from the lesser petrosal nerve.

Trigeminal (fifth cranial) nerve. The trigeminal nerve has a complicated structure. It is not only the sensory nerve of the face and head, but it also sends motor fibers to the muscles of mastication. It has extensive central connections with reflex arcs associated with cranial nerves III to XII.

> Motor root
>   Muscles of mastication
>   Tensor tympani muscle
>   Tensor veli palatine muscle
> Sensory root
>   Ophthalmic branch (V_1)
>   Maxillary branch (V_2)
>   Mandibular branch (V_3)
> Mesencephalic root
>   Proprioceptive from muscles of mastication

Motor nucleus and root. The masticator is the motor portion of the trigeminal nerve. Its nucleus is located cephalad to the facial nerve nucleus near the floor of the cerebral aqueduct of Sylvius. The fibers are distributed with the mandibular nerve and innervate the muscles that move the mandible and the muscles of mastication: the masseter, the temporalis, the internal pterygoid, the mylohyoid, the anterior belly of the digastric, and the external pterygoid. In addition, motor fibers supply the tensor tympani muscle, which tenses the eardrum, and the tensor veli palatine muscle, which stretches out the soft palate.

The mesencephalic root of the trigeminal nerve is situated between the main sensory and the motor nuclei. Fibers of this root are distributed with each of the main divisions of the trigeminal nerve. In the act of biting, impulses pass to the mesencephalic root. It has been postulated that proprioceptive fibers in the extraocular muscles terminate in the mesencephalic nucleus, but this has not been demonstrated.

Sensory nuclei. The principal sensory nucleus of the trigeminal nerve is located near the point of entry of the sensory root into the pons; it lies near the lateral surface of the pons close to the margin of the inferior cerebral peduncle. Functionally, it appears related to tactile impulses.

The nucleus of the spinal trigeminal tract extends down to the second cervical segment of the spinal cord and becomes continuous with the substantia gelatinosa of the dorsal horn. It is functionally associated with the sensation of pain and temperature.

The sensory root is composed of fibers that arise in the semilunar (gasserian) ganglion together with a few fibers from the ciliary ganglion and possibly from other ganglia. The sensory root extends from the posterior border of the semilunar ganglion to the pons. As it leaves this ganglion, it pierces the dura mater under the attached border of the tentorium, which contains the superior petrosal sinus at this point. It lies on the trochlear nerve and then crosses over the facial and auditory nerves as they pass to enter the internal auditory foramen. It is then related to a groove in the medial aspect of the petrous portion of the temporal bone lateral to the abducent nerve.

The sensory root of the trigeminal nerve enters the brain on the lateral surface of the pons about midway between its anterior and posterior margins. Inside the pons it divides into ascending and descending tracts. The thick ascending fibers terminate almost immediately in the principal sensory nucleus. The thin descending fibers are adjacent to the nucleus of the spinal trigeminal tract.

Semilunar ganglion. The semilunar ganglion is a crescent-shaped mass of cells lying in the Meckel cave, which is a cleft located between layers of dura mater in the middle fossa of the skull on a depression on the anterosuperior surface of the petrous bone. At its anterior concave aspect the semilunar ganglion receives three branches: the ophthalmic division (V_1), the maxillary division (V_2), and the mandibular division (V_3).

The *ophthalmic division* (V_1) may be outlined as follows:

> Frontal nerve
> Lacrimal nerve
> Nasociliary nerve
>   Long (sensory) root of ciliary ganglion
>   Long ciliary nerves
>   Posterior ethmoidal nerves
>   Infratrochlear nerves: superior and inferior palpebral nerves
>   Anterior ethmoidal nerves
>   Interior nasal nerves: medial and lateral nasal nerves
>   External nasal nerves

The ophthalmic is the smallest division of the semilunar ganglion. It is located in the lateral wall of the cavernous sinus. Just posterior to the sphenoid fissure it divides into the frontal, the lacrimal, and the nasociliary nerves. The frontal and lacrimal nerves enter the orbit above the ligament of Zinn, whereas the nasociliary branch enters through the ligament and accompanies the ophthalmic artery as it passes over the optic nerve and under the superior rectus muscle to the medial wall of the orbit (Fig. 1-47).

The *frontal nerve* is located in the roof of the orbit between the levator palpebrae superioris muscle and the periosteum. It terminates in the supraorbital and supratrochlear nerves. The supraorbital nerve leaves the orbit through the supraorbital notch and supplies the forehead, scalp, and upper eyelid. Its terminal branches are the medial and lateral frontal nerves. The supratrochlear nerve contains fibers from the medial scalp, eyelid, and conjunctiva that enter the orbit near the trochlea.

The *lacrimal nerve* follows the upper border of the lateral rectus muscle accompanied by the lacrimal artery. Its superior branch terminates as the lateral palpebral nerve, supplying the skin and conjunctiva of the upper and lower eyelids. The inferior branch receives a twig from the zygomaticotemporal branch of the maxillary division (V_2) of the trigeminal nerve, which may be secretory to the lacrimal gland.

The *nasociliary nerve* has much the same course as the ophthalmic artery and provides the only sensory innervation of the globe. The long (sensory) root of the ciliary ganglion is given off at the superior orbital fissure and runs to the ciliary ganglion.

Two long ciliary nerves arise from the nasociliary nerve as it crosses above the optic nerve. They pierce the sclera with the short ciliary nerves and accompany the long posterior ciliary arteries anterior to the ciliary plexus. The fibers are mainly sensory and are combined with sympathetic fibers to the dilatator pupillae muscle. The other branches of the nasociliary nerve have the regional distribution indicated in their nomenclature.

Autonomic nervous system

The autonomic nervous system is a subdivision of the motor portion of the nervous system that carries impulses to smooth muscles, cardiac muscle, and glands. In contrast to skeletal muscle, in which a single neuron extends from the central nervous system to the muscle fiber, the autonomic nervous system is composed of a two-neuron chain. The first, or preganglionic neuron, has its cell body in the central nervous system and synapses in a ganglion with postganglionic neurons. The second, or postganglionic neuron, has its cell body in an autonomic ganglion and terminates in smooth muscle, cardiac muscle, or glands.

The autonomic nervous system is composed of two parts: (1) visceral efferent fibers in cranial nerves III, VII, IX, X, and XI and sacral nerves II, III, and IV, which comprise the parasympathetic portion (craniosacral division); and (2) visceral efferent fibers of thoracic and lumbar nerves, which comprise the sympathetic system (thoracolumbar division).

Parasympathetic nervous system. The visceral efferent branch of the oculomotor nerve arises from cell bodies located in the Edinger-Westphal nucleus. Together with the inferior division of the oculomotor nerve, the axons pass with the branch to the inferior oblique muscle and form the preganglionic motor root (short) of the ciliary ganglion. Here synapse is made with the cells of postganglionic fibers, which pass with the short ciliary

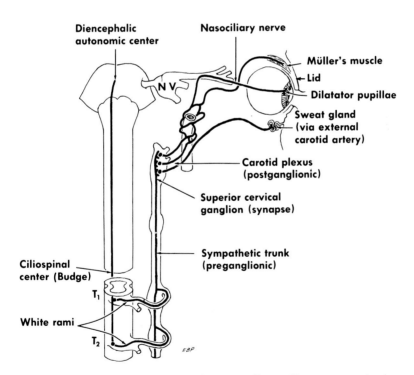

Fig. 1-48. Sympathetic nervous system of the eye. Afferent fibers synapse in the superior cervical ganglion. Postganglionic fibers then pass to the sweat glands of the face and eyelids along the external carotid artery. Other branches extend intracranially with the internal carotid artery and pass with the ophthalmic artery into the orbit. Vasomotor fibers are distributed by the short ciliary nerves to blood vessels in the choroid. Fibers to the dilatator pupillae muscle do not pass through the ciliary ganglion and are carried to the globe by the long ciliary branches of the ophthalmic division of the trigeminal nerve.

nerves to innervate the ciliary and sphincter pupillae muscles.

Sympathetic nervous system. The sympathetic nervous system (Fig. 1-48) has centers located in the hypothalamus and the medulla: (1) the superior ciliospinal center and (2) the inferior ciliospinal center (of Budge). The *superior ciliospinal center* is located near the nucleus of the hypoglossal nerve. The *inferior ciliospinal center* (of Budge) is located in the upper portion of the spinal cord. Sympathetic efferent fibers arise in the anterior lateral columns that leave the spinal cord in the ventral roots of thoracic I to lumbar II spinal nerves. These fibers pass with the anterior rami lateral to the vertebral column until they leave the anterior rami in the white ramus communicans. The white rami turn at right angles at the vertebral column to form the sympathetic nerve trunk, which extends from the base of the skull to the tip of the coccyx. Within the trunk are ganglia in which synapse is made with peripheral postganglionic sympathetic nerves.

The ganglia at the level of cervical I, II, and III spinal nerves fuse to form a superior cervical ganglion. Most of the preganglionic fibers making synapse in the superior cervical ganglion have left the spinal cord at the level of the first two thoracic nerves and have coursed upward in the sympathetic nerve trunk.

Postganglionic fibers from the superior cervical ganglion are widely distributed. The internal carotid branch extends intracranially with fibers distributed to the internal carotid artery and the cavernous plexus. These fibers provide nearly all of the sympathetic nerve branches to the eye and the orbit. Fibers for sweating of the face, however, are distributed with the external carotid artery.

Sympathetic nerve fibers pass through the ciliary ganglion without synapse. They are mainly vasomotor and are distributed by the short ciliary nerves to the uveal blood vessels.

Fibers to the dilatator pupillae muscle are mainly carried to the globe by the two long ciliary nerves that are given off by the nasociliary nerve and do not pass through the ciliary ganglion.

Supranuclear centers

The supranuclear centers of the cranial nerve nuclei to the eyes control reflex and voluntary ocular movements and are concerned with conjugate movements of the two eyes, such as eyes right, eyes left, eyes up, and eyes down.

Voluntary control and regulation of ocular movements that are not dependent on visual stimuli are functions of the frontal motor cortex in areas designated as 8 alpha, 8 beta, and 8 gamma, located at the posterior end of the second frontal convolution. Stimulation of these areas causes both eyes to turn to the side opposite the area stimulated. Extirpation of the frontal lobe causes the eyes to turn to the same side. Fibers from the frontal cortex reach the cranial nerves of the brain stem through the corticobulbar pathway that courses through the internal capsule. The fibers either enter the appropriate nuclei directly or course in the medial longitudinal fasciculus.

In movements in which the eyes follow a moving object (pursuit movement, p. 109), the supranuclear centers are in the occipital lobe. Stimulation of the occipital lobe causes conjugate deviation to the opposite side. The connections of visual centers in the occipital lobe with cranial nuclei are by corticotectal fibers to the superior colliculi, by corticotegmental fibers to centers for lateral gaze, and by corticotectal fibers that are involved in vertical gaze. The corticotegmental fibers, which end in the abducent nuclei of the opposite side, are involved in lateral gaze. Midbrain lesions tend to cause vertical defects of gaze (Parinaud syndrome, p. 527), and pontine lesions produce horizontal defects.

The frontal motor cortex and the occipital lobe on the same side are connected to each other. The frontal area is dominant, but if both frontal lobes are lost, the lack of voluntary eye movements is compensated for by voluntary head movements in response to visual stimuli arising from the occipital area (oculomotor apraxia).

In addition to those noted, other supranuclear centers are located in the cerebellum, basal ganglion, and extrapyramidal systems.

EMBRYOLOGY

The optic primordium and optic sulcus appear at the eight-somite state (22 to 23 days postovulation), and thereafter any adverse environmental influences cause ocular developmental abnormalities. In general, genetic or exogenous factors that influence development early in embryonic life cause such severe defects that the fetus seldom survives. Thus ocular defects seen clinically arise relatively late in ocular development.

The eye originates from neural and surface ectoderm and from mesoderm. Both the neural and pigment layers of the retina develop from neural ectoderm, and both layers continue anteriorly to give rise to the ciliary epithelium and the pigmented epithelium of the iris and its sphincter and dilatator muscles. The neuroglial and neural portions of the optic nerve originate from neural ectoderm.

The surface ectoderm gives rise to the lens, the epithelium of the cornea, the conjunctiva, and the eyelid together with the epithelium of their glandular structures. The mesoderm gives rise to the corneal endothelium and stroma, the sclera, the iris stroma, the extrinsic muscles of the eye, and the blood vessels and bones of the orbit (Table 1-2).

After fertilization of the ovum, a solid cluster of cells forms, the morula (Fig. 1-49, A). This develops into the blastula (Fig. 1-49, B), a hollow sphere containing a central cavity, the blastocele. The outer

Table 1-2. Primordia of ocular structures

Surface ectoderm	Mesoderm	Neural ectoderm
Lens	Corneal stroma	Sensory retina, retinal pigment epithelium
Corneal epithelium	Corneal endothelium (mesothelium) and Descemet membrane	Ciliary body epithelium, pigmented and nonpigmented
Conjunctival epithelium	Blood vessels	Pigmented epithelium of iris
Cilia	Sclera	Sphincter pupillae muscle, dilatator pupillae muscle
Epithelium, tarsal glands	Choroid	Neurologic and neural portions of optic nerve
Epithelium, Zeis and Moll glands	Conjunctival stroma	Melanocytes
Epithelium, lacrimal and accessory lacrimal glands	Episclera	
Epithelium, lacrimal passages	Tenon capsule	
	Iris stroma	
	Extrinsic eye muscles	
	Ciliary muscles	
	Bones of orbit	
	Vitreous	
Eyelid*		Bruch membrane†
Zonule (tertiary vitreous)*		

*From surface ectoderm and mesoderm.
†From neural ectoderm and mesoderm.

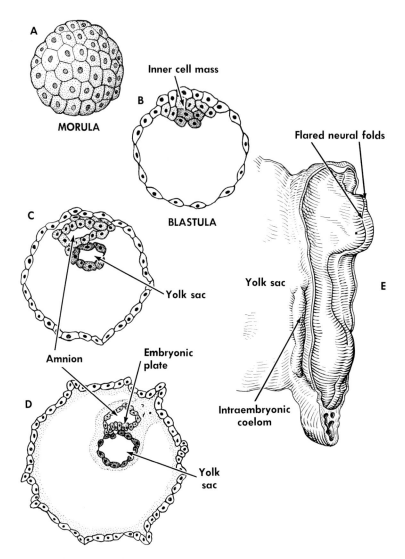

Fig. 1-49. A, Morula. **B,** Blastula containing the inner cell mass. **C,** Outer wall of the blastula is destined to form the placenta; the inner cell mass adjacent to the wall of the blastula gives rise to the amnion; the remaining cells form the yolk sac. **D,** Embryo develops at the area of contact between the amnion and the yolk sac. **E,** Amnion is cut away to show the neural folds at the anterior extremity of the neural plate.

wall of the blastula forms the placenta. The cells in one section of the inner wall form the embryo, amnion, and yolk sac (primitive gut or archenteron) (Fig. 1-49, C). The embryo develops from the embryonic plate at the area of contact between the amnion and the yolk sac (Fig.

1-49, D). It consists of two layers: a dorsal ectoderm and a ventral entoderm connected to the inner wall of the blastula by a body stalk. A primitive streak, followed by a groove, develops on the ectodermal surface and provides an axial symmetry to the embryonic plate. From the area of the

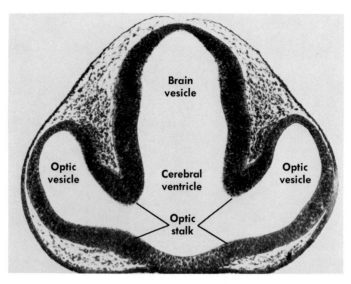

Fig. 1-50. Optic vesicles at 28 postovulation days. (×70.) (With permission from O'Rahilly, R.: Exp. Eye Res. **21:**93, 1975. Copyright by Academic Press Inc. [London] Ltd.)

groove, intraembryonic mesoderm appears and divides the plate into three layers.

In the dorsal ectoderm anterior to the primitive streak, a neural groove (longitudinal groove) and, by cell proliferation, the neural (medial) plate develop. At the anterior extremity of the neural plate, marked development of ectoderm forms two parallel folds (the neural folds) (Fig. 1-49, *E*). The neural folds are first recognizable 18 days postovulation and are prominent by 3 weeks. The optic primordium and optic sulcus appear in the neural fold on each side of the forebrain at about 22 to 23 days, when the embryo has eight pairs of somites and is about 2 mm maximum in length. At 24 days, the optic sulcus has become the optic vesicle. The anterior portion of the primitive brain consists of a cerebral vesicle separating lateral optic vesicles (Fig. 1-50).

After about the twenty-eighth postovulation day, the retinal disk appears in the wall of the optic vesicle, and the lens disk appears in the surface ectoderm. Within a few days, the retinal disk becomes invaginated to form the optic cup, and the retinal fissure is delineated. The lens disk becomes indented to form the lens pit (Fig. 1-51).

By the thirty-sixth postovulation day, the vitreous body begins to form, and melanin pigment appears in the outer wall of the optic cup destined to be the retinal pigment epithelium. The lens pit has closed to form the lens vesicle surrounded by its capsule. The restored surface ectoderm constitutes the epithelium of the future cornea. The lens body appears with early lens fibers, and the hyaloid artery enters the lentiretinalis space through the retinal fissure. By the forty-second postovulation day, the thicker inner layer of the optic cup begins to differentiate, and the cavity of the lens vesicle becomes obliterated by primary lens fibers. By the fifty-sixth day (Fig. 1-52), the ganglion cells of the retina give rise to the optic nerve fibers. The nerve fiber layer of the retina appears, and nerve fibers grow into the brain. The

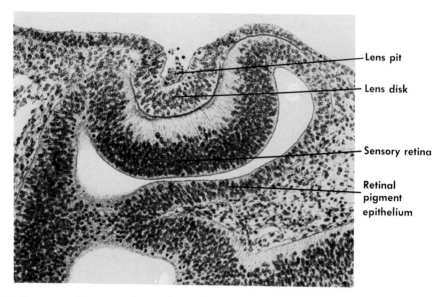

Lens pit

Lens disk

Sensory retina

Retinal
pigment
epithelium

Fig. 1-51. Optic cup at 32 postovulation.days. The sensory retina has a nucleus-free zone. Invagination of the lens disk has resulted in the appearance of a linear pit. (×210.) (With permission from O'Rahilly, R.: Exp. Eye Res. **21**:93, 1975. Copyright by Academic Press Inc. [London] Ltd.)

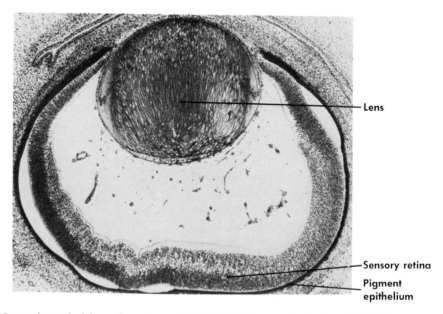

Lens

Sensory retina

Pigment
epithelium

Fig. 1-52. Eye at the end of the embryonic period. (×65.) (With permission from O'Rahilly, R.: Exp. Eye Res. **21**:93, 1975. Copyright by Academic Press Inc. [London] Ltd.)

mesothelium of the anterior chamber, the substantia propria of the cornea (Fig. 1-53), and the pupillary membrane develop. The scleral condensation is more apparent. Secondary lens fibers and the secondary vitreous body are forming. The embryo has a crown length of 30 mm, and the optic cup is approximately 1.5 to 2 mm in diameter.

Failure of the optic cup to invaginate results in a congenital cyst in which the orbit contains a large cyst with traces of nerve elements rather than an eye.

Invagination of the optic vesicle involves not only the lateral surface but also its inferior surface and the distal end of the optic stalk, so that a linear cleft or fissure forms on its posterior surface. This cleft is the retinal, or embryonic, fissure and is sometimes called the choroidal fissure. The retinal fissure provides a bypass for blood vessels and optic nerve fibers that enter and leave the optic vesicle so they do not pass around the lateral margin. Defects in the region of the ret-

inal fissure result in colobomas that may involve the 6 o'clock meridian of the optic nerve, the retina, the choroid, the ciliary body, and the iris.

During the 17- to 20-mm stage (7 weeks), the nose develops by fusion of the median nasal processes with each other and with the lateral nasal processes to form the frontonasal process. Failure of this fusional process results in the median cleft face syndrome.

THE EYE
Outer coat

The sclera. The sclera originates as a condensation of mesenchyme surrounding the anterior portion of the optic cup and then extends posteriorly. During the fourth month collagenous fibers extend posteriorly, and by the fifth month a continuous fibrous coat envelops the globe.

The cornea. The corneal epithelium is formed by the surface epithelium, from which the lens placode detaches itself. Mesodermal fibers give rise to the cor-

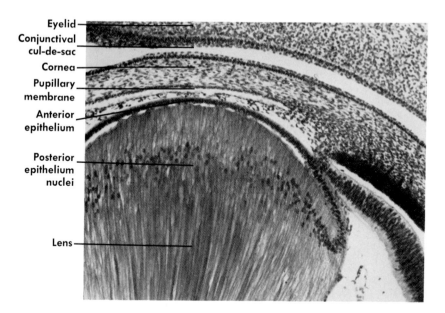

Fig. 1-53. Cornea and lens at the end of the embryonic period. (×135.) (With permission from O'Rahilly, R.: Exp. Eye Res. **21**:93, 1975. Copyright by Academic Press Inc. [London] Ltd.)

Eyelid
Conjunctival cul-de-sac
Cornea
Pupillary membrane
Anterior epithelium
Posterior epithelium nuclei
Lens

neal stroma and later to the corneal mesothelium (endothelium) and the Descemet membrane. The mesenchymal stream of the stroma provides the primary pupillary membrane, which is then vascularized.

Medial coat

The choroid. The choroid originates from the mesoderm surrounding the primary optic vesicle. All of its layers can be recognized by the fifth month. Pigment develops relatively late, first near the entrance of the posterior ciliary artery branches and then extending forward. At 6 weeks it is highly vascular, and the tissue is spongy. The choroid corresponds to the pia mater and arachnoid of the brain; anteriorly, it differentiates into the connective tissue and muscle of the ciliary body and the stroma of the iris. Uveal pigment is derived from the optic neural crest and is present initially in the peripapillary area and then extends forward.

At the anterior edge of the secondary optic cup, the inner sensory and outer pigmentary layers fuse together to form the following structures: (1) the ciliary epithelium (pars ciliaris retinae), with an inner nonpigmented layer that is a continuation of the neural layer and a pigmentary layer that is the continuation of pigmented epithelium, and (2) further anteriorly, the iris epithlium (pars iridica retinae) together with the sphincter and dilatator pupillae muscles.

The ciliary body. The ciliary body is formed by a fusion of the optic cup and the adjacent mesoderm. The ciliary processes are derived from the pigmented and nonpigmented epithelium of the primitive retina, and the capillaries are derived from mesenchyme. The ciliary muscle grows in from mesoderm located between the sclera and the ciliary ectoderm. Longitudinal fibers are formed

about the fourth month, and the circular portion is formed at the end of the sixth month. The attachment of the longitudinal fibers to the scleral spur establishes an anterior chamber angle. Secretion by the ciliary epithelium and outflow through the trabecular meshwork begin about the sixth or seventh month.

The iris and pupil. The iris is derived from both the ectoderm of the optic cup and the adjacent mesenchyme. The surface pattern of the iris in postnatal life closely reflects its embryologic origin. The most anterior extremity of the optic cup is visible as the pupillary frill. The sphincter pupillae muscle and dilatator pupillae muscle of the pupil are derived from neural ectoderm and, with the arrectores pilorum muscles, are the sole muscles in the body of ectodermal origin. Mesoderm first grows over the surface of the optic cup to form the anterior stromal layers up to the iris. Until the third month of embryonic life, the margin of the optic cup extends only a short distance beyond the equator of the lens. About the fourth month the cup grows forward with an attachment to the mesoderm. The mesoderm in the pupillary area then atrophies as far back as this attachment, which forms the collarette. The collarette is concentric with the pupillary margin and marks the position of the minor vascular circle of the iris.

Inner coat

Retinal pigment epithelium. The outer layer of the optic cup forms the retinal pigment epithelium. Initially, it is some four to six cells thick (32 postovulation days), but with cytolysis of these cells the pigment epithelium becomes deeply pigmented and a single cell-layer thick. This cytolysis may influence the stratification of the sensory retina. Inasmuch as the sensory retina grows at a different rate, the two layers are not in apposition until stratification of the sensory retina is complete.

Sensory retina. The sensory portion of the retina develops from the inverted portion of the optic cup. It consists, as does the neural tube, of three zones (ependymal, mantle, and marginal) limited by a terminal bar net on one side and by a basement membrane on the other. Because of formation of the optic cup by invagination, the basement membrane is on the vitreal surface and the terminal bar net is on the surface closest to the retinal pigment epithelium. The terminal bar net forms the external limiting membrane located at the level of the photoreceptor inner segment. The basement membrane provides the internal limiting lamina of the retina.

The ependymal zone develops cilia that project into the vesicle between the inner and outer walls of the optic cup; these develop into cone and rod outer segments. The marginal zone develops into the nerve fiber layer (and a transient, nonnucleated layer of Chievitz). The central mantle layer develops into the primitive neuroepithelium, which is divided into an outer and inner neuroblastic layer. The outer neuroblastic layer contains nuclei of rods and cones and bipolar and horizontal cells. The inner neuroblastic layer contains ganglion cells, amacrine cells, and Müller cells. Development proceeds from the posterior pole toward the periphery. The specialized area of the macula lutea begins in the third month, but its development proceeds slowly. Not until the sixth month is there a thinning of ganglion cells, and anatomic differentiation continues after birth. Inasmuch as central vision does not fully develop until the third to the fifth year, it is evident that functional differentiation lags behind anatomic differentiation.

Lens. The optic vesicle, as it extends laterally, is covered by surface ectoderm that becomes thickened into several layers, the lens placode. A groove or pit appears in this placode, forming a vesicle that becomes cut off from the surface ectoderm and forms the lens (Figs. 1-51 and 1-52). Lens fibers are laid down concentrically from the periphery, and their ends meet to form suture lines. The nuclei form the nuclear bow, and new lens fibers develop through life from the equator, the tips growing toward the front and back poles of the lens, adding layer after layer around the core.

The surface neural ectoderm is cytolyzed, and this causes the stimulation of the tissue to form the lens. Death of ectoderm cells and their subsequent autolysis are stimulants that cause the formation of new lenses in adult rabbits and mice whose lenses have been removed.

Vitreous body. The vitreous body is classically described as consisting of primary vitreous (the hyaloid vasculature system and the fibers that subsequently bridge it), secondary vitreous (the main mass of vitreous), and tertiary vitreous (the zonule). Strict distinction is not justified, and early in the fetal period the primary vitreous body is encroached by the secondary vitreous, which seems to originate from mesoderm.

The choriocapillaris arises from the mesoderm surrounding the primary optic vesicle, and during the fifth month the three vascular layers are present.

BLOOD SUPPLY

The fetal fissure extends to about the anterior one third of the optic stalk. About the end of the first month (when the fetus is 7 to 8 mm), an arterial plexus below the optic cup consolidates into (1) a hyaloid artery that enters the optic nerve and cup through the fissure and (2) a small annular vessel that ramifies on the rim of the cup and eventually becomes the choroid.

The hyaloid artery forms a network of

vessels covering the back of the lens (tunica vasculosa lentis) and filling the vitreous body (vasa hyaloidea propria). The hyaloid system disappears about the fifth month.

The vascular return of the entire hyaloid system is by the capsulopupillary membrane that covers the lens from the equator to the edge of the pupil. As the hyaloid system atrophies, the pupillary membrane is supplied by the long posterior arteries. It continues to develop until early in the sixth month, when the arteries begin to atrophy and disappear.

At about 14 to 15 weeks of intrauterine life (70 to 110 mm), mesenchymal cells appear in the vicinity of the hyaloid artery. They proliferate into the optic disk and subsequently invade the nerve fiber layer of the retina. The mesenchymal cells differentiate into endothelial cells that form solid chords, which gradually canalize to become capillaries. Thus, arteries and veins arise from capillaries and not the reverse. The growth progresses from the optic disk, and only at birth have the blood vessels reached the ora serrata, an important factor in the retinopathy of prematurity.

A wide variation in orbital blood vessels occurs, mainly because of failure of early branches to disappear. Portions of the pupillary membrane commonly persist over the pupillary aperture, and persistence of the hyaloid artery is common. It appears to arise from the optic disk and extends a variable distance into the vitreous cavity, sometimes as far as the lens. It may form a small opacity (the Mittendorf dot) on the posterior lens capsule. The Bergmeister papilla is a glial sheath that surrounds the first one third of the hyaloid artery. It may persist in the adult as a small tuft of tissue replacing the physiologic optic cup.

The optic stalk provides the neuroglial supporting structures of the optic nerve. The nerve fibers consist of axons of ganglion cells located in the inner layer of the retina together with fibers extending from the brain to the retina. The sheaths and septa of the optic nerve develop from mesoderm.

EYELIDS

The eyelids are derived from both mesoderm and surface ectoderm. The upper eyelid develops in medial and lateral parts from the frontonasal process. The mesodermal portion of the lower eyelid arises from an upgrowth of the maxillary process. The covering ectoderm gives rise to the skin on the outside and the conjunctiva on the inside. The eyelids grow together and fuse at approximately 9 weeks, and the eyes do not reopen until the seventh month. The tarsal plate and muscular tissues of the eyelid are derived from mesoderm; their glands and cilia arise from ectoderm.

LACRIMAL APPARATUS

The lacrimal gland arises from the ectoderm forming the conjunctival surface of the eyeball. Once formed, it receives connective tissue septa and supporting structures from the mesoderm.

The lacrimal passages develop in a cleft between the lateral nasal and maxillary processes. This cleft is converted into a tube by canalization of a solid rod of ectodermal tissue cells found beneath the surface, and these epithelial cells form the lacrimal passages. The lacrimal puncta do not open into the eyelid margins until just before the eyelids separate during the seventh month. The lower ends of the nasolacrimal ducts frequently do not open into the nose until birth or shortly thereafter.

BIBLIOGRAPHY

Beard, C., and Quickert, M. H.: Anatomy of the orbit, ed. 2, Birmingham, 1977, Aesculapius.

Hamming, N. A., Apple, D. J., Gieser, D. K., and Vygantas, C. M.: Ultrastructure of the hyaloid vasculature in primates, Invest. Ophthalmol. **16:** 408, 1977.

Howard, R. O., Boue, J., Deluchat, C., and others: The eyes of embryos with chromosome abnormalities, Am. J. Ophthalmol. **78:**167, 1974.

Kaufman, H. E., and Katz, J. I.: Pathology of the corneal endothelium, Invest. Ophthalmol. **16:** 265, 1977.

Kuwabara, T.: The maturation of the lens cell; a morphologic study, Exp. Eye Res. **20:**427, 1975.

LaVail, M. M.: Rod outer segment disk shedding in rat retina; relationship to cyclic lighting, Science **194:**1071, 1976.

Mausolf, F. A.: The anatomy of the ocular adnexa; guide to orbital dissection, Springfield, Ill., 1975, Charles C Thomas, Publisher.

O'Rahilly, R.: The prenatal development of the human eye, Exp. Eye Res. **21:**93, 1975.

Torczynski, E., and Tso, M. O. M.: The architecture of the choriocapillaris at the posterior pole, Am. J. Ophthalmol. **81:**428, 1976.

Tripathi, R. C.: Applied physiology and anatomy; tears, cornea, conjunctiva and ocular adnexae. In Ruben, M., editor: Contact lens practice; visual, therapeutic and prosthetic, London, 1975, Ballière Tindall.

Tripathi, R. C.: The functional morphology of the outflow systems of ocular and cerebrospinal fluids, Exp. Eye Res. **25:**65, 1977.

Warwick, R., editor: Eugene Wolff's anatomy of the eye and orbit, ed. 7, Philadelphia, 1977, W. B. Saunders Co.

Yamada, E., and Shikanos, S., editors: Electron microscopic atlas in ophthalmology, Philadelphia, 1972, J. B. Lippincott Co.

Chapter 2

PHYSIOLOGY AND BIOCHEMISTRY OF THE EYE

The human eye is by no means the best of all possible eyes. Its visual acuity is exceeded in birds, some of which have two foveas. Phenomena caused by polarized light may be appreciated by humans under special conditions, but we are unable to utilize the polarized light of the sky for orientation as bees do. Although sensitivity of the human eye increases markedly with dark adaptation, many nocturnal animals have a lower threshold to light.

Despite its inferiority for specific functions, the human eye provides vision in a wide variety of conditions. Humans have fairly good visual acuity both far and near. Color vision is well developed, and the human eye can adapt to light and dark over an intensity range of 100,000 to 1. The location of the eyes in the front of the head and the decussation of half of the nerve fibers from each retina lead to a retinal correspondence so that an object may be seen with depth and solidity (stereoscopic vision).

THE CORNEA

The cornea is a transparent tissue composed mainly of stroma with a regularly arranged epithelium on its outer surface and a single layer of endothelial cells lining its inner surface (p. 7). The anterior surface is bathed with tears, whereas the endothelium of the posterior surface is immersed in the aqueous humor.

The corneal stroma consists of collagen fibers of unusually uniform diameter gathered together in lamellae arranged at right angles to each other. They are enmeshed in a cementlike substance consisting of acid mucopolysaccharides (glycosaminoglycans), chondroitin, chondroitin-4-sulfate (chondroitin A), chondroitin-6-sulfate (chondroitin C), and keratin sulfate. The transparency of the stroma is intimately related to the metabolism of the epithelium and the endothelium, both of which must be intact to prevent stromal edema.

Because the central cornea is avascular, it must derive oxygen from the atmosphere and metabolic materials by diffusion from the pericorneal capillaries, from the aqueous humor, and from the tears. Only the peripheral cornea receives adequate nutrients from the bloodstream.

Transparency. The cornea transmits electromagnetic radiation (p. 98) having a wavelength* of between 300 nm in the ultraviolet and 2,500 nm in the infrared.

---

*The wavelength of electromagnetic energy is designated as nanometers (one billionth of a meter; m × 10^{-9}). Old units included Angstrom units (one ten-billionth of a meter; m × 10^{-10}) and millimicrons, which are the same as nanometers.

Transmission is about 80% at 400 nm and nearly 100% at 500 to 1,200 nm. There are two areas of absorption beyond 1,200 nm, but transmission is otherwise high between the long wavelengths. Radiation with wavelengths of more than approximately 1,000 nm is not absorbed by the visual photopigments of the retinal-photoreceptors and does not cause sensory stimulation. However, it is absorbed by the retinal pigment epithelium and dissipated as heat. Ultraviolet radiation below 365 nm is partially absorbed by the cornea; the rest is absorbed by the lens and does not reach the retina unless the intensity is very high. At high intensities the retina is stimulated by ultraviolet at 317 nm and infrared at 1,000 nm. In the visible range of the electromagnetic spectrum (approximately 380 nm to 760 nm), the cornea transmits nearly 100% of the light. This high transmission indicates that (1) the cornea does not contain particles such as pigment that absorb or reflect light and (2) the lamellar structure of the cornea is transparent.

The transparency of the cornea arises from its avascular anatomic structure and from a dynamic balance between salt and water maintained by an endothelial pump that controls corneal dehydration (deturgescence).

The anatomic factors include the absence of blood vessels and pigment in the cornea, the regular arrangement of the epithelial and endothelial cells, and the paucity of cells in the stroma. Additionally, the epithelial cells are not keratinized, and the anterior surface of tears forms a regular refracting surface. The endothelial cells and Descemet membrane do not reflect light at their interface, because they each have the same index of refraction. The collagen fibrils of the corneal stroma are oriented in a two-dimensional lattice, and the distance between each fiber is approximately equal (Fig. 2-1). The fibers are separated by less

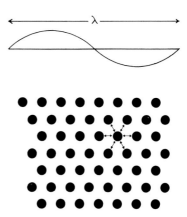

Fig. 2-1. The lattice structure of the cornea explains its transparency. Arrows between the fibrils indicate the system of forces that are supposed to maintain the regularity of the structure. The wavelength of light above is drawn to the same scale as the lattice. (From Maurice, D. M.: J. Physiol. [Lond.] **136:**263, 1957.)

than one wavelength of light and are so arranged that only forward scattering occurs. That portion of the light scattered by the lattice itself is eliminated by destructive interference. This mechanism of corneal transparency is unique. In other transparent tissues, such as the lens and corneal epithelium, the transparency occurs because of the uniform index of refraction of the cellular components.

Relative dehydration of the stroma is necessary for transparency. Each corneal lamella contains about 65% of the water it is capable of binding. A button of cornea with the stroma exposed swells to about three times its normal thickness and becomes translucent. If the endothelium is poisoned with ouabain, cyanide, or iodoacetate, similar swelling occurs.

This deturgescence is maintained by the epithelium, which is largely impermeable to water, and by an endothelial transport system. The endothelial system pumps fluid from the corneal stroma to the aqueous humor. Endothelial cells have a resting potential of about −14 millivolts relative to the aqueous humor (0 mV) and the stroma (1.0 mV). The negative charge within the endothelial system is the opposite of what would be expected of an electrogenic cation (Na^+) transport system. The explanation may be an anion pump involving bicarbonate with a bicarbonate-activated adenosine triphosphatase (HCO_3 ATPase) mechanism.

In the choroid plexus, gallbladder, and small intestine, H^+ is pumped into the intracellular spaces, and sodium and bicarbonate enter the cell passively. Subsequently, sodium is pumped out of the cell in a reaction catalyzed by sodium-potassium adenosine triphosphatase (Na-K ATPase).

In the mechanism involving bicarbonate, two thirds are considered to originate in the corneal stroma, and one third is provided by the endothelial cells converting exogenous carbon dioxide to bicarbonate. A cornea with sclera attached so the stroma is not in direct contact with fluid survives much longer in the laboratory when placed in bicarbonate Ringer's solution free of carbon dioxide than when placed in saline solution. Whatever the mechanism, the important observation is that corneal deturgescence is maintained by an active endothelial action that pumps fluid from the corneal stroma into the aqueous humor. Corneas for transplant survive longer in a tissue-culture medium enriched with oxidized glutathione, possibly because it influences adenosine triphosphate energy.

Epithelial defects cause subepithelial edema, and endothelial defects cause stromal edema. The anterior condensation of the corneal stroma (Bowman layer) apparently limits the extent of the edema.

Permeability. The peripheral cornea may maintain its metabolism by means of the capillary network at the corneoscleral limbus. The central cornea, however, depends for its nutrition on substances penetrating either the endothelium or the epithelium. Any substance reaching the epithelium must be water soluble so as to penetrate the film of tears covering the cornea. The epithelium constitutes the principal barrier of the cornea to ions. The zonula occludens and adherens and macula occludens and adherens make it impermeable to ions and other lipid-insoluble substances. The cornea is readily permeable to lipid-soluble substances, presumably because the cell membranes are composed of a lipoprotein. To pass through the stroma and endothelium, the compounds must be water soluble.

Metabolism. The cornea requires energy to maintain its deturgescence, provide its metabolic needs, and provide for epithelial cell renewal. Energy in the form of adenosine triphosphate is provided by the degradation of glucose from the aqueous humor and oxygen from the atmosphere. Inasmuch as most cells are located in the epithelium, this is the major site of metabolism.

Glucose is first phosphorylated to glucose-6-phosphate so that it may be utilized. This step requires the enzyme hexokinase, which is inhibited by its own product, glucose-6-phosphate. The glucose-6-phosphate is used in one of several metabolic pathways.

1. In glycolysis (Embden-Meyerhof pathway), which requires no oxygen, the glucose-6-phosphate is converted to two molecules of glyceraldehyde-3-phosphate, which is converted to two molecules of pyruvate. In the absence of oxygen the pyruvate is converted to two molecules of lactic acid and excreted into the precorneal tear film.

2. In the presence of oxygen the pyruvate is first decarboxylated to acetylcoenzyme A and, by a series of enzymatic reactions in the tricarboxylic acid cycle (Krebs or citric acid), is converted to carbon dioxide and water. This is the major cellular source of energy from glucose and molecular oxygen.

3. Glucose-6-phosphate may be degraded (phosphogluconate pathway, pentose phosphate pathway, or hexose monophosphate shunt) to 5-carbon sugars. The D-ribose-5-phosphate generated by the pathway is used in the nucleic acid synthesis required by the corneal epithelium.

About 65% of glucose-6-phosphate in the cornea is metabolized by glycolysis and the remainder by way of the phosphogluconate pathway. The enzymes of the tricarboxylic acid cycle are located in the epithelium but not in the stroma. Thus, when the corneal epithelium is deprived of oxygen by means of a contact lens, an epithelial edema develops (Sattler veil). This reflects the inability of glycolysis alone to support epithelial metabolism and the inadequacy of the oxygen supply from the corneoscleral limbus vasculature. If the epithelium of the cornea is removed and a contact lens applied, the stroma and endothelium remain transparent almost indefinitely.

Wound healing. After laceration or freezing of the cornea, repair takes place in the epithelium, stroma, and endothelium. Loss of corneal epithelium causes enlargement and flattening of adjacent uninjured epithelial cells within an hour. These cells develop pseudopodia and migrate into the denuded area to provide a new layer that is one cell thick and covers the denuded area. This is followed by mitosis and thickening of the epithelial cell layer and, after 6 weeks, by adhesion of the basement membrane of the epithelium to the underlying stroma. The migration is influenced only by severe injury, but mitosis is inhibited by many compounds commonly used in the treatment of eye disease and injury: sulfonamides, anesthetics, antibiotics, and lanolin ointment.

Injury to the Bowman layer causes scar formation. Inasmuch as the Bowman layer is a condensation of the corneal stroma, wound repair is similar in both layers. Repair is effected by multiplication of undamaged corneal cells and keratocytes together with migration of either fibroblasts from the blood or monocytes transformed into fibroblasts. New mucopolysaccharide synthesis begins after 24 to 48 hours and is well established by the fifth day. Chondroitin sulfate predominates, and only late in the healing process is it replaced with the usual keratin sulfate. Stromal healing is not initiated until the defect is covered with epithelium.

Endothelial healing is by mitotic multiplication in lower animals, but in humans, healing is by endothelial cells spreading to cover the defect. Inasmuch as damaged cells are not replaced, stromal and epithelial edema occurs (bullous keratopathy) if there are too few remaining cells to cover the injured area.

In the early methods of corneal transplant, the donor cornea became hydrated, and the swelling caused a watertight wound, permitting the anterior chamber to re-form. Now, the same effect is achieved by multiple sutures. Corneal grafts always "take." A hypersensitivity reaction is manifested not by expulsion of the donor graft but by loss of transparency, swelling, and vascularization of the graft. Presumably because of its avascularity, the normal cornea participates minimally in the immune processes of the body. Nonetheless, hypersensitive reactions may occur more often in recipients of corneal grafts with keratoconus (avascular) who have HLA-B12 or HLA-B27 histocompatibility antigen groups. When the cornea is vascularized, its participation in immune processes seems to be proportionate to the degree of vascularization.

TEARS

The anterior surface of the eye is moistened by tears formed by the lacrimal gland and the accessory lacrimal glands of Krause and Wolfring (p. 57). The accessory glands constitute some 10% of the mass of the main gland. The glands contain many plasma cells that appear to be independent of antigenic stimulation, as is the lymphoid tissue in the gut. The major flow of tears is along the eyelid margin and in the conjunctival fornices. Periodic involuntary blinking spreads the tears over the surface of the globe and causes a pumping action of the lacrimal drainage system.

Orbicularis oculi fibers attach around the puncta, and other fibers insert into the fascia of the lacrimal sac. Blinking draws the puncta nasally, shortening the canaliculi, and forces tears into the lacrimal sac. Contraction of the orbicularis oculi expands the lacrimal sac, creating a partial negative pressure to suck in tears. The pumping action of the orbicularis oculi muscle is essential for normal tear drainage.

The corneal epithelium is covered by a relatively stagnant layer of tears, the precorneal tear film. This is composed of three layers (Fig. 2-2): (1) a thin anterior oily layer derived from the meibomian glands, (2) a middle aqueous layer derived from the lacrimal glands, and (3) a thin mucoid layer arising from the goblet cells of the conjunctiva. The oily layer retards the evaporation of tears and provides a smooth and regular anterior optical surface. The mucoid layer wets the microvilli of the corneal epithelium and must be intact to retain the precorneal film.

The average normal secretion of tears is between $0.5\mu l$ and $2.2\mu l$/min. The maximum capacity of the cul-de-sac is about $30\mu l$, so that tears overflow if the rate of drainage does not increase with increasing rate of secretion. Once the rate of tear secretion exceeds $100\mu l$/min, overflow occurs.

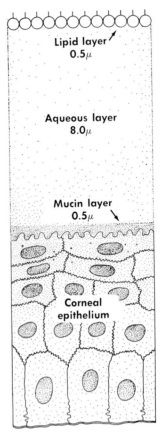

Fig. 2-2. Schematic representation of the precorneal tear film. The mucin is a wetting agent that provides a hydrophilic surface to the hydrophobic corneal epithelium.

With the eyes open and the precorneal oily film intact, a maximum of $0.85\mu l$ of tears is evaporated each minute, and the remainder pass through the lacrimal passages. The evaporation causes the tears to become slightly hypertonic, so that there is an osmotic flow of water from the anterior chamber, through the cornea, to the tear film. When the eyes are closed, the precorneal tear film is in osmotic equilibrium with the aqueous humor, no osmotic flow occurs, and the corneal stroma thickens.

Collection of tears to determine their

composition is complicated by evaporation and by dilution resulting from stimulation. The concentration of chloride, sodium, urea, and phosphate is approximately the same as in plasma, whereas the sugar content is markedly less.

There is a relatively large amount of protein, averaging between 1 to 2 gm/100 ml. The concentration is lower in the aged than in the young. The protein is composed of 30% albumin, 40% globulins, and 30% lysozyme (muramidase), an enzyme.

Lysozyme (muramidase) is an antibacterial enzyme widely distributed in nature—egg is the commercial source. Its activity is limited to lysis of the mucopolysaccharide coating of a few nonpathogenic gram-positive bacteria. Additionally, a local ocular secretory antibody can be stimulated by virus inoculation of the conjunctiva.

IgA, the main immunoglobulin of the tears, is synthesized by subconjunctival plasma cells and lacrimal plasma cells. Epithelial cells manufacture a secretory IgA, complement, lysosome, and other serum factors that cause bacteriolysis. IgA also inhibits the adherence of bacteria to mucosal surfaces, thus limiting colonization.

Tears are secreted in response to (1) reflex stimuli and (2) psychic stimuli. Reflex tearing is mediated through stimulation of the fibers of the ophthalmic division of the trigeminal nerve (N V). Irritation of the cornea, conjunctiva, and nasal mucous membranes results in tear secretion. Application of heat to the tongue and mouth and uncomfortable retinal stimulation by bright lights cause reflex tearing. Normal moisture of the eye may be entirely maintained by the accessory lacrimal glands; secretion of tears constitutes an emergency or psychic response.

Clinically, tear formation is measured by hooking a piece of filter paper 5 mm wide over the middle portion of the lower eyelid and determining the millimeters of wetting that occur in 4 minutes (p. 233). The filter paper irritates the conjunctiva, and the response indicates reflex tearing rather than normal secretion. If the eye is first anesthetized with a topical anesthetic, filter-paper wetting then more closely corresponds to basic tear secretion. A more accurate method is measurement of the dilution of a dye, usually fluorescein, which also causes some reflex tearing. These tests indicate less tear formation after the age of 50 years, but the results may be interpreted as decreased reflex sensitivity rather than decreased tear formation.

AQUEOUS HUMOR

The aqueous humor contributes to the maintenance of intraocular pressure and supports the metabolism of the lens, which does not have a blood supply and thus has mainly an anaerobic metabolism. Additionally, aqueous humor contributes to the nutrition of the cornea. It is formed by both secretion and diffusion by the epithelium of the ciliary processes. The fluid thus formed is elaborated by the nonpigmented epithelial cells of the ciliary body that are closest to the posterior chamber. Once compounds are secreted, their concentration is modified by water and chloride diffusion into the posterior chamber. Sodium is the chief cation of the aqueous humor and enters the eye mainly by secretion. Water is believed to follow the sodium by diffusion. The aqueous humor formed in the posterior chamber flows through the pupil into the anterior chamber, with a minimal amount flowing posteriorly through the zonule to the vitreous cavity. The composition of the aqueous humor in the anterior chamber is modified by diffusion of water from blood vessels in the iris stroma. The aqueous humor leaves the eye through the trabecular meshwork, passing to the canal of Schlemm and then to veins in the deep scleral plexus (Fig. 2-3). The normal flow-rate of aqueous humor is approximately $2\mu l$/min.

The aqueous humor of the posterior chamber differs in composition from the aqueous humor of the anterior chamber. In humans, posterior chamber aqueous humor contains chloride and ascorbate in excess of that of plasma and the anterior chamber aqueous humor. There is a deficiency of bicarbonate. In animals with large lenses, chloride is deficient, and there is an excess of bicarbonate, which is presumably required to buffer the lactic acid resulting as the end prod-

uct of glycolysis in the absence of oxygen in the large lens.

In vitro, the ciliary processes transport organic ions out of the eye. There are at least three separate systems: a hippuran, an iodipamide, and an iodide system. Additionally, prostaglandins are actively transported out of the eye, although this transport may utilize one of the first two systems rather than an additional one.

Inhibition of carbonic anhydrase (p. 126) decreases the secretory activity of the ciliary epithelium by about two thirds. The carbonic anhydrase inhibitors have become important compounds in the management of glaucoma (p. 401). Sodium- and potassium-activated adeno-

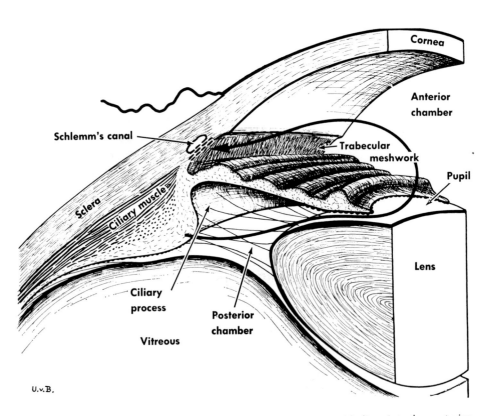

U.v.B.

Fig. 2-3. Aqueous humor is secreted by the nonpigmented ciliary epithelium into the posterior chamber. It flows through the pupil into the anterior chamber and leaves the anterior chamber through the trabecular meshwork, which opens into the canal of Schlemm.

sine triphosphatase (ATPase) is involved in electrolyte secretion into the posterior chamber. The cardiac glycosides, which inhibit ATPase, thus decrease the secretion of aqueous humor and have been used experimentally in the management of glaucoma. Interference with the sodium transport mechanism, metabolic poisoning of the ciliary epithelium, and reduction of the temperature of the ciliary body to 19° C also decrease secretory activity.

The major difference between the aqueous humor and blood plasma is in the low protein concentration in the aqueous humor. The aqueous humor of humans contains about 25 mg/100 ml of protein, mainly orosomucoid, transferrin, albumin, and IgG. The concentration of proteins in the aqueous humor varies with their molecular size, and the blood-aqueous barrier is thought to have a pore diameter of about 104 nm. If the ciliary body epithelium or the blood vessels of the iris are damaged through injury or through the release of prostaglandin, the aqueous humor has the same composition as plasma, and there is no difference in the concentration between the serum and the plasma.

INTRAOCULAR PRESSURE

The interior pressure of the eye must exceed that of the surrounding atmosphere to prevent collapse. The normal intraocular pressure is between 10 and 20 mm Hg greater than atmospheric pressure. There is a 1 to 2 mm Hg variation in intraocular pressure with each heartbeat caused by fluctuation in the intraocular vascular volume, and there are slower variations in the intraocular pressure with respiration. The intraocular pressure normally fluctuates 2 to 5 mm Hg daily.

The two main factors concerned with the maintenance of intraocular pressure are (1) the rate of secretion of the aqueous humor and (2) the ease with which the

aqueous humor passes through the trabecular meshwork to the canal of Schlemm and into the collecting channels of the canal. Some 75% of the resistance to outflow is in the trabecular meshwork. The ease with which the fluid exits is indicated as the coefficient of the facility of outflow (C) and in normal eyes is more than $0.20 \mu l/min/mm$ Hg of pressure within the eye. It is measured clinically by tonography (p. 395).

Many additional factors contribute to the intraocular pressure. Variations are usually quickly compensated, so that the intraocular pressure is affected only momentarily. The pressure in the episcleral veins connecting to the canal of Schlemm is somewhat less than 10 mm Hg. If this pressure is markedly increased, there is a reflux of blood into the canal of Schlemm and increased resistance to outflow. The intraocular arterial and venous pressure and the volume of the arteries usually remain constant. Markedly increased venous pressure, as occurs in the Valsalva maneuver, is accompanied by a marked increase in intraocular pressure because of intraocular venous dilation. The intraocular pressure rapidly returns to normal when the Valsalva maneuver is stopped. Increased osmotic pressure of the blood brought about by administration of glycerol, mannitol, or urea (p. 127) decreases the intraocular pressure. Decreased osmotic pressure of the blood induced by intravenous saline solution or by drinking a large quantity of water on an empty stomach causes a modest increase in intraocular pressure. The elasticity of the cornea and the sclera remains relatively constant but is an important factor in the measurement of the intraocular pressure by tonometry.

The intraocular pressure is directly measured by a sensitive transducer introduced to the interior of the eye in a manner that avoids disturbance of the flow of aqueous humor and the vasculature. This is done mainly in experimental animals and is done in humans only before enucleation of the eye because of disease. Clinically, the ocular tension is measured by means of a tonometer (p. 171) that determines the resistance of the surface of the globe to a change in shape. There are two main types of tonometers: (1) contact types, which measure ocular tension by mechanical indentation (Schiøtz), by electronic indentation (Mackay-Marg), or by flattening of the cornea (Goldmann applanation, which requires a biomicroscope, or the hand-held types of Draeger or Perkins); and (2) noncontact types, which flatten the cornea with a pulse of air. The applanation tonometer of Langham and McCarthy also uses an airstream but touches the eye.

THE LENS

The lens is derived either from surface ectoderm or from stimulation of the optic vesicle by cytolysis of the surface ectoderm. The lens is covered by a homogeneous capsule and has epithelium only beneath the anterior capsule.

New lens fibers are synthesized throughout life by cells that have their nuclei in the equatorial region. These new fibers increase the weight of the lens from some 100 mg at birth to 250 mg at the age of 65 years. The latest formed fibers near the surface of the lens (cortex) surround the older fibers that have lost their nuclei and are compressed toward the central region of the lens. The lens is held in position behind the pupil by means of zonular fibers. These fibers relax with contraction of the ciliary muscle, and the lens becomes more spherical (accommodation).

Transparency. The lens transmits almost 80% of electromagnetic energy between 400 and 1,000 nm. Its transparency arises because of its acellularity and because all of its parts have nearly the same index of refraction. The single layer of epithelial cells beneath the anterior capsule is not thick enough to interfere with transparency, and these are the sole nuclei in the visual axis.

Despite the homogeneity of the lens structure, its total index of refraction is greater than any single portion. This results from a concentric, onionlike structure in which older central layers have a greater index of refraction than the surrounding younger layers.

The total refractive power of the lens is thus much greater than one would anticipate from its external curvature, thickness, and the index of refraction of individual layers. In a simplifying assumption in physiologic optics, the lens is considered to be composed of a central core with a high index of refraction that has a layer with a lower index of refraction on either side.

Metabolism. The crystalline lens of the experimental animal is used widely to study protein synthesis and cataract induction and is an excellent source of membranes. The animal lens, though, differs from the human lens in many respects. The bovine, rabbit, and rat lens grows fast at first but slows down; thus, in the second half of a lifespan there is little increase in weight. In contrast, the human lens grows slowly throughout life. The nucleus of the rabbit and cow lens reaches about 50% dry weight, but the human lens maintains a water content of about 65% throughout life. It is only in the human and primate lens that there is a change in shape with accommodation. The concentric rings of the human lens, called "zones of discontinuity," have no counterpart in other mammalian lenses. In middle life the color of the lens slowly yellows, thus decreasing the amount of blue and violet light that reaches the retina. Some of the yellow color may be from low molecular weight derivatives of tryptophan found only in the human and primate lens. They are fluorescent and absorb ultraviolet light maximally at the 360- to 368-nm wavelength. The bovine, rabbit, or rat lens does not metabolize tryptophan.

The lens fibers are composed almost entirely of soluble and insoluble proteins. Fractionation of water-soluble lens proteins yields four fractions: α-, β_{Heavy}-, β_{Light}-, and γ-crystallin. The α-crystallin is formed before birth and consists of related proteins of differing size but composed of the same sort of polypeptides. The β-crystallin is composed of at least two major fractions, β_H and β_L, and is formed throughout life. Human lens protein is more labile than that of other species, and the β-crystallin of higher primates differs from that of nonprimate mammals in lacking one of the precipitative bands present in the nonprimates. In addition to the water-soluble proteins, the urea-soluble and water-insoluble fraction (albuminoid) increases with age. This may give rise to the yellowish color of the aging lens.

In aging, macromolecules of protein are formed that have a high molecular weight and contain large amounts of calcium. There is an increase in negatively charged components within the lens during aging. Protein aggregates of large molecular weight scatter light to produce an opacity. Heavy molecular weight aggregates represent some 10% to 15% of the total soluble protein of normal human lenses at 72 years of age. Molecular weight may be greater than 1.5×10^8.

About 85% of the glucose metabolism of the lens is by means of glycolysis in which the 6-carbon glucose molecule is degraded to two molecules of 3-carbon lactic acid. In the process, adenosine triphosphate is generated from adenosine diphosphate and phosphate. The first step in the process is the conversion of glucose, phosphate, and adenosine diphosphate to glucose-6-phosphate, a reaction catalyzed by the enzyme hexokinase. Hexokinase is present in a limited amount in the lens and limits the amount of glycolysis. The glucose-6-phosphate is then cleaved to two molecules of glyceraldehyde-3-PO_4, which is converted to lactate. The lactate chiefly diffuses into the anterior chamber.

About 15% of the glucose-6-phosphate formed is degraded through an aerobic phosphogluconate pathway (pentose phosphate pathway or hexose monophosphate shunt) to form ribose-5-phosphate and carbon dioxide. The ribose-5-phosphate is then available for nucleic acid synthesis. Additionally, this reaction generates reducing power in the cytoplasm in the form of reduced nicotinamide-adenine dinucleotide phosphate (NADPH; also called reduced triphosphopyridine nucleotide [TPNH] or coenzyme II [obsolete]). This reducing power is required for the hexokinase reaction and also the aldose reductase reaction, which is an important pathway in sugar cataracts, as well as for providing reduced glutathione.

In many respects the lens behaves as a single large cell. Thus it maintains a high intracellular potassium content although surrounded by aqueous humor and vitreous humor, both of which have a high sodium content. The lens epithelium maintains this gradient and actively transports sodium out of the lens by an Na^+-K^+ ATPase pump. Glycolysis provides the necessary ATP energy. The lens transports and accumulates potassium, amino acids, and ascorbic acid. It synthesizes inositol (a completely hydroxylated cyclohexane) and glutathione. With interference in lens metabolism, sodium and water accumulate in the lens, and it loses potassium, glutathione, amino acids, and inositol.

Cataract. Any loss of transparency is called a cataract. Cataract may occur with (1) hydration of the lens fibers and (2) transformation of the normally transparent lens fiber protein to a protein that is opaque. Three mechanisms cause cataract: (1) damage to the lens capsule that modifies its membrane properties, (2) change of lens fiber protein synthesis by interference with mitotic activity at the equator by means of irradiation or poisons, and (3) increased lens hydration.

In the normal lens, active sodium extrusion and relative impermeability of the lens membrane to sodium counteract osmotic forces that tend to drive water into the lens. A nearly mature cataract is almost impermeable to sodium and to this water accumulation, but, as further opacification occurs, the sodium-extruding mechanism progressively fails. In humans both the Mg^{2+} and the Na^+-K^+ dependent ATPase activities are considerably decreased in cataractous lenses. However, the magnesium concentration in cataracts is greater than the equilibrium value.

When excessive glucose is present in the lens, the enzyme aldose reductase coupled to NADPH, derived from the phosphogluconate shunt, reduces the glucose to the alcohol D-glucitol (L-sorbitol). Sugar alcohols, or polyols, do not penetrate membranes well and accumulate to high levels, drawing water into the lens and causing swelling of the lens fibers. This in turn leads to stretching of the lens capsule along with secondary electrolyte imbalance and loss of amino acids. Currently, major attention is directed to aldose reductase in the study of experimental cataract inasmuch as aldose reductase is inhibited by many compounds. The flavonoids, derived from citrus peels, currently are popular inhibitors in experimental animals. These studies, which implicate aldose reductase in experimental sugar cataracts, lead to speculation as to whether this enzyme is involved in the neuropathy, nephropathy, and retinopathy of human diabetes mellitus. High concentrations of aldose reductase have been found in the Schwann cells of peripheral nerves, in the pericytes of the retinal blood vessels, and in the kidney papillae. In mice with hereditary cataracts, there is a deficiency of Na-K ATPase, which leads to electrolyte imbalance.

THE VITREOUS BODY

The vitreous body is a transparent hydrogel that fills the vitreous cavity. It is composed mainly of water (98% to 99.5%); collagen provides a framework, and a high level of hyaluronic acid provides its gel properties. It is firmly attached to the ciliary body and the retina in the region of the ora serrata and to the periphery of the optic disk. It is composed of (1) a cortical tissue layer whose surfaces are condensed to form an anterior hyaloid adjacent to the lens and a posterior hyaloid in intimate contact with the inner limiting membrane of the retina and (2) a vitreous body proper.

The *cortical tissue* is approximately 100μ thick and surrounds the vitreous body proper. It contains fine fibrils composed of collagen, an accumulation of proteins, a high concentration of hyaluronic acid, and a few cells. The collagen fibrils run approximately parallel to the surface of the vitreous body, and up to the age of 20 years they attach to the basement membrane of the retina and the ciliary body. Thereafter such attachments are found only in the anterior one third of the eye.

The *vitreous body proper* is a true biologic and chemical gel. Its framework is composed of fine collagen fibrils (Fig. 2-4). The spaces between the fibrils (the interfibrillar spaces) are filled with hyaluronic acid (N-acetylglucosamine and D-glucuronic acid). It occurs in tissues with a high water content and forms a molecular network in the vitreous.

The vitreous body has no metabolic ac-

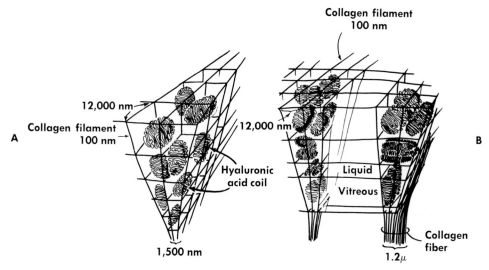

Fig. 2-4. Schematic drawing of fine structure of the vitreous gel showing fibrous network reinforced with hyaluronic acid molecules. **A,** Structural units are distributed randomly. **B,** There has been partial collapse of the network and the formation of a liquid pool. (From Balazs, E. A.: Molecular morphology of the vitreous body. In Smelser, G. K., editor: Structure of the eye, New York, 1961, Academic Press, Inc.)

tivities that use glucose to produce energy, but cells in the cortical layer convert glucose to hyaluronic acid. The significance is not known.

THE RETINA

The optic cup consists of two layers: (1) the outer layer, which forms the retinal pigment epithelium and is one cell-layer thick, and (2) the inner layer, which gives rise to the sensory layer consisting of the photoreceptor cells, and the supporting glia. The microvilli of the retinal pigment epithelium surround the outer segments of rods and the slender cones in the central retina. There are no junctions, but the complex is enmeshed in a mucopolysaccharide synthesized by the photoreceptor cell. All metabolites of the outer retina pass through the retinal pigment epithelium, and the external limiting membrane (p. 30) of Müller cells marks the division between metabolic support by the choriocapillaris through the retinal

pigment epithelium and support by the central retinal artery branches. The base of retinal pigment epithelium has binding sites for the specific protein that transports vitamin A. Additionally, it contains the enzymes necessary for the visual cycle.

The rods and cones are the light-sensitive elements of the sensory retina. The rods serve vision at low levels of illumination (scotopic vision), whereas the cones are effective at medium and high levels of illumination (photopic vision) and in color vision. The cones are concentrated in the fovea centralis where rods are absent but are also scattered in the peripheral retina. The rods are the main photoreceptor in the periphery (Fig. 2-5).

The outer segments of rods and cones are constantly removed by the phagocytic action of the pigment epithelium cells. In this way the outer segments undergo constant renewal by the inner segment of the visual cell with a much more active turn-over rate for rod outer segments than cone outer segments. Cone membranes are phagocytized at evening and synthesized during the night, whereas rod membranes are phagocytized at morning and synthesized during the day.

The outer segment (nearest the retinal pigment epithelium) of each rod and cone is composed of about 700 protein-lipid disks containing light-sensitive pigments (Fig. 2-6). The inner segment contains a dense concentration of mitochondria. The axons of the rods and cones synapse with bipolar cells and horizontal cells to form a portion of the outer plexiform

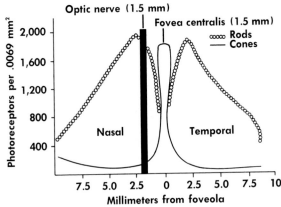

Fig. 2-5. Distribution of rods and cones in the human eye. Cones are concentrated in the fovea centralis, where there are no rods. Rods are the main photoreceptors in the periphery. (Redrawn from Østerberg, G.: Acta Ophthalmol. [Suppl.] [Kbh.] **6**:1, 1935.)

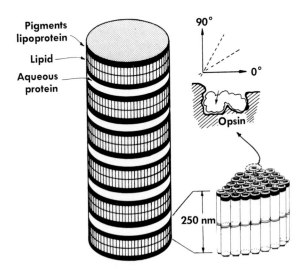

Fig. 2-6. Protein lipid disks of the photoreceptor outer segment. They number about 700 and are about 250 nm thick. Each disk contains 1 molecule of photosensitive pigment. (From Wolken, J. J.: J. Opt. Soc. Am. **53**:1, 1963.)

layer. The axons of the bipolar cells synapse with amacrine cells and with dendrites of the ganglion cells in the inner plexiform layer. The axons of the ganglion cells join to form the optic nerve and extend to the brain (Fig. 1-33 and p. 39).

The cell bodies and neurons of the retina are closely invested with astroglia and the glia of Müller cells. These form an elaborate plexus so that the retina has no true extracellular space.

The human sensory retina contains about 120 million rods and 6 million cones. The optic nerve contains somewhat more than 1 million fibers. However, the distribution of optic nerve fibers to receptors is not uniform. In the center of the fovea, the approximately 200,000 cones are connected to at least that many optic nerve fibers. In the far periphery, however, there may be as many as 10,000 rods connected in clusters to a single nerve fiber with considerable overlapping, so that a point of light may stimulate several clusters at once.

Metabolism of the retina is intimately related to its special function and may be divided into two parts: (1) general metabolism required for the maintenance of cell integrity and (2) specialized reactions related to photoreception and nerve impulse transmission.

General metabolism. Retinal function is dependent on a continuous supply of glucose from the bloodstream. In humans, the blood supply from the choriocapillaris nurtures the outer layers of the retina and branches of the central retinal artery, the inner layers. Both systems must be intact for normal function. In rats, interruption of the blood supply for as short a period as 6 minutes causes irreversible retinal degeneration. The retina has an unusually high rate of aerobic metabolism.

It is believed that glucose diffuses from the choriocapillaris of the choroid, is then converted into glucose-6-phosphate, possibly by the pigment epithelium, and finally diffuses down the neuron. The enzymes of the phosphogluconate pathway are concentrated in the rod and cone nuclei and provide the ribose needed for RNA synthesis.

The enzymes of the glycolytic pathway are mainly concentrated in the inner layers of the retina. Müller cells contain the enzymes required for glycogen synthesis and degradation. Additionally, these cells contain the enzymes required for the tricarboxylic acid cycle.

Photochemistry of vision. When that portion of the electromagnetic spectrum constituting light (400 to 700 nm) is absorbed by the pigment of the retinal photoreceptor cells, a photochemical product is generated that initiates a graded electrical potential. The potential is amplified and modulated in the retina and is propagated to the brain, where perception occurs. So that continued stimulation is

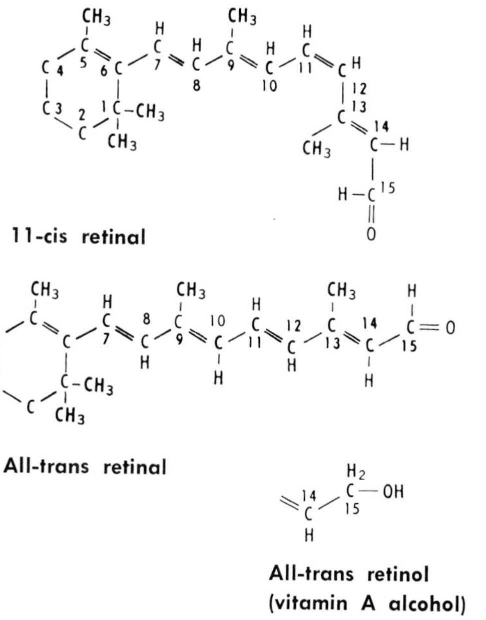

11-cis retinal

All-trans retinal

All-trans retinol
(vitamin A alcohol)

Fig. 2-7. The 11-*cis* isomer of retinal (vitamin A aldehyde) and the all-*trans* isomer.

possible, the pigment of the photoreceptor cells must be constantly renewed. So that the nervous impulse stops after cessation of the stimulus, the chemical reaction initiating the nervous impulse must stop simultaneously.

Human photoreceptors contain at least four light-absorbing conjugated proteins (opsins), each tightly bound to 11-*cis*-retinal, the aldehyde of vitamin A_1 (Fig. 2-7). Rhodopsin (visual purple [obsolete]) is the photopigment of rods and has a maximum absorption at about 507 nm and an absorption spectrum similar to the light-sensitivity curve of the eye in dim light. The cones contain three different photopigments that have a maximum absorption at about 440 nm (blue-sensitive), 535 nm (green-sensitive), and 570 nm (red-sensitive). In each the prosthetic group is 11-*cis*-retinal.

Retinol (vitamin A, an alcohol) contains four carbon-carbon double bonds in its side chain (Fig. 2-6). It must be utilized in the retina in its aldehyde form (retinal), and only when the 11-12 position is *cis* and the other three are *trans* is it conjugated with opsin. When the pigment absorbs light, the bound 11-*cis*-retinal undergoes an isomerization to all-*trans*-retinal with a substantial change in shape (Fig. 2-7). This isomerization of retinal is followed by a series of chemical reactions ending in the disassociation of the bleached photopigment to yield free opsin and all-*trans*-retinal, which initiates a graded potential. It is postulated that light absorption also changes the shape of the opsin molecule so that it alters the permeability of the disk outer segments.

The outer segment membrane of photoreceptor disks has a high Na^+ permeability. The change in shape of rhodopsin (and retinal) releases Ca^{2+} sequestered within the disk and closes the Na^+ channels in the membrane with a decreased flow of Na^+ and hyperpolarization of the plasma membrane, thus triggering a graded nervous potential. Ouabain, an Na-K ATPase inhibitor, stops the reaction.

For additional photosensitive pigment to be synthesized, the all-*trans*-retinal must be isomerized to 11-*cis*-retinal. This occurs either by exposure to light in the photoreceptors or by a sequence of reactions (Fig. 2-8) catalyzed by two enzymes in the retinal pigment epithelium and the myoid of the inner segment of the photoreceptors.

All-*trans*-retinol is vitamin A_1 and is transported in the blood complexed to a specific retinol-binding protein (proalbumin). The bases of the retinal pigment epithelium cells have specific receptor sites for the complex where the vitamin A is released to the cell and the carrier protein excluded. Dietary sources of vitamin A are from both the vitamin

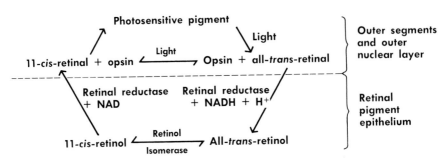

Fig. 2-8. The visual cycle. NADH is reduced nicotinamide adenine dinucleotide.

and from carotenoids, particularly carotene, which are converted into vitamin A by enzymatic reactions in the intestinal mucosa and liver.

Synaptic transmission in the retina. Synaptic transmission in the retina is both by direct contact and by secretion of neural transmitters that are released by the axon and react with receptors on the outside of the cell membrane of dendrites; this leads to a change in electrical potential across the membrane. A high concentration of cyclic nucleotide phosphodiesterase is found in the outer segments of the retina, strongly indicating that cyclic AMP is involved inasmuch as the enzyme degrades cyclic AMP into a physiologically inactive form of AMP. Among the neural transmitters in the retina, dopamine, γ-aminobutyric acid, glycine, and taurine usually exert a depressant action on retinal neurons, whereas glutamate and aspartate can either excite or depress retinal neurons, depending on their concentration.

Axoplasmic transport. Axoplasmic transport is the flow of substances from the nerve cell body distally through its axon. A flow also occurs into the dendrite. Axoplasmic transport occurs in two components: a slow component at a rate of approximately 1 mm a day and a fast component that is some one hundred times faster. Most materials studied travel at both rapid and slow rates. However, glycoproteins and sulfated mucopolysaccharides are transported almost completely by the rapid component. Rapidly transported material is largely in the membrane or particulate form that includes synaptic vessels, mitochondria, and smooth endoplasmic reticulum. The slow component consists mainly of soluble protein.

The eyes of birds and goldfish have been the site for study of this phenomenon, because the material may be injected into the vitreous cavity in close proximity to ganglion cells and because complete crossing of optic fibers at the chiasm allows for passage of the radioactive-labelled material to the contralateral optic tract and tectum. Rapidly transported substances appear to involve the circumferential portion of the axons, whereas slow flow progresses within the core of the axon. Rapid transport may be responsible for the movement of substances required at synaptic terminals, including the enzymes necessary for synthesis or destruction of transmitter substances. Slow components act to maintain and replenish substances necessary for structural integrity of the axon.

Rapid axoplasmic transport is inhibited by anoxia, by metabolic inhibitors such as sodium cyanide and dinitrophenol, and by local anesthetics. Increased intraocular pressure may impede axonal flow, particularly the slow transport.

The retinal cotton-wool spot (histologically a cytoid body) is causally related to focal ischemia from arteriolar occlusion, which gives rise to localized swelling of the axons of ganglion cells. The swollen nerve fiber of the retinal cotton-wool spot microscopically contains aggregations of mitochondria, dense bodies, vesicles, and granules. Possibly, the cotton-wool spot arises from axonal ischemia in the retina because of orthograde and retrograde interruption of axon transport with an aggregation of organelles on either side of the lesion.

Neural activity. Of the 3,000,000 or so fibers that enter the primate brain, some two thirds arise from the eye. Six of the twelve cranial nerves are necessary for optimum performance of the eye as a visual organ. William James (1892) proposed "that the main function of the peripheral part of the retina is that of sentinels which when beams of light move over them cry 'who goes there' and call the fovea to the spot."

Vision is thus divided into surround (or ambient) vision, which is mediated primarily by the peripheral retina and provides information concerning spatial localization, and focal vision, mediated primarily by the central retina, which subserves form, perception, identification, and color vision. The peripheral aspects of vision achieve spatial orientation in the peripheral retina with large ganglion cells (mainly Y- and transient cells) and Y nerve fibers, which may be connected not only with the cortex but with the superior colliculus. Focal vision is sustained through the fovea, using cones, small ganglion cells, and neurons (mainly X- and sustained cells) and extending particularly to the lateral geniculate body and then to the visual cortex.

Ganglion cells may be divided into two types on the basis of their response to a receptive field. The receptive field consists of the information gathered by a group of photoreceptors as transmitted to the ganglion cells. Receptive fields are organized in a concentric manner, having a central region surrounded by a ring-shaped outer zone.

There are two types of receptive fields: (1) those in which illumination of the center causes stimulation of the ganglion cell and illumination of the periphery causes inhibition in the ganglion cell (an on-center, depolarizing type of receptive field) and (2) a reverse type of receptive field) in which illumination of the center causes inhibition of the ganglion cell and illumination of the periphery causes stimulation (an off-center, hypopolarizing receptive field). It appears that some ganglion cells in the retina do not have concentric "on" and "off" zones but have the two zones coincident.

Receptive fields are not constant in size, and they are larger in the dark-adapted eye than in the light-adapted eye. They are larger in the peripheral than in the central retina. They change in size and shape and alter in their stimulatory and inhibitory components with the state of light adaptation.

The neural circuitry within the retina is exceedingly complex. The signal from rods is received by rod bipolars and by horizontal cells. Cones stimulate two types of bipolars—flat and invaginating—and also *a* and *b* horizontal cells. Amacrine cells possibly serve bipolar and ganglion cells related solely to rods.

In lower species, neural function is further complicated by the existence of at least three and perhaps more classes of ganglion cells. The classification extends from retina to cortex and consists of X-cells, Y-cells, and W-cells. The X-cells have sustained responses to stimuli, axon conduction velocities of 9 to 14 m/sec, and are in greatest concentration in fovea centralis. The Y-cells have transient responses to stimuli, axon conduction velocities of 29 to 39 m/sec, and respond to rapid motions. The W-cells appear to respond both to the beginning and to the ending of a flash of light throughout their entire receptive field.

The retinal neural activity is considerably integrated in lower species. In the frog, some receptive fields are responsive to small, dark, moving objects (bug detectors) but not to large or stationary objects. Thus the frog's retina integrates the signal useful in capturing food. The mud puppy retina has three distinct properties. The average luminance affects receptor cells, and the luminance in the cells surrounding this is integrated by horizontal cells that connect with photoreceptors, other horizontal cells, and bipolar cells. Movement or change in luminance is integrated by amacrine cells, which connect to other amacrine cells, ganglion cells, and bipolar cells. The electrical output from the ganglion cells through the optic nerve consists of light-sensitive output and change-sensitive output (Fig. 2-9). In more complex

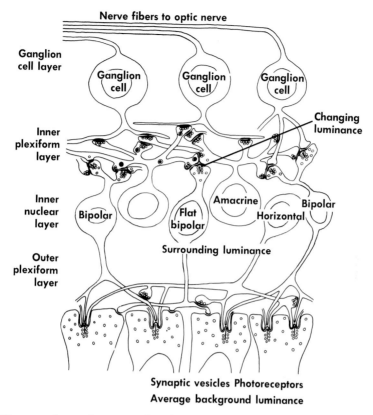

Fig. 2-9. Diagram of synaptic contacts found in vertebrate retinas. In the outer plexiform layer, processes from bipolar and horizontal cells penetrate into invaginations in the receptor terminals. The processes of flat polar cells make superficial contacts on the bases of some receptor terminals. Horizontal cells make conventional synaptic contacts on bipolar dendrites and other horizontal cell processes. In the inner plexiform layer, bipolar terminals may contact one ganglion cell dendrite and one amacrine process at a ribbon synapse or may contact amacrine cell processes. Amacrine processes in all retinas make synapses of the conventional type back onto bipolar terminals (reciprocal synapse). (From Dowling, J.: Invest. Ophthalmol. **9:**655, 1970.)

retinas there is less integrative function in the retina; most integration is in the brain.

The spiked discharges from retinal ganglion cells are further integrated in the lateral geniculate body. The images from the two eyes may be reinforced in binocularity to cause a more vigorous response or may be inhibited with a diminished response in the absence of binocular vision. The lateral geniculate body contains color-coded cells that are organized to deal with both color and brightness information.

The complexity and capacity of the visual cortex is emphasized by its size: 20 square feet by $\frac{1}{10}$ inch if flattened out. The major portion of the striate cortex is concerned with form vision; in monkeys 1° of foveal vision is represented 6 mm linearly at the cortex.

Form-sensitive cortical cells are described as "simple," "complex," and "hypercomplex." "Simple" cells are arranged into excitatory and inhibitory regions separated by boundaries that are straight and parallel, and they are related to the X- (simple) system. Their fields may be mapped with stationary retinal stimuli. "Complex" cells (related mainly to the Y-system) appear to be combinations of simple cells that respond particularly to moving edges on the retina with directional sensitivity. "Hypercomplex" cells respond only to moving stimuli on the retina and are most potently stimulated by the ends of lines, line segments, and corners. Again, the signal may be inhibited or reinforced. Unlike the retinal receptive fields, which are round, the cortical fields are linear.

These studies constitute one of the most exciting topics in physiology today. The factors to be measured seem endless: color vision, binocularity, dark adaptation, connections and processing in the central brain, fine anatomy of the visual system, and the ontogeny and embryology of visual development. However, the experiments are complicated, the number of cells is large, and far more work is required before we will know how we see.

VISUAL MECHANISMS

Electromagnetic spectrum. Electromagnetic radiation consists of massless particles called photons that mediate the transfer of energy. Photons travel 3×10^8 m/sec in a vacuum and have a sinusoidal oscillation and an associated electromagnetic field. Physical processes such as absorption and emission of electromagnetic radiation are most easily understood in terms of photons themselves, whereas processes such as diffraction, polarization, and interference are best understood by considering the associated electromagnetic field.

The energy carried by a photon is inversely proportional to the wavelength of the associated electromagnetic field.

Thus, green light (535 nm) has less energy than blue light (440 nm). The wavelengths vary from many kilometers for low-frequency radio waves to a minute fraction of a micron for high-energy gamma radiation. A small group of photons are absorbed by photosensitive pigments of the eye and appreciated as visible light. Those photons with energy corresponding to wavelengths of between 400 and 700 nm pass through the cornea, the lens, and the other ocular media until absorbed by the photosensitive pigment in the rods and cones. This initiates a chemical change and triggers the visual impulse. Photons with greater or lesser energy are usually not absorbed by the rods and cones and are therefore not seen. Photons with energies of tens of kilovolts (x-rays) cause the sensation of green light in a dark-adapted eye. Cosmic rays cause minute flashes of light that were first described by those who journeyed into outer space.

Action of light on the eye. When that portion of the electromagnetic spectrum known as visible light (400 to 700 nm) is absorbed by the visual pigment in the rods and cones, a nervous impulse arises that is transmitted to the brain and causes a subjective sensation.

It has been found experimentally that equal amounts of radiant energy of different wavelengths do not produce equal visual sensations. Thus, $1/1,000$ watt of green light appears bright to an observer, whereas $1/1,000$ watt of blue light appears dim. Luminous units express the amount of radiant light energy in terms of the production of the sensation of brightness in the observer. Luminous energy is radiant energy corrected for the sensitivity of the retina to different wavelengths. Since individuals show slight differences, luminous units are expressed in terms of the average of many observers (the standard observer). Photopic, or cone, luminosity function (V_λ) represents the sensitivity of a light-adapted human eye. It has a maximum sensitivity at 555 nm. Scotopic luminosity function ($V_\lambda^!$) represents the sensitivity of the dark-adapted human eye and has a maximum sensitivity at 507 nm (rhodopsin). When viewed in dim illumination, a colored object appears to have no color. As illumination is increased, the object appears colored. This change from achromatic to chromatic vision reflects the change from scotopic (rod) vision to photopic (cone) vision. The change in luminosity function is called the Purkinje shift (Fig. 2-10).

Dark adaptation. The increase in sensitivity of the eye to detection of light that occurs in the dark is called dark adaptation. The pupil dilates, and there are both neural (largely unknown) and biochemical changes in the retina. In darkness, after exposure to bright light that bleaches the visual photopigments, there is an initial hundredfold increase in sensitivity following an exponential time course that reaches a plateau after 5 to 9

minutes. This initial phase is attributed to regeneration of photosensitive pigments in the cones. Thereafter, there is a thousandfold to ten-thousandfold increase in sensitivity following a slower exponential time course that reaches a plateau in 30 to 45 minutes (Fig. 2-11). This second phase is attributed to regeneration of rhodopsin in the rods. In addition to photoreceptor pigment regeneration, there are changes in retinal summation and inhibition that cause further increased sensitivity. The rapidity of dark adaptation is delayed by prolonged exposure to bright light (thus the increased danger of driving at night after a day in bright sunshine).

When fully dark adapted, the retina is about 10,000 times more sensitive to light than when light adapted. Additionally, the dilation of the pupil in decreased light makes the total increase in sensitivity about 100,000 times greater than in the light-adapted eye.

The dark-adapted retina is most sensitive in the region 15° to 20° from the

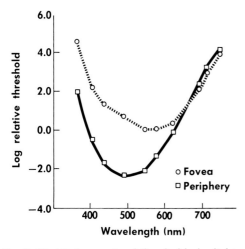

Fig. 2-10. Minimum visual thresholds for light of different wavelengths at the fovea and the periphery of the retina. Thresholds for the fovea are higher (requiring a greater light intensity for perception) and shifted toward the red end (longer wavelength) of the spectrum.

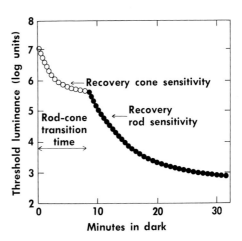

Fig. 2-11. The dark-adaptation curve. Time course of dark adaptation has a plateau at approximately 5 to 9 minutes. Initial portion of curve is the smallest light intensity that will stimulate cones. Rods reach their maximum sensitivity after approximately 30 to 45 minutes.

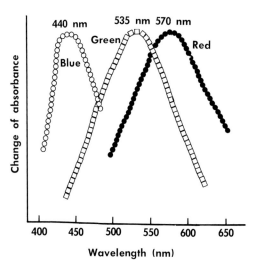

Fig. 2-12. Absorption by long wavelength–sensitive cones (red-sensitive), middle wavelength–sensitive cones (green-sensitive), and short wavelength–sensitive cones (blue-sensitive). (Redrawn from Marks, W. B., Dabelle, W. H., and MacNichol, E. F.: Science **143:**1181, 1964.)

fovea. In the fully dark-adapted eye a visual sensation can be evoked by the activity of approximately seven rods, each being stimulated by the absorption of a single photon. The variation in sensitivity in different parts of the retina probably reflects differences in the number of photoreceptors and their neural summation mechanism rather than differences in the sensitivity of the photoreceptor itself.

Light adaptation. Exposure of the dark-adapted eye to bright light results in a marked decrease in sensitivity involving two changes: (1) a neural process that is completed in about 0.05 second and (2) a slower process, apparently involving the uncoupling of retinal and opsin in rhodopsin, occurring in about 1 minute. The neural mechanism occurs regardless of the area of the retina stimulated, whereas the photochemical mechanism involves only the region of stimulation. In the light-adapted eye the rhodopsin is bleached, the pupil is constricted, there is a shift of luminosity to the yellow-red end of the spectrum, and hydrogen ion con-

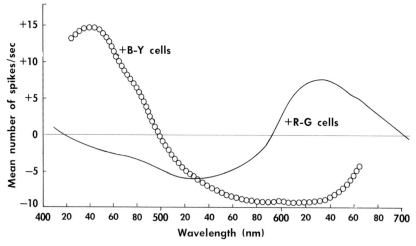

Fig. 2-13. Mean spectral response curves for cells in the lateral geniculate body that show an increase in firing to retinal stimulation by blue light (+B) and decreased firing to retinal stimulation by yellow light (−Y). Such cells are designated +B−Y cells. Red-sensitive (+R) and green-inhibition (−G) cells are also shown (+R−G). In addition there are +Y−B and +G−R cells. The curves have been corrected for a spontaneous rate. (Redrawn from DeValois, R. L., Abramov, I., and Jacobs, G. H.: J. Opt. Soc. Am. **56:**966, 1966.)

centration (pH) of the retina shifts from 7.3 to 7.0.

Color perception. Light is the visible portion of the electromagnetic spectrum. The sensation of color arises from stimulation of particular cones by light. There are three classes of cones (Fig. 2-12) in the human retina. Long wavelength–sensitive cones have a peak sensitivity in the region of 570 nm. These cones have often been called red-sensitive cones. Middle wavelength–sensitive cones have a peak sensitivity in the region of about 535 nm, corresponding to green-sensitive cones. Short wavelength–sensitive cones have a peak sensitivity of about 440 nm, constituting blue-sensitive cones, which are substantially fewer (5%) than middle and long wavelength–sensitive cones. Color perceptions are based on differential stimulation of these three types of cones. The sensation of white arises when all three types are simultaneously stimulated each to a specific degree. Yellow is produced by the stimulation of green- and red-sensitive cones.

When red and blue-green or yellow and blue are mixed, they do not produce an intermediate hue but give the sensation of gray, achromatic. Such pairs of colors are called complementary colors. The messages received by the three classes of cones are further coded in the lateral geniculate body. Cells in the lateral geniculate body are stimulated by one color and inhibited by another color (Fig. 2-13). Thus four types of opponent-process cells in the lateral geniculate body are classed according to the region of the spectrum in which they show peak activity. A cell that shows an increase in firing to retinal stimulation by long wavelengths (red) and a decrease in firing to wavelengths in the middle of the spectrum (green) is designated as $+R-G$. A cell that increases activity at the middle of the spectrum (green) and decreases activity at long wavelengths (red) is called

$+G-R$. The other two types of cells are $+B-Y$ and $+Y-B$, designating the blue and the yellow portions of the spectrum.

Current theories of color perception hold that the initial events at the retinal level are trichromatic. The information is then integrated in the lateral geniculate body according to the opponent-process scheme.

Defective color perception. Defective color perception may be hereditary and appears at birth or in adolescence. Acquired color defects arise from diseases of the cones or their connections in the retina, optic nerve, or brain. Hereditary defective color perception occurs because one or more of the retinal photopigments is absent or abnormal, or it follows cone degeneration. A person with normal color vision has all three cone pigments in a normal proportion (a trichromat). If only two cone pigments are present, the person is a dichromat, or if only one pigment is present, a monochromat.

X chromosome–linked color defects may be divided into those types in which there is an abnormality but not a complete absence of one of the cone pigments (anomalous trichromacy) and those types in which one of the cone pigments is absent (dichromacy). Visual acuity is normal, the defect is present at birth, and the condition is not progressive. The types are designated according to the pigment involved: protan (first), the red-sensitive pigment; deutan (second), the green-sensitive pigment; and tritan (third), the blue-sensitive pigment.

In protanomaly there is an abnormality in the red-sensitive pigment and poor red-green discrimination, and the red end of the spectrum appears dimmer than it does in normal individuals. In deuteranomaly there is an abnormality in the green-sensitive pigment and poor red-green discrimination, but the red end of the spectrum appears nearly as bright as it does to normal individuals.

A dichromat with an X chromosome–linked defect has but two cone pigments and is differentiated from the corresponding anomalous trichromat by tests involving color and brightness matching. Dichromats are classed as protanopes (absence of red-sensitive pigment) and deuteranopes (absence of green-sensitive pigment). Probably both protanopes and deuteranopes see red, yellow, and green as yellow.

About 7% of American and European men are protans or deutans in some degree. Less than 1% of women show either defect.

Tritan defects are transmitted as an autosomal dominant defect and probably do not involve cone pigments.

Table 2-1. Types of hereditary defective color perception

I. Congenital
  A. Anomalous trichromatism (abnormality of one photosensitive pigment)
    1. Protanomaly (red)
    2. Deuteranomaly (green)
    3. Tritanomaly (blue; possibly never occurs)
  B. Dichromatism
    1. Protanopia (absence of red photopigment)
    2. Deuteranopia (absence of green photopigment)
    3. Tritanopia (absence of blue photopigment; ganglion cell disease?)
  C. Achromatopsia
    1. Typical (reduced visual acuity and nystagmus)
      a. Complete (rod monochromacy)
      b. Incomplete
        (1) Autosomal recessive
        (2) X chromosome–linked (blue cone monochromacy)
    2. Atypical (normal vision)
      a. Complete (cone monochromacy)
        (1) Protanoid
        (2) Deuteranoid (red cone monochromacy)
      b. Incomplete (pseudomonochromacy)
II. Developmental
  A. Progressive cone degenerations
  B. Generalized cone-rod dystrophies
  C. Generalized rod-cone dystrophies

The general term *cone degeneration,* or achromatopsia, describes individuals born with severely deficient color perception or those who develop a specific degeneration of cones after birth, usually during adolescence. There are two types present at birth: typical, associated with reduced visual acuity and nystagmus, and atypical, associated with normal visual acuity. Either may be complete or incomplete (Table 2-1). The developmental types are associated with organic changes in the photoreceptors; these changes are confined to the cones in either the fovea centralis or the periphery. Vision, which is usually good initially, deteriorates, and there are severe color vision defects and impaired photopic electroretinography. The condition may progress until the defects are so severe that exact diagnosis is not possible.

Resting potential. The cornea in humans is positive in relation to the back of the eye, and there is a difference in potential of several millivolts. The resting potential is thus a dipole with the cornea positive. The resting potential is dependent on the retinal pigment epithelium, and it is approximately two times greater in the light-adapted eye than in the dark-adapted eye.

Electro-oculography. When electro-oculography is used, the increase in potential with light adaptation is measured so as to evaluate the condition of the retinal pigment epithelium. Electrodes are placed at each canthus (Fig. 2-14), and the changes in the potential between these electrodes are recorded as the eyes move

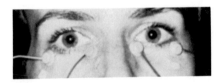

Fig. 2-14. Arrangement of electrodes for recording the electro-oculogram.

(Fig. 2-15). The average amplitude of the resting potential in light and dark adaptation is measured as the eyes turn a standard distance to the right and the left. If the light intensity and the period of dark adaptation are adequate, the ratio of the maximum amplitude obtained in the light (light peak) to the minimum amplitude obtained in the dark (dark trough) is normally greater than two, whereas the ratio is less than two in patients with disorders of the retinal pigment epithelium.

Electroretinography. When the retina is stimulated with light, an action potential is superimposed on the resting potential. The record is obtained by placing an active electrode on the cornea, usually one embedded in a corneal contact lens, with saline solution bridging the gap between the electrode and the cornea, and an indifferent electrode on the forehead. The small voltage is amplified and usually photographed from the face of an oscilloscope (electroretinogram [ERG]). The retina is stimulated with light after either dark (scotopic) or light (photopic) adaptation. After the stimulus, there is a latent period and then an initial negative deflection known as the a-wave, followed by a positive deflection designated as the b-wave (Fig. 2-16). The a-waves are thought to reflect photoreceptor activity. The origin of b-waves is less clear. They probably arise from cells in the inner nuclear layer, most likely from a cell that undergoes depolarization when the retina is stimulated. The intracellularly recorded

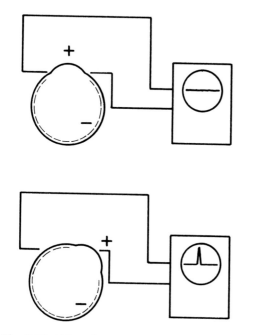

Fig. 2-15. When the eye is turned, the electrode closest to the cornea becomes positive, and a deflection is induced in the recording system.

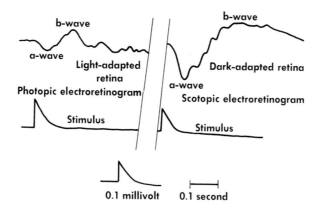

Fig. 2-16. Components of normal ERG with high-intensity stimuli showing photopic, or light-adapted, response and scotopic, or dark-adapted, response.

responses of Müller (glial) cells most closely match the b-wave.

The b-wave usually exceeds the largest amplitude of the a-wave by a factor of at least 1.5. The duration of the entire response is usually less than 250 milliseconds. The value for the b-waves is generally between 75 and 200 microvolts for photopic response and between 250 and 450 microvolts for scotopic response. The ERG is a mass response of the entire external layer of the retina. The record varies with the state of adaptation of the retina, the color of the light used in adaptation, and the intensity and color of the light used for stimulation.

Pathologic responses are described as supernormal, subnormal, negative, or absent. When a large area of the retina is damaged or diseased, the ERG is subnormal. When the entire retina is involved, there is no ERG response.

Visual-evoked potential. Stimulation of the retina with light changes the electrical activity of the cerebral cortex; this is called visual-evoked potential (VEP). The VEP is recorded from electrodes placed on the scalp (either on the midline or over the right and left occipital regions) and on the forehead.

With most stimuli the VEP is too small to be separated from other cerebral electrical activity, so a number of successive responses are averaged. The cerebral electrical activity is not related to any stimulus; thus it averages zero. The VEP electrical activity is synchronized with the presentation of the stimulus, and its average provides an index of the neural activity that follows a light impulse. Patients with inflamed or demyelinated optic nerves have decreased VEP amplitudes and latencies most pronounced when high-frequency stimuli are used. Initially of interest chiefly to investigators, the technique is becoming a valuable diagnostic tool in the assessment of optic nerve diseases, transmission of the visual impulse through the optic tracts and radiation, and cerebral disease.

IMAGE-FORMING MECHANISMS

Refraction. When a ray of light passes from one transparent medium to another, its velocity is either decreased in a more dense medium or increased in a less dense medium. If the medium is bounded by surfaces that are not perpendicular to the ray of light, then, in addition to the change in velocity, the emerging ray has a different direction than the entering ray. This change in direction of light is called refraction. It is proportionate to the sine of the angle formed by the light ray, the surface of the refracting medium, and the velocity of light in this medium. (The index of refraction is the ratio of the velocity of light in a vacuum to

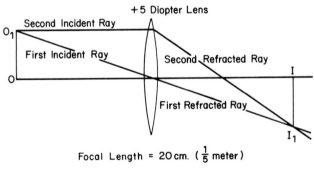

Focal Length = 20 cm. ($\frac{1}{5}$ meter)

Fig. 2-17. Parallel rays for object O_1-O form image I-I_1 at $\frac{1}{5}$ m from a 5-diopter lens.

the velocity of light in the medium. The greater the change in the velocity of the light as it passes from one medium to another, the greater will be its refraction.) Usually, rather than stating this angle and the index of refraction, the refractive power of a lens (Fig. 2-17) is described as the distance from its surface that the rays come to a focus (the focal length) or as the reciprocal of this distance in meters (diopters). Thus, if the focal length of a lens is 20 cm ($\frac{1}{5}$ m), its dioptric power is 5.

Refractive surfaces. A ray of light entering the eye is refracted by the cornea and then, after passing through the aqueous humor, by the lens. The anterior surface of the cornea is the main refractive surface of the eye. The refractive power of the cornea is approximately 43 diopters. The anterior and posterior surfaces of the lens are convex, but inasmuch as the lens is immersed on either side in fluids with similar indexes of refraction, it has less refractive power than the cornea. Optically the lens behaves as though it were composed of a series of concentric lenses, so that its total index of refraction is greater than any individual portion of the lens. With accommodation, in a youthful eye the refractive power of the lens increases from about 19 to 33 diopters because of the change in its thickness and curvature.

Refractive error. A refractive error (p. 431) is determined by two factors: (1) the refractive power of the cornea and the lens and (2) the length of the eye. Usually there is a remarkable correlation between the refractive power and the length of the eye. Most individuals have a refractive power almost exactly appropriate to cause parallel rays of light to fall upon the retina. The normal eye varies in length from about 22 to 27 mm, and the total refractive power of the normal eye at rest thus varies from about 52 to 63 diopters. Failure of the refractive power of the anterior

segment to be correlated with the length of the eye results in an error of refraction.

Accommodation. Accommodation is the process by which the refractive power of the anterior lens segment increases so

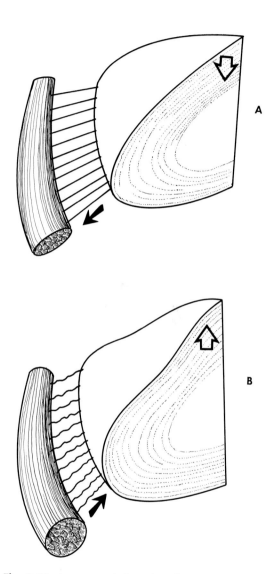

Fig. 2-18. Accommodation. **A,** When the ciliary muscle is at rest, the zonule is contracted, and the refractive power of the lens is minimal. **B,** When the ciliary muscle contracts, the zonule is relaxed, and the inherent elasticity of the lens causes it to increase in thickness and power of refraction.

that a near object may be distinctly imaged upon the retina. The increased refractive power results from increased thickness of the lens and increased convexity of the central portion of its anterior surface in response to contraction of the circular portion (mainly) of the ciliary muscle. This muscle is attached to the lens capsule through zonular fibers. When the muscle is relaxed its diameter is maximal, the zonular fibers are taut, and the lens is not accommodated. Contraction reduces the diameter of the circular muscle and relaxes the zonular fibers (Fig. 2-18). This relaxation permits the lens to become thicker and more spherical, producing a greater refractive power.

Because of the elasticity of its anterior capsule, the lens tends to assume a more spherical shape. The anterior surface of the lens, particularly its central portion, becomes more markedly curved, and the anterior pole of the lens moves forward so the lens increases in thickness in its center.

The stimulus to accommodation is maintenance of a clear retinal image. One may imagine a continuous feedback mechanism in which the brain signals the amount of accommodation required and, through stimulation of the short ciliary branches of the oculomotor nerve, constricts or relaxes the circular muscle so

that the eye almost instantly adjusts to provide clear vision at whatever distance.

With aging, the lens capsule becomes less elastic and the lens nucleus becomes harder and less compressible, so that the lens can become less spherical with relaxation of the zonule. This results in a gradual loss of accommodation. The process begins shortly after birth and continues thereafter until about the age of 50 years, when only one diopter of accommodation remains. This condition is known clinically as presbyopia. The process is mainly the result of changes in the lens, but there may be decreased strength of the ciliary body musculature with aging.

Accommodation and convergence of the two eyes normally occur together. The change in convergence that accompanies a change in accommodation is termed accommodative convergence. A lack of correspondence between accommodative convergence and accommodation may result in strabismus (p. 412).

EXTRAOCULAR MUSCULAR MECHANISMS

Each eye is moved by six extraocular muscles. Normally their action is so sensitively adjusted that each eye is directed to the same object in space.

When the eye is directed straight ahead, it is said to be in the primary posi-

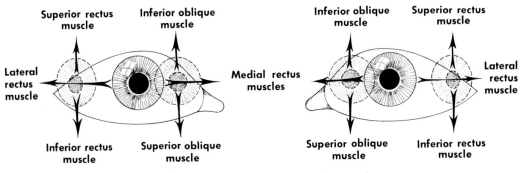

Fig. 2-19. Action of the six extraocular muscles.

tion. If it is directed upward, downward, laterally, or medially, it is said to be in a secondary position. If it is directed in an oblique position (up and in or down and in), it is said to be in a tertiary position.

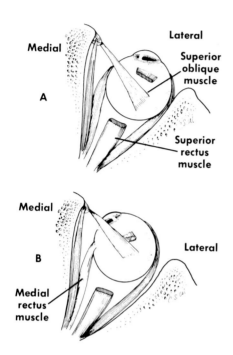

Fig. 2-20. The superior rectus muscle is removed to expose the reflected portion of the superior oblique muscle. **A,** With eye directed straight ahead (primary position), the main action of the superior oblique muscle is intorsion. **B,** When eye is turned medially, the main action of the superior oblique muscle is to turn the eye downward. When eye is turned laterally (not shown), the superior oblique muscle aids in the abduction.

The medial rectus muscle (N III) has the single action of turning the eye medially (adduction) (Fig. 2-19). The lateral rectus muscle (N VI) has the single action of turning the eye laterally (abduction). The remaining four extraocular muscles, the cyclovertical muscles, have different actions depending on the position of the globe (Table 2-2). When the eye is directed straight ahead, the superior oblique muscle (N IV) turns the globe around an anteroposterior axis so that a point on the corneoscleral limbus in the 12 o'clock position turns medially (Fig. 2-20, *A*) (intorsion). If the eye is directed laterally, the superior oblique muscle steadies the globe in this abducted position. If the eye is directed medially, the superior oblique muscle depresses the eye (Fig. 2-20, *B*). The action of the other muscles is shown in Table 2-2 and Fig. 2-19.

Duction. The movement of one eye from one position to another is called duction (Fig. 2-21). The muscles of one eye that work together in duction are called synergists in that function. In adduction the medial rectus muscle is aided by the superior and inferior recti muscles, whereas in abduction the superior and inferior oblique muscles are synergists of the lateral rectus muscle. In elevation the superior rectus and the inferior oblique muscles are synergistic, and in depression the inferior rectus and the superior oblique muscles are synergistic. In intorsion the superior oblique and superior

Table 2-2. Action of ocular muscles

Adduction (in)	Abduction (out)	Intorsion	Extorsion
Medial rectus muscle	Lateral rectus muscle	Superior oblique muscle	Inferior oblique muscle
Superior rectus muscle	Superior oblique muscle	Superior rectus muscle	Inferior rectus muscle
Inferior rectus muscle	Inferior oblique muscle		
Elevation in adduction	*Elevation in abduction*		
Inferior oblique muscle	Superior rectus muscle		
Depression in adduction	*Depression in abduction*		
Superior oblique muscle	Inferior rectus muscle		

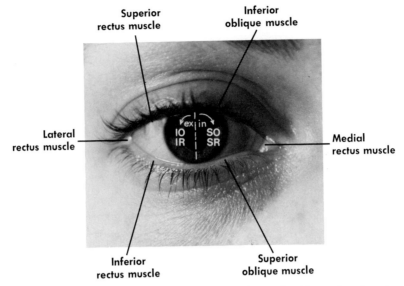

Fig. 2-21. Ductions of the eye showing the main muscle involved in each action. *In* refers to intorsion by superior oblique and superior rectus muscles. *Ex* refers to extorsion by the inferior oblique and inferior rectus muscles.

rectus muscles are synergists, and in extorsion the inferior rectus and inferior oblique muscles are synergists. Each extraocular muscle is opposed by an antagonist that has the opposite action in a particular position. Thus the antagonist of the medial rectus muscle is the lateral rectus muscle. When the eye is elevated by the superior rectus muscle, its antagonist is the inferior rectus muscle.

An innervational impulse flows to the active muscle while the innervational impulse is inhibited to the muscle's antagonist (Sherrington's principle of reciprocal innervation).

Version. The simultaneous movement of eyes from the primary position to a secondary position is called version: (1) eyes right—dextroversion, (2) eyes left—levoversion, (3) eyes up—sursumversion, and (4) eyes down—deorsumversion. The muscles of two eyes primarily responsible for directing the eyes in version movements are yoke muscles. Thus in turning the eyes to the right, the right

lateral rectus muscle is yoked to the left medial rectus muscle. Each superior rectus muscle is yoked to the contralateral inferior oblique muscle, and each inferior rectus muscle is yoked to the contralateral superior oblique muscle.

In version movements, an equal innervational impulse flows from the cerebral oculogyric centers to each muscle involved in the action (Hering's law). Thus with both eyes turned to the right, the right lateral rectus and the left medial rectus receive equal innervational stimulus.

This equal innervation is important in the diagnosis of a paretic muscle (p. 523). Thus, if the paretic muscle is on the right side and the right eye is used for fixing (as might be accomplished by covering the left eye), the nerve impulse required to hold the right eye in position is greater than it would be if the muscle was normal. Inasmuch as the impulse is directed equally to the left eye, the left eye yoke muscle will receive an excessive innervational impulse and the eye will deviate. The deviation of the left eye will thus be greatest when the paretic right eye is used for fixation. If the nonparetic left eye fixes, a normal innervation impulse is relayed to the paretic right eye and its deviation is minimal.

Vergence. Vergence is the term applied to simultaneous ocular movements in which the eyes are directed to an object in the midbody plane, that is, somewhere in front of the nose. The term is applied to convergence, in which the eyes rotate inward toward each other, or to divergence, in which they rotate outward simultaneously. Vertical (sursumvergence) and torsional vergences are uncommon.

The locations of convergence and divergence centers are not known, although many assume them to be present, inasmuch as convergence and divergence paresis is observed clinically. The nucleus of Perlia has long been considered the center for convergence. Convergence palsy occurs in midbrain disease, and the convergence center is assumed to be located in this region. Divergence paresis may occur following head injury associated with perceptual deafness, and the center is postulated to be located in the midbrain near the acoustic nerve nucleus.

Ocular movements. The two basic types of eye movements are saccadic and vergence. *Saccadic movements* are involved in version or duction, and they may reach an angular velocity of 500° of arc/sec. They are also called following reflexes and are involved in movements of an eye when the fovea follows a moving target. They also constitute the fast phase of opticokinetic and vestibular nystagmus. Saccadic movements are typically found during reading. *Vergence movements* are designed to maintain the fovea of each eye fixed upon an object of attention located approximately directly in front of the eyes. Their average velocity is about

8° to 20° of arc/sec. On the basis of the difference in velocity in saccadic and vergence movements, it has been suggested that saccadic movements involve large muscle fibers innervated by coarse myelinated nerves and that vergence movements involve small, specific muscle fibers innervated by thin, nonmedullated autonomic nerve fibers. Saccadic and vergence movements play a part in a variety of movements related basically to (1) maintaining the eyes in a forward position despite movements of the head and body and (2) bringing an image from the peripheral retina to the fovea or maintaining it on the fovea of either one or both eyes.

The eyes maintain a horizontal position, despite movements of the head, by means of postural reflexes originating in the neck muscles and in each labyrinth. Thus, when the chin is depressed on the chest, an innervational impulse stimulates the elevators of the two eyes and inhibits the depressors, and the eyes remain directed ahead. Elevation of the chin causes the opposite reaction (the depressors are stimulated, and the elevators inhibited). If the head is tilted to either shoulder, torsion occurs so that the 12 o'clock meridian rotates and the vertical meridian of the cornea remains vertical, assuming the tilting of the head is less than 20°.

If the fovea is fixed on a *steady target,* three types of movement occur: (1) those with a frequency of 30 to 70/sec and an amplitude of 20 seconds, (2) those with an irregular frequency of about 1 every second and an amplitude of 3 minutes (saccade, or flick movements), and (3) irregular drafts of about 6 minutes. The fine high-frequency movements permit new retinal receptors to be stimulated during the latent period so that the image does not disappear. The saccadic, or flick, movements tend to correct either drift or previous saccade.

If the fovea is fixed on a *moving target* with an angular velocity of less than 30°/sec, the eye follows the target almost exactly (pursuit or tracking movement). With greater velocity, an irregular type of saccadic movement results, with overcorrection and correction.

Fusional movements are vergence movements directed toward the maintenance of a single perception by keeping the retinal image on receptors having the same visual direction.

The near reaction is related to convergence involving the visual response to the awareness of the nearness of an object. It may occur without visual clues when an individual converges for the distance he believes the object to be, basing his judgment on sound or touch.

Electrical phenomena. There is continuous electrical activity in the extraocular muscles during a waking state. Moving the eye into the major field of action of a muscle causes a marked increase in the number and frequency of electrical discharges of the muscle involved. Accompanying this is a reduction in activity of the antagonistic muscle (Sherrington's principle).

The ocular muscles do not exhibit the electrical phenomena of fatigue. Sleep, however, reduces the electrical activity of the extraocular muscles to zero. During dreaming there are bursts of electrical activity and ocular movements (rapid eye movements, REMs). During sleep, the eyes are usually directed upward and outward in the Bell phenomenon. During general anesthesia, anatomic-mechanical factors position the eyes in the anatomic position of rest in which there is no muscle tone, so that the eyes are somewhat divergent.

THE IRIS AND PUPIL

The iris is a delicate diaphragm originating from the anterior extremity of the optic vesicle and the adjacent mesoderm. The iris surrounds a central aperture, the pupil, and contains the sphincter pupillae muscle (N III) and the dilatator pupillae muscle (sympathetics), which are smooth muscles arising from the ectoderm of the primitive optic vesicle.

The pupil regulates the amount of light entering the eye, increases the depth of focus of the eye, and minimizes spherical and chromatic aberrations of the eye and the astigmatism caused by oblique pencils of light.

Pupillary reflexes

Direct light reflex. When the amount of light falling upon the eye is increased, the pupil constricts. There is a latent period of about 0.18 second, and maximum contraction occurs about 1 second after the start of the stimulus. There is considerable variability in the state of the pupil thereafter unless the stimulus is maintained. The pupil may dilate again and then constrict, or it may remain constricted.

Light falling upon one eye and causing pupillary constriction also causes the pupil of the fellow eye to constrict simultaneously and to a similar degree—the *indirect* or *consensual light reflex.*

The pupillary reflex to light (Fig. 2-22) is a true reflex. The receptors for the pupillary response are the retinal photoreceptors. The afferent fibers responsible for conducting pupillary impulses from the retina to the brain do not synapse in the lateral geniculate body but pass through its medial border by way of the brachium of the superior colliculus into the pretectal nucleus, which is located at the junction of the diencephalon and the tectum of the midbrain. Fibers synapse here and pass to the Edinger-Westphal nucleus on both the same and opposite sides. From the Edinger-Westphal nucleus, pupillary constrictor fibers pass with the inferior division of the oculo-

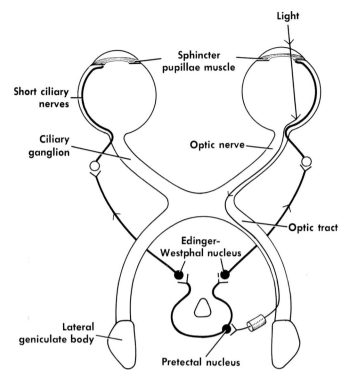

Fig. 2-22. Pathway of the light reflex. The pupillomotor fibers do not synapse in the lateral geniculate body but pass in the brachium conjunctiva to synapse with the pretectal nucleus. Intercalated neurons pass to the Edinger-Westphal nucleus (N III). Visceral efferent preganglionic fibers pass in the oculomotor nerve (N III) to the ciliary ganglion, where synapse is again made. Postganglionic fibers pass in 6 to 20 short ciliary nerves to the sphincter pupillae muscle. Thus, when one retina is stimulated by light, both pupils constrict simultaneously and equally.

motor nerve to the ciliary ganglion. Here they synapse with the postganglionic fibers, which pass by the short ciliary nerves to the sphincter muscle.

Near reaction (miosis). When an individual directs his eyes to and focuses on a nearby object, there is accommodation (lens), convergence, and pupillary constriction. The near reaction, miosis, is one of synkinesis, or an associated movement involving the common innervation of the medial rectus muscle and the sphincter pupillae muscle by the inferior branch of the oculomotor nerve.

Eyelid closure reaction (orbicularis muscle reflex). The eyelid closure reaction does not occur consistently. When effort is made to close the eyes by contraction of the orbicularis muscle (N VII), the pupil on the side of closure may constrict. This reaction indicates the close association between the third and the seventh cranial nerves.

Trigeminal reflex. Continued stimulation of trigeminal nerve from irritation of the cornea, conjunctiva, or skin of the face causes constriction of the pupil. Reflex dilation of the blood vessels of the iris also causes pupillary constriction.

Psychic reflex. Emotional states, such as fear, may cause dilation of the pupil. There is simultaneous stimulation of the sympathetic nerves and inhibition of the parasympathetic nerves.

BIBLIOGRAPHY

Armington, J. C.: The electroretinogram, New York, 1974, Academic Press, Inc.

Bonting, S. L., editor: Transmitters in the visual process, Oxford, England, 1976, Pergamon Press, Inc.

Campbell, C. J., Koestner, C. J., Rittler, M. C., and Tackaberry, R. B.: Physiological optics, New York, 1974, Harper & Row, Publishers, Inc.

Davson, H., editor: The eye; visual function in man, ed. 2, vols. 1-6, New York, 1975, Academic Press, Inc.

Duncan, G., and Bushell, A. R.: Ion analyses of human cataractous lenses, Exp. Eye Res. **20:**223, 1975.

Heller, J., and Bok, D.: A specific receptor for retinal binding protein as detected by the binding of human and bovine retinal binding protein to pigment epithelial cells, Am. J. Ophthalmol. **81:**93, 1976.

Hodson, S.: The endothelial pump of the cornea, Invest. Ophthalmol. **16:**589, 1977.

Lemp, M. A.: Cornea and sclera, Arch. Ophthalmol. **94:**473, 1976. (Superb review of corneal wound healing.)

Minckler, D. S., Tso, M. O. M., and Zimmerman, L. E.: A light microscopic, autoradiographic study of axoplasmic transport in the optic nerve head during ocular hypotony, increased intraocular pressure, and papilledema, Am. J. Ophthalmol. **82:**741, 1976.

Moses, R. A., editor: Adler's physiology of the eye; clinical application, ed. 6, St. Louis, 1975, The C. V. Mosby Co.

Obstbaum, S. A., and Podos, S. M.: Axoplasmic transport, editorial, Invest. Ophthalmol. **13:**81, 1974.

Pannbacker, R. G., and Lovett, K.: Localization of cyclic nucleotide phosphodiesterase activity within the bovine photoreceptor cell, Invest. Ophthalmol. **16:**166, 1977.

Spencer, W. H.: Drusen of the optic disk and aberrant axoplasmic transport, Am. J. Ophthalmol. **85:**1, 1978.

Van Horn, D. L., Sendele, D. D., Seidemann, S., and Buco, P. J.: Regenerative capacity of the corneal endothelium in rabbit and cat, Invest. Ophthalmol. **16:**597, 1977.

Verriest, G., editor: Modern problems in ophthalmology. Vol. 17: Color vision deficiencies, Basel, Switzerland, 1976, S. Karger.

Yanoff, M., and Fine, B. S.: Ocular pathology; a text and atlas, New York, 1975, Harper & Row, Publishers, Inc.

Young, R. W.: Visual cells and the concept of renewal, Invest. Ophthalmol. **15:**700, 1976.

Chapter 3

PHARMACOLOGY

Many different drug actions may be observed within the eye. The effects of cholinergic or adrenergic stimulation or blockade of the pupillary musculature are easily observed, as is the hypersensitivity of denervation. Many anti-inflammatory and anti-infective agents are available for topical administration, and unusually high tissue concentrations may be obtained. Toxic reactions range in severity from dermatitis medicamentosa of the eyelids to glaucoma induced by topical corticosteroids or mydriatics to permanent alteration of the fundi with impaired vision induced by phenothiazines.

DRUG ADMINISTRATION
Systemic route

Medications instilled in the conjunctival sac enter the aqueous humor mainly through the cornea, and their effects are limited to the anterior segment. If the lens is absent, minor amounts may be distributed posteriorly. The amount is sometimes large enough to cause cystoid central retinal edema, as may occur after prolonged topical instillation of epinephrine in the aphakic eye. The ocular tissue concentration of drugs administered systemically parallels that of other tissues with one important difference: the vitreous body, aqueous humor, and lens lack blood vessels. The blood-aqueous barrier is comparable in many respects to the blood-brain barrier, and the ciliary epithelium has a secretory activity similar to that of the choroid plexus. Drugs that are either ionized or lipid insoluble, or both, are largely excluded from the intraocular extracellular space. Lipid-soluble drugs enter the eye in proportion to their lipid solubility. The tight junctions of the endothelium of the retinal and iris capillaries limit the diffusion of drugs in general and lipid-insoluble substances particularly. The fenestrated choriocapillaris and ciliary body capillaries permit the passsage of relatively large molecules, but the tight junctions of the retinal pigment epithelium and its anterior extension, the pigmented ciliary body epithelium, minimize further intraocular penetration. Severe inflammation damages the blood-aqueous barrier, and compounds that do not enter the normal eye in high concentrations enter with ease and are distributed as in other body tissues and fluids.

The ciliary body epithelium extrudes organic ions from the posterior aqueous humor into the blood by a transport process similar to that in the renal tubule and choroid plexus. Uric acid and drugs such as the penicillins are actively transported out of the posterior chamber by the nonpigmented ciliary epithelium, and this transport is inhibited by probenecid.

The concentration of some drugs, such

as the phenothiazines in cells containing melanin, leads to a high level in the retinal pigment epithelium. This may cause toxic reactions in the sensory retina, but alternatively, the stabilization of cell lysosomes by this group of drugs may interfere with phagocytosis of photoreceptor outer segments.

Local route

Drugs may be applied to the eyelids or anterior globe in aqueous or viscous solutions or suspensions, in ointments, as fine powders, by application on cotton pledgets, by drug-impregnated contact lenses, by injection, by mechanical pumps, or by membrane release systems. In contrast to the tissue concentration after systemic administration, the ocular concentration after topical administration is extremely high. However, dilution of the drug by the tears, overflow onto the cheek, and excretion through the nasolacrimal system limits effectiveness, as does improper instillation. Several ingenious constant delivery systems that provide continuous release of medications over a long period are useful in the management of glaucoma.

Placing the drug under a contact lens or applying saturated cotton pledgets to the eye ensures prolonged contact and enhances penetration. A soft contact lens may be soaked in a compound, and when the lens is placed in contact with the cornea, it gradually releases the drug. This has been done with pilocarpine in glaucoma management.

Subconjunctival or sub-Tenon retrobulbar injection is popular for the administration of antibiotics and corticosteroids. A high tissue concentration is maintained for a long period. Some surgeons inject an antibiotic subconjunctivally at the end of an intraocular operation to ensure a high concentration of antibiotic in the aqueous humor. Injections into the anterior chamber of the vitreous body are limited to a few antibiotics and are largely reserved for infections that threaten destruction of the globe.

Maximal effectiveness of topical preparations requires proper instillation. The patient is instructed to look upward, and the skin of the lower eyelid is grasped and drawn outward to create a pouch be-

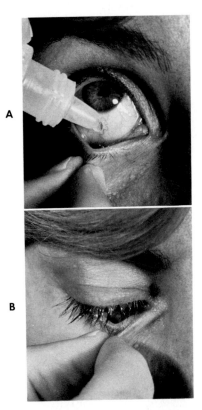

Fig. 3-1. **A,** The proper method of instillation of eye drops in the eye. The lower eyelid is drawn away from the globe, the patient is instructed to look upward, and the drop is delivered into the pouch. **B,** The patient is then instructed to look downward, and the skin of the eyelid is slowly released. The patient should be warned not to squeeze the eye. The eyelids may then be gently closed for 2 minutes. Increased concentrations may be provided in a particular region by having the patient tilt the head in the direction of desired effect.

tween the eyelid and the globe. The drug is then instilled in the pouch without touching the eyelids with the container. The patient is instructed to look down and to close the eye without squeezing (Fig. 3-1). Increased viscosity of the vehicle minimizes dilution and prolongs contact. Thus medications may be prescribed in oils, ointments, methyl cellulose, and other viscous vehicles.

Membrane release systems. These systems provide continuous release of a predetermined amount of a drug over a 5- to 7-day period. Ocusert R (pilocarpine) is commonly available for glaucoma treatment. It provides a continuous but much lower drug concentration, which produces the same effects as topical instillation and usually minimizes side effects of pilocarpine treatment in individuals with active accommodation. Daily inspection is required to be certain the device has not been inadvertently lost.

Corneal penetration. Compounds enter the anterior chamber mainly through the cornea. The tight junctions of the epithelium are the chief barrier to water-soluble, polar compounds. Lipid-soluble compounds pass through the epithelium. When the epithelium is diseased or damaged, penetration by water-soluble, polar compounds into the anterior segment is increased. Local anesthetics, wetting agents, massage, and abrasion damage the epithelium and enhance penetration. To penetrate the stroma, the drugs must be water soluble. Thus the highest intraocular concentrations follow administration of compounds that are both water and lipid soluble.

The medication must have a greater affinity for the cornea than for the vehicle. If the medication has a greater affinity for the vehicle, it will not be released and will remain in the vehicle rather than be absorbed into the eye.

Topical preparations. Many factors relate to the effectiveness, safety, and comfort of topically applied eye medications: sterility, hydrogen ion concentration, tonicity, physiologic activity, stability, toxicity, surface tension, and compatibility. In recent years, to ensure sterility, nearly all commonly used medications are prepared commercially and thus require quality control and Food and Drug Administration approval. When high concentrations of antibiotics are required for topical use, antibiotics not usually available as ophthalmic preparations may be prepared by mixing the product intended for intravenous use with an artificial tear vehicle.

Sterility. To prevent inactivation by heating, many compounds intended for ocular use are filtered through a micropore filter. This ensures the initial sterility required by interstate commerce, but the solution is easily contaminated once the container is opened. The physician should regard a solution in an unsealed container as contaminated.

The adenovirus causing keratoconjunctivitis (p. 263) may be transmitted by means of contaminated eye anesthetic solutions. Fluorescein solution is liable to contamination by *Pseudomonas aeruginosa*, and it may introduce the organism when used in the diagnosis of corneal abrasions. To avoid infection, fluorescein should be instilled only from a sterile individual container or should be applied by means of a filter paper strip that has been saturated with fluorescein and then sterilized. It must never be used from a stock bottle.

Eyecups are usually contaminated and may cause recurrent infections. Eyedroppers are easily contaminated by touching the eyelids or the conjunctiva, and they may then contaminate a stock bottle. Plastic "squeeze" bottles in which most commercially available medications are now distributed are far more difficult to contaminate than bottles with eyedroppers.

AUTONOMIC DRUGS

The autonomic nervous system may be divided into parasympathetic (or cholinergic) and sympathetic (or adrenergic) systems. Drugs affecting these systems may be divided into cholinergic-stimulating (agonist) and cholinergic-blocking (antagonist) agents and adrenergic-stimulating (agonist) and adrenergic-blocking (antagonist) agents.

Acetylcholine is the cholinergic neurohumoral transmitter, and norepinephrine (noradrenaline, arterenol) is the main adrenergic neural transmitter. Acetylcholine is inactivated by the enzyme cholinesterase, whereas norepinephrine is largely inactivated by reuptake by the axon that released it (90%) or by the ezyme catechol-O-methyl transferase. The amount of norepinephrine stored in the axon of the synaptic junction is limited by norepinephrine inactivation by monoamine oxidase.

The sphincter pupillae and ciliary muscles are innervated by postganglionic parasympathetic efferent fibers of the short ciliary nerve branches of the oculomotor nerve (N III) that have synapsed in the ciliary ganglion. The dilatator pupillae muscle is innervated by the long ciliary nerves carrying postganglionic fibers of the sympathetic nervous system that have synapsed in the superior cervical ganglion. The sphincter pupillae and ciliary muscles belong principally to the cholinergic system, whereas the dilatator pupillae muscle belongs to the adrenergic system. Cholinergic stimulation of the sphincter pupillae muscle causes constriction of the pupil (miosis) (Table 3-1). Cholinergic stimulation of the ciliary muscle increases accommodation. Cholinergic blockade dilates the pupil (mydriasis) and relaxes the ciliary muscle, causing decreased accommodation (cycloplegia).

Adrenergic stimulation causes dilation of the pupil, whereas adrenergic blockade causes pupillary constriction. The ciliary muscle may have minor adrenergic innervation with stimulation decreasing accommodation. The more prominent cholinergic effects obscure adrenergic effects.

Cholinergic compounds

The neurohumoral theory of nerve transmission postulates that acetylcholine is the neurohumoral transmitter responsible for (1) synaptic transmission at all autonomic ganglia (including the sympathetic ganglia and the adrenal medulla),

Table 3-1. Drugs acting predominantly on the cholinergic (parasympathetic, acetylcholine effector) nervous system

---

I. Cholinergic-stimulating compounds
   A. Displacement of acetylcholine from axonal terminal
      1. Carbachol
      2. Tetraethylammonium (also a blocking agent)
   B. Mimicking of acetylcholine at postsynaptic receptor
      1. Muscarinic-type receptors
         a. Pilocarpine
         b. Muscarine
         c. Arecoline
         d. Methacholine (Mecholyl)
      2. Nicotinic-type receptors
         a. Nicotine
         b. Pilocarpine
         c. Arecoline
   C. Inhibition of enzymatic breakdown of acetylcholine
II. Cholinergic-blocking compounds
   A. Interference with acetylcholine synthesis
      1. Hemicholinium
   B. Prevention of acetylcholine release
      1. Botulinus toxin
   C. Blockade of transmitter at postsynaptic receptor
      1. Muscarinic-type receptors
         a. Atropine (smooth and cardiac muscles)
      2. Nicotinic-type receptors
         a. Nicotine (autonomic ganglia and motor endplates of skeletal muscle)
         b. d-Tubocurarine (same as nicotine)
         c. Hexamethonium (autonomic ganglia)
         d. Decamethonium (motor endplates of skeletal muscle)

---

(2) some synaptic transmission in the central nervous system, (3) activation of skeletal muscles innervated by spinal nerves, (4) activation of smooth and cardiac muscles innervated by postganglionic parasympathetic nerves, and (5) activation of sweat glands and arrectores pilorum muscles, which are innervated by postganglionic sympathetic nerves.

Acetylcholine affects two types of choline receptors: (1) muscarinic receptors (blocked by atropine) located in smooth and cardiac muscles and exocrine gland cells, and (2) nicotinic receptors (blocked by large doses of nicotine) in autonomic ganglia cells and the motor endplates of skeletal muscle. d-Tubocurarine blocks nicotinic receptors in both locations, but hexamethonium blocks only those located in autonomic ganglia and decamethonium blocks only those located in the motor endplates of skeletal muscle (Table 3-1).

Acetylcholine is synthesized by the neuron and stored at the site of activity in small synaptic vesicles. Acetylcholine is formed by combination of acetylcoenzyme A (arising from pyruvate) and choline; the final step is acetylation of choline catalyzed by choline acetyltransferase (acetyl acetylase). Release of acetylcholine at the synaptic vesicle depolarizes the postsynaptic membrane and transmits the nervous impulse. The released acetylcholine is inactivated in time periods that range from 1 millisecond to 1 second by the enzyme cholinesterase, which permits repolarization of the membrane and transmission of the next impulse.

There are two types of cholinesterase: (1) specific acetylcholinesterase, which occurs in neurons, neuromuscular functions, and erythrocytes, and (2) nonspecific cholinesterase, or pseudocholinesterase, which is found in plasma and many tissues and is probably synthesized by the liver. Nonspecific cholinesterase

inactivates long-chain choline esters as well as acetylcholine. Specific acetylcholinesterase inactivates acetylcholine only. It is the main cholinesterase of the iris and the lens.

Cholinergic drugs are compounds that mimic the action of acetylcholine on effector cells or at synapses. The action may be brought about directly by compounds chemically related to acetylcholine or by those such as pilocarpine that act directly on smooth muscle. Indirect stimulation occurs when the activity of acetylcholine is prolonged by inactivating the cholinesterase that normally hydrolyzes it. Such compounds are called anticholinesterases and are commonly classified as reversible if their action is relatively short or as irreversible if it is long.

Cholinergic-stimulating drugs. Most direct-acting cholinergic drugs are chemically related to acetylcholine and are so potent and have such marked effects when systemically administered that their therapeutic uses are limited. They cause vasodilation; decreased heart rate and blood pressure; stimulation of the salivary, lacrimal, sweat, and gastric secretions; and increased tone of the gastrointestinal, urinary, and bronchiolar musculature.

When instilled in the conjunctival sac, choline esters cause dilation of the conjunctival and uveal arterioles, constriction of the pupil, and increased permeability of the blood-aqueous barrier. Most of the compounds penetrate the intact cornea poorly.

The direct-acting cholinergic drugs used in ophthalmology include the following compounds.

Acetylcholine. Acetylcholine (1:100) may be injected into the anterior chamber to constrict the pupil after cataract extraction. The toxicity of acetylcholine is low because it is so rapidly destroyed by cholinesterase. The cholinesterase in the cornea rapidly inactivates it so that after topical administration no acetylcholine enters the anterior chamber.

Methacholine. Methacholine (Mecholyl) is not commercially available.

Carbachol. Carbachol (Carcholin, Doryl), 0.75% to 3.0%, must be combined with a wetting agent to penetrate the cornea. It is not hydrolyzed by cholinesterases and is so potent that it is not used systemically. Frequently this drug is substituted for pilocarpine in patients who have developed a tolerance to pilocarpine.

Pilocarpine. Like acetylcholine, pilocarpine acts directly on glandular and smooth muscle receptors, that is, structures innervated by postganglionic cholinergic nerves. It is effective in producing pupillary constriction even though the ciliary ganglion has been blocked. It causes pupillary constriction, stimulates the ciliary muscle to increase accommodation, and increases the permeability of the trabecular meshwork. In some patients it decreases aqueous secretion. Its chief value is in the treatment of glaucoma, for which it is used topically in a 1% to 4% solution. It is stable, penetrates the cornea well, and is the most popular drug for the treatment of glaucoma and to reverse the effects of mydriatics. It is prescribed in the minimum concentration that will prevent progression of the glaucoma and is seldom instilled more frequently than once every 4 hours. In open-angle glaucoma the increased permeability of the trabecular meshwork is its most useful function, whereas in angle-closure glaucoma the pupillary constriction is most important. Systemic toxicity is rare, although a contact allergy of the eyelids and conjunctiva or lens opacities may develop after long-term use.

Anticholinesterase drugs. Anticholinesterase drugs permit the accumulation of acetylcholine by inactivating cholinesterase. There are three main types of anticholinesterase compounds: (1) physostigmine (eserine), a tertiary amine with a urethane group; (2) neostigmine (Prostigmin), a quaternary ammonium compound; and (3) organophosphates. The first two are classified as reversible cholinesterase inhibitors. The organophosphates inactivate cholinesterase irreversibly.

Administration of anticholinesterase compounds causes widespread cholinergic stimulation. There is constriction of gastrointestinal, urinary, and bronchiole muscles. Skeletal muscle is weakened and fibrillates. Salivation, lacrimation, and sweating increase together with increased pulmonary secretions. Central nervous system symptoms range from giddiness to coma and convulsions.

The sphincter pupillae and ciliary muscles contract so that the pupil is miotic and accommodation is increased. The drugs do not constrict the pupil after retrobulbar anesthesia or if the eye has no parasympathetic innervation and hence no acetylcholine. The organophosphates cause more marked dilation of the conjunctival and ciliary blood vessels as well as increased permeability of the blood-aqueous barrier than do physostigmine or neostigmine.

Physostigmine. Physostigmine (eserine) was the first miotic used in the treatment of glaucoma (1876). It is used in an aqueous solution of the salicylate salt in a concentration of 0.25% to 1% or as a 0.25% ointment. Usually it is given only at bedtime to supplement the instillation of pilocarpine. Prolonged use causes conjunctival irritation.

Neostigmine. Neostigmine (Prostigmin) was synthesized as an analogue of physostigmine. It is used in the treatment of glaucoma as a 5% solution every 4 to 6 hours and systemically in the treatment of myasthenia gravis. It penetrates the cornea poorly and is used rarely.

Edrophonium chloride (Tensilon), an analogue of neostigmine, has a systemic action of 2 or 3 minutes. It is injected intravenously in doses of 2 to 5 mg in the diagnosis of myasthenia gravis (p. 568).

Organophosphates. Echothiophate iodide (Phospholine Iodide) is an organophosphate in which a quaternary ammonium compound has been substituted. It is extremely active against nonspecific cholinesterases. Echothiophate iodide is used locally every 12 hours in a 0.06% to 0.25% solution. It causes intense miosis and spasm of the ciliary muscle.

All organophosphates are contraindicated in angle-closure glaucoma (p. 404), bronchial asthma, gastrointestinal spasm, vascular hypertension, myocardial infarction, and Parkinson disease. Long-term use of echothiophate iodide may cause iris cysts in children. It inactivates the Na^+-K^+ ATPase of the specific cholinesterase of the lens capsule and may cause water vesicles in the anterior portion of the lens.

Despite the long list of contraindications, echothiophate iodide has proved to be particularly effective in open-angle glaucoma, aphakic glaucoma, and accommodative esotropia (p. 418).

Local instillation of echothiophate iodide (and other organophosphates) depletes systemic pseudocholinesterases. Thus, if succinylcholine is used as a muscle relaxant in the course of general anesthesia, the succinylcholine is not inactivated, and there may be dangerously prolonged apnea. Additionally, the compounds can cause abdominal distress that may be mistaken for an acute surgical emergency.

Reactivators of cholinesterase. Severe toxicity from anticholinesterase compounds in drugs, chemical warfare agents, and insecticides occurs because of the accumulation of acetylcholine. Atropine (2 to 20 mg, intravenously or intramuscularly) antagonizes acetylcholine at muscarinic receptor sites. Pralidoxime (1 gm at maximum rate of 500 mg/minute, intravenously) reactivates acetylcholinesterase, particularly at the motor endplate of skeletal muscle.

Cholinergic-blocking drugs

The action of acetylcholine in nerve transmission may be blocked at (1) the motor endplate of postganglionic parasympathetic nerve fibers in smooth and cardiac muscle—these structures are stimulated by muscarine and blocked by the atropine group of drugs; (2) the autonomic ganglia of both the parasympathetic and the sympathetic nervous system—nicotine in small doses stimulates ganglionic transmission, the action being opposed by ganglionic-blocking agents, whereas nicotine in large doses is a ganglionic-blocking agent; and (3) both the motor endplate of skeletal muscle and the central nervous system.

Atropine group. In general, these drugs prevent the action of acetylcholine at postganglionic nerve endings in smooth muscle, cardiac muscle, and exocrine glands. Systemic administration increases the heart rate and decreases sweating, lacrimation, salivary secretion, gastric secretion, gastrointestinal motility, and tone. Many of the compounds have a depressant effect on the central nervous system and can cause confusional psychosis.

The ocular effects of the atropinelike drugs are mainly dilation of the pupil through paralysis of the sphincter pupillae muscle and decrease of accommodation through paralysis of the ciliary muscle. The duration of these effects varies with different compounds.

Systemic administration has less effect than local administration because of decreased concentration of the componds at the effector sites in the eye. Systemically administered atropine has a greater pupillary effect than the atropinelike compounds used for their antispasmodic action on the gastrointestinal tract.

Atropine and related compounds reduce the permeability of blood vessels of the iris and the ciliary body; consequently, they are used in inflammations of the iris and ciliary body to reduce vascular permeability and to dilate the pupil and paralyze accommodation. The paralysis of accommodation places the inflamed ciliary muscles at rest and minimizes pain.

On local instillation, the atropinelike compounds developed as gastrointestinal antispasmodics have varying degrees of mydriatic and cycloplegic activity. Systemic administration in younger persons may cause an annoying decrease in accommodation. Many patients with ill-defined gastrointestinal complaints for whom atropinelike antispasmodics are prescribed also have unsuspected open-angle glaucoma (p. 398).

Members of the atropine group of drugs used in ophthalmology include atropine, scopolamine, homatropine, eucatropine (Euphthalmine), cyclopentolate hydrochloride (Cyclogyl), and tropicamide (Mydriacyl).

Atropine. Atropine is the principal alkaloid of belladonna. It is used in a 0.5% to 4% aqueous solution, in an ointment, or in a castor oil base to minimize the possibility of systemic absorption. It causes pupillary dilation that begins in about 15 minutes and persists 10 to 12 days. Paralysis of accommodation begins at 20 to 30 minutes after instillation and persists 3 to 5 days. Atropine is widely used in the treatment of anterior uveitis and keratitis and in the refraction of children, particularly those with strabismus. In inflammatory condition it may be used every 1 to 6 hours. For refraction in children it is commonly instilled in an ointment base three times daily for 3 days, and examination is on the fourth day.

Scopolamine. This drug is closely related to atropine but has a shorter duration of action (2 to 3 days) on both pupillary dilation and accommodative paralysis. It is frequently substituted for atropine, which may cause conjunctival irritation or contact allergy when prolonged mydriasis and cycloplegia are used in conditions such as retinal separation or uveitis.

Homatropine. This synthetic, atropine-like compound is used mainly to paralyze accommodation for refraction. It is used in a 1% to 5% aqueous solution, and it produces mydriasis and cycloplegia for 12 to 36 hours.

Eucatropine (Euphthalmine). This is a synthetic compound that has a mydriatic action without cycloplegic effects. It is used almost exclusively to dilate the pupil in a provocative test in patients suspected of having primary angle-closure glaucoma.

Cyclopentolate. Cyclopentolate (Cyclogyl) is an atropinelike compound that causes mydriasis and cycloplegia; there is a return to normal usually within 6 hours. It is used almost exclusively in refraction. Instillation causes a pronounced burning sensation for a few seconds. In susceptible elderly patients, local use may cause temporary psychosis.

Tropicamide (Mydriacyl). This cholinergic-blocking drug causes a more rapid paralysis of accommodation and quicker recovery than any other such compound. If the drug is used in a 1% concentration instilled at least two times at 5-minute intervals, maximum cycloplegia occurs in about 20 minutes. Its effect usually disappears within 2 to 4 hours. It causes more pupillary dilation than other cholinergic compounds and is often combined with phenylephrine for ophthalmoscopy.

Ganglionic-blocking drugs. These compounds block the transmission of impulses across both sympathetic and parasympathetic autonomic ganglia. They are used in the treatment of hypertensive cardiovascular disease to reduce peripheral resistance by decreasing sympathetic tone to vascular beds. They are also useful in vasospasm therapy and in producing a controlled hypotension in general anesthesia.

The ocular side effects of ganglionic blockade constitute their main ophthalmic interest. The conjunctival blood vessels and the pupil are dilated. The volume of tears and the amount of accommodation decrease. The intraocular pressure decreases slightly, apparently because of a decreased secretion of aqueous humor. The decrease is accompanied by an increased resistance to the exit of aqueous humor through the trabecular meshwork. Increased intraocular pressure does not occur because of the reduced aqueous secretion.

Neuromuscular-blocking drugs. These compounds may be effective in the spinal cord and subcortical centers or at the motor endplates of skeletal musculature. Curare is a competitive neuromuscular-blocking agent that combines with choline receptor sites and blocks the transmitter action of acetylcholine. Succinylcholine depolarizes the motor endplate by an unknown mechanism.

The main ophthalmic application of this group of drugs is in general anesthesia in which the administration of *d*-tubocurarine chloride causes relaxation of the extraocular musculature, which is desirable in cataract extraction. Succinylcholine produces a short period of muscular relaxation but also extraocular muscular contraction before paralysis develops. Its use is therefore contraindicated in intraocular surgery and in ocular lacerations because of the increased intraocular pressure.

Adrenergic compounds

The catecholamines (norepinephrine, dopamine, and epinephrine) are the neurohumoral transmitters responsible for the stimulation of the majority of structures innervated by postganglionic sympathetic nerves (Table 3-2). (The arrectores pilorum muscles and sweat glands are exceptional in having acetylcholine as the postganglionic effector substance.) Norepinephrine (noradrenalin or levarterenol) is the major transmitter at most postganglionic sympathetic impulses; dopamine is the major transmitter in the extrapyramidal system; and epinephrine is the major hormone in the adrenal medulla.

The initial step in catecholamine synthesis is the hydroxylation of phenylalanine to tyrosine. Tyrosine is hydroxylated to dopa, a key compound in synthesis of catecholamine and certain "false transmitters" used therapeutically. Dopa is catalyzed to dopamine by the enzyme L-aromatic acid decarboxylase (dopa decarboxylase). Dopamine is converted to norepinephrine by the enzyme dopamine β-hydroxylase. Methylation of norepinephrine yields epinephrine. Norepinephrine is mainly confined to postganglionic fibers, whereas epinephrine is localized to chromaffin cells of the adrenal medulla.

There are two types of adrenergic receptor cells: (1) alpha receptors, which are mainly excitatory to smooth muscle and gland cells but cause relaxation of intestinal smooth muscle; and (2) beta receptors, which are differentiated into two types: beta$_1$ in the heart and small intestine and beta$_2$ in the bronchi, vascular beds, and uterus. Generally, the effect of sympathomimetic drugs is excitatory on alpha receptors and inhibitory on beta receptors, but this is not always true. Thus, epinephrine stimulation of alpha receptors in blood vessels causes constriction, and stimulation of beta receptors causes dilation; however, alpha stimulation usually predominates.

The norepinephrine released from the sympathetic nerve vesicle is almost com-

Table 3-2. Compounds acting predominantly on the adrenergic nervous system

I. Stimulation
  A. Direct
    1. Both alpha- and beta-adrenergic receptors
      a. Epinephrine
      b. Ephedrine
      c. Dopamine
      d. Amphetamine
    2. Mainly alpha-adrenergic receptors
      a. Norepinephrine
      b. Phenylephrine (Neo-Synephrine)
      c. Hydroxyamphetamine (Paredrine)
      d. Methenamine
      e. Methoxamine
    3. Mainly beta$_1$-adrenergic receptors
      a. Isoproterenol (Isuprel)
    4. Mainly beta$_2$-adrenergic receptors
      a. Salbutamol (Albuterol)
      b. Metaproterenol (Alupent)
      c. Terbutaline (Bricanyl)
      d. Fenoterol (Berotec)
  B. Indirect
    1. Potentiation of catecholamine action
      a. Postganglionic denervation
        (1) Surgical
        (2) Pharmacologic: reserpine, guaneth-
            idine, subconjunctival 6-hydroxy-
            dopamine
    2. Promotion of release of transmitter
      a. Tyramine
      b. Guanethidine
      c. Amphetamine
    3. Prevention of uptake of transmitter
      a. Cocaine
      b. Imipramine
    4. Inhibition of monoamine oxidase
      a. Tranylcypromine
      b. Pargyline
    5. Inhibition of catechol-O-methyl transferase
      a. Pyrogallol
      b. Quercetin

II. Blockade
  A. Direct
    1. Both alpha- and beta-adrenergic receptors
      a. Labetalol
    2. Mainly alpha-adrenergic receptors
      a. Dibenamine
      b. Ergot alkaloids
      c. Phenoxybenzamine (Dibenzyline)
      d. Tolazoline (Priscoline)
      e. Phentolamine mesylate (Regitine)
      f. Phenothiazines
      g. Yohimbines
    3. Both beta$_1$- and beta$_2$-adrenergic receptors
      a. Propranolol (Inderal)
      b. Dichloroisoproterenol (partial)
      c. Pronethalol
      d. Timolol
    4. Mainly beta$_1$-adrenergic receptors
      a. Practolol
      b. Atenolol
    5. Mainly beta$_2$-adrenergic receptors
      a. Butoxamine
  B. Indirect
    1. Impaired synthesis transmitter
      a. Block with alpha-methyl-p-tyrosine
      b. Synthesize "false transmitter" from alpha-
          methyldopa (Aldomet)
    2. Prevention of release of norepinephrine at
       synaptic terminal
      a. Bretylium
      b. Iproniazid
    3. Depletion of transmitter
      a. Reserpine
      b. Guanethidine (initial release and then de-
          pletion)
    4. Autonomic ganglia of adrenergic nervous
       system
      a. Ganglionic-blocking agents acting on
          sympathetic ganglia such as superior cer-
          vical ganglion
      b. Central nervous system depressants

pletely (90%) inactivated by reuptake by the terminal that released it. The remainder diffuses into the circulation or is inactivated by the enzymes catechol-O-methyl transferase and monoamine oxidase.

Not all of the adrenergic receptors in the human intraocular musculature have been determined. The dilatator pupillae and sphincter pupillae muscles of the monkey eye contain mainly alpha-adrenergic receptors. Thus, stimulation of alpha receptors in the iris musculature provides antagonistic actions, but the larger number of receptors in the dilatator muscle causes pupillary dilation. The trabecular meshwork contains mainly alpha receptors, and stimulation increases the facility of outflow. The ciliary epithelium contains mainly beta receptors, and

Table 3-3. Ocular effects of autonomic drugs

	Effect on secretion	Effect on aqueous outflow	Effect on intraocular pressure	Accommodation (ciliary muscle)	Sphincter pupillae muscle	Dilatator pupillae muscle
Cholinergic agonist	±	Increase	Decrease	Increase	Miosis	
Cholinergic antagonist	±	±		Decrease	Mydriasis	
Alpha-adrenergic agonist	±	±	Decrease			Mydriasis
Beta-adrenergic agonist	Decrease	±	Decrease			
Alpha-adrenergic antagonist	±*		±			
Beta-adrenergic antagonist	±†	±	Decrease			Slight mydriasis

*Beta-adrenergic predominance.
†Alpha-adrenergic predominance.

stimulation inhibits secretion of aqueous humor.

Adrenergic-stimulating compounds. Ophthalmic interest in these drugs is concerned with stimulation of alpha- and beta-adrenergic receptors by topical administration. When the few molecules involved in neurohumoral transmission are considered, the number instilled in therapy and diagnosis appears enormous. Phenylephrine stimulates alpha receptors, isoproterenol stimulates beta receptors, and epinephrine stimulates both alpha and beta receptors (Table 3-3). The ocular effects (but not the systemic) are minimal after systemic administration.

Topical instillation of adrenergic-stimulating compounds causes (1) pupillary dilation, (2) increased facility of outflow of aqueous humor through the trabecular meshwork, (3) decrease secretion of aqueous humor by the ciliary epithelium, and (4) vasoconstriction of the conjunctival blood vessels.

Epinephrine. Epinephrine (adrenaline) penetrates the cornea poorly, and pupillary dilation requires instillation of a 1% or stronger solution. In denervation hypersensitivity (p. 126) when the postganglionic sympathetic fibers to the dilatator muscle have been interrupted, a 0.1% solution will dilate the pupil. One-quarter percent to 2% epinephrine is used in the treatment of glaucoma to increase the outflow of aqueous humor through the trabecular meshwork and to decrease aqueous humor production. In glaucoma therapy, epinephrine is usually combined with a cholinergic-stimulating drug such as pilocarpine. In ocular hypertension, topical 1% epinephrine is used without pilocarpine.

In some individuals the epinephrine produces black, localized, isolated subconjunctival deposits of adrenochrome in the conjunctiva or cornea. It may cause a reversible maculopathy when used topically in aphakic patients for treatment of glaucoma.

Phenylephrine hydrochloride. Phenylephrine hydrochloride (Neo-Synephrine), an almost exclusive alpha receptor stimulator, is effective for pupillary dilation. It penetrates the cornea well and is commonly used to dilate the pupil for examination of the ocular fundus. It may cause severe vascular hypertension in individuals past 60 years of age who are using drugs that cause sympathetic denervation with subsequent hypersensitivity to the alpha receptor–stimulating effects of phenylephrine. Cerebrovascular accidents have been attributed to this hypertension. Phenylephrine is sometimes used in combination with cholinergic-blocking agents to enhance pupillary dilation in the treatment of uveitis. It is available in 1%, 2.5%, and 10% solutions. The 10% solution should not be instilled in individuals more than 60 years old.

Phenylephrine is the preferred agent for dilating the pupil to study the ocular fundus because it can be easily neutralized with cholinergic drugs. It may prevent the formation of cysts of the pupillary pigment epithelium in children in whom anticholinesterase preparations are used to minimize accommodation in accommodative esotropia (p. 412).

Norepinephrine. Norepinephrine (levarterenol) is not as potent when administered topically as it is at the postganglionic nerve terminal. It acts predominantly on alpha-adrenergic receptors and has a feeble effect on beta receptors. Experimental topical administration reduces intraocular pressure but may cause severe hypertension in susceptible persons.

Isoproterenol. Isoproterenol (Isuprel) acts almost exclusively to stimulate beta receptors. It decreases aqueous humor secretion and reduces intraocular pressure about as effectively as epinephrine. However, in the 5% concentration used topically it causes tachycardia and palpitation. Unlike epinephrine, it does not cause constriction of conjunctival vessels and is readily absorbed systemically.

Other adrenergic-stimulating drugs. Hydroxyamphetamine hydrobromide (Paredrine) and other amphetamines cause variable amounts of pupillary dilation when instilled into the conjunctival sac. With the exception of hydroxyamphetamine hydrobromide, which is a less effective dilating agent than phenylephrine, they are not used in clinical ophthalmology.

Potentiation of catecholamines. The action of norepinephrine on a receptor is mainly terminated by its reentry into the sympathetic axons from which it was released. The action of norepinephrine is prolonged by cocaine and protriptyline, which interferes with the axonal uptake.

Epinephrine and norepinephrine are partially inactivated by the enzyme catechol-O-methyl transferase. This enzyme is inhibited by pyrogallol and by quercetin, which therefore permit the accumulation of norepinephrine and epinephrine and prolong their physiologic effects. These compounds are of pharmacologic interest mainly; their activities are not comparable to those of the anticholinesterase compounds in the cholinergic nervous system.

Monoamine oxidase is concerned with the metabolites of epinephrine and norepinephrine resulting from the action of catechol-O-methyl transferase. If monoamine oxidase is inhibited, there is an accumulation of norepinephrine in the brain and elsewhere. This may occur because the accumulation of end products of metabolism inhibits the inactivation of norepinephrine. The mechanism is not known.

Adrenergic-blocking agents

The adrenergic nervous system may be blocked at several levels. In many instances the pharmacologic actions are obscured by side effects, and the adrenergic blockade is not conspicuous. Adrenergic blockade may occur at the following levels: (1) interference with catecholamine synthesis; (2) blocking the effect of catecholamines on effector cells—there may thus be alpha-, beta$_1$-, and beta$_2$-blocking agents; and (3) prevention of the initial storage and subsequent release of norepinephrine.

In addition to these primary agents, there are a number of secondary adrenergic-blocking compounds. Blocking acetylcholine activity at the level of autonomic ganglia decreases adrenergic stimulation. Central nervous system depressants also block adrenergic actions.

Systemically administered compounds that inhibit postganglionic sympathetic nerves at effector sites produce orthostatic hypotension and nasal stuffiness, and some cause pupillary constriction. They cause reduction of intraocular pressure, presumably through reduced ciliary body secretion.

Interference with catecholamine synthesis. Dopa is catalyzed to dopamine by dopa decarboxylase. The synthesis of dopamine and subsequently norepinephrine can be blocked by compounds that inhibit decarboxylase.

Alpha-methyldopa (Aldomet) is converted by dopa decarboxylase to alpha-methyl norepinephrine, a "false neurotransmitter," and the systemic level of norepinephrine is reduced. Topical administration does not affect the intraocular pressure in experimental animals. Systemic administration reduces the arterial blood pressure, and there is a parallel but transient reduction in intraocular pressure.

Blockade of adrenergic receptors. Agents that block adrenergic receptors are used mainly in the management of vascular hypertension, cardiac arrhythmias, and angina pectoris. Labelol, which blocks both alpha and beta receptors, has been used in the treatment of vascular hypertension. Most other members of the group block predominantly either alpha- or beta-adrenergic receptors.

Blockade of alpha-adrenergic receptors. Many compounds block alpha-adrenergic receptors and are available for clinical study. The main members of the group are phenoxybenzamine (Dibenzyline), ergot alkaloids, tolazoline (Priscoline), and phentolamine mesylate (Regitine Mesylate). Dibenamine, which is similar to but less potent than phenoxybenzamine, has been used experimentally in the treatment of angle-closure glaucoma. Retrobulbar tolazoline causes vasodilation, particularly of the central retinal artery.

Blockade of beta-adrenergic receptors. Compounds that block beta-adrenergic receptors are used widely in cardiology. Generally they are contraindicated in bronchial asthma. Topical administration of timolol, which blocks both beta$_1$- and beta$_2$-adrenergic receptors, reduces intraocular pressure for 12 to 24 hours.

Timolol is still being investigated and is not clinically available in the United States. Instillation of a 0.1% to 0.5% solution lowers intraocular pressure in open-angle glaucoma for 12 to 24 hours. The effect is enhanced by epinephrine. There is no increase in outflow, and its action is presumably by reduction of the secretion of aqueous humor. Its action is perplexing inasmuch as both beta receptor stimulation and blockade reduce intraocular pressure.

Practolol, a beta blocker used in the treatment of vascular hypertension, causes a disorder comparable to the oculomucocutaneous syndrome (p. 568), a complication not seen with other compounds in this group.

Interference with catecholamine storage. Several compounds interfere with the storage of catecholamines in the synaptic cytoplasmic vesicles. Generally these compounds cause an initial release of stored norepinephrine and thereafter diminish the amounts of norepinephrine available for endogenous release into the tissues.

Reserpine. Reserpine is one of the alkaloids of *Rauwolfia serpentina*. It causes the release and inhibits the binding of norepinephrine in synaptic vesicles and thus mimics the systemic effects of a sympathectomy. The tranquilizing effects are the result of a similar effect on serotonin binding. It causes a slight decrease in intraocular pressure, but the mechanism is unknown.

Guanethidine. Guanethidine (Ismelin) causes an initial depletion of norepinephrine in the nerve fiber, blocks its neuronal release, and blocks the reuptake of catecholamines by the axon. Additionally, it sensitizes adrenergic receptor sites. After depletion of the catecholamines, denervation hypersensitivity occurs. Local instillation of a combination of 0.5% guanethidine and 1% epinephrine is used to treat open-angle glaucoma in young patients, with the guanethidine potentiating the pharmacologic effects of epinephrine.

Denervation hypersensitivity

When a structure innervated by postganglionic autonomic nerves loses its nerve supply, a marked decrease occurs in either cholinesterase or catechol-O-methyl transferase at the synaptic junction. The denervated structure is therefore far more sensitive to exogenous neurohumoral transmitter than when it is normally innervated. Thus in the Adie pupil (p. 285), an abnormality that likely involves the ciliary ganglion or postganglionic cholinergic nerves, the pupil is constricted by the instillation of 0.1% pilocarpine, which does not affect the normal sphincter pupillae muscle—it normally constricts only with instillation of a 1% concentration.

6-Hydroxydopamine causes a reversible destruction of sympathetic nerve terminals. Anterior segment chemical sympathectomy with 6-hydroxydopamine potentiates the effect of epinephrine in the treatment of open-angle glaucoma. If there is interference with the sympathetic pathway between the superior cervical ganglion and the dilatator pupillae muscle, as occurs in Horner syndrome (p. 285), the pupil dilates on instillation of 0.1% epinephrine. There is no effect on the normally innervated pupil.

PROSTAGLANDINS

Prostaglandins form a family of compounds that are structurally related, cyclic, oxygenated, unsaturated 20-carbon fatty acids, divided into primary E and F types and secondary A, B, and C types derived from the E type. A sequential group of reactions grouped as prostaglandin synthetase catalyze their formation, which is blocked by aspirin. Prostaglandins are essential for normal fertility. They inhibit the enzyme adenyl cyclase, decrease gastric secretion, are potent vasodilators, increase capillary permeability, and stimulate the adrenal cortex, the thyroid gland, and the islets of Langerhans.

Release of aqueous humor from the eye (keratocentesis), stroking the iris, or trauma to the eye causes synthesis of prostaglandin E within the eye. There is a breakdown of the blood-aqueous barrier that results in an increase in protein in the aqueous humor, ciliary injection, and miosis. Prostaglandin E tends to inhibit release of norepinephrine and depress adrenergic receptors, but prostaglandin F has opposite effects. Prostaglandins also act as neurohumoral transmitters.

9$^\Delta$-TETRAHYDROCANNABINOL

Marijuana smoking reduces intraocular pressure in humans as does oral or intravenous administration of 9$^\Delta$-tetrahydrocannabinol, its active principle. Additionally, smoking marijuana dilates conjunctival blood vessels and decreases tearing and the rate of blinking. Recent synthetic compounds lower ocular pressure without the tachycardia, hypotension, and euphoric effects of marijuana. After oral or topical administration intraocular pressure is reduced about one third. The mode of action is unknown but may involve beta-receptor blockade with decreased ciliary body secretion or inhibition of prostaglandin synthetase with increased effectivity of norepinephrine. Clinical experiments in humans indicate the action to be in the secretory phase of ocular pressure rather than the outflow phase.

CARBONIC ANHYDRASE INHIBITORS

Carbonic anhydrase is an enzyme that catalyzes the equilibrium between carbonic acid and carbon dioxide. The enzyme is widely distributed in (1) erythrocytes, where it functions in the exchange of carbon dioxide in capillaries; (2) the renal tubule cell, where it functions in the exchange of intracellular hydrogen for tubular sodium; (3) the epithelium of the ciliary body, where it functions in the secretion of aqueous humor; (4) the choroid plexus, where it functions in the secretion of cerebrospinal fluid; and (5) the gastric mucosa and the pancreas.

Inhibitors of carbonic anhydrase were synthesized after it was observed that the systemic administration of sulfonamides caused an acidosis because of loss of sodium bicarbonate to the urine and failure of the exchange of cellular hydrogen for tubular sodium. Despite the widespread distribution of carbonic anhydrase in the tissues of the body, the effects of enzyme inhibition are largely renal. With some of the agents, however, there is decreased secretion of aqueous humor and cerebrospinal fluid. Decreased secretion of aqueous humor occurs even in the absence of renal effects and is apparently the result of interference with secretory activity of the ciliary body in an unknown manner.

Effective drugs in this group reduce the secretion of aqueous humor from 50% to 60%. There is a concomitant reduction in intraocular pressure. The most commonly used agent is acetazolamide (Diamox). Because of side effects, a number of other compounds have been substituted for acetazolamide.

Acetazolamide. Acetazolamide (Diamox) is the most widely used carbonic anhydrase inhibitor in ophthalmology. In patients with open-angle glaucoma the usual dosage is either 125 or 250 mg orally every 6 hours (not four times daily) or 250 or 500 mg every 12 hours in sustained-release tablets. The ocular effect is observed 1 to 2 hours after oral administration, and the maximum effect persists for 3 to 5 hours. It may be used intrave-

nously in patients with angle-closure glaucoma. The secretion of aqueous humor is reduced but never stopped, and it is evident that only mechanisms of secretory activity involving carbonic anhydrase are concerned (p. 86). A variety of side effects may occur. Myopia (p. 434), aplastic anemia, exfoliative dermatitis, and other reactions observed with sulfonamide derivatives occur rarely. Paresthesia, with numbness and tingling in the extremities, and anorexia are common. There is a slight tendency to renal lithiasis, gout, blood dyscrasias, and depression; confusion may occur in the elderly. Side effects may necessitate the substitution of another carbonic anhydrase inhibitor.

Ethoxzolamide (Cardrase), dichlorphenamide (Daranide), and methazolamide (Neptazane) are carbonic anhydrase inhibitors that may be substituted for acetazolamide. Their side effects are similar to those caused by acetazolamide, but occasionally one may be substituted to provide equal tension-lowering effects and less patient discomfort.

OSMOTIC AGENTS

If the osmotic pressure of the blood is increased, fluid is drawn from the vitreous body, and the intraocular pressure is decreased. The increased osmotic pressure of the blood is usually maintained for only a short time, and within 4 to 6 hours the intraocular pressure returns to its previous level. The osmotic pressure of the blood is increased in ophthalmic practice when it is desirable to decrease the intraocular pressure and volume for a relatively short period, as in the following: (1) in angle-closure glaucoma to reduce the intraocular pressure so the sphincter pupillae muscle will respond to miotics, (2) immediately before surgery to reduce intraocular pressure, (3) in retinal detachment surgery to reduce intraocular volume to aid in scleral wound closure, and (4) in orbital surgery to reduce orbital volume.

Mannitol. Mannitol is the alcohol of the sugar mannose and is pharmacologically inert. It is excreted by filtration through the renal glomeruli and is minimally reabsorbed by the tubules. It induces marked systemic dehydration. Mannitol is administered intravenously in a 20% solution in a dose of 1.0 to 2.0 gm/kg of body weight. Use before surgery usually requires urethral catheterization because of diuresis. The maximum fall in intraocular pressure occurs within 1 hour, and it returns to pretreatment levels after about 4 hours. The acute expansion of extracellular fluid volume may cause cardiac decompensation in vulnerable persons. Hypersensitivity rarely occurs. Reduction of intracranial pressure may cause headache.

Glycerol. Glycerol is a trivalent alcohol that contributes to glyceride and phosphatide molecules. It is metabolized to carbon dioxide and water by the tricarboxylic acid cycle. (Insulin is not required in its metabolism.) In oral administration of a 50% solution in lemon juice in doses of 1.0 to 1.5 gm/kg of body weight, it decreases intraocular pressure within 30 to 60 minutes; pretreatment levels return within 4 to 5 hours.

Side effects are few. Usually headache does not occur, and diuresis is not marked. Nausea and vomiting may prevent its long-term use.

Topical glycerol does not reduce intraocular pressure but is used to reduce corneal edema in glaucoma to make gonioscopy possible.

Isosorbide. Isosorbide (Hydronol) is a dihydric alcohol formed by the removal of two molecules of water from glucitol (sorbitol). It is given orally in a 50% ginger-flavored solution. In a dosage of 1 to 2 gm/kg of body weight, the intraocular pressure reaches a minimal value 1 to 2 hours after administration and remains

depressed for 5 to 6 hours. Side effects are uncommon, but the drug has not been thoroughly studied.

Miscellaneous agents. Ascorbate, ethanol, and sucrose produce an osmotic vitreous-blood gradient with reduction of intraocular pressure. Additionally, alcohol inhibits the antidiuretic hormone and induces diuresis. Ingestion of large amounts of ethanol 8 to 12 hours before examination may produce abnormally low tonometric values in glaucoma patients.

DYES

Fluorescein and rose bengal are used to stain breaks in the continuity of the epithelium of the cornea or conjunctiva and for a variety of diagnostic tests. Sodium fluorescein is used in 2% alkaline solution. Because of the possibility of contamination with *Pseudomonas aeruginosa*, it should be instilled either from a single-dose container or by means of a strip of sterile filter paper saturated with dye. The dye is instilled in the conjunctival sac, and after 1 minute the excess dye is washed away. The corneal stroma stains bright green in areas of diseased or absent corneal epithelium. Foreign bodies embedded in the cornea are surrounded by a bright green ring. The intensity of staining is accentuated if 2% cocaine ophthalmic solution is instilled in the eye or if the eye is illuminated with a cobalt blue filter to stimulate fluorescence.

Fluorescein is also instilled in the eye to demonstrate the dilution that occurs when anterior aqueous humor escapes from a postoperative fistula, a penetrating wound, or a conjunctival bleb following glaucoma filtration surgery. It is used to demonstrate areas of contact ("touch") between the lens and the cornea or sclera in the fitting of contact lenses. Applanation tonometry is based on the appearance of the fluorescein pattern when pressure is applied to the eye. The rate of disappearance of fluorescein through the nasolacrimal passages is used to estimate their patency (p. 234).

Intravenous sodium fluorescein is combined with serial fundus photography to study the dynamics of the retinal circulation (p. 177). Two to 5 ml of a 10% to 25% solution is injected rapidly into the brachial vein, and fundus photographs are taken. Nausea may occur with the injection. Fluorescein is excreted in the urine for the following 24 to 48 hours (and prevents testing of urine for sugar). Allergic reactions vary in severity from urticaria to a shocklike state. Coma, cardiac arrest, and myocardial infarction have been reported. The drug should not be used in individuals with a history of drug sensitivity. When angiography is performed, an emergency tray and oxygen should be readily available. Administration of the fluorescein through a small indwelling catheter permits the administration of drugs in the event a severe reaction should develop.

Intravenous administration is followed by the appearance of fluorescein in the aqueous humor, a method of measuring aqueous flow. Similarly, if fluorescein is allowed to remain in contact with the surface of the globe, it enters the anterior chamber, and its disappearance rate can be used to gauge the outflow of aqueous humor.

Rose bengal (1%) stains devitalized cells better than fluorescein, which has an affinity for the corneal stroma. Rose bengal's principal application is demarcation of devitalized conjunctival epithelium in keratoconjunctivitis sicca (p. 268).

Both fluorescein and rose bengal stain soft contact lenses, which must be removed before instillation of the drugs.

LOCAL ANESTHETICS

The small size of the eye and the accessibility of its nerve supply make possible most adult ocular surgery with local anesthesia. The conjunctiva and cornea are readily anesthetized by means of topically instilled agents, of which cocaine, the prototype, has been succeeded by tetracaine (Pontocaine, 0.5%), benoxinate (Dorsacaine, 0.4%), and proparacaine (Ophthaine, 0.5%). Infiltration or block anesthesia is readily achieved with skillfully administered procaine (Novocain) or lidocaine (Xylocaine).

Topical anesthetics are used for procedures such as tonometry or removal of corneal foreign bodies. The severe pain of corneal abrasions, ultraviolet keratitis, and corneal foreign bodies is quickly relieved. Inasmuch as these agents are potent sensitizers that delay corneal epithelization, they should not be prescribed for analgesia.

Infiltration anesthesia is used mainly in the region of the eyelids for the excision of local lesions. Simultaneous motor and sensory block is obtained by injecting the anesthetic agent in the region of the orbital portion of the orbicularis oculi muscle (van Lint technique) to prevent eyelid closure in intraocular surgery.

Blockade of the eyelid musculature is provided by infiltrating fibers of the temporal branch of the seventh nerve as they pass anterior to the temporomandibular articulation (O'Brien technique). Blockade of the motor nerve supply to the extraocular muscles and sensory block of the nerve supply to the globe are obtained by retrobulbar injection of anesthetic solution posterior to the globe in the region between the lateral rectus muscle and optic nerve. This blocks the nerve supply to all of the extraocular muscles except the superior oblique muscle; it blocks the ciliary ganglion so the pupil dilates; and it anesthetizes the entire globe. Other sensory blocks follow injections of anesthetic agents in the region of the supra- and infratrochlear nerves at the superior medial angle of the orbit; the infraorbital nerve, either in its orbital course or as it emerges through the infraorbital foramen to the face; and the lacrimal and zygomaticofacial nerves as they exit from their respective foramina.

Epinephrine (1:100,000) prolongs anesthesia by inducing vasospasm in the injected area with slower absorption. It is contraindicated in patients with coronary artery disease or thyrotoxicosis and in halothane anesthesia.

ANTI-INFECTIVE AGENTS

Several factors modify the use of anti-infective agents in ocular infections. Frequent local instillations of antibiotics or sulfonamides provide unusually high concentrations in the superficial tissue. Compounds that have severe adverse effects when administered systemically often may be useful when instilled locally. Heavy metals such as zinc sulfate are still used in astringent eye drops, and silver nitrate is not surpassed by any other agent in the prophylaxis of gonorrheal ophthalmia. To prevent intraocular infection, some ophthalmic surgeons inject an antibiotic subconjunctivally at the end of an intraocular surgical procedure. However, some nonmicrobial ocular inflammations mimic infections, and anti-infective agents are sometimes erroneously prescribed. Similarly, the difficulty in distinguishing microbial inflammation from other inflammations has led to the widespread use of topical preparations containing a combination of an anti-infective agent and a corticosteroid.

Many compounds instilled in the conjunctival sac cause either an allergic or irritative contact dermatoconjunctivitis. Prolonged use of antibiotics (particularly tetracyclines) combined with corticosteroids predisposes to superinfection, particularly with fungi. A fungal invader must be considered in any persistent conjunctival or corneal inflammation. Local anti-infective agents are diluted rapidly by tears, and they must be instilled at 1- or 2-hour intervals to assure adequate local tissue concentration.

The blood-aqueous barrier limits the penetration of many anti-infective agents into the ocular fluids from the systemic circulation. However, intraocular inflammation impairs the blood-aqueous barrier, so adequate concentrations follow systemic administration of drugs that do not ordinarily enter the eye. Injection of the anti-infective agent into the subconjunctival space, sub-Tenon space, or retrobulbarly is generally limited to those instances in which high local concentration is required. Intraocular injection of antibiotics is limited to disastrous infections in which the damage that may be caused by the agent is balanced by the destructiveness of the disease.

Sulfisoxazole and sulfacetamide are the most useful sulfonamides for topical therapy. These two agents rarely cause local hypersensitivity. As with other sulfonamides, their action is inhibited by pus. The penicillins, cephalosporins, and streptomycin cause hypersensitivity reactions so frequently that topical application is contraindicated. Chloramphenicol is useful, and topical instillation does not cause aplastic anemia in susceptible individuals. Neomycin, bacitracin, and polymyxin B are widely used topically, particularly in combination (Neosporin). Gentamicin is effective.

The sulfonamides are useful in trachoma and inclusion conjunctivitis. They are used as an adjunct to pyrimethamine in systemic toxoplasmosis.

Endophthalmitis after intraocular surgery causes such rapid destruction of the eye that ophthalmic surgeons use antibiotics prophylactically. Preoperatively, gentamicin, Neosporin, or erythromycin are often used topically to reduce the bacterial content of the conjunctiva. Gentamicin, carbenicillin, chloramphenicol, or aqueous penicillin combined with streptomycin are injected subconjunctively at the time of surgery so that the aqueous humor of secondary formation will contain a high concentration of antibiotics. Alternatively, an antibiotic such as ampicillin may be administered before surgery so that it enters the eye in a high concentration as the blood-aqueous barrier is damaged by the opening of the anterior chamber.

To be effectively managed, intraocular infection necessitates prompt diagnosis and therapy. Subconjunctival and systemic therapy is used. Until the causative organism(s) is identified, the most efficacious agents appear to be carbenicillin, cephalexin, lincomycin, gentamicin, and chloramphenicol.

Antibiotics

Antibiotics are compounds produced by some microorganisms or prepared synthetically that inhibit the growth (bacteriostatic) or destroy (bactericidal) microorganisms in dilute solution. They are effective through one of several mechanisms. They may (1) inhibit biosynthesis of the cell wall (penicillins, cephalosporins, bacitracin, vancomycin, cycloserine, and ristocetin), (2) inhibit protein synthesis (tetracyclines, chloramphenicol, erythromycin, streptomycin, and lincomycin), or (3) alter cell wall permeability (polymyxin B, colistin, amphotericin B). Some antibiotics have more than one action, and it is not possible to tell which of the actions is more important.

The use of antibiotics is complicated by bacterial resistance, hypersensitivity reactions, toxicity, alteration of normal microorganismal flora, peripheral neuritis, and hematologic complications. Staphylococcic penicillinase destroys the antibiotic. The beta-lactamases of many gram-negative bacteria inactivate the penicillins. In some instances spontaneous mutations give rise to enzymatic changes that permit microbial resistance. Many gram-negative bacteria contain a resistance transfer factor that may transmit resistance to other bacteria.

Cutaneous hypersensitivity varies in severity from contact dermatitis (especially with penicillin and streptomycin) to purpura erythema multiforme and exfoliative dermatitis. Systemic hypersensitivity may be manifested by fever, serum sickness, and (rarely) anaphylactic shock (mainly with penicillin).

Renal toxicity may be produced by a variety of antibiotics (cephaloridine, neomycin, polymyxin B, colistin, gentamicin, kanamycin, vancomycin, and amphotericin). Eighth nerve damage has occurred after administration of streptomycin, and auditory damage may follow administration of vancomycin, kanamycin, neomycin, and gentamicin. Renal impairment with decreased excretion may cause exceptionally high levels of these agents in the blood.

Alteration of normal bacterial flora is particularly common after the use of tetracyclines. Topical instillation combined with corticosteroids is a frequent factor in superinfection of the cornea with fungi (p. 264). Systemic administration may be associated with overgrowth of *Candida albicans* in the mouth, pharynx, and bowel, and there may be tetracycline-resistant *Proteus, Pseudomonas,* and *Staphylococcus* organisms in the bowel. Tetracyclines may stain developing teeth and are contraindicated before emergence of second dentition.

Failures with the use of antimicrobial agents arise from (1) use in conditions not caused by microorganisms; (2) failure to identify causative organism and to use appropriate antimicrobial agent in proper dosage; (3) use in conditions caused by organisms not susceptible to agents; (4) continued use after bacterial resistance has developed, toxic or allergic reactions have developed, or superinfection has occurred; and (5) use of improper combinations.

Penicillins. Penicillins may be divided into those prepared by fermentation and those synthesized by conjugation of various side chains to 6-amino-penicillinic acid obtained from penicillin fermentation media. They impair bacterial cell wall synthesis in those organisms accessible to the penicillin agent. Their use is governed by three main disadvantages: (1) degradation by gastric acid so that some cannot be used orally, (2) destruction by the enzyme penicillinase, and (3) relatively high incidence of hypersensitivity reactions. One group of the semisynthetic penicillins (methicillin, oxacillin, nafcillin, cloxacillin) resists the action of penicillinase and is used mainly in the treatment of infections by penicillinase-producing staphylococci. Penicillins are actively transported out of the eye by the ciliary epithelium and do not cross the intact blood-aqueous or blood-retina barrier (p. 87).

All of the penicillins cause hypersensitivity reactions that may range in severity from urticaria to anaphylaxis to delayed hypersensitivity reactions. The penicillins are all cross-reactive, and a patient sensitive to one will be sensitive to other penicillins although not always to the same extent. Patients are more sensitive to the natural penicillins than to the semisynthetic derivatives.

Penicillin G is the penicillin of choice in the treatment of syphilis and infections caused by streptococci (including the pneumococci), meningococci, gonococci, anthrax, and actinomycetes. It is available in a crystalline form for intramuscular or intravenous use and in a repository form (procaine penicillin G or benzathine penicillin G). Penicillin V may be given orally.

The penicillinase-resistant penicillins available for parenteral use include methicillin, oxacillin, and nafcillin. Oxacillin and nafcillin are most active, but methicillin is less bound to serum protein so that more may be available to enter the eye. Methicillin may cause reversible bone marrow depression and interstitial nephritis. In severe systemic infection (such as orbital cellulitis caused by gram-positive cocci), a penicillinase-resistant penicillin should be used as initial therapy pending identification and susceptibility testing of the agent.

In hospitals where methicillin-resistant strains of *Staphylococcus aureus* are prevalent vancomycin may be substituted.

Ampicillin, amoxicillin, and carbenicillin are not penicillinase resistant but have increased activity against some gram-negative bacilli. They are more active than penicillin G against streptococci, *Neisseria*, and clostridia. Additionally, they are active against several gram-negative species, such as *Escherichia*, *Haemophilus influenzae*, and *Proteus*. Most strains of *Klebsiella* and all strains of *Pseudomonas* are resistant to ampicillin and amoxicillin. Carbenicillin has an antibacterial range similar to that of ampicillin with an important added activity against some strains of *Pseudomonas aeruginosa*. Gentamicin, which is also used in *Pseudomonas* infections, should never be mixed in the same bottle with carbenicillin, which inactivates aminoglycosides.

A history of adverse reactions to penicillin in the past may be more important than the results of various tests to anticipate allergic reactions. Skin testing may be hazardous, but test material is available to learn if immediate-type allergy is present. If the results are positive, penicillin should be used with great caution, if at all. Additionally, there may be cross allergy to the penicillins and the cephalosporins.

Cephalosporins. Cephalothin (Keflin), cephapirin (Cefadyl), cefazolin (Ancef,

Kefazol), and cephaloridine (Loridine) are bactericidal against many gram-positive cocci, including penicillinase-producing staphylococci and some gram-negative rods. They are often drugs of choice in patients sensitive to penicillin, although they too may cause sensitive reactions. Cephalothin may cause a positive Coombs test for erythrocyte antibodies. Cephaloridine may cause renal damage.

Aminoglycosides. This group of drugs includes streptomycin, neomycin, kanamycin (Kantrex), gentamicin, tobramycin, amikacin, and paromomycin. These differ widely in clinical effectiveness, but all may cause auditory (VIII) nerve and renal damage.

Neomycin. Neomycin is bactericidal against staphylococci and gram-negative bacteria excluding *Pseudomonas* species. It is widely used topically in ophthalmology, often combined with polymyxin B. Localized hypersensitivity occurs frequently but may be masked by corticosteroid given concurrently.

Gentamicin. Gentamicin is bactericidal for *Pseudomonas*, *Proteus*, and other gram-negative bacteria as well as for *Staphylococcus*. It is effective against bacteria resistant to other aminoglycoside antibiotics such as neomycin. It is commonly used as a topical agent in ophthalmology.

Tetracyclines. Tetracycline (Achromycin) and the substituted tetracyclines, including chlortetracycline (Aureomycin), oxytetracycline (Terramycin), demeclocyline (Declomycin), and minocycline (Minocin), are essentially bacteriostatic and inhibit a broad range of gram-positive and gram-negative bacteria in addition to *Mycobacterium tuberculosis*, *Rickettsia*, *Chlamydia*, and the agent (Eaton) of primary atypical pneumonia, *Mycoplasma pneumoniae*. The compounds penetrate the intact blood-aqueous barrier poorly. Resistant strains develop during therapy. After suppression of susceptible micro-flora, the superimposition of resistant strains has developed.

Tetracyclines are usually administered orally and may give rise to nausea, vomiting, and diarrhea. Outdated tetracycline may cause reversible tubular dysfunction indistinguishable from the Fanconi syndrome. Discoloration of developing teeth and fatal hepatic necrosis in pregnant women have been reported. Demeclocycline causes photosensitivity in some individuals. A number of tetracyclines are available for local use. The compounds have a low antigenicity, and sensitivity reactions are uncommon.

Polypeptides. This group includes bacitracin, polymyxin B, and colistin (polymyxin E). Bacitracin has an antibacterial spectrum similar to penicillin but rarely causes hypersensitivity reactions. It is usually combined with neomycin and polymyxin B for topical instillation. Pending identification of the organism, bacitracin is often the agent of choice for topical application in gram-positive cocci infections. Polymyxin B and colistin are active against gram-negative organisms and are particularly useful in *Pseudomonas* infections. Polymyxin B and colistin are nephrotoxic and are rarely used systemically. Generally their use has been superseded by gentamicin and carbenicillin.

Chloramphenicol. Chloramphenicol (Cloromycetin) is a potent inhibitor of microbial protein synthesis by blocking the polypeptide linkage and messenger RNA–ribosome complex. It is used primarily for anaerobic infections, *Haemophilus influenzae* meningitis, and infections caused by *Salmonella typhi*. It is rapidly and completely absorbed from the gastrointestinal tract and is not impaired by simultaneous administration of food or antacids. It penetrates well into all tissues, including the brain, cerebrospinal fluid, and aqueous humor. High intraocular concentrations follow systemic use. Its most important toxic effect is bone marrow suppression, which occurs either in a dose-related form or as an idiosyncratic reaction. Severe granulocytopenia is rare if treatment with the drug is discontinued when the white blood cell count decreases to less than 4,000/cu mm. Retrobulbar neuritis (p. 367) and peripheral neuritis may occur in patients with cystic fibrosis who receive systemic chloramphenicol for more than 12 weeks.

Chloramphenicol is used widely for topical administration in ocular infections. The likelihood of inducing an idiosyncratic aplastic anemia by this route is remote. Chloramphenicol is particularly useful in the initial treatment of endophthalmitis before identification of the causative organism.

Erythromycin. Erythromycin is effective against gram-positive microorganisms and is well tolerated. It is used particularly in patients who are allergic to the penicillins. The drug is often used in topical preparations in ophthalmology.

Lincomycin. Lincomycin (Lincocin) is effective against gram-positive bacteria, including penicillinase-producing strains of *Staphylococcus*. It is primarily bacteriostatic but may be bactericidal in a dosage range up to 30 times that required to produce bacteriostasis. It may be administered orally, intravenously, and intramuscularly. High intraocular levels are obtained. Diarrhea is the major toxic manifestation of oral administration.

Vancomycin. Vancomycin is effective against gram-positive bacteria. It is used intravenously in severe staphylococcal infections and endocarditis when the causative agent is resistant to the usual antibiotics. It is locally irritating and causes thrombophlebitis and (in large doses) eighth nerve disease.

Sulfonamides

The sulfonamides are bacteriostatic agents that prevent susceptible microorganisms from synthesizing folic acid from para-aminobenzoic acid by substrate competition. Sulfonamides have a limited usefulness in ophthalmology as topical agents and are used systemically in the management of chlamydial infections (p. 221) and as an adjunct of pyrimethamine in systemic toxoplasmosis (p. 468). When resistance develops to one sulfonamide, then cross-resistance to all derivatives is observed. Similarly, cross-sensitivity occurs, and therefore no sulfonamide is safe once a patient demonstrates a hypersensitivity reaction to any derivative.

Most sulfonamides are fairly insoluble, and therapeutic concentrations are not obtained with most compounds when used locally. Two compounds are used locally in ophthalmology: sulfacetamide (Sulamyd) and sulfisoxazole (Gantrisin).

Sulfacetamide. Sulfacetamide (Sulamyd) is used in 10% and 30% solutions and 10% ointment. It is probably the most useful of the sulfonamide compounds for local use. It is minimally antigenetic, and hypersensitivity reactions are rarely observed.

Sulfisoxazole. Sulfisoxazole (Gantrisin) is used locally in a 4% solution. A white precipitate of the drug may gather at the canthus. Other sulfonamides should not be used for local therapy.

Corticosteroid combinations

A variety of antibiotics and sulfonamides for topical use have been combined with corticosteroids for the treatment of conjunctival and eyelid inflammations. Such a combination should provide greater therapeutic effects and safety than either component alone. The FDA advisory panel on ophthalmic preparations accepted antibiotic-corticosteroid preparations for the treatment of (1) mixed staphylococcal marginal blepharitis, (2) blepharoconjunctivitis with primary or secondary replicating organisms, (3) marginal corneal ulcers related to staphylococcal infection, and (4) post-surgical trauma.

For the most part, such combinations are not indicated. The corticosteroids reduce local tissue immunity, induce increased resistance to the outflow of aqueous, and may lead to the development of glaucoma in susceptible eyes. The combination of a corticosteroid and an antibiotic may facilitiate the development of a fungal keratoconjunctivitis. Fixed combinations do not permit the administration of the two drugs in different concentrations or at different time intervals. The effects of the antibiotic on the microorganism may also be obscured by the anti-inflammatory action of the corticosteroid.

Oculomycosis chemotherapy

The available antifungal drugs reach fungistatic but rarely fungicidal levels in the tissue. Thus the objective of antifungal treatment is to inhibit fungal growth over a long period until the individual's immune mechanism excludes the fungus. Often chemotherapy is combined with removal of the infected tissue by vitrectomy or keratoplasty. Diabetes and alcoholism must be carefully controlled.

Three groups of agents are used in antifungal therapy: (1) polyenes (amphotericin B, nystatin, natamycin [pimaricin]); (2) imidazoles (clotrimazole, miconazole, econazole, and thiabendazole); and (3) flucytosine. Not all compounds are clinically available in the United States.

Amphotericin B. Amphotericin B inhibits a wide variety of fungi as well as protozoa, flatworms, snails, and higher algae, but not bacteria. The drug is administered intravenously and causes mild renal damage in total doses between 5 and 10 gm and severe damage in total doses of more than 10 gm. If the blood urea nitrogen level exceeds 40 mg/100 ml, the drug should be discontinued until the level falls to normal. It has been used lo-cally in concentrations of 2.5 to 10 mg/ml in 5% glucose solution.

Nystatin. Nystatin is administered topically in a concentration of 100,000 units/ml of commercial diluent in demonstrated fungus infections of the anterior ocular segment. Its main value is in the treatment of superficial *Candida* infection, and it is ineffective in cutaneous dermatophyte infections. It is not absorbed from the gastrointestinal tract, and its toxicity is such that it cannot be used intravenously. It is insoluble in saline solution and is administered as a suspension.

Natamycin (pimaricin). This drug is used topically as a 5% suspension in propylene glycol or as an ointment. It has a fairly broad spectrum and is more useful in superficial fungus infections than the topical agents previously described. Systemically it may be administered orally in doses of 400 mg daily. Doses in excess of this cause diarrhea and vomiting.

Clotrimazole, miconazole, and econazole. These agents are used systemically and locally. Clotrimazole is as effective as the polyenes but activates inhibitory enzymes in the liver after one or two weeks' administration. In Great Britain, a 1% ointment is used topically for prophylaxis in injuries and for initial treatment of *Aspergillus* and *Candida* species infections. It is not effective against *Fusarium* species. Miconazole and econazole do not induce inactivation by liver enzymes but are irritating when applied topically.

Flucytosine. Flucytosine (5-fluorocytosine) is a pyrimidine active against *Candida* and *Cryptococcus* species. It is used experimentally in a 1% solution.

Other agents. Actinomycetes are bacteria, and infections caused by them respond to the penicillins and sulfonamides. Nocardiosis is responsive to the sulfonamides and streptomycin. Potassium iodide is used in the therapy of sporotrichosis.

Virus chemotherapy

Chemotherapy of ocular virus infections is concerned mainly with keratitis caused by herpes simplex type 1. Only idoxuridine and vidarabine are commercially available in the United States.

Idoxuridine. Idoxuridine (IDU, 6-iodo-2-deoxyuridine) closely resembles thymidine and is incorporated into the viral DNA in place of thymidine. This gives rise to a DNA that is functionally deficient, which presumably will not form effective virus particles. Additionally, the altered DNA may cause a defective messenger RNA and may lead to the synthesis of enzymes incapable of producing viral DNA. The main usefulness of IDU in ophthalmology remains in its topical application for corneal herpes simplex. In disease limited to the epithelium, the drug is not superior to mechanical removal of the diseased epithelium, but with extension of the infection to the geographic type, IDU is markedly superior.

Vidarabine. Vidarabine (adenine arabinoside, AraA) is an antimetabolite with antiviral activity against a variety of DNA viruses, such as herpes simplex types 1 and 2, cytomegalic virus, varicella-zoster virus, and vaccinia virus, but little or none against RNA viruses. Generally, it is more potent than IDU and is active against IDU-resistant viruses. It appears to act by inhibiting DNA synthesis but does not prevent virus attachment to, or penetration into, the cell, nor does it act as a competitive inhibitor of nucleosides.

Trifluorothymidine. Trifluorothymidine (F_3T) resembles IDU but is incorporated far more extensively into viral DNA than into cellular DNA, allowing for selective antiviral activity. F_3T is significantly superior to IDU in the therapy for herpetic corneal ulcers. It has less toxicity, greater potency, and greater effectiveness against IDU-resistant strains of the virus.

Interferon. Interferon is a nontoxic species-specific protein with broad action mainly against RNA viruses and less extensively against DNA viruses, such as herpes simplex. It inhibits virus replication (p. 458) through its action on the cells, not on the virus. Currently, interferon instilled topically into the conjunctival sac twice daily prevents recurrence of herpes infection individuals susceptible to inflammation.

Photodynamic inactivation. Photodynamic inactivation is a process in which certain dyes, such as neutral red and proflavine, are bound irreversibly to the herpesvirus, causing its inactivation when exposed to fluorescent light. However, the photodynamically inactive virus may retain enough genetic information to mutate into malignant cells, and this therapy is not recommended.

Heavy metals

Mercuric chloride is used locally, mainly in an ointment base. Nitromersol (Metaphen) is used in a 1:2,500 ointment in the conjunctival sac. Silver nitrate is used as a 1% solution in Credé's prophylaxis of ophthalmia neonatorum (p. 221). It precipitates protein, including that of bacteria, and reacts with the sodium chloride of tissues to form insoluble silver chloride. The silver proteinate salts have largely been abandoned in ophthalmic therapeutics. Zinc sulfate is specific for the diplobacillus of Morax-Axenfeld (p. 220), but antibiotics are superior for this purpose. Zinc sulfate is used as an astringent in many collyria and nonspecific eye preparations of nonspecific eye disabilities.

CORTICOSTEROIDS

The adrenal gland consists of the medulla and the cortex. The medulla secretes mostly epinephrine and possibly a small amount of norepinephrine. The adrenal cortex produces three types of steroids: (1) the androgenic steroids, which are concerned with the development of secondary sex characteristics; (2) the mineralocorticoids, mainly aldosterone and desoxycorticosterone, which are concerned with fluid and electrolyte metabolism; and (3) the glucocorticoids, mainly corticosterone and hydrocortisone, which act on the metabolism of carbohydrates, proteins, fats, electrolytes, and water. The glucocorticoids are strongly anti-inflammatory, inhibit the manifestation of cell-mediated immunity in humans, and stabilize lysosomal enzymes.

Corticosteroids are mainly effective in suppressing the manifestations of inflammation without affecting the cause of inflammation. Thus the drugs are most useful in self-limited or intermittent disease processes by permitting the decrease of acute inflammatory disease until remission occurs. Relatively high doses and long-term administration may be required to suppress inflammation. Long-term systemic administration is associated with numerous side effects that limit their usefulness. Ocular complications may be seen following topical, retrobulbar, or systemic administration of the compounds.

The most common ocular complication of topical administration is secondary open-angle glaucoma (p. 399), which may cause severe loss of vision combined with typical excavation of the optic disk and visual field defects. Posterior subcapsular cataracts may occur after topical administration, but they are more common in patients with connective tissue disorders who receive high doses of corticosteroids for a long period. Patients with rheumatoid arthritis are particularly prone to cataract formation. Cataracts rarely occur in patients with ulcerative colitis or asthma who receive similar doses. Retrobulbar administration of corticosteroids may cause a disastrous progression of toxoplasmosis retinochoroiditis after initial improvement. This course

is not seen in individuals who receive concomitant sulfadiazine and pyrimethamine therapy alone or in those who receive systemic corticosteroids rather than retrobulbar corticosteroids.

Local tissue immunity confines most herpes simplex inflammation of the cornea (p. 261) to the corneal epithelium. Topical corticosteroids reduce local tissue immunity, and the virus infects additional epithelium and may cause stromal necrosis. The anti-inflammatory effect of the corticosteroids is such that the eye is less injected and more comfortable. Unwittingly the patient may use excessive amounts of corticosteroid, and this results in eventual rupture of the cornea.

Fungus infections were a rarity until the widespread use of topical corticosteroids combined with antibiotics. A mycotic infection must be suspected in any corneal ulceration that persists after long-term treatment with these compounds.

Topical instillation of corticosteroids delays fibroblastic regeneration. Generally, the local tissue concentration is inadequate to interfere with wound healing after systemic administration. However, the abdominal striae seen in Cushing disease are evidence that systemic corticosteroids interfere with wound healing. Topical corticosteroids in small amounts after cataract extraction and corneal transplant do not appear to affect wound healing adversely. Topical corticosteroids may also cause a mild blepharoptosis and pupillary dilation.

Long-term systemic administration may suppress immunity to *Candida* species, toxoplasmosis, cytomegalic inclusion, and *Herpesvirus hominis*. These organisms may cause widespread intraocular inflammation, necrotizing angiitis, and loss of vision. Similar disorders after immunosuppression are seen in the course of Hodgkin disease, lymphatic leukemia, and tumor radiation therapy.

Considerable caution must be exercised in the treatment of ocular disorders with long-term corticosteroids. A maintenance dose of 200 mg or less of prednisone every other morning does not seem to have serious side effects.

In addition to those described, side effects associated with long-term corticosteroid administration include peptic ulcer, perforation of the stomach and intestine, gastrointestinal hemorrhage, osteoporosis, psychosis, nitrogen depletion, diabetes mellitus, myopathy, sodium retention with edema, vascular hypertension, potassium depletion, and avascular bone necrosis. Side effects also include gain in weight, fat distribution of the Cushingoid type, acne, hirsutism, amenorrhea, cutaneous striae, and increased tendency to bruise. Retinal microaneurysms as well as papilledema have been described.

Corticosteroids may intensify a vasculitis, and withdrawal may be associated with a nonspecific conjunctivitis. Despite these contraindications, the corticosteroids remain a most useful group of drugs.

CHELATING AGENTS

Chelating agents form complexes with heavy metals and reverse their binding to body tissues. Those of ophthalmic interest include edathamil, deferoxamine, and penicillamine.

Edathamil (ethylenediaminetetraacetate [EDTA]). The calcium in band keratopathy (p. 256) or alkalis may be removed from the cornea by bathing in 0.01 mole sodium EDTA for 15 to 20 minutes. In band keratopathy the corneal epithelium must be removed initially, since EDTA does not penetrate it.

Deferoxamine. Deferoxamine (desferrioxamine mesylate) is specific for iron and may remove corneal rust stains. It is applied topically in a 10% solution in methylcellulose. Deferoxamine is not effective in the removal of blood staining the cornea.

Penicillamine. Penicillamine is a chelating agent for copper, mercury, zinc, and lead and promotes their excretion in the urine. It is well absorbed in the intestinal tract and is used in the treatment of hepaticolenticular degeneration (p. 488). In the course of such treatment, the pathognomonic Kayser-Fleischer ring of the cornea may disappear. Additionally, systemic penicillamine is of value in the therapy of scleromalacia perforans (p. 277).

COMPLICATIONS OF TOPICAL ADMINISTRATION OF DRUGS

A surprising number of ocular conditions are either induced, persistent, or aggravated because of overtreatment with drugs used locally. Inasmuch as many eye diseases are self-limiting, there is no indication for the local instillation of medication in the absence of exact diagnosis.

Mechanical injury. Patients and attendants instilling medications into the eye by means of an eyedropper or squeeze bottle should be instructed to place the long axis parallel to the eyelid margin so that if the patient lunges forward, he will not be struck by the side of the container. Patients should be reassured that the conjunctival sac holds but a single drop and the exact measurement of a single drop is not necessary because the excess medication overflows. However, because medications are costly, patients should be taught how to instill them effectively.

Pigmentation. Prolonged instillation of various compounds may cause pigmentation of the conjunctiva and the eyelids. Persistent instillation of silver preparations causes argyrosis. Metallic silver is deposited in the conjunctiva, particularly in the fornices, where it causes a slate-gray color. Microscopically, it arises from minute, closely packed dots of gray-black matter of metallic silver. There is no effective treatment.

Mercury preparations such as ammoniated mercury or yellow oxide of mercury may cause a similar type of pigmentation from mercury deposition if used for a long period.

Epinephrine used locally over a long period may cause a black pigmentation of the eyelid margins that looks like eye makeup. More common is a sharply defined, rounded black area of adrenochrome pigmentation arising from the oxidation of epinephrine to adrenochrome in the conjunctiva or cornea. There are no symptoms, and the deposits disappear after the medication is stopped.

Ocular injury. Many compounds may cause direct ocular injury on instillation. Silver nitrate in concentrations of more than 5% may cause necrosis of the cornea. To be assured of using only 1% silver nitrate in Credé's prophylaxis, one should use the wax ampules distributed for this purpose. Physicians who cauterize umbilical cords with silver nitrate find silver nitrate sticks safer to use than strong solutions.

A variety of compounds may cause minute epithelial defects of the cornea, which produce a foreign body sensation. Compounds that denature the protein of the corneal epithelium, such as ethanol and benzalkonium chloride (Zephiran), are common offenders. These may be brought to the eye on instruments used for minor ocular surgery. Local anesthetics are often dispensed in a stronger solution for use on nasal and oral mucous membranes rather than for the eye. Instillation of these stronger solutions may cause a white precipitate in the superficial corneal epithelium; the precipitate usually disappears when irrigated with distilled water.

Cocaine solutions are markedly hypotonic to the tears and cause desiccation of the corneal epithelium, which may then be removed easily. Cocaine is an excellent local anesthetic, and its use in surgery is sometimes desirable because it produces local vasoconstriction and moderate dilation of the pupil. Many believe

that the ease with which the corneal epithelium is removed following its use constitutes an overwhelming disadvantage.

Sensitivity reactions. Nearly any compound that is applied frequently to the eyelids and the conjunctiva causes a contact dermatitis and conjunctivitis. Repeated instillation of drugs such as pilocarpine, which is required in the treatment of glaucoma, may irritate the conjunctiva or cause a local hypersensitivity with many follicles evident in the lower eyelid.

Contact dermatitis of the skin characterized by an erythematous, desquamating, irritable lesion localized to the eyelid may be caused by a number of compounds. Adhesive tape, nail polish, and cosmetics are particular offenders. Previously, sulfonamides (particularly sulfathiazole), penicillin, and streptomycin were common offenders. Locally applied antihistamines may cause reactions that may be unrecognized inasmuch as the compounds have been prescribed for a preexisting reaction. Local anesthetics are also a common cause of dermatitis medicamentosa.

Delay of corneal epithelization. Small defects in the cornea heal by sliding of adjacent epithelium; large defects heal by mitosis and sliding of adjacent epithelium (p. 83). Many of the compounds used in ocular therapeutics delay mitosis but have no effect on epithelial sliding. Particular offenders are anesthetic solutions and ointments containing lanolin.

Pupillary constriction. Compounds causing miosis may give rise to a number of minor and major complaints. The extreme miosis produced by the organophosphates combined with edema of the ciliary body may cause angle-closure glaucoma in susceptible individuals (p. 404). Extreme miosis has been considered a cause of retinal detachment and traction of the zonular fibers that insert in the anterior retina.

Constriction of the pupil in patients

with minor lens opacities may cause a severe visual impairment that is not present when the pupil is of normal size. The reduction in vision presents a difficult problem in the management of glaucoma in patients with cataract and may necessitate a sector iridectomy, although the patient's glaucoma is adequately controlled with medication and the cataract is not sufficiently opaque to require surgery otherwise. In children in whom miotics are used in the treatment of accommodative strabismus, cysts may form at the pupillary margin involving the pigment epithelium. The use of phenylephrine immediately following the instillation of the miotic prevents the development of cysts. In young individuals, spasm of accommodation occurs with compounds that cause miosis and may give rise to a severe myopia.

Systemic reactions to local instillation. Atropine, pilocarpine, sympathetic amines, or cholinesterase inhibitors through the conjunctiva, the mucous membranes of the nose, or the lacrimal passages may give rise to characteristic systemic pharmacologic responses. Such reactions are more common with these drugs than with others inasmuch as 1 drop of the ophthalmic preparation (0.15 ml) may be comparable to, or exceed, the therapeutic systemic dose (Table 3-4).

Drugs should be prevented from entering the nasolacrimal duct by maintaining pressure over the inner corner of the closed eyelids for 2 minutes after instillation. Atropine and scopolamine are often administered either in an oily solution or in ointment to minimize systemic absorption. Even though this is done, systemic absorption from the conjunctiva and aqueous humor may cause toxicity.

Atropine poisoning develops quickly, and there is dryness and burning of the mouth and difficulty in talking and swallowing. There is also intense thirst. The pupils are dilated, and accommodation is paralyzed. The skin becomes flushed, hot, dry, and a high fever develops. Treatment is symptomatic—reduce the fever with ice packs or sponging and, if necessary, maintain respiration with a respirator.

Cyclopentolate hydrochloride (Cyclogyl) (p. 120) may cause a temporary psychosis in susceptible elderly patients.

Pilocarpine poisoning occurs commonly in the management of angle-closure glaucoma in which a high concentration of the drug is instilled frequently. Sweating and the flow of saliva are stimulated, and vomiting may occur. These are all effects commonly attributed to angle-closure glaucoma.

Anticholinesterase agents, particularly the organophosphates, significantly depress the erythrocyte cholinesterase levels. Systemic absorption may cause diarrhea, abdominal cramps, and the signs and symptoms of an acute abdominal or other gastrointestinal disturbance. On occasion, these signs have led to unnecessary laparotomy. Children receiving these compounds, particularly echothiophate iodide (Phospholine Iodide), may become irritable and cross; their be-

Table 3-4. Therapeutic dose of eye medications

	Dose	
	1 drop	**Therapeutic systemic dose**
1% atropine	0.75 mg	0.6 mg
4% pilocarpine	3.0 mg	5.0 mg
0.25% echothiophate iodide (Phospholine Iodide)	0.16 mg	Too toxic for systemic therapy
10% phenylephrine	7.5 mg	5.0 mg

havior problems result from chronic cholinesterase poisoning. Children with Down syndrome are particularly sensitive to echothiophate iodide. Patients using organophosphates should be advised to inform their other physicians of the drug they are using. The use of succinylcholine during general anesthesia in a cholinesterase-depleted individual may lead to dangerously prolonged apnea.

Instillation of 10% solutions of phenylephrine in elderly individuals may give rise to increased blood pressure, which sometimes causes a cerebrovascular accident and cardiac arrhythmias with extrasystole. There may be extreme sensitivity (of denervation) if the individual is receiving compounds causing adrenergic blockade. Generally, at the University of Chicago Hospitals 2.5% phenylephrine is the maximal concentration used in individuals more than 60 years old.

OCULAR REACTIONS TO SYSTEMIC ADMINISTRATION OF DRUGS

The eye may be involved in a variety of reactions following the systemic administration of drugs. Occasionally, ocular reactions do not occur in experimental animals, and severe eye lesions may be produced before the relationship between the eye abnormality and the drug is suspected.

Alcohol. In large doses, ethyl alcohol, a central nervous system depressant, causes an esophoria with an accompanying diplopia that the intoxicated individual may not recognize. The condition known as alcohol amblyopia is solely a nutritional deficiency with an accompanying optic neuropathy that causes reduced visual acuity with a central scotoma (p. 162). It arises because of reduced food intake and a lack of vitamins, particularly the B-complex group. In its early stages it may be corrected by an adequate diet and the administration of large doses of vitamin B, even though excessive use

of alcohol continues. Ethanol also decreases intraocular pressure, chiefly through systemic dehydration.

Methyl alcohol may cause fatal acidosis accompanied by abdominal pain, vomiting, and signs of severe intoxication. In patients who survive, severe primary optic atrophy and blindness may occur. The acidosis must be combated by the administration of bicarbonate. Ethyl alcohol in large doses competes successfully with methyl alcohol for metabolic sites and may prevent blindness.

Most central nervous system depressants may give rise to muscle weakness along with diplopia and, on occasion, blurred vision. In some instances these compounds aggravate preexisting ocular defects or cause nystagmus. The eye signs are usually reversible after reduced intake of the medication.

Chloroquine. Chloroquine is an antimalarial agent commonly used for the treatment of lupus erythematosus, arthritis, and other connective tissue disorders. Prolonged administration of high doses may give rise to a keratopathy, myopathy, or retinopathy. Generally, the total chloroquine dose must exceed 100 gm, and the drug must be used for more than a year before a retinopathy develops. The drug may be retained in the body for years after its use has been discontinued, and the retinopathy may develop several years later.

Chloroquine keratopathy is a reversible deposition of chloroquine in the cornea. Minute whitish dots distributed in a whorl pattern can be observed with the slit lamp. Patients complain of "glare," ill-defined blurring of vision, and iridescent vision, the halo surrounding lights being identical to that in glaucoma. The condition is entirely reversible on discontinuation of the drug, and it may disappear spontaneously even if the drug is continued.

Chloroquine retinopathy is a severe

pigmentary degeneration of the retina that may progress to blindness. Initially there is a minute degree of pigment clumping in the central retinal area. A characteristic "bull's eye" or "doughnut" retinal lesion develops that may be incomplete. This is followed by stippling or hyperpigmentation of the fovea centralis, surrounded by a clear zone of depigmentation, which in turn is circled by another ring of pigment. In the end stages there is widespread retinal atrophy, pigment clumping, and threadlike retinal vessels.

Quinine. Quinine in excessive doses has long been known to cause damage to the retinal ganglion cells and associated constriction of the retinal arterioles. Idiosyncratic reactions may follow administration of even minute amounts of quinine (as little as that contained in quinine water), and constriction of the visual field to a central area 5° to 10° in diameter may also occur. There may be associated deafness and other signs of central nervous system damage. Quinine is often mixed with heroin, and drug users may develop typical quinine poisoning. The abnormality is usually reversible, but continued ingestion of quinine may cause irreversible constriction of the visual fields, impaired dark adaptation, and loss of visual acuity.

In rare instances severe atrophy of the pigment epithelium of the iris may follow quinine amblyopia. The pupils do not react to light in the area of iris atrophy (p. 293). The condition is presumably caused by ischemia of the anterior uvea.

Ethambutol. Ethambutol is an oral chemotherapeutic agent widely used in therapy of pulmonary tuberculosis. The main ocular complication of long-term use is an optic neuritis that occurs in about 2% of those treated. Visual acuity should be measured before treatment is started and then monthly during the first months of treatment. Patients must be alerted to note any loss of vision. The optic neuritis

(p. 367) produces typical signs of reduced visual acuity and color vision and a central scotoma. More rarely, a peripheral neuritis causes peripheral visual field defects. The neuritis is reversible when the drug is discontinued, and vision improves over a period of weeks. After recovery, the use of the drug may be reinstituted without recurrence of the optic neuritis.

Digitalis. Digitalis toxicity may be associated with disturbed vision in which objects may appear to be covered with frost or having a pale yellow color or in which flashing lights may be present. Usually, visual symptoms are associated with nausea, vomiting, and bradycardia at high dosage levels, but they may occur in patients using the drug in a therapeutic range. A similar xanthopsia has been attributed to systemic effects of chlorothiazide and also to aspidium (male fern).

Oral contraceptives. The agents most commonly used for oral contraceptive therapy are progesterone and estrogen in combination or in sequence. These may cause occlusive vascular disease in susceptible patients. Women who smoke or who have vascular hypertension, migraine, or vascular disease are thought to be especially vulnerable. Brain infarction may be associated with ocular signs, depending on the area of the brain involved. Papilledema and optic neuritis (papillitis or retrobulbar neuritis) appear to occur more commonly in women using contraceptive therapy than in others. Retinal hemorrhages may be seen. The indications for using oral contraceptives must be carefully weighed. A patient should not receive them for long periods without medical supervision. They should be discontinued in the event of thromboembolic disease, neurologic disease, or suggestion of liver damage.

Some contact lens wearers develop an intolerance to the lenses while taking oral contraceptives. Often this is characterized by photophobia, increased irritation caused by the lenses, and prolonged recovery from corneal edema that may occur when wearing the lenses.

Induced refractive errors. Many compounds increase the refractivity of the eye through either a spasm of a ciliary muscle or increased refractive power of the lens. The sulfonamides and related compounds, particularly acetazolamide (Diamox), may increase the refractive power of the lens. All of the anticholinesterase compounds may cause ciliary spasm and miosis. Many insecticides are anticholinesterases, and spasm of accommodation combined with pupillary constriction has been described. Increased refractive power or sustained accommodation reduces hyperopia or increases myopia.

The ganglionic-blocking agents used in the treatment of vascular hypertension cause a decrease in accommodation that many patients in the younger age groups find extremely annoying. This may be associated with the dilation of the conjunctival blood vessels, giving the appearance of conjunctivitis. The loss of accommodation may have to be corrected by means of bifocal lenses. The conjunctival injection may be alleviated slightly by local instillation of a vasoconstrictor, such as 1:1,000 epinephrine.

Optic atrophy. Many compounds have been reported to cause optic atrophy. These include chloramphenicol, streptomycin, sulfonamides, and isoniazid. Tryparsamide, a pentavalent arsenical previously used in the therapy of central nervous system syphilis, has a direct toxic effect on the optic nerve.

Hypercarotenemia. Carotenoids are pigments, the molecule of which usually contains 40 carbon atoms. They are of ophthalmic interest because each molecule is composed of two molecules of vitamin A, which forms the visual pigments. Carotenoids contribute to the yellow-colored xanthomas and atheromas associated with hyperlipidemia. Excessive ingestion of plants containing carotenoids (2 or more quarts of carrot juice daily for 1½ years) may give rise to a yellow-orange pigmentation of the skin that starts in the nasolabial folds and palms of the hands and gradually spreads over the entire body. The conjunctiva is diffusely pigmented and has a yellowish color similar to that seen in jaundice.

Vitamin A. Prolonged high doses of vitamin A may give rise to a deposition of the vitamin A pigment (carotenosis) in the skin and in the conjunctiva; this simulates the appearance of jaundice. Papilledema and retinal hemorrhages have also been reported.

Hypovitaminosis A is the leading cause of childhood blindness in many underdeveloped countries. The children often develop severe keratomalacia without preexisting Bitot spots. The disease heals with scarring and may be distinguished from trachomatous scarring by its onset between the ages of 1 and 6 years (p. 221).

BIBLIOGRAPHY

Bloomfield, S. E., Dunn, M. W., Miyata, T., and others: Soluble artificial tear inserts, Arch. Ophthalmol. **95:**247, 1977.

Cogan, D. G.: Immunosuppression and eye disease, Am. J. Ophthalmol. **83:**777, 1977.

Ellis, P. P.: Ocular therapeutics and pharmacology, ed. 5, St. Louis, 1977, The C. V. Mosby Co.

Fraunfelder, F. T.: Drug-induced ocular side effects and drug interactions, Philadelphia, 1976, Lea & Febiger.

Fraunfelder, F. T.: Extraocular fluid dynamics; how best to apply topical ocular medication, Trans. Am. Ophthalmol. Soc. **74:**457, 1976.

Fraunfelder, F. T., and Scafidi, A. F.: Possible adverse effects from topical ocular 10% phenylephrine, Am. J. Ophthalmol. **85:**447, 1978.

George, F. J., and Hanna, C.: Ocular penetration of chloramphenicol, Arch. Ophthalmol. **95:**879, 1977.

Geraci, J. E.: Vancomycin, Mayo Clin. Proc. **52:**631, 1977.

Goodman, L. S., and Gilman, A.: The pharmacological basis of therapeutics, ed. 5, New York, 1975, Macmillan, Inc.

Grant, W. M.: Toxicology of the eye, ed. 2, Springfield, Ill., 1974, Charles C Thomas, Publisher.

Hanna, C., Fraunfelder, F. T., Cable, M., and Hardberger, R. E.: Effect of ophthalmic ointments on corneal wound healing, Am. J. Ophthalmol. **76:** 193, 1973.

Hardberger, R. E., Hanna, C., and Goodart, R.: Effects of drug vehicles on ocular uptake of tetracycline, Am. J. Ophthalmol. **80:**133, 1975.

Havener, W. H.: Ocular pharmacology, ed. 3, St. Louis, 1974, The C. V. Mosby Co.

Hyndiuk, R. A., Hull, D. S., Schultz, R. O., and others: Adenine arabinoside in idoxuridine unresponsive and intolerant herpetic keratitis, Am. J. Ophthalmol. **79:**655, 1975.

Jones, B. F.: Principles in the management of oculomycosis, Am. J. Ophthalmol. **79:**719, 1975.

Kaback, M. B., Podos, S. M., Harbin, T. S., Jr., and others: The effects of dipivalyl epinephrine on the eye, Am. J. Ophthalmol. **81:**768, 1976.

Kitazawa, Y., Nose, H., and Horie, T.: Chemical sympathectomy with 6-hydroxydopamine in the treatment of primary open-angle glaucoma, Am. J. Ophthalmol. **79:**98, 1975.

Kupferman, A., and Leibowitz, H. M.: Topical antibiotic therapy of staphylococcal keratitis, Arch. Ophthalmol. **95:**1634, 1977.

Laties, A. M., Neufeld, A. H., Vegge, T., and Sears, M. L.: Differential reactivity of rabbit iris and ciliary process to topically applied prostaglandin E (dinoprostone), Arch. Ophthalmol. **94:**1966, 1976.

Leopold, I. H., editor: Symposium on ocular therapy, vols. 1-7, St. Louis, 1966-1974, The C. V. Mosby Co.

Leopold, I. H., and Burns, R. P., editors: Symposium on ocular therapy, vols. 8-9, New York, 1976, John Wiley & Sons, Inc.

Mackool, R. J., Muldoon, T., Fortier, A., and Nelson, D.: Epinephrine-induced cystoid macular edema in aphakic eyes, Arch. Ophthalmol. **95:**791, 1977.

Oakley, D. E., Weeks, R. D., and Ellis, P. P.: Corneal distribution of subconjunctival antibiotics, Am. J. Ophthalmol. **81:**307, 1976.

Pavan-Langston, D.: Clinical evaluation of adenine arabinoside and idoxuridine in the treatment of ocular herpes simplex, Am. J. Ophthalmol. **80:** 495, 1975.

Pavan-Langston, D., and Foster, C. S.: Trifluorothymidine and idoxuridine therapy of ocular herpes, Am. J. Ophthalmol. **84:**818, 1977.

Place, V. A., Fisher, M., Herbst, S., and others: Comparative pharmacologic effects of pilocarpine administered to normal subjects by eyedrops or by ocular therapeutic systems, Am. J. Ophthalmol. **80:**706, 1975.

Podos, S. M.: Prostaglandins; nonsteroidal anti-inflammatory agents in eye disease, Trans. Am. Ophthalmol. Soc. **74:**637, 1976.

Pollack, I. P.: Effect of L-norepinephrine and adrenergic potentiators on the aqueous humor dynamics of man, Am. J. Ophthalmol. **76:**641, 1973.

Sonntag, J. R., Brindley, G. O., and Shields, M. B.: Effect of timolol therapy on outflow facility, Invest. Ophthalmol. **17:**293, 1978.

Thompson, R. L.: The cephalosporins, Mayo Clin. Proc. **52:**625, 1977.

Wilkowske, C. J.: The penicillins, Mayo Clin. Proc. **52:**616, 1977.

Wilson, W. R.: Tetracyclines, chloramphenicol, erythromycin, and clindamycin, Mayo Clin. Proc. **52:**635, 1977.

Zimmerman, T. J., and Kaufman, H. E.: Timolol; a beta-adrenergic blocking agent for the treatment of glaucoma, Arch. Ophthalmol. **95:**601, 1977.

PART TWO

History taking and examination of the eye

Chapter 4

HISTORY AND INTERPRETATION

Every well-trained physician, whatever his specialty, should be able to examine the eye quickly and be assured that the eyes do not cross, the pupils constrict to light, visual fields are intact, and the optic disk is not swollen or atrophic.

The practitioner should be reassured in knowing that glasses have nothing to do with the health of the eyes and that the wearing of incorrect glasses cannot harm the eyes. At worst, incorrect glasses may blur vision and cause discomfort that may lead to a headache. The eyes are meant to be used, and there is no way that they can be worn out by use. Reading in dim light may be difficult and uncomfortable and may even cause headache, but this does not harm the eyes. The distance at which material is held has no effect on the eyes, although it may be related to discomfort. Headache is usually not caused by the eyes, and certainly organic types of headaches, such as migraine, cluster headaches, and other specific types, never originate from the eyes.

There are a number of important ob-

SOME ELEMENTARY PRINCIPLES OF EYE CARE

Reading in dim light does not harm eyes.

Bright light does not harm eyes. Sunglasses are not necessary.

Excessive use of eyes does not harm them, and "bad eyes" are not the result of overuse.

Sitting too close to television does not harm eyes.

Too strong, too weak, or wrongly ground glasses do not harm eyes.

Contact lenses neutralize refractive errors but do not abolish them.

The eyes clean themselves, and eye drops are not required.

Headaches usually do not occur because of eyestrain. Organic headaches such as migraine never do.

Healthy eyes do not require annual examination.

An eye with open-angle glaucoma does not appear abnormal.

Cataract extraction is indicated only if the opacity interferes with activities.

Persistent watering of an infant's eye suggests either congenital glaucoma or blocked tear duct.

Chemicals must be irrigated immediately from eyes with no delay to measure vision.

Table 4-1. Symptoms of eye disease

I. Disturbances of vision
   A. Decreased visual acuity
      1. Near
      2. Distance
   B. Abnormal color vision
      1. Hereditary: bilateral
      2. Acquired: often unilateral
   C. Abnormal visual field
      1. Unilateral asymmetric defects in retinal and optic nerve diseases
      2. Bilateral symmetric defects in diseases at or posterior to chiasm
   D. Defective dark adaptation
   E. Iridescent vision ("halos")
   F. Floaters
   G. Photopsia
      1. Unilateral: retinal stimulus other than light
      2. Bilateral: visual hallucination
         a. Unformed: occipital lobe origin
         b. Formed: temporal lobe origin
   H. Objects appear smaller (micropsia) or larger (macropsia) than they actually are
      1. Fovea centralis abnormality
   I. Cortical blindness: bilateral lesions of occipital cortex
   J. Perceptual blindness: lesions of angular gyrus of parieto-occiptal fissure
   K. Diplopia (double vision)
      1. Physiologic
      2. Monocular: local disturbance of one eye
      3. Near only: convergence abnormality
      4. Distance only: divergence abnormality
      5. Varying with eye or head movements: ocular muscle weakness
II. Pain in one or both eyes or in the head
   A. Superficial foreign body sensation
   B. Deep pain within the eye
   C. Headache
   D. Burning, itching, "tired" eyes
   E. Photophobia (abnormal ocular sensitivity to light)
III. Abnormal secretion from eyes
   A. Lacrimation (excessive tear production)
   B. Epiphora (defective tear drainage)
   C. Mucus
   D. Pus
   E. Dry eyes
IV. Physical signs described by the patient as symptoms
   A. Red eye
      1. Conjunctival injection
      2. Ciliary injection
      3. Subconjunctival hemorrhage
   B. New growths
   C. Abnormal position of eyes or eyelids
   D. Protrusion of globe
   E. Widened palpebral fissure
   F. Narrowed palpebral fissure
   G. Pupillary abnormality

---

servations in ophthalmology. Any child who has an eye that constantly crosses after the age of 6 months requires specialized examination with pupillary dilation. There should be no delay because the child is not old enough to cooperate in the examination. Reading problems in children are not caused by an abnormality of the eyes, and eye exercises will not correct disorders of reading. Ocular abnormalities have no causative role in reading problems except insofar as reduced visual acuity impairs ability to recognize letters.

The eye is a remarkably sturdy organ. The pupil constricts when excess light enters it. Thus sunglasses may make things more comfortable, but no harm comes from not wearing them. Similarly, tears function so efficiently that it is not necessary to use eye drops. Once it has been determined that a pair of eyes are healthy, annual examinations are not necessary unless symptoms such as severe pain in the eyes, loss of vision, double vision, or sudden showers of floaters occur.

Contact lenses only neutralize refractive errors and do not correct them. However, if incorrect contact lenses are worn, the shape of the eye may be temporarily changed, and there may be a period in which vision seems to have been improved by the contact lens. The conjunctiva prevents contact lenses from getting behind the eye.

With age, each person loses accommodation (presbyopia, p. 437). If the individual was myopic (nearsighted) before the onset of presbyopia, he will be able to read without glasses, even though presbyopic. Similarly, if an individual develops a nuclear sclerosis (cataract, p. 379), he may have a period of being able to see near work without lenses. Reading without lenses after the age of 50, though, indicates that one was either nearsighted previously or is developing cataract.

A cataract is located behind the pupil and develops nearly universally. The indication for its extraction is the effect of the impaired vision on the normal activities of the individual. Inasmuch as the lens is located behind the iris, it is not peeled off but is surgically extracted.

Unfortunately, eyes with open-angle glaucoma, a common cause of visual loss, appear to be normal; there is no way of diagnosing glaucoma without measuring the intraocular pressure, although in advanced glaucoma the characteristic excavation of the optic disk (cupping) will indicate the cause.

The main symptoms of ocular abnormality include the following: (1) disturbances of vision, (2) pain in one or both eyes or in the head, and (3) abnormal secretion from the eyes.

DISTURBANCES OF VISION

A visual abnormality may arise because of (1) a defect in image formation, (2) an interference with impulse transmission in the visual pathways, and (3) an abnormality in the visual perceptual centers. A defect in image formation is caused by an abnormality within the eye itself. Both eyes may be involved, but often one eye is more severely affected. The cause is a refractive error and not an organic disease if vision is corrected to normal by lenses. If transmission of the nervous impulse is interrupted anterior to the chiasm, only one eye is involved. If there is interference at the chiasm or posterior to it, both eyes will always be involved. Visual perceptual defects often produce bizarre patterns of inability to recognize objects. The physician must learn, therefore, whether the defect involves one or both eyes, if it is corrected with lenses, and if it involves distance or near vision, or both. Furthermore, he must determine if the visual loss is transient or permanent, if it involves central or peripheral vision, and if the vision itself is normal with visual phenomena such as floaters superimposed. If the visual defect disappears when the patient wears correcting lenses, it should be evident that a refractive error is the most likely cause of symptoms. There are many people who require lenses but do not wear them. They describe a variety of unusual, apparently inexplicable ocular symptoms, all of which would be relieved by corrective lenses. Attempts to provide relief by other means are seldom successful.

Some individuals who have psychologic disorders with ocular manifestations have accumulated many spectacles, none of which relieves their symptoms. They may be convinced another pair of glasses will help and are reluctant to recognize the psychologic basis of their complaints.

Symptoms that involve near vision when the distance vision is normal (or vice versa) are most suggestive of a refractive error. One or both eyes may be involved.

Diagnosis of the cause of sudden, persistent, unilateral decrease of vision is based on the appearance of the external eye. The external eye is abnormal in keratitis, iridocyclitis, and angle-closure glaucoma. In vitreous hemorrhage, retinal artery or vein closure, or optic neuritis, the eye appears normal. Periodic visual loss, varying from slight haziness to no light perception and lasting for a few seconds to minutes (amaurosis fugax: transient blindness; transient ischemic attack), may result from spasm of the ophthalmic artery in occlusive disease of the internal carotid artery or from abnormalities of the aortic arch (p. 531). Gradual unilateral loss of vision occurs with corneal opacities, glaucoma, cataract, vitreous opacities, retinal detachment, central retinal degeneration, or intraocular inflammation.

Sudden loss of vision involving both eyes is uncommon. Inquiry usually indicates that vision failed first in one eye and that the sudden loss described was noted by the patient when vision in the fellow eye decreased. Both eyes may be involved in the diseases that cause sudden unilateral loss of vision, but this occurs rarely. A sudden bilateral decrease of vision is most suggestive of a conversion reaction, the toxic effects of drugs, or poor observation.

Gradual loss of vision in both eyes may result from nearly any ophthalmic disorder. Generally, if visual acuity is decreased and peripheral vision is intact, the disorder is anterior to the chiasm. If peripheral vision is decreased in each eye, the disorder may be at or posterior to the chiasm.

Color vision. Color vision is a cone function (p. 101). A deficiency in color perception is inherited in approximately 7% of men and 0.5% of women. It is transmitted as an X chromosome–linked abnormality. Visual acuity in these individuals is normal, but color perception is depressed to a varying degree. Acquired unilateral depression of color sense occurs in diseases affecting the cone function of one eye, such as central retinal degeneration and optic nerve disease. Loss of visual acuity parallels the loss of color discrimination. Bilateral acquired depression in color vision may occur in malnutrition and after the ingestion of toxic drugs. Opacities of the ocular media, particularly those involving the cornea (leukoma) or lens (cataract), may cause depression but not loss of color vision.

Color perception is disturbed in a variety of diseases of the optic nerve and fovea centralis as well as in nutritional disturbances. The occurrence of glucose-6-phosphate dehydrogenase deficiencies associated with hemolytic anemia and red-green color blindness in the inhabitants of Sardinia has excited geneticists and hematologists. It seems likely that in years to come sensitive color vision tests will move from the laboratory to routine clinical use.

Peripheral vision. The retinal periphery

contains rods mainly, but cones are scattered throughout (p. 92, Fig. 2-5). A visual field defect may occur in many abnormalities of the retina, optic nerve, and optic pathways. If the abnormality is anterior to the chiasm, the defect is unilateral. Disorders affecting the chiasm or visual pathways involve both eyes. When one eye is involved in retinal or optic nerve disease, the patient frequently describes the sensation of a curtain falling over a portion of the visual field. When both eyes are involved, the patient may be unaware of the defect.

Defects in the visual fields are usually described as central (within 30° of fixation point) or peripheral. Localized areas of defective vision surrounded by areas of normal vision are called scotomas. Peripheral defects are described as temporal, nasal, superior, and inferior. It should be recalled that the visual field is a projection of visual function opposite to the areas of the retina involved (p. 41). A temporal visual field defect reflects light stimuli to the nasal retina. A superior field defect involves the inferior retina. Thus a superior temporal field defect indicates failure to see objects projected on the inferior nasal retina.

Night blindness. Patients who have an organic disease with night blindness often do not complain of this defect. Conversely, some patients who do not have organic ocular disease may have many complaints concerning poor vision in reduced illumination. Night blindness is caused by pigmentary degenerations of the retina, optic nerve disease, glaucoma, or vitamin A deficiency occurring in cirrhosis of the liver or because of inadequate nutrition. The defect often involves poor recovery of vision during night driving after the headlights of an oncoming car shine in the patient's eyes. Vision that is poorer in bright illumination than in dim illumination occurs in cone degenerations and in toxic involvement of the optic nerve.

Iridescent vision. This term is applied to the halos or rainbow seen surrounding bright lights when there is diffusion by the ocular media. The most common cause is subepithelial edema of the cornea, which may follow a rapid increase in intraocular pressure. Prolonged wearing of hard contact lenses and swimming in fresh water with the eyes open also cause corneal edema. Pus floating across the cornea in conjunctivitis may cause iridescent vision that is corrected by rapid blinking. Corneal degeneration (dystrophy) and cataract may also cause the symptom.

Entoptic phenomena. These are structures visualized within the eye. Floaters are translucent specks of various shapes and sizes that float across the visual field. They can be seen only when the eye is open. Commonly the patient observes them when looking at a bright blue sky or a brilliantly illuminated pastel-colored wall. All individuals have small fixed remnants of the hyaloid vascular system in the vitreous body (muscae volitantes) seen as small dots that dart away as one tries to fix them. Lens opacities may cause floaters that do not move (fixed). Leukocytes from inflammation of the retina or uvea may cause floaters, but usually such large numbers are present that vision is generally depressed. A sudden shower of floaters may occur in the periphery of the visual field with a vitreous hemorrhage. This may be the initial symptom of hole formation preceding retinal separation. The location of the floaters may be helpful in locating the retinal hole. The sudden appearance of a moderately large floater is the main symptom of vitreous detachment. Rarely, a patient learns inadvertently to observe the leukocytes in his own capillaries and becomes concerned about the flecks that disturb his reading.

Photopsia. These are visual perceptions arising in the absence of light stimuli. The term is applied to such visual phenomena as specks, rings, lightning flashes, and luminous bodies that are observed when the eyes are closed. When monocular, the condition is caused by a retinal stimulus (inadequate stimulus) other than light. It occurs in retraction of the vitreous upon the retina or with pressure upon the closed eye. Visual hallucinations (bilateral photopsia) are divided into formed and unformed types. Visual hallucinations from the occipital cortex and association areas produce static light and stars, whereas hallucinations from the parastriate area 18 may produce luminous sensations of colored flashes and rings. Hallucinations from the parieto-occipital cortex center on objects, people, and animals. In addition to the visual illusions, there may be preservation of the visual image in time (palinopia) or in space (visual illusory spread), impaired visual recognition (visual agnosia), defective visual localization, errors in naming color, or defective perception of color.

Hallucinations from the temporal cortex may be scenes recalled from experience or may consist of landscapes, prairie fires, or seascapes, usually with repetitive activity and a minimum of detail. Visual hallucinations may be associated with auditory hallucinations.

Micropsia and macropsia. Micropsia, or perceiving images to be smaller than actual size, arises from an abnormality of image formation at the fovea or from disorders of the temporal cortex. Edema, tumors, and hemorrhages in the central retinal region may cause the cones to be spread farther apart and give rise to micropsia.

Macropsia is an abnormality in which objects appear larger than they actually are. It arises from edema, tumors, and hemorrhages in the foveal region that may cause the cones to be pressed closer together.

Cortical blindness. Cortical blindness is an abnormality in perception arising from bilateral impairment of the visual cen-

Table 4-2. Visual acuity in visually handicapped persons (better eye with best possible correction)*

Common definition	Snellen index	Practical test	Legal significance
No light perception (total blindness)	—	Cannot see light	Totally blind
Light perception only	Less than 1/60 (3/200)	Unable to see hand movement at 1 meter	Satisfies all criteria for legal blindness†
Form and motion	Less than 2/60 (6/200)	Hand movement visible, but unable to count fingers at 1 meter	Total disability for Social Security Administration
Travel vision	Less than 3/60 (10/200)	Unable to read newspaper headlines	Legal blindness
Minimal reading	Less than 6/60 (20/200)	Reads headlines, but not 14-point (4.7 mm) type	Maximum acuity for legal blindness for Internal Revenue Service and most state industrial commissions
Partially seeing (borderline)	More than 6/60 (20/200), but less than 6/24 (20/70)	Cannot read 10-point (3.4 mm) type without marked difficulty	Not legally blind, but eligible for some services

*After Wheeler, P. C.: Mo. Med. **64:**315, 1967.
†Legal blindness also present if visual field is constricted to 20° or less.

ters of the occipital cortex (area 17). It is characterized by a loss of the visual sensation with retention of the pupillary reaction to light. The patient may not be conscious of his loss of vision.

Perceptual blindness. Perceptual blindness is an abnormality caused by lesions in the angular gyrus of the parieto-occipital fissure in which individuals are unable to recognize objects visually (agnosia) but are able to recognize objects by touch or other sensory portals. An individual so afflicted will be unable to recognize a key when looking at it but will readily recognize it when touching it. Defects related to this condition include alexia (inability to read), agraphia (inability to write), and dyslexia (distrubance in the ability to read). These abnormalities may be highly selective and permit the patient to recognize numbers but not letters, or to recognize printed matter but not written script, and the like.

Blindness. The definition of blindness differs, but generally a person is considered legally blind when his best visual acuity with lenses in the better eye is 6/60 (20/200) or less when the peripheral visual field is constricted to within 20° (Table 4-2). The chief causes of blindness in the United States are glaucoma, unoperated cataract, and retinal disorders, mainly proliferative diabetic retinopathy and central retinal degeneration.

The physician managing a blind patient must avoid any hint of condescension and must learn that the patient's interpretation of his voice and actions are the major factors in reassurance. A person talking to a blind individual should identify himself by name, should not shout, should always give detailed verbal directions and not visual signals, and should always warn the patient before touching him. Blind persons prefer to grasp the arm of a guide rather than having their assistant grasp them.

A surprising number of blind individuals are not aware of the agencies and services available to promote their adjustment and independence. Information may be obtained from the American Foundation for the Blind, 15 West 16th Street, New York, N.Y. 10011.

Diplopia. Diplopia, or double vision, occurs whenever the visual lines (p. 412) are not directed simultaneously to the same object. Unilateral diplopia is a curiosity in which light rays are split by an opacity in the cornea or lens so that a single object is imaged twice on the retina. Frequently the images are so blurred that the patient notices the defect only under exceptional visual conditions.

Physiologic diplopia is a normal phenomenon in which objects not within the area of fixation are seen double. Usually it does not impinge on the consciousness. It is easily demonstrated by looking at a near object with attention directed to a distant object, which then appears doubled. Such physiologic diplopia contributes to parallax, which enables one to judge the distance of objects.

Diplopia is a cardinal sign of weakness of one or more of the extraocular muscles (p. 523). Characteristically, the separation of images increases in the field of action of the extraocular muscle(s) involved. Diplopia can occur only if binocular vision has developed. The absence of diplopia thus does not guarantee that a paresis of an extraocular muscle is not present. Diplopia may also occur without muscle weakness if there is displacement of the globe so that the visual lines cannot be directed simultaneously to the same object.

PAIN

Pain and aches in the region of the eye or in the head may be difficult to interpret and require considerable clinical skill in evaluation. Some patients are phlegmatic about pain, the severity of which would be disabling to others. Moreover, pain is a subjective sensation, and considerable insight into a patient's temperament is required for evaluation.

A superficial foreign body sensation may be caused by a lesion in the eyelid, a foreign body on the cornea or the conjunctiva, inflammation of the cornea or the conjunctiva, or loss of conjunctival or corneal epithelium. A local anesthetic instilled in the conjunctival sac usually eliminates the sensation of a superficial foreign body but not that caused by inflammation of the conjunctiva and the cornea. If the eyelid is drawn away from the globe, the sensation caused by a foreign body on the tarsal conjunctiva will be eliminated, whereas the sensation caused by a foreign body on the cornea will continue. Patients invariably localize a foreign body sensation to the outer portion of the upper eyelid irrespective of its location.

Deep, severe pain within the eye may be present in a variety of disorders. The most important causes, inasmuch as they require immediate attention, are inflammations of the ciliary body and rapid increase in the intraocular pressure, such as that occurring in angle-closure glaucoma. In each of these instances, the eye is red and vision is decreased.

Many relatively minor ocular abnormalities manifest themselves by burning, itching, and uncomfortable eyes. These symptoms may arise from an inadequately corrected refractive error, fatigue, conjunctival irritation, and chronic conjunctivitis (p. 225). Mild, nonspecific inflammation of the eyelids or the conjunctiva without obvious signs may cause ocular discomfort, particularly when the eyes are used intensively. Minor ocular irritation arising from prolonged use of the eyes is mainly without significance.

The interpretation of headache as a symptom of ocular disease requires familiarity with its causes. Headaches that are relieved by salicylates are usually not caused by serious organic disease. Uncorrected errors of refraction or wearing incorrect lenses does not cause severe incapacitating headaches. Headaches that are present on awakening in the morning are not caused by excessive use of the eyes the previous night.

One should determine whether a headache is intermittent or continuous, its location in the head, and other associated signs. An aura followed by severe unilateral headache (hemicrania), nausea, and vomiting is suggestive of migraine. A headache aggravated by straining and associated with vomiting without nausea is suggestive of an internal hydrocephalus. A severe frontal headache associated with paralysis of ocular muscles is suggestive of an infraclinoid aneurysm of the internal carotid artery (p. 533).

Tic douloureux gives rise to a characteristic excruciating pain in the region of distribution of the sensory branches of the trigeminal nerve. Usually the history of episodic pain of a similar type alerts one to the nature of the disorder. Zoster ophthalmicus may give rise to severe retrobulbar pain, which may precede the cutaneous vesiculation by several days. Often the cause of the pain is not recognized until the typical eruption occurs in the area of distribution of the ophthalmic nerve. Postzoster neuralgia may be extremely disabling in the elderly.

Photophobia is a reflex in which light stimulating the retina causes constriction of the pupil and pain. The term is widely used to indicate any discomfort arising from bright light, such as the reflection of a great amount of light from the sky or an unpleasant contrast between light and dark areas. Glare is the term given to excessive light directed into the eyes from a reflecting surface. A common sign of ocular neurosis is excessive sensitivity of the eye to light.

Patients with cone degenerations often have an aversion to bright light first noted by the examiner when he attempts oph-thalmoscopy. Inquiry will then indicate that the patient prefers activities in dim illumination. There may be a reduction in visual acuity as the amount of illumination increases.

ABNORMAL SECRETION

It is sometimes possible to diagnose an ocular disease by observing the nature of an abnormal secretion from the eyes (p. 220). Pus is found in the conjunctival sac in mucopurulent conjunctivitis. The lashes are frequently agglutinated to each other by drying pus, and it may be difficult to open the eyes in the morning. A foamy secretion at the inner canthus is produced by *Corynebacterium xerose,* which lives solely on desquamated epithelium. A stringy secretion with excoriation of the canthus characterizes the inflammation caused by the diplobacillus of Morax-Axenfeld. A tenacious, stringy secretion occurs in allergic inflammation of the conjunctiva.

A distinction is made between lacrimation, in which there is an excessive production of tears, and epiphora, in which there is overflow of a normal amount of tears secondary to closure of some portion of the lacrimal drainage system. Lacrimation arises from those diseases that cause reflex secretion of tears, whereas epiphora arises from an abnormality of the drainage system (p. 233). Persistent tearing of one or both eyes of an infant is a cardinal sign of congenital glaucoma. There is an associated corneal edema. Tearing in infancy may occur because of failure of the nasolacrimal duct to open as it normally does about the third week of life. Tearing also occurs in photophobia, in inflammations of the cornea and conjunctiva, and reflexly in inflammations of the ciliary body.

Decreased tear formation gives rise to drying of the eyes (keratoconjunctivitis sicca). This occurs in Sjögren syndrome (p. 563), in vitamin A deficiency, and in cicatrizing lesions of the conjunctiva that close the orifices of the lacrimal glands. Erythema multiforme, trachoma, and chemical burns are the chief causes of such scarring.

READING DEFECTS

Reading is an integrated skill that is important in intellectual maturation. Inasmuch as children develop at different rates, not all are ready to begin reading at the same age. Thus some children learn to read slowly but read well at an older age. Defective vision, refractive errors, defective fusion, and muscle imbalance have no causative role except insofar as reduced visual acuity makes it difficult for the child to interpret symbols.

Basically there are two main types of reading disorders: (1) general reading backwardness and (2) specific learning disability, or developmental dyslexia. General reading backwardness affects both boys and girls and is found in children who have other learning problems. Abnormal neurologic findings are common, and disorders of motor, constructional, and speech function are frequent. The condition is often seen in children from large families and deprived social classes. Specific reading disability is three times as common in boys as in girls, is rarely associated with a neurologic or other abnormality, and occurs in children who are average or superior in other areas of learning, such as mathematics. Essentially, the reading skills and related areas of vocabulary and speech function are disproportionately lower than their other learning skills and their chronologic age.

Individuals with reading problems are characterized by (1) poor word recognition with inability to pronounce words or to identify unfamiliar words, (2) poor comprehension with difficulty in deriving literal and implied meanings and in drawing conclusions and then following directions, and (3) difficulty in developing vocabulary and a slow reading rate. In addition to the defect in reading, there may be delay in learning to tell time, gross inaccuracy in spelling, and muddled serial thinking. This is followed in later life by a relatively restricted vocabulary, great difficulty in fluent expression of ideas on paper with acceptable standards of syntax and punctuation, and often a lifelong reluctance rather than an incapacity to read.

Specific reading disability (developmental dyslexia) is defined by the World Federation of Neurology as "difficulty in learning to read despite conventional instruction, adequate intelligence and sociocultural opportunity. It is dependent upon fundamental cognitive disabilities which are frequently of constitutional origin."

As indicated in Table 4-3, there are many causes of reading problems. The family physician plays a key role in managing the disorder. Early recognition of a

Table 4-3. Contributing factors and causes of reading deficiencies

I. Sociopsychologic
  A. Defects in teaching
  B. Deficiencies in cognitive stimulation
  C. Deficiencies in motivation
    1. Associated with social pathology
      a. Poverty
      b. Cultural deprivation
    2. Associated with psychopathology ("emotional")
II. Psychophysiologic
  A. Mental retardation
  B. Cerebral palsy
  C. Seizure disorders
  D. Hearing deficits
  E. Progressive neurologic disorders
III. Learning-disorder syndromes
  A. Developmental hyperactivity (short attention span; impulsivity)
  B. Minimal brain dysfunction
  C. Specific learning disabilities
  D. Perceptual deficits
  E. Developmental dyslexia (specific reading retardation)

condition by the teacher is of importance inasmuch as it is much more easily corrected if special teaching is begun at the age of 6 or 7 years. The physician may wish psychologic consultation to be certain intelligence is not impaired; an auditory screening test is usually all that is required. A neurologist may be enlisted to exclude mild forms of neurologic abnormalities. There is no adequate evidence to indicate that visual training, such as ocular muscle exercises, ocular pursuit, or neurologic organizational training (for example, laterality training and balance board or perceptual training), is of value. Intense, specialized, structured instruction in reading skills in an uncluttered, unornamented, nondistracting classroom aid all but a few if instruction is begun early enough.

A reading problem may arise because of a deficiency in memory skills, in processing not only letters but geometric forms and abstract forms. The large amount of information perceived by the visual system persists in a raw perceptual form called *visual information storage* for about 0.25 second. During this period, subjects actively code and transfer this information into more permanent storage called *short-term storage*. Testing of 12-year-olds with reading defects indicates a normal visual information storage, but a gross defect in processing visual information into short-term storage. This suggests that those with a reading disability have some problem in the encoding, organizational, or retrieval skills that normally follow the initial stage of visual information storage. It appears not to involve verbal and linguistic processes primarily, although inability to recognize and pronounce words follows from the reading defect.

Cerebrovascular disease affecting the angular and supramarginal gyri on the opposite side of the dominant hand may cause loss of ability to read in previously normal individuals. If all ability is lost, the condition is classed as alexia; if the difficulty is partial, the condition is classed as neurologic dyslexia or acquired dyslexia. The severity and the nature of the defect vary markedly in ability to read letters while retaining ability to read numbers, ability to recognize words in large type but not in small type, and the like. Color perception may be affected (acquired dyschromatopsia). Often there is severe involvement of large areas of the brain, and exact diagnosis is not possible.

PERIODIC EYE EXAMINATION

Examination of the newborn infant should include inspection of the eyelids and the external eye. The pupils should react to light, and ophthalmoscopic examination should indicate a red reflex with no opacities of the media. A careful practitioner will view the optic disk and the area immediately adjacent to it. In eyes that are not constantly parallel after the age of 6 months or that cross thereafter, a complete eye examination including cycloplegic refraction is indicated.

Vision should be measured in each eye no later than the third year inasmuch as strabismic or anisometropic amblyopia may be corrected if detected at this age. A complete eye examination with cycloplegic refraction is desirable before beginning grammar school, in the fourth grade, and before beginning high school, college, and graduate school. If an abnormality is discovered, more frequent examinations may be necessary. Young adults who are without symptoms and who do not have a refractive error may be examined every 5 years. If correcting lenses are worn, they should be examined every 2 years. After the age of 45 years, examinations should be done every 2 years.

A complete eye examination should include examination of the anterior segment of the eye and the eyelids with a biomicroscope; the ocular fundus should be inspected with a direct ophthalmoscope, and the peripheral fundus studied with an indirect ophthalmoscope by means of scleral depression. The intraocular pressure should be measured with a tonometer. The visual fields should be estimated by confrontation or other screening method, and if there is any question of an abnormality, they must be carefully measured with a perimeter (p. 162). The muscle balance, including convergence and divergence, must be measured for both near and far. The visual acuity should be measured for near and far and the refractive error determined.

Particular attention must be directed to ocular signs of systemic disease. Effective treatment is available for many ocular conditions in their early stages, and it is disheartening to see individuals with reduced vision arising from abnormalities not detected in their early stages. Similarly, many systemic diseases are first evident in the eyes. In the Framingham Eye Study, over 25% of those who were found to have eye changes characteristic of diabetic retinopathy had no previous diagnosis or treatment for diabetes.

BIBLIOGRAPHY

Bettman, J. W.: Ophthalmology; the art, the law, and a bit of science, Birmingham, Ala., 1977, Aesculapius Publishing Co.

Goldberg, H. K., and Schiffman, G. B.: Dyslexia, New York, 1972, Grune & Stratton, Inc.

Kini, M. M., Leibowitz, H. M., Colton, T., and others: Prevalence of senile cataract, diabetic retinopathy, senile macular degeneration, and open-angle glaucoma in the Framingham Eye Study, Am. J. Ophthalmol. 85:28, 1978.

Localization of visual hallucinations, Br. Med. J. 2: 147, 1977.

Morrison, F. J., Giordani, B., and Nagy, J.: Reading disability; on information-processing analysis, Science 196:77, 1977.

Chapter 5

FUNCTIONAL EXAMINATION OF THE EYES

The different functions of the eye are evaluated by many tests. The cone function of the fovea centralis is assessed usually by measurement of the ability to distinguish the shape of symbols such as letters. This is designated as visual acuity. It is measured for both near and far, with and without the best possible correction of any refractive error (p. 431). Because only cones participate in color vision and because they are concentrated in the fovea, the measurement of color recognition also measures foveal function. The function of the peripheral retina, which contains mainly rods, is measured by estimation of the peripheral visual field.

Any reasonably complete physical examination should indicate (1) that vision is approximately normal and equal in each eye for near and far, each eye being measured separately, (2) that the peripheral visual field of each eye is intact on gross testing, (3) that the ocular movements are normal, (4) that both pupils constrict with direct stimulation of the retina by light, and (5) that the optic disks are flat and of normal color.

Such an examination is not a complete eye examination but can be performed quickly and will exclude many different serious diseases.

VISUAL ACUITY

Measurement of visual acuity is essentially an assessment of the function of the fovea centralis. It involves the discrimination of small details within and between objects. The test object must be so constructed that each portion of it is separated by a constant interval. By custom, this interval has become 1 minute of arc, and the test object is one that subtends an angle of 5 minutes of arc. A variety of test objects have been constructed on this principle, so that an angle of 5 minutes is subtended at distances varying from a few inches to many feet.

Visual acuity is designated by two numbers. The first indicates the distance separating the test object from the patient; the second indicates the distance at which the test object subtends an angle of 5 minutes. Until recently, in the United States these numbers were usually given in inches or feet, whereas in Europe the designation is in meters.

The most familiar test objects are letters or numbers (Figs. 5-1 and 5-2). Such tests have the disadvantage of requiring a literate and cooperative observer. Additionally, they vary in their recognizability. Thus L is the easiest letter in the alphabet to recognize, and B is the most difficult. A broken ring (Fig. 5-3), in

158

which the break in the ring subtends a 1-minute angle and the entire ring subtends a 5-minute angle, eliminates this variability. Similarly, the letter E may be arranged so that it faces in different directions (the illiterate E) (Fig. 5-3). The checkerboard design (Fig. 5-3) is so arranged that when the target is too small for the checkerboard to be discriminated, all four squares appear uniformly gray. These test objects can be used to test illiterates and persons not familiar with the Western alphabet. A variety of pictures have been designed for testing children.

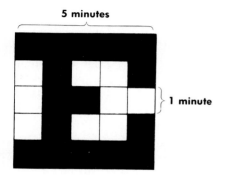

Fig. 5-1. Construction of the Snellen (1862) letter to subtend an angle of 5 minutes; each part subtends an angle of 1 minute. Letters constructed without serifs are recommended by nearly all investigators.

The measurement of visual acuity involves many complex factors not necessarily related to the ability to see test objects. Visual acuity varies with motivation, attention, intelligence, and physical variants. The testing situation in many physicians' offices differs considerably (as does the patience of the examiner).

Devices that project test symbols on a screen permit test distances of more than 3 meters (10 feet) but less than 6 meters (20 feet). Letters are proportionately reduced for the situation, but visual acuity appears to be better when the test distance is less than 6 meters. When a mirror is used, vision may be poorer than when measured in a 6-meter lane.

An isolated letter is recognized easier than a series of letters. This is particularly true in individuals with amblyopia (p. 426), who may have vision as good as 5/12 (20/50) when measured with isolated letters and as poor as 6/60 (20/200) when the letters are placed in a series. The visual acuity scores improve if the individual is given an unlimited time to recognize the letters, and they decrease when the letters are presented rapidly.

The measurement of visual acuity in a manner that may be consistently reproduced involves attention to a number of complex physical and psychic details. These are controlled only in experimental situations. The maximum visual acuity

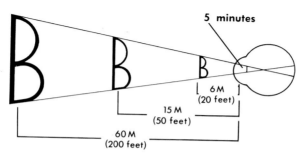

Fig. 5-2. Test letters subtending an angle of 5 minutes at varying distances from the eye. (Not to scale.)

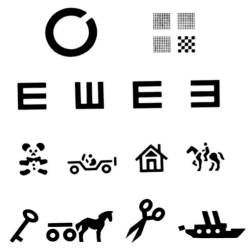

Fig. 5-3. Test objects used in testing visual acuity. Top line illustrates the Landolt broken ring and the Goldmann checkerboard. In successive lines are shown the illiterate E (without serifs), the Henry F. Allen preschool vision test, and the Østerberg chart.

is that in which the individual correctly recognizes 51% of the test symbols presented in a definite time interval. If a portion of the test objects is not recognized, it is customary to indicate the best vision minus the number of letters missed, such as 6/9−2. However, because the number of letters on the 6/9 line is not indicated, this is not particularly meaningful.

Despite the variations that occur in the measurement of visual acuity, it is a relatively accurate clinical test of function and, when normal, indicates the following: (1) that myopia is not present or, if present, is of minor degree or has been compensated by partially closing the eyelids; (2) that any hyperopia present has been compensated by accommodation; (3) that the cornea and lens and ocular media are relatively clear in the visual axis, permitting an image to be formed on the retina; (4) that the fovea centralis is relatively intact, as are its nervous connections to the brain; and (5) that per-

ception by the higher visual centers is intact.

The largest symbol used in the United States subtends an angle of 5 minutes at a distance of 60 meters (200 feet). Symbols then subtend a 5-minute angle at distances of 30 (100), 20 (60), 10 (30), and 6 (20) meters. If the individual is unable to recognize the largest test symbol, he should be brought closer to it, and the distance at which he recognizes it should be recorded. Thus, if he recognizes the test symbol that subtends a 5-minute angle at 60 meters when he is 4 meters away, the visual acuity is recorded as 4/60 (12/200). This is not a fraction but indicates two measurements: the test distance and the size of the symbol.

Special symbols that subtend a 5-minute angle at distances as far as 400 meters are available for measuring individuals with reduced vision. If an individual cannot recognize any symbol, however close, then one determines the distance at which he is able to count fingers, and this is recorded as counting fingers at 20 centimeters, 1 meter, and so on (CF at 1 meter). If he is unable to count fingers, the distance at which he can recognize hand movements is recorded (HM at x meters). If he is unable to recognize hand movements, a small penlight is used to indicate whether he can project the direction from which light is entering the eye. This is recorded as light projection. If he is unable to project the direction of light, it is determined whether or not he can perceive light. (To avoid confusion, one must spell out perception or projection and not abbreviate as LP.) Only in the absence of perception of light is the eye recorded as blind. Because blindness has a variety of legal and sociologic definitions, many examiners record such an eye as having no light perception (NLP) rather than blind. Tests for visual acuity are carried out in each eye separately and then with both eyes open.

The preceding discussion unfortunately suggests that the measurement of visual acuity is a complicated, time-consuming, difficult-to-interpret maneuver. Rather, it is rapidly performed, simple, and requires minimal equipment. Vision should be measured without the patient wearing lenses appropriate for the distance, because it is nonproductive to measure distance vision while the patient is wearing reading glasses.

Measurement of near vision is by no means as accurate as that of distance vision. For the most part, the distance at which near vision is tested is not recorded, and one records the smallest type that can be recognized irrespective of the distance. The standard test distance is considered to be 33 cm (13 inches). Test symbols subtending a 5-minute angle at various distances are used.

Many individuals have never had visual acuity measured in each eye separately. Sometimes the first indication that vision is decreased in one eye is a trifling eye injury or disease. If the physician has not measured the vision before inspecting or manipulating the eye, the patient may wrongfully accuse the physician of causing the decreased vision. In an emergency it is not necessary to have specific testing equipment available. One may gauge the visual acuity by using a telephone book or a newspaper and recording the smallest print that can be recognized with each eye.

It is desirable to measure the visual acuity of children sometime during their third year to detect strabismic or sensory amblyopia (p. 426) and to recognize the presence of severe refractive errors. Picture charts, the illiterate E, or the broken ring may be used. A rotating drum with alternating strips of black and white that induce rhythmic back-and-forth movement of the eyes (opticokinetic nystagmus, p. 537) is used to measure vision objectively. This is the usual method of measuring visual acuity in experimental animals. A strip of cloth 66 by 7 cm may have a series of 5-cm circles of a different color sewn on it. Movement of the strip in front of the eyes induces an opticokinetic nystagmus in infants and indicates vision adequate for subsequent normal schooling.

Pinhole test. Measurement of visual acuity with the patient viewing test symbols through a small opening in an opaque shield rapidly indicates whether reduced vision is caused by an error of refraction (and is thus correctable with lenses) or by some other abnormality. Vision is improved when a refractive error is present, because only rays that are nearly parallel to the visual axis, and thus not refracted, are seen. Usually, if vision is improved using a pinhole, a correcting lens will provide even better vision. Exceptionally, in keratoconus (p. 257) the visual improvement cannot be duplicated. In cataract (p. 377) and vitreous opacities (p. 358), the pinhole reduces rather than improves vision.

VISUAL FIELDS

The function of the retinal periphery is assessed by measurement of the peripheral field of vision. This may be measured accurately by means of several instruments, or it may be estimated by means of the confrontation test. The confrontation test grossly measures the visual field, and although the test results are normal, a defect may still be detected by more sensitive methods of examination. The confrontation test is carried out as follows.

The examiner sits facing the patient at a distance of 1 m in an area with good illumination. The patient is asked to close one eye, usually by holding the eyelid closed with his fingers. The examiner closes his own eye that is directly opposite the closed eye of the patient. Thus, if the patient closes his right eye, the examiner closes his left eye. The examiner then places his hand midway between the subject and himself, bringing his hand slowly in from the periphery with one, two, or three fingers extended. The patient is instructed to tell the examiner when he can see and count the number of fingers in his field of vision. When the patient and the examiner have normal vision, each should recognize the number of fingers at the same time. Usually one tests the temporal and nasal fields and the fields above and below each eye in turn. Confrontation testing may also be carried out by substituting a hat pin with a 3- or 5-mm white tip. In children, the examiner may stand behind the child, who has one eye occluded, and bring his hand into the nasal and temporal fields from behind the child's head.

Visual field screening. Visual field screening may be done conveniently by means of a Harrington-Flocks visual field screener. This consists of a screen on which dots of various sizes in different parts of the visual field are flashed for one tenth of a second. The device is valuable in detecting those defects resulting from glaucoma and from neurologic involvement of the optic nerve and visual pathways.

Two main groups of test equipment have been developed for precise measurement of the visual field: perimeters and tangent screens.

Perimeters. Perimeters are constructed in such a manner that the eye is at the center of rotation of a hemisphere that has a radius of curvature of 33 cm. Some consist of an arc of a circle that is rotated, whereas others are constructed as a hemisphere (Fig. 5-4, *A*). In the simplest devices the test object is moved on the end of a wand into the field of view, and in more elaborate perimeters it is projected (Fig. 5-4, *B*). The testing distance of 33 cm remains constant, and the size and color of the test object as well as the contrast of the projected test object with the surrounding background may be varied. The line connecting the points at which a test object may be just recognized is called the peripheral isopter. It is recorded as (1) the size, such as 1, 2, 3, 10 mm; (2) the test distance; (3) the color; and (4) the contrast. Accurate determination of visual fields is time-consuming, and frequently it is superficially and inaccurately done. Conversely, the disease that necessitates the examination may also impair the patient's attention and consciousness so that only the grossest responses can be obtained.

Tangent screens. Because photoreceptors are concentrated near the fovea centralis and the optic disk contains the ganglion cell axons, determination of field defects within 30° of the fixation point is important. Visual fields within this area are usually measured using a tangent screen (Fig. 5-4, *C*) (tangent because it is a plane tangent to the arc of a perimeter). A tangent screen is usually covered with black felt, and the test is conducted 1 or 2 m from the eye. Test objects varying in size from 1 to 50 mm are used. The peripheral isopter, the blind spot, and various scotomas may be demonstrated. For the most part, testing with the tangent screen presents a smaller stimulus to the patient, and the results are more accurate than when the perimeter is used. Similarly, a greater degree of cooperation on the part of the patient is required.

The Amsler test involves the use of a pattern consisting of a 20-cm square divided into 5-mm squares. The patient looks at the center of the square and projects any defect in the visual field onto the square. It is a sensitive method of assessing abnormalities of the fovea centralis that are so slight as not to be detected by the usual methods of perimetry.

Visual field defects. Defects in the visual field are usually described as central or peripheral. A central field defect, a scotoma, is surrounded by a seeing area.

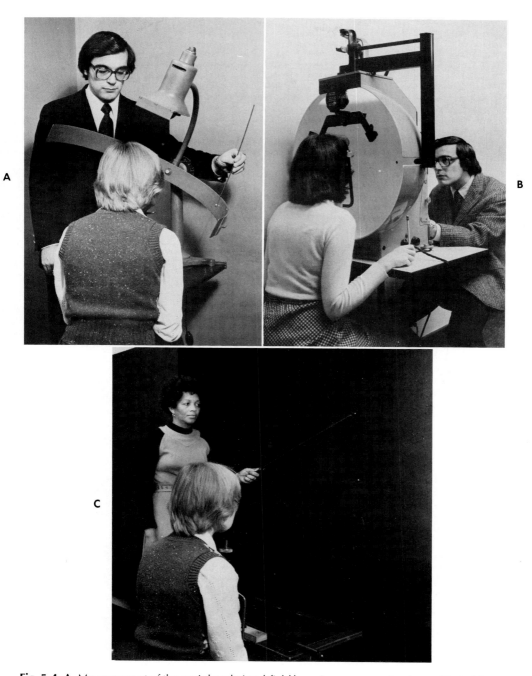

Fig. 5-4. A, Measurement of the peripheral visual field by using an arc perimeter and test object on a wand. Each eye is measured separately. **B,** Measurement of the visual field by using a hemisphere with a projected test object and control of the surrounding illumination (Goldmann). **C,** Measurement of the central visual field by means of a tangent screen.

Central scotomas involve the fixation point (Fig. 5-5), and paracentral scotomas involve an area adjacent to the fixation point. Central scotomas characterize diseases involving the fovea centralis and the papillomacular bundle of nerve fibers in the optic nerve. Centrocecal scotomas (Fig. 5-6) involve both the physiologic blind spot and the fixation point and are characteristic of toxic diseases of the optic nerve. Annular scotomas form a circular defect around the fixation point and are particularly common in diseases that first manifest themselves at the equator of the eye, particularly retinal pigmentary degenerations. Arcuate (arched) scotomas involve a bundle of nerve fibers and characterize the field defect of glaucoma.

Reference is always to the blind portion of the visual field. Hemianopia means half-blindness (Gr. *hemi*, half; *an*, negative; *ope*, vision). A right hemianopia indicates a right half-blindness (Fig. 5-7) and must involve impulses from the left half of the retina. Homonymous hemianopia indicates involvement of the right

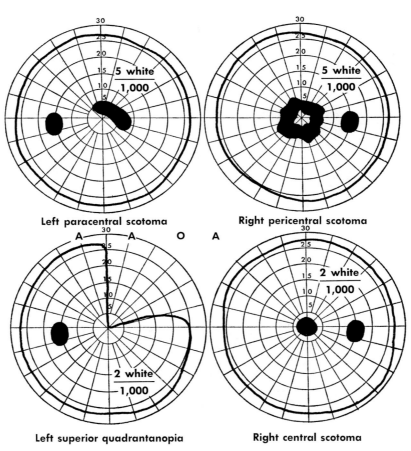

Left paracentral scotoma

Right pericentral scotoma

Left superior quadrantanopia

Right central scotoma

Fig. 5-5. Various types of central field defects. The blind spot is temporal to the point of fixation. The left visual field is to the left of the viewer and the right visual field to the right. The designation 5 white/1,000 indicates that the test was done by using a 5-mm white test object at 1,000 mm.

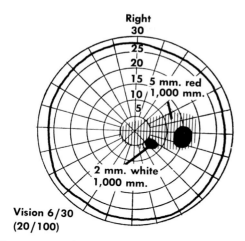

Fig. 5-6. Centrocecal scotoma with an absolute scotoma (in black) surrounded by a relative scotoma (in lines).

or left portion of each visual field and thus interference with impulse transmission posterior to the optic chiasm (Fig. 5-7). (The term "heteronymous" is not used; a bitemporal hemianopia such as that in chiasmal disease is, however, heteronymous.)

COLOR VISION TESTING

Good color vision is especially important in industry, school, and vehicle operation, but often color vision testing is neglected. The tests used clinically are relatively gross and too insensitive to detect small changes but nonetheless may be unusually helpful to the individual. Color vision abnormalities occur as a hereditary defect in about 7% of men and 0.5% of women. They are transmitted as an X chromosome–linked abnormality.

Autosomal defects in color vision occur

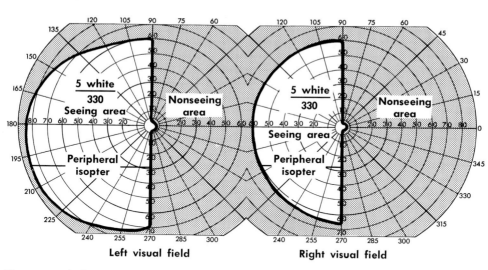

Fig. 5-7. Right homonymous hemianopia measured on a perimeter. The hemianopia always designates the blind portion of the field. The designation 5 white/330 indicates that the test was done by using a 5-mm white test object at 330 mm. The limits of the seeing area (isopters) are the heavy black lines, which enclose the visual field. The field defect results from a loss of transmission of the stimulus from the left half of each retina. Because both eyes are involved, the defect must be posterior to the decussation. Defects exactly similar in size, shape, severity, and extent are congruous defects and involve identical fibers posterior to the lateral geniculate body.

in congenital achromatopsias and in cone degenerations. In retrobulbar neuritis (p. 368) there may be early severe depression of color vision. In foveal degeneration caused by vascular disease (p. 345), separation (p. 347), and other acquired disorders, the decrease in color vision parallels the loss of visual acuity.

The least accurate test for detecting color deficiency involves the matching of yarns (Holmgren test) or recognizing red and green lanterns. Color plates are available in which numbers are outlined in the primary colors and surrounded by confusion colors. The color-deficient individual is unable to see the figure that is recognized quickly by a person with normal color appreciation. More sensitive tests of color vision involve the use of the Nagel anomaloscope, in which the hue and saturation of yellow are matched by mixtures of red and green. The Farnsworth-Munsell test of hue discrimination consists of 84 chips of color that are matched in terms of increasing hue.

Color perception is disturbed in a variety of diseases of the optic nerve and fovea centralis as well as in nutritional disturbances. Testing has an important role in the diagnosis of total color blindness. Sensitive color vision tests are now used routinely in the clinical evaluation of cone degenerations and other foveal disorders.

BIBLIOGRAPHY

Keeney, A. H.: Ocular examination; basis and technique, St. Louis, 1976, The C. V. Mosby Co.

Chapter 6

PHYSICAL EXAMINATION OF THE EYES

A skilled physician studies his patients constantly and unobtrusively for the physical basis of their symptoms. In the initial meeting the physician should note the diameter and shape of the head and the position of the eyes. Gross variations in the insertion of the canthal ligaments are observed easily, and the obliquity of the palpebral fissure is readily evident. Simple observation reveals wrinkling of the forehead because of photophobia or an attempt to elevate the upper eyelid in blepharoptosis. Good illumination is required, but close inspection is not necessary to reveal jaundice or injection of the conjunctival vessels. The position of the eyelid margins in relation to the eye as well as any discomfort in holding the eyes open should be evident.

Entropion (p. 202) or ectropion (p. 203) is usually evident without the eyelid margins. In the course of visiting with the patient the physician should observe whether the eyes move in unison and whether the movements are full.

More careful inspection may be carried out by means of a small penlight, which provides a concentrated beam of light upon the eye. Better visualization of details may be obtained if good illumination is combined with inspection through a +20 diopter convex lens (Fig. 6-1). This lens may also be used for indirect ophthalmoscopy and for inspection of skin lesions. Better magnification is provided by a binocular loupe that magnifies three to five times.

EXTERNAL EXAMINATION

Examination is carried out in a systematic manner beginning with the skin of the eyelids and continuing inward. The examiner first notices the symmetry and width of the palpebral fissures and the position of the eyes. The eyelids usually conceal the corneoscleral limbus in the 12 and 6 o'clock meridians. Proptosis (p. 240) or retraction of the upper eyelid in thyroid ophthalmopathy (p. 505) is often first manifested by exposure of a narrow rim of sclera above or below the corneoscleral limbus. Subtle proptosis and keratoconus (p. 257) are most easily appreciated by viewing the contact of the cornea with the lower eyelid from above and behind the patient. The examiner stands behind the seated patient and looks over his brow (Fig. 6-2). By drawing the upper eyelids upward, any difference in prominence of the two eyes is easily noted. In keratoconus the cornea distorts the lower eyelid outward (Munson sign).

Eyelid margin. The eyelashes (cilia) and the eyelid margin are inspected for

167

the characteristic scaling of squamous blepharitis (p. 210). Abnormalities in position of the eyelid margin are also noted at this time. Intermittent entropion may be demonstrated if the patient

squeezes his eyelids closed and then opens them. Particular attention is directed to the position of the puncta in relation to the lacrimal lake at the inner canthus (p. 58). The inferior punctum should not be seen when the eyes are rotated upward. A frequent cause of tearing is slight eversion of the puncta. Sties involve the eyelid margin, whereas chalazia usually appear in the deeper substance of the eyelid.

Conjunctiva. The bulbar conjunctiva may be inspected directly. The caruncle is evident as a minute pink mass of tissue at the inner canthus. The semilunar fold is not markedly evident unless the conjunctiva is inflamed. The superior and inferior portions of the bulbar conjunctiva are inspected easily by having the patient look upward and downward while the eyelids are drawn apart.

Eversion of the upper eyelid. Inspection of the upper tarsal conjunctiva requires eversion of the upper eyelid. While the patient looks down, the lashes of the upper eyelid are grasped by the examiner between the thumb and the index finger.

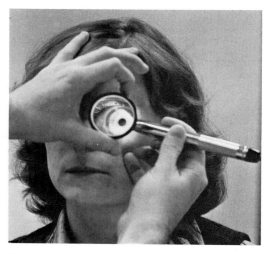

Fig. 6-1. Use of a penlight and a +20 diopter convex lens to study details of the anterior segment.

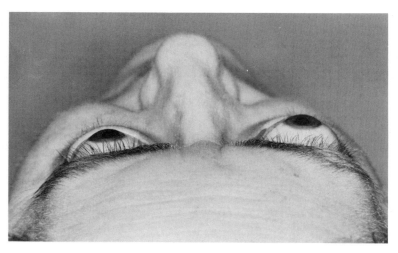

Fig. 6-2. Inspection of prominence of eyes by standing behind the patient, looking over the brow from above and behind, and elevating the upper eyelids. Note the proptosis of the right eye.

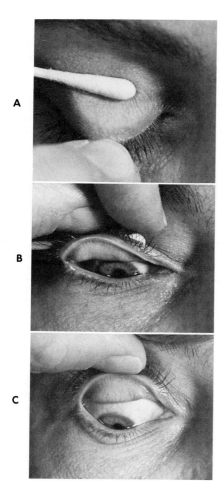

The eyelid is drawn gently outward to break the suction between the eyelid and the globe. The eyelid is then everted on a toothpick or applicator placed on the palpebral sulcus (Fig. 6-3). The tarsal conjunctiva is exposed, and the meibomian glands perpendicular to the eyelid margin may be seen through the transparent tarsal conjunctiva. Sometimes a small portion of the lacrimal gland may be seen at the outer canthus.

Eversion of the lower eyelid. Inspection of the lower eyelid is performed easily. The patient looks upward, and the eyelid is drawn downward by the examiner's index finger applied to its orbital portion (Fig. 6-4). The lower tarsus is not nearly as wide as the upper tarsus. With the exception of trachoma (p. 222) and vernal catarrh (p. 223), nearly all conjunctival inflammations are more marked in the inferior fornix than in the superior fornix.

Cornea. Attention is directed to the diameter and the clarity of the cornea. A cornea with a horizontal diameter of more than 12 mm may suggest congenital glaucoma or megalocornea (see Fig. 12-1). Extremely small corneas in the adult are suggestive of microcornea, with which

Fig. 6-3. Eversion of the upper eyelid. The patient is instructed to look downward, and the lashes of the upper eyelid are grasped between the thumb and index finger. **A,** A cotton-tipped applicator is placed at the level of the tarsal fold. **B,** The eyelid is then folded back on the cotton-tipped applicator while the patient continues to look downward. **C,** The applicator is then removed, and the details of the tarsal conjunctiva are inspected. The superior conjunctival fornix can be further studied if the eyelid is doubled over a speculum applied to the skin after single eversion.

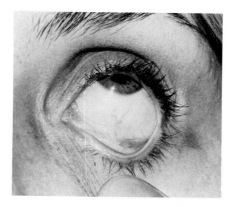

Fig. 6-4. Eversion of the lower eyelid by drawing the margin downward as the subject looks upward.

hyperopia and angle-closure glaucoma occur.

The evaluation of corneal clarity involves several factors. The anterior surface of the cornea should be smooth, regular, and mirrorlike. The iris pattern should be distinctly seen in all regions. Corneal blood vessels should not be present. In corneal edema, the cornea has a diffuse ground-glass appearance. Marked opacities are usually evident, but magnification is required for less severe defects. Corneal vascularization may be superficial or deep and may involve the entire cornea or merely a segment of it. Deep vascularization may be appreciated solely as a loss of corneal clarity; magnification is required to see the individual blood vessels. The corneoscleral limbus may be involved in corneal arcus, particularly in elderly individuals or in those with lipid disturbances. Staining of the cornea with fluorescein solution (sterile) (p. 128) may be required to demonstrate areas where epithelium is deficient.

Corneal sensitivity. The sensory innervation of the cornea is derived from the nasociliary branch of the ophthalmic division of the trigeminal nerve (N V) through the long ciliary nerves. Corneal sensitivity is tested clinically by means of a cotton-tipped applicator with a wisp of cotton drawn to a point. The patient is instructed to look directly ahead, and the cornea is touched with the cotton wisp. With normal innervation, an eyelid closure reflex follows almost immediately. Care must be taken not to touch the eyelashes or the eyelid margins with the cotton wisp and not to stimulate eyelid closure by allowing the patient to see the wisp. A different cotton-tipped applicator should be used for each eye.

Corneal sensitivity is reduced in herpes simplex inflammations of the cornea, following herpes zoster involving the nasociliary branch of the ophthalmic division of the trigeminal nerve, and in

adenovirus disease of the cornea. Corneal sensitivity may be reduced in lesions at the apex of the orbit, which may also be associated with involvement of motor nerves to the eye. Corneal anesthesia is an important sign in cerebellopontine angle tumors.

Anterior chamber. Normal aqueous humor is acellular and transparent. Even in severe uveal inflammations, good magnification is required to see inflammatory cells and a Tyndall phenomenon (flare) in the anterior chamber. Rarely, blood in the anterior chamber (hyphema) obscures the view of the iris. A severe leukocytic reaction may cause pus to collect in the inferior portion of the anterior chamber (hypopyon).

The depth of the anterior chamber is estimated as the distance between the posterior surface of the cornea and the front surface of the iris. Usually it measures 3 mm or more. If the iris appears to be convex and to parallel the posterior corneal surface and if the depth of the anterior chamber is less than 2 mm, there is a danger of angle-closure glaucoma (p. 404). Directing the beam of a penlight from the temporal side of the eye across the anterior chamber may demonstrate a narrow angle, since the iris may bow forward and cast a shadow on the opposite nasal side.

If a shallow anterior chamber is present, attention should be directed particularly (1) to episodes of blurring or fogging of vision or severe pain in an eye following movies, television, or prolonged darkness and (2) to occasional halos around lights (iridescent vision). Migraine, impending cerebral aneurysm rupture, or other diseases causing hemicrania may be erroneously diagnosed in patients with periodic attacks of angle-closure glaucoma.

Iris and pupil. The iris crypts and collarette should be clearly visible. Inability to see them suggests a corneal opacity, cells in the aqueous humor, or an iritis. A difference in color of the irises of the two eyes suggests the possibility of uveal inflammation, tumor, or an anomaly in the sympathetic innervation of the dilatator pupillae muscle, as occurs in Horner syndrome. A retained intraocular foreign body containing iron causes the iris to become brown. An absence of some portion of the iris (coloboma) may be surgical or congenital. Absence of the crystalline lens removes support from the iris, which becomes tremulous, a condition known as iridodonesis.

Attention is directed to the shape, size, reaction, and equality of the pupils. If the pupil is adherent to the cornea (adherent leukoma) or to the lens (posterior synechiae), it will not be circular. Minor inequalities in pupillary diameter, as occur in Horner and Adie syndromes and in Argyll Robertson pupils (p. 285), are often not diagnosed because of inadequate observation.

The direct pupillary response to light is measured by directing the light of a penlight into the eye and observing the pupillary constriction (p. 110). Each eye is measured separately. The pupillary response to convergence is not of diagnostic importance if the direct pupillary light reflex is present.

Lens. The transparent lens is observed by the image reflected from its anterior surface. Cataract may cause a gray, opaque appearance in the pupillary aperture. The lens is evaluated by means of the biomicroscope, but opacities are evident on ophthalmoscopic examination.

Ocular movements. The patient is instructed to look to the right, left, up, and down. Full movements indicate integrity of the third, fourth, and sixth cranial nerves. The patient is then directed to look at a penlight held about 13 inches in front of his eyes. Normally the image reflected from the cornea is approximately in the center of the pupil. The presence or absence of a phoria or tropia is determined by the cover test (p. 414) and using a small figure instead of a penlight.

Biomicroscopic examination. The ophthalmic slit lamp consists of a microscope that has approximately the same power as a laboratory dissecting microscope. Additionally, it projects a bright light beam shaped like a rectangle. When transmitted through the cornea or lens, the rectangle is seen as a parallelogram, and the examiner is able to appreciate the depth at which the abnormalities occur.

MEASUREMENT OF INTRAOCULAR PRESSURE

Intraocular pressure is directly measured by means of a cannula within the eye that is connected to a suitable transducer and amplifier. Such testing has been carried out in humans before removal of an eye because of disease, usually tumor. It must be done carefully so as not to disturb the normal pressure equilibrium of the eye by the loss of aqueous humor around the cannula or by excessive manipulation of the eye.

Clinical testing of the ocular tension is carried out by means of indentation tonometry, as is done with a Schiøtz tonometer (Figs. 6-5, *A*, and 20-1), or by applanation tonometry that requires a biomicroscope (Fig. 6-5, *B*). Noncontact tonometers measure tension by means of the deformation of the light reflex from the cornea caused by a puff of air.

The examiner palpates the eye through closed eyelids to estimate whether the eye is extremely hard or unusually soft (tactile tension). In practice the patient is instructed to look downward. The examiner then rests the fingers of both hands on the forehead and gently exerts alternate pressure on the globe through the upper eyelids with each index finger. The pressure should be directed to the globe and not to the orbit. The tension is estimated by the resistance encountered.

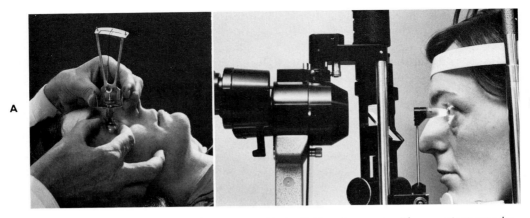

Fig. 6-5. A, Measurement of ocular tension with the Schiøtz tonometer. The examiner must be careful not to exert pressure on the globe through the eyelids. **B,** Measurement of the ocular tension with a Goldmann applanation tonometer. This method is more sensitive than Schiøtz tonometry, but it requires an expensive biomicroscope.

An extremely soft eye characterizes diabetic acidosis and penetrating injuries of the eye (a condition in which this measurement is contraindicated). Extremely high tensions occur most commonly in angle-closure and secondary glaucoma. Usually vision is markedly reduced. Accurate tension cannot be estimated in the intermediate ranges, and palpation is not recommended for determining the ocular tension.

CORNEAL STAINING

Epithelial defects of the cornea may be demonstrated by instillation of a 2% fluorescein solution (p. 128). The stroma in areas not covered by epithelium stains a brilliant green color. Fluorescein is a valuable agent in the diagnosis of foreign bodies, abrasions, and inflammations of the cornea, but it must be used solely as a sterile solution or as a sterile strip of filter paper stained with fluorescein solution and then dried.

Rose bengal (2%) is valuable for demonstrating loss of conjunctival and corneal epithelium in keratoconjunctivitis sicca (p. 268). It causes considerable discomfort. A local anesthetic used before its instillation causes minute epithelial defects that may be incorrectly interpreted.

Both dyes stain soft contact lenses and should not be used while lenses are worn.

RED EYE

Red eye is a cardinal sign of ocular inflammation. It is customarily divided into ciliary and conjunctival injection (Table 6-1).

Ciliary injection involves branches of the anterior ciliary artery that becomes dilated in inflammations of the cornea, iris, and ciliary body and in angle-closure glaucoma. Each of these conditions is associated with loss of vision and frequently with pain deep within the eye.

Conjunctival injection involves mainly the posterior conjunctival blood vessels that extend from the peripheral marginal arcade in the eyelid and anastomose with the anterior ciliary arteries at the corneoscleral limbus. The posterior conjunctival vessels are most numerous in the conjunctival fornix and are injected in conjunctival inflammations. There is never a loss of vision, and there is ocular discomfort

Table 6-1. Red eye

	Conjunctival injection	Ciliary injection
Blood vessels	Posterior conjunctival	Anterior ciliary
Location	Superficial conjunctiva, arise from marginal arcade in eyelids	Deep conjunctiva, extend anterior from rectus muscle insertion to superficial and deep corneal plexus
Appearance	Vessels superficial, red, removable with conjunctiva, most numerous in fornix, fade toward corneoscleral limbus	Vessels deep, violet, immovable, most numerous at corneoscleral limbus, fade toward fornix
1:1,000 epinephrine	Constricts vessels, "whitens" conjunctiva	No effect
Diseases	Conjunctivitis	Keratitis, iridocyclitis, angle-closure glaucoma
Associated signs	Cornea clear, pupil and iris normal, vision undisturbed, eye uncomfortable	Cornea cloudy, pupil distorted, iris pattern muddy, vision reduced, eye painful

rather than frank pain. Because the posterior conjunctival blood vessels are superficial, they are redder than the ciliary arteries, which are violet. The posterior conjunctival blood vessels move with the conjunctiva and are bleached on local instillation of 1:1,000 epinephrine.

Subconjunctival hemorrhage occurs with the rupture of a small blood vessel beneath the conjunctiva and causes a bright red blotch of blood beneath the conjunctiva that frequently alarms the patient. The condition is nearly always unilateral, and the hemorrhage absorbs spontaneously. It is caused for the most part by the same mechanisms that cause black-and-blue spots elsewhere. A subconjunctival hemorrhage that involves the entire bulbar conjunctiva following head injury is a serious sign and suggests either rupture of the posterior globe or a fracture of one of the bones of the orbit.

OPHTHALMOSCOPY

Inspection of the interior of the eye with the pupil dilated is fundamental to diagnosis and permits visualization of the optic disk, arteries, veins, retina, choroid, and media. There are three methods of viewing the ocular fundus: (1) direct ophthalmoscopy, by which a magnification of about 15 diameters is obtained; (2) indirect ophthalmoscopy, by which a larger field is obtained, but with magnification of 4 to 5 diameters; and (3) biomicroscopy combined with a lens to neutralize corneal refracting power.

Pupillary dilation. Adequate ophthalmoscopic examination of the ocular fundus requires dilation of the pupils. Without pupillary dilation, the optic disk and surrounding area (about 15% of the fundus) may be visualized (often with difficulty). With direct ophthalmoscopy and pupillary dilation about one half of the fundus may be seen. Examination of the entire fundus requires indirect ophthalmoscopy combined with pupillary dilation and scleral indentation.

For ophthalmoscopy in infants, pupils are dilated by using 2½% phenylephrine combined with 1% cyclopentolate. In individuals between 3 and 60 years of age, 10% phenylephrine may be combined with 1% tropicamide. Phenylephrine eye drops should not be used in individuals with vascular hypertension or in those receiving drugs that cause adrenergic blockade. After the age of 60 years 2½% phenylephrine may be combined with tropicamide. At the conclusion of ophthalmoscopic examination, 1% pilocarpine is instilled, and the examiner must be assured the pupils are beginning to constrict before he discharges the patient.

Caution is required in dilating the pupils of patients with shallow anterior chambers to avoid precipitating an attack of angle-closure glaucoma. There is greater danger, however, of missing significant ocular or systemic disease by failing to dilate the pupils than there is of precipitating glaucoma by dilation. The pupils should not be dilated if the patient has had an intraocular lens implant during cataract surgery. Soft contact lenses should be removed before instillation of dilating medications.

Direct ophthalmoscopy. Direct ophthalmoscopy (Fig. 6-6) provides an upright image of the retinal structures that is magnified about 15 times. Maximal pupillary dilation makes it possible to study the ocular fundus as far as an area slightly anterior to the equator—the area between the equator and the ora serrata cannot be seen. The maximum resolving power is about 70μ, and objects smaller than this, such as capillaries, small hemorrhages, or microaneurysms, are not seen. The illumination by the modern direct ophthalmoscope is so bright that some translucent structures, particularly opacities in the media, may not be seen, and other features, such as copper-wire arteries, do not have the color described in classic reports.

Technique. The patient is examined in a dimly illuminated or dark room. A fixation light is provided so that the patient does not look at the ophthalmoscope light. It is preferable to examine the patient while he is seated. If the examiner wears correcting lenses constantly, he should become accustomed to wearing them when learning to do ophthalmoscopy. Patients who have more than 5 diopters of refractive error ease visualization if they wear their lenses during ophthalmoscopy.

The examiner examines the patient's right eye with his own right eye and the patient's left eye with his own left eye. The ophthalmoscope is held in the corresponding hand. The examiner sits or stands to the side of the eye to be examined. The head of the ophthalmoscope is steadied in the mediosuperior margin of the examiner's bony orbit. His index finger is used to change lenses. The examiner's free hand rests at his side.

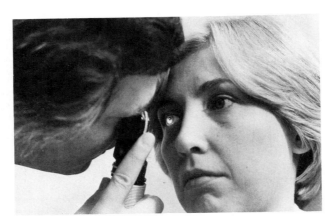

Fig. 6-6. Direct ophthalmoscopy of a patient's right eye. The examiner uses his right eye for observation. The ophthalmoscope is held steady in the right bony orbit and held in the right hand when the right eye is studied; the index finger is used to change lenses.

Usually it is not necessary to elevate the patient's eyelid for an adequate view.

The texture and detail of the retina and the blood vessels are appreciated by constantly focusing the ophthalmoscope lens for superficial and deep views, much as one adjusts a microscope when studying a tissue section.

Accessories such as slits, special filters, colored lenses, and reticules are seldom useful to the novice ophthalmoscopist, and when used by the experienced examiner, they are usually combined with special attachments.

A +10 diopter lens is rotated onto the viewing aperture of the ophthalmoscope, and the patient looks at a fixation object. The examiner directs the ophthalmoscopic light into the eye at a distance of about 20 cm. A red fundus reflex will be observed. Any opacities in the ocular media will stand out as black silhouettes against a red background. Keeping his attention directed to the red reflex, the examiner gradually approaches the patient's eye while steadily decreasing the power of the ophthalmoscope lens. Once fundus details are seen, a blood vessel is followed to its origin at the optic disk, and the systematic examination usually begins with the optic disk.

Indirect ophthalmoscopy. Indirect ophthalmoscopy (Fig. 6-7) is carried out by means of a mirror with a central perforation. Light is directed into the eye, and the emerging rays are observed through the opening in the mirror. The image formed by the emerging rays is observed by means of a convex lens of +10 to +20 diopter power. A binocular indirect ophthalmoscope worn on the examiner's head permits him to use his hands to depress the sclera near the ora serrata in order to observe the extreme retinal periphery. Thus the entire retina from the disk to the ora serrata may be inspected. The indirect ophthalmoscope provides an inverted image that is magnified about

five times. The field of observation is much larger than that seen with the direct ophthalmoscope, and a stereoscopic image may be seen with the binocular instrument. The maximum resolving power is about 200μ, and small hemorrhages or microaneurysms are not seen. The stereoscopic image of the binocular instrument combined with parallax permits detection and appreciation of details not evident with the direct ophthalmoscope. This method of ophthalmoscopy is particularly useful when there are opacities in the media.

Biomicroscopy. The biomicroscope may

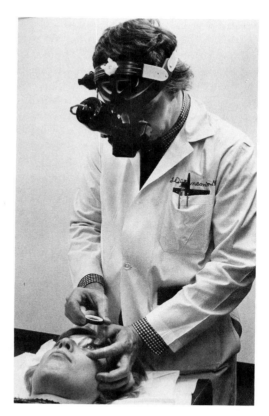

Fig. 6-7. Indirect opthalmoscopy using a binocular ophthalmoscope. This method provides visualization of the ocular fundus as far as the ora serrata.

be combined with a −55 diopter concave lens to neutralize the corneal refraction for study of the retina. Its particular value is increased magnification combined with oblique illumination for more accurate estimation of the depth of lesions. The contact lens may be fitted with mirrors so that, with adequate pupillary dilation, it is possible to study the retinal periphery.

THE FUNDUS

The red background of the fundus results from the blood in the choriocapillaris of the choroid, the visibility of which varies with the amount of melanin in the retinal pigment epithelium. The pigment usually parallels the complexion of the individual. In lightly pigmented persons, choroidal veins can be seen. The arteries supplying the choroid go almost directly to the choriocapillaris, and the major portion of the choroid is composed of freely anastomosing veins (p. 15) that are the ophthalmoscopically visible choroidal vessels. In some patients the contrast between choroidal pigment and blood viewed through a moderately pigmented retinal epithelium gives rise to a tessellated or tigroid fundus.

The optic disk is about 1.5 mm in diameter. The diameter of the disk is the standard unit of measurement in the fundus. The disk appears to be approximately the same size in most patients. Marked enlargement in the size of the disk suggests a conus or a posterior staphyloma. The disk appears smaller than normal when the lens is absent (aphakia).

The disk has a pale pink color, except for the physiologic cup (Fig. 20-3), which is nearly white. The edges of the disk are usually flat and sharp, but not uncommonly the nasal margin is less distinct than the temporal margin. Pigment may be visible, particularly on the temporal side, sometimes as a continuous arc and at other times as linear streaks concentric with the disk. This is called the choroidal ring and is of no pathologic significance. Slightly more uncommon is an arc of stark white tissue on the temporal side of the disk, a scleral ring, which may occur in degenerative myopia. It is often combined with a choroidal ring.

The physiologic cup of the optic disk is a funnel-shaped depression of varying size and shape. In some cases it is located nearly at the center of the disk, and grayish areas of the lamina cribrosa are evident. In other eyes it has a more oblique course. The ratio of the horizontal diameter of the cup to the horizontal diameter of the disk is of significance in glaucoma (p. 396). Irrespective of the position of the physiologic cup, there is always a rim of nerve tissue between the cup and the edge of the disk in the healthy eye. Occasionally, the area usually occupied by the physiologic cup is filled with glial tissue that may extend for a short distance over the arteries and the veins. This glial tissue should not be mistaken for vascular sheathing.

The bifurcation of the central retinal artery into its superior and inferior branches may be observed on the surface of the optic disk or slightly within the optic cup. The central vein usually bifurcates a little deeper within the optic nerve and has a pulsation nearly synchronous with the heart. When this physiologic pulsation is not present, it may be elicited by a very slight increase in intraocular pressure induced by pressing the globe with the index finger through the eyelids. In the healthy eye the central retinal artery does not pulsate, and the occurrence of pulsation indicates either an extremely high pulse pressure, as occurs in aortic regurgitation, or an increased intraocular pressure. Each of the papillary branches of the central artery divides into a nasal and a temporal branch. These branches do not have a continuous muscle coat or an internal elastic lamella and are thus arterioles

(p. 32). In the healthy eye the walls of the vessels are never visible. Instead, the column of blood is observed through a transparent tube.

The retinal arterioles have a smaller diameter than the venules, the usual ratio of arteriole to venule being 3:4 or 2:3. A broad, bright streak is reflected from the convex surface of arterioles. The reflection from venules is much narrower and not nearly as bright. The oxygenated blood is much brighter red in the arterioles than in the veins. In a complete examination of the fundus, the superior and inferior temporal and nasal arteries are followed as far to the periphery as they can be seen.

In the usual ophthalmoscopic examination, final attention is directed to the central retina (Fig. 6-8). This is about 6 mm in diameter and anatomically corresponds to an area in which the ganglion cell layer is more than one cell nucleus thick. The fovea centralis is stituated about 2 disk diameters (3 mm) temporal to the optic

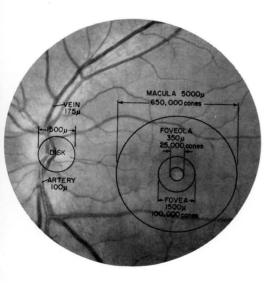

Fig. 6-8. Posterior pole of the left retina. (In illustrations of the left retina, the optic nerve is to the observer's left.)

disk. Usually pupillary dilation is required for careful examination of this area inasmuch as pupillary constriction is marked when the fovea is illuminated. Within the fovea centralis is the foveola, which measures 400μ to 500μ in diameter and corresponds to the capillary-free area of the central retina. The temporal blood vessels arch above and below the central retina.

The area surrounding the fovea centralis extending to the temporal vessels above and below and about 3 mm on either side has a yellowish pigmentation in primates. It is best observed in a sectioned eye, and it persists for about 15 minutes after the eye has been deprived of its blood supply. The area is called the macula lutea (yellow spot), and thus the posterior pole is frequently loosely called the "macula."

FLUORESCEIN ANGIOGRAPHY

Fluorescein angiography plays an important role in ophthalmoscopic diagnosis. Unlike light ophthalmoscopy, in which light is reflected from the column of blood within the blood vessel, the fluorescein emits light so that the entire diameter of a vessel can be seen. After the intravascular injection of a solution of 10% sodium fluorescein, ophthalmoscopy using a blue filter to excite the fluorescence (fluorescein angiography) is useful in detecting leaking capillaries, but the absence of a permanent record limits its value. Photography of the ocular fundus during fluorescein angiography, however, provides much information concerning vascular obstructions, neovascularization, microaneurysms, abnormal capillary permeability, and defects of the retinal pigment epithelium.

For fluorescein angiography, sensitive black-and-white film is used, and a filter is placed in front of the light source to furnish blue light, which excites the fluorescence. The emitted light is green, and a green filter is placed in front of the film carrier. A control photograph is first made to record intrinsic fluorescence of the fundus. Then 5 ml of a 10% solution of sodium fluorescein solution is rapidly injected into the antecubital vein. Patients experience a hot flash and sometimes nausea; equipment to manage an occasional severe allergic reaction adequately must be on hand. The fluorescein is excreted in the urine and feces during the subsequent 48 hours.

The fluorescein may be seen coursing through the retinal arteries 10 to 13 seconds after injection (Fig. 6-9, A). If the patient is blond or albino, the filling of the choriocapillaris gives a background mottled appearance except in the central retina, where the lipofuscin of the retinal pigment epithelium blocks fluorescence. During capillary filling there is a nearly simultaneous laminar type of flow in the veins, so that the dye first appears to be in the peripheral portion of the vessels (Fig. 6-9, B). Finally, the veins and arteries are both filled with the dye. One minute after injection the vessels still fluoresce slightly, and choroidal veins may be seen as black segments against a slight scleral fluorescence (Fig. 6-9, C).

Abnormal vascular permeability permits the pooling of fluorescein in the choroid, retina, or vitreous, and such areas may fluoresce for several hours after the injection. The accurate localization of such "leaks" may allow treatment by

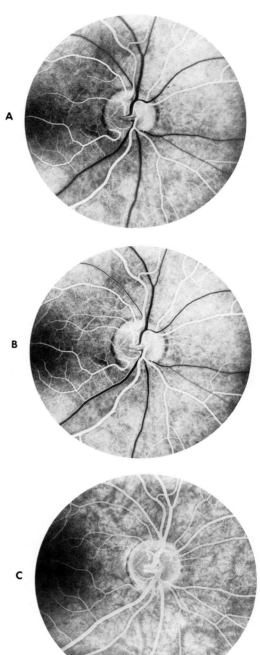

Fig. 6-9. Fluorescein angiography of the right fundus. **A,** The arterial phase after fluorescein injection. The mottled background fluorescence results from filling of the choroid. **B,** The early venous phase. There is filling of some capillaries of the retina, and a laminar flow is evident in the veins. The choriocapillaris is filled, causing a background fluorescence. **C,** The late venous phase. The retinal vessels fluoresce less markedly and contain fluorescein diluted by mixing in the blood. The choroidal veins may be seen as black lines contrasting with scleral fluorescence.

means of xenon or laser photocoagulation.

ULTRASONOGRAPHY

Sound waves with frequencies of more than 18,000 Hz are used in the diagnosis of both intraocular and orbital tumors. The ultrasound is reflected toward its source when it encounters a change in elasticity or density of the medium through which it is passing. This reflected vibration (echo) is converted into an electrical potential by a piezoelectrical crystal and displayed on a cathode ray oscillograph.

Two types of ultrasonography are used. The A-scan measures the time or distance of changes in acoustic impedance from the transducer as well as acoustic density. The change is shown as a spike on the tracing. It is particularly useful in evaluating the density of intraocular tumors to suggest the histologic type. The B-scan moves in a linear fashion across the eye, and any change in acoustic impedance is shown as an intensification on the line of the scan that builds up a picture of the eye and the orbit (Fig. 6-10).

COMPUTED TOMOGRAPHY

Computed tomography (Fig. 6-11) has largely supplanted conventional roentgenography in the diagnosis of orbital disease. Additionally, intraocular masses can be visualized. A crystal detector is substituted for conventional film, and the skull is scanned through 180° in a path 1 cm wide. The signal from the detector undergoes Fourier analysis to produce a picture some 100 times more accurate

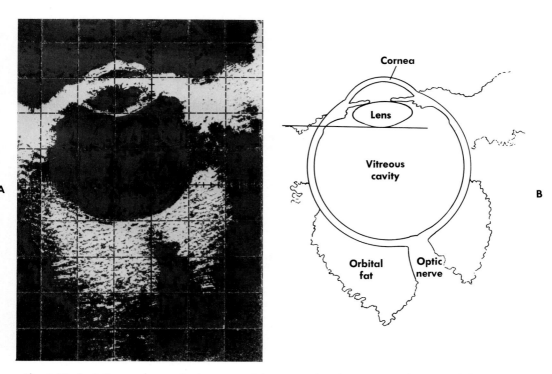

Fig. 6-10. A, A B-scan demonstrating parts of the eye and optic nerve. **B,** The parts of the eye demonstrated.

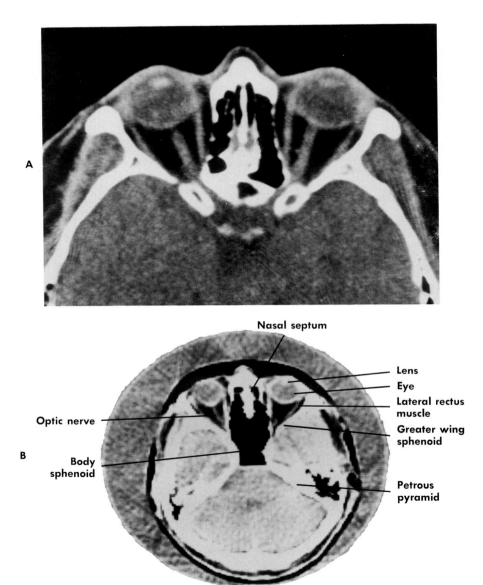

Fig. 6-11. A, Computed tomography of the orbit. The eye, optic nerve, and medial and lateral recti muscles are clearly seen, well outlined by the radiolucent orbital fat. The radiodense area within the anterior portion of each eye is the crystalline lens. This section was prepared with the AS&E scanner, which uses 600 detectors and forms an image with a 512 × 512 matrix. (Courtesy Sadek K. Hilal, Professor of Radiology, Neurological Institute, New York.) **B,** The bony landmarks of computed tomography.

han conventional roentgenograms. The orbits can be contrasted, and the globe, optic nerve, fat, and various tumors are outlined because of their differences in tissue density. The examination is augmented by the intravenous injection of soluble contrast material that increases the density of vascularized orbital lesions.

BIBLIOGRAPHY

Arger, P. H., editor: Orbit roentgenology, New York, 1977, John Wiley & Sons, Inc.

Baker, H. L., Jr., Kearnes, T. P., Campbell, J. K., and Henderson, J. W.: Computerized transaxial tomography in neuro-ophthalmology, Am. J. Ophthalmol. **78:**285, 1974.

Bronson, N. R. II: Contact B-scan ultrasonography, Am. J. Ophthalmol. **77:**181, 1974.

Bronson, N. R. II, Fisher, Y. L., Pickering, N. C., and Trayner, E. M.: Ophthalmic contact B-scan ultrasonography for the clinician, Westport, Conn., 1976, Intercontinental Publications, Inc.

Coleman, D. J., Lizzi, F. L., and Jack, R. L.: Ultrasonography of the eye and orbit, Philadelphia, 1977, Lea & Febiger.

Jack, R. L., Hutton, W. L., and Machemer, R.: Ultrasonography and vitrectomy, Am. J. Ophthalmol. **78:**265, 1974.

New, P. F. J., and Scott, W. R.: Computer tomography of the brain and orbit (EMI scanning), Baltimore, 1975, William & Wilkins Co.

Schatz, H., Burton, T. C., Yannuzzi, L. A., and Rabb, M. F.: Interpretation of fundus fluorescein angiography, St. Louis, 1977, The C. V. Mosby Co.

PART THREE

Diseases and injuries of the eye

Chapter 7

INJURIES OF THE EYE

Prompt and appropriate care of common injuries may prevent much visual disability and, in some instances, the necessity for major corrective surgery. If the patient's general physical condition permits, one should attempt to learn whether vision is present and whether the eye is grossly distorted. Every effort must be made to prevent marked squeezing of the eyelids by the patient or pressure on the globes by the examiner.

Except in chemical burns, when immediate dilution is imperative, vision should be measured in each eye as carefully as conditions will permit. Many patients do not realize they have defective vision in one eye until there is injury, and they may wrongfully accuse the physician of damage that has existed for many years. It is not necessary to use a testing chart—a newspaper or a telephone book will indicate how much vision is present. If the vision is markedly impaired, finger counting, hand motion, and light projection and perception may be tested (p. 160).

If the cornea is lacerated and there is distortion of the pupil or inability to see the iris, or if scleral lacerations are present, both eyes should be covered with a large dressing with no pressure on the globe. The patient should be given parenteral analgesics for pain (aspirin should *not* be used) and should be evacuated supine upon a litter to a facility for special care.

If the globes are intact, additional treatment is indicated.

If the patient is anesthetized for nonocular injuries, eyelid and conjunctival debris may be carefully irrigated away by using a sterile irrigating solution, preferably Ringer or normal saline solution. This should be followed by the generous topical application of sterile solutions of an ophthalmic antibiotic. Wounds of the face and eyelids should not be debrided. The eye should not be occluded or patched.

FOREIGN BODIES
Cornea

Foreign bodies on the surface of the cornea constitute about 25% of all ocular injuries. A history of the injury and the probable character of the foreign body help in its detection and removal.

The symptoms vary from little or no discomfort to severe pain. Usually there is a sensation of a foreign body that the patient localizes, inaccurately, to the outer portion of the upper eyelid. There may be associated tearing, photophobia, and ciliary injection.

The foreign body may be seen by careful inspection of the cornea, preferably aided by magnification with a loupe or a magnifying glass. Sterile 2% fluorescein solution instilled in the eye stains and demarcates the foreign body in the cornea. Corneal foreign bodies should be removed entirely to permit re-epithelization and to relieve pain. Topical anesthesia must be used to prevent pain and eyelid closure during removal.

An attempt should be made to remove the foreign body by means of irrigation. A bulb-type syringe or a hypodermic syringe without a needle is used with sterile saline solution as the irrigating fluid. Foreign bodies that are not hot when they strike the eye usually may be removed by directing a stream of fluid against the foreign body so as to float it off the cornea. This method is often used by physicians' assistants.

If the foreign body cannot be removed by irrigation, it usually cannot be removed by means of a cotton-tipped applicator, which removes much normal epithelium and is, therefore, undesirable. Less injury is caused if the foreign body is lifted gently out of the corneal substance by means of a sharp instrument. Ophthalmologists often use a biomicroscope to provide adequate illumination and magnification, but good visualization can be obtained with a binocular loupe. A sterile spud designed for this purpose or, in an emergency, a 25- to 27-gauge hypodermic needle fitted to a 2-ml syringe may be used. The instrument is held tangent to the cornea so that the cornea will not be perforated if the patient lunges forward. The spud gently elevates the foreign body off the cornea. If a ferrous metal has been embedded for several days, a rust ring may remain after the removal of the main portion of the foreign body; this is removed in the same manner as the foreign body. If it cannot be removed easily at the first attempt, frequently it can be lifted out entirely 24 hours later when leukocytes have softened the surrounding corneal tissue.

After removal of a corneal foreign body, a solution (not ointment) of a sulfonamide such as sulfacetamide or an antibiotic mixture such as polymyxin B sulfate (Neosporin) is instilled. A dressing is applied to the eye to immobilize the eyelids and prevent discomfort resulting from blinking. The dressing is not required if it causes discomfort. In the absence of keratitis, local medications to cause pupillary dilation are not used. If marked ciliary congestion and photophobia are present or if the removal of the foreign body has been particularly difficult, a cycloplegic such as 5% homatropine is instilled. Atropine causes prolonged pupillary dilation and cycloplegia and is usually not indicated. Inasmuch as a foreign body may introduce microorganisms into the cornea, the eye should be inspected for infection each day until the area no longer stains with sterile fluorescein. Foreign bodies that injure only the corneal epithelium do not cause a scar. Scarring follows injuries to the Bowman membrane or to the substantia propria.

Conjunctiva

Foreign bodies of the conjunctiva can always be removed with irrigation, a spud, or a cotton-tipped applicator.

Foreign bodies frequently lodge on the upper tarsal conjunctiva at its peripheral margin. The upper eyelid must be everted (p. 169) to remove them. The physician must be prepared to remove the foreign body when he everts the eyelid, because the foreign body may be dislodged and difficult to locate again if the eyelid is released.

Intraocular

Intraocular foreign bodies follow injuries in which small particles penetrate the cornea or the sclera. Large foreign bodies cause marked disruption of the globe and so much associated injury that the eye is destroyed and eventually enucleation may be required. Foreign bodies composed of vegetable material such as wood or plants may introduce infection that causes a severe purulent panophthalmitis to occur within hours. Many intraocular foreign bodies are small and are sterilized by the heat caused by their high velocity. They mainly consist of small bits of metal, glass, plastics, and similar material. Their nature varies with the types of industry and recreation of the locality.

The diagnosis and treatment depend on the following factors.

1. *Size of the foreign body.* A foreign body must have a minimal density and size to be demonstrated by means of roentgen-ray examination. A number of special techniques have been developed to diagnose and localize foreign bodies by means of roentgen rays. These have been supplemented by devices for locating metal that indicate also whether or not the foreign body is magnetic. Computed tomography may be most helpful.

2. *Magnetic properties.* Only nickel and iron may be removed by means of a magnet, and for this reason it is important to determine whether the tool or other material from which the foreign body originated is magnetic.

3. *Tissue reaction.* Many plastics, stainless steel, and glass do not oxidize, and other materials such as aluminum hydroxide oxidize slowly and if retained cause minimal damage to the eye. Often such foreign bodies are not removed. Iron slowly oxidizes within the eye and combines with the protein of the intraocular tissues (siderosis) to form an irreversible ferrous compound that results in gradual loss of vision of the eye. The electroretinographic response of the eye is reduced before there is a decrease in visual acuity or a change in the appearance of the retina and foreign body. Unlike siderosis, the tissue reaction caused by retention of copper particles (chalcosis) is reversible if the particle is removed. However, copper is much more rapidly injurious to the eye. An intraocular foreign body must always be considered in

any patient with uveitis in whom there is a history of injury. Rarely, a foreign body is enmeshed in scar tissue, metallic ions are not released within the eye, and retention of the foreign body causes no symptoms.

4. *Location within the eye.* Foreign bodies in the anterior chamber may be directly observed, although gonioscopy is required to see them in the chamber angle recess. Small metallic foreign bodies within the lens may be tolerated for a long period. However, severe injury to the lens capsule leads quickly to cataract formation. Foreign bodies in the vitreous body and retina are often obscured by hemorrhage but sometimes may be demonstrated by means of ophthalmoscopy, particularly by using the indirect ophthalmoscope.

Retained foreign bodies must be suspected in all instances of perforating wounds of the eye. If the point of entry is extremely small, high magnification may be required to see the wound in the cornea or the iris. Minute wounds in the sclera are nearly invisible. Roentgenograms or computed tomography (p. 179) of the orbit is indicated in all such injuries to assure absence of foreign bodies.

Once the presence of a foreign body has been established within the eye, removal is indicated unless the trauma of surgery is more severe than the damage caused by retention of the foreign body. The foreign body is initially localized by means of roentgen rays. The corneoscleral limbus approach is used for anterior segment foreign bodies. Foreign bodies in the posterior ocular segment are removed through the sclera at the pars plana. In removal through the sclera, the foreign body is first localized and the sclera exposed in the quadrant nearest the foreign body. An electronic metal localizer is then used to refine the localization of the foreign body, and a scratch incision is made in the sclera close to it. A suture is placed in the incision but left untied and looped out of the field. A magnet is then applied, and the foreign body is removed. The suture is tied quickly. The incision is then surrounded by cryotherapy.

Nonmagnetic foreign bodies are removed by a combination of vitrectomy and suction or by foreign body forceps through the pars plana.

Early removal is important inasmuch as foreign bodies may become enmeshed in fibrin and may be difficult to remove after the lapse of a long period. However, it is probably better to delay treatment until specialized facilities are available than to attempt removal without the benefit of diagnostic devices.

LACERATIONS
Eyelids

Lacerations of the eyelids are divided into two groups: (1) those that are parallel to the eyelid margin and hence do not gape and (2) those that involve the eyelid margin and are drawn apart by traction of the fibers of the orbicularis oculi muscle (Fig. 7-1, A). Eyelid margin lacerations involving the inner one sixth of the eyelid sever the canaliculus and are particularly troublesome to repair (p. 57). Children's eyelids are often heavily lacerated by dog bites and scratches. If no tissue is missing, surgical correction can be surprisingly effective (Fig. 7-1, B).

All wounds of the eyelid must be meticulously cleaned with soap and water. Care must be taken not to irritate the conjunctiva and the cornea. Even though markedly contused and damaged, skin is not excised from the laceration, because the excellent blood supply assures survival.

Lacerations parallel to eyelid margins require no specialized treatment and are closed with fine sutures. The laceration is parallel to the normal skin folds, and no conspicuous defect results.

Vertical lacerations are divided into those involving the outer five sixths of the eyelid (ciliary) margin and those involving the inner one sixth of the eyelid (lacrimal) margin, which avulse the canaliculi leading to the tear sac.

Ciliary margin. In those lacerations involving the outer five sixths of the eyelid

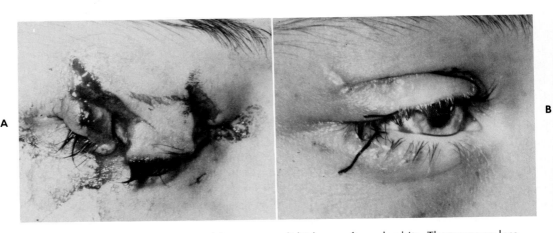

Fig. 7-1. A, Multiple lacerations of the upper eyelid 3 hours after a dog bite. There was no loss of tissue. **B,** Repaired eyelid 7 days later. The long sutures are in the gray line of the eyelid margin.

margin, the key to successful repair is the placement of the first suture through the gray line of the eyelid to unite both edges of the laceration with the eyelid margin in the proper plane (Fig. 7-2). Once the eyelid margin is closed properly, the remainder of the eyelid can be closed in layers, using catgut sutures for the tarsus and silk for the skin. The sutures are not tied on the conjunctival surface of the tarsus where they will irritate the cornea. Unless other injuries are so serious that treatment must be delayed, it is better not to procrastinate, for a delay of even 24 hours may be followed by retraction of the wound edges, and major plastic surgery may be required for repair.

Lacrimal margin. Lacerations of the inner one sixth of the eyelid in which the canaliculus is severed require (1) placement of a stent through the canaliculus in the hope that it will remain patent, (2) closure of the laceration, and (3) prevention of traction by the mass orbicularis oculi muscle located lateral to the laceration. The stent, usually a stainless steel

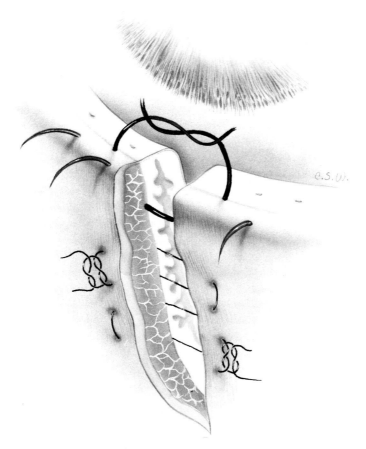

Fig. 7-2. Repair of a laceration of the eyelid by means of a suture through the gray line. The suture is usually double-armed, and each needle enters the tissue through the laceration and emerges through the gray line. Once the eyelid margin is approximated without a notch, the skin may be closed with interrupted silk sutures. It is not necessary to close the conjunctiva.

rod, must be left in place 10 to 21 days. Simple closure of an eyelid laceration causes a typical notched defect of the eyelid margin and constant tearing. Even with highly expert repair, it may not be possible to unite the avulsed ends of a lacerated canaliculus, and additional surgery may be required to correct tearing.

Lacerations of the inner one third of the upper eyelid may damage the trochlea of the superior oblique muscle. This may be followed by either paresis of the superior oblique muscle or a contracture that impairs elevation of the eye when adducted.

Conjunctiva

Lacerations of the bulbar conjunctiva that do not involve the globe are rarely severe enough to require closure. With such injuries, the physician must be certain there is no associated laceration of the sclera. Usually the lacerated conjunctiva is surrounded by an area of subconjunctival hemorrhage, and the laceration is evident as a white, crescentic area. Fluorescein will stain the margins of the laceration. The eye is uncomfortable, but there is no loss of vision.

Cornea

Lacerating wounds of the cornea, unless of a puncture type, are followed by prolapse of the iris, which closes the wound. A characteristic teardrop distortion of the pupil is present. In severe lacerations there may be frank prolapse of the iris, ciliary body, lens, and vitreous body, causing a completely disorganized globe.

Once the diagnosis of a perforating wound of the globe has been established, further examination should be made only by those responsible for surgical correction. Corneal lacerations are frequently associated with retained intraocular foreign bodies, traumatic cataract, secondary glaucoma, infection, and late complications, so that treatment should be carried

out by those able to manage the responsibility of the aftercare. First aid is limited to the diagnosis of the condition. A delay of up to 24 hours is preferable to inexpert examination. A broad-spectrum antibiotic is administered systemically in large doses. Tetanus toxoid, 0.5 ml, should be given if the patient has been previously immunized. A booster dose is not necessary if the patient has been immunized within 10 years or received a booster dose within 10 years, or within 3 years if the wound is severe and conducive to anaerobic infection. If immunization has been done within the year, tetanus toxoid is not indicated.

The history of the injury and examination of the eye frequently suggest whether a foreign body is retained. Careful roentgen-ray study may indicate metallic foreign bodies. Local anesthesia may be adequate for repair, but if there has been severe trauma, general anesthesia is preferable. Rapid induction is necessary so that there will be no struggling, which increases the intraocular pressure and enhances prolapse of intraocular contents. Succinylcholine must not be used as a muscle relaxant, because it causes a transient increase in the intraocular pressure.

The method of repair depends on the severity of the injury. When the corneal laceration is sharply defined, it is closed with direct appositional sutures. When the wound edges are contused or when there has been a loss of corneal tissue, immediate corneal transplantation is done by using preserved cadaver cornea. The corneal wound edges are sutured after the prolapsed iris is either excised or replaced in the eye. Inasmuch as the tissue may introduce infection into the eye, many surgeons favor iridectomy despite the resulting cosmetic defect. More severe injuries involving the lens and vitreous are treated by immediate reconstruction of the anterior segment with lens removal and excision of vitreous. The laceration is then meticulously repaired with fine sutures. Such eyes must be carefully observed and removed if the potential for vision does not outweigh the danger of sympathetic ophthalmia.

Sclera

Careful inspection of corneal lacerations is necessary, because they may extend into the sclera and be covered by intact conjunctiva. Involvement of the ciliary body invariably leads to some loss of the vitreous body combined with damage to the zonule of the lens. Such lacerations are much more likely to produce severe damage to the eye than those involving only the cornea. To repair, the lacerated area is exposed by dissecting the cut edges of the conjunctiva and Tenon capsule from the scleral laceration. The first suture is placed exactly at the corneoscleral limbus. Prolapsed uveal tissue is then excised, and the laceration is closed with interrupted sutures. The conjunctiva is closed separately.

If the lens has been injured, it is removed, and a partial anterior vitrectomy may be performed by introducing a small-bore vitrectomy instrument into the eye through the laceration.

SYMPATHETIC UVEITIS

Sympathetic uveitis (sympathetic ophthalmia) is a rare, bilateral, diffuse, granulomatous inflammation of the entire uveal tract that usually follows perforation of the eye. The etiology is unknown, but the disease may be an autoimmune hypersensitivity reaction to uveal pigment. Histologically there is a diffuse inflammation of the uvea but not of the choriocapillaris or sensory retina. Lymphocytes and epithelial cells occur almost exclusively with uveal pigment phagocytized by the epithelioid cells. Epithelioid cells accumulate between the retinal pigment epithelium and Bruch membrane (Dalen-Fuchs nodules).

Most cases develop within 3 months of injury, although it may take from 5 days to many years. The injured eye (the exciting eye) exhibits a torpid, persistent, granulomatous type of uveitis that is then followed by a similar uveitis in the fellow eye (the sympathizing eye). The inflammation may be suppressed by corticosteroids or other immune suppression, which may have to be continued for many months or years. Enucleation of the exciting eye is futile once the fellow eye has become inflamed. Sympathetic ophthalmia does not occur if the injured eye is removed within 7 to 14 days after the injury. Inasmuch as sympathetic ophthalmia does not occur immediately after an injury, irrespective of the severity of the ocular damage, it is never necessary to enucleate an injured eye as an emergency procedure.

CONCUSSION INJURIES

Apparently minor blunt trauma to the eye and orbit may result in surprisingly severe injury. Hemorrhage into the eyelids is in itself usually of little import but may be associated with fractures of the orbital bones. Usually these may be diagnosed by observing the asymmetry of the face and by gently palpating the orbital structures.

A severe subconjunctival hemorrhage and a persistently soft globe after a severe contusion suggest the possibility of a rupture of the posterior sclera. If the hemorrhage involves the entire conjunctiva with bleeding into the eyelids, there is possibly a fracture of a wall of the orbit.

The cornea may be abraded in contusion injuries, but this is usually not serious and heals quickly. The sphincter pupillae muscle may be ruptured, and if so, the pupil is semidilated and does not react to light or accommodation (iridoplegia). In relatively minor contusion injuries there may be minute ruptures of the sphincter so that the pupil is no longer round. In more severe injuries the outer edge of the iris may be torn from its insertion to the scleral spur, giving rise to iridodialysis. This may be so minute as to be visible only with a gonioscope, or it may involve a major portion of the insertion of the iris. An extensive iridodialysis is repaired by suturing the peripheral edge of the iris into a corneoscleral wound. Correction is not indicated unless the iridodialysis is extensive or if diplopia is present because of the additional pupil.

Contusion of the globe may cause rupture of a portion of the zonule of the lens, causing the lens to become subluxated (p. 376). The vitreous body bulges into the anterior chamber through the ruptured area. The lens is seldom markedly displaced, and it is rarely necessary to remove it. Curiously, lens subluxation is most common in individuals with syphilis. As years pass, the lens may become opaque. A transient lens opacity may also occur immediately after a blunt injury to the globe.

Glaucoma may develop 10 to 20 years after ocular contusion. The glaucoma resembles open-angle glaucoma except that it is monocular. Gonioscopic examination indicates that a sector of the anterior chamber angle is much deeper (angle recession) than other regions. Often the patient no longer recalls the injury. Blunt contusion of the eye may be the main cause of monocular open-angle glaucoma in the adult. It is a secondary type of open-angle glaucoma.

·Contusion may cause the release of a large amount of pigment into the anterior chamber, and this may give rise to the appearance of an iritis. There are no keratic precipitates, and posterior synechiae do not form.

Choroidal and retinal hemorrhage, edema, and necrosis following blunt trauma are discussed elsewhere (pp. 309 and 352).

Traumatic hyphema

Contusion injuries of the globe frequently are followed by frank bleeding into the anterior chamber. This blood usually does not clot and, with bed rest, settles at the most dependent portion of the anterior chamber, and a fluid meniscus forms (Fig. 7-3). Frequently the original hyphema, which may be relatively minor, is followed by more severe bleeding 24 to 48 hours after the original injury. A secondary glaucoma may occur immediately or many years later. Aspirin should never be used in treatment, because secondary hemorrhage is far more frequent after aspirin administration.

If the anterior chamber is not entirely filled with blood, spontaneous recovery will probably take place if there is no secondary hemorrhage, irrespective of the treatment. Binocular patching, sedation, and bed rest are often effective. After 96 hours, corticosteroids may be used locally to minimize the traumatic uveitis. If a recurrent hemorrhage occurs that does not fill the anterior chamber, similar treatment is effective.

Secondary glaucoma developing when the anterior chamber is only partially filled with blood is likely the result of vasodilation and is treated by means of systemic acetazolamide. Oral glycerol or intravenous mannitol usually do not reduce pressure permanently.

Secondary glaucoma developing when the anterior chamber is filled with blood often causes blood staining of the cornea. The posterior stroma is infiltrated with hemosiderin, giving rise to a deep yellowish-greenish opacity of the cornea. Clearing occurs at the periphery, but a central corneal opacity remains. The blood must be removed from the anterior chamber when the intraocular pressure does not respond to acetazolamide and is persistently increased or when the chamber is completely filled with black blood. An incision large enough for drainage is more desirable than flushing fluid

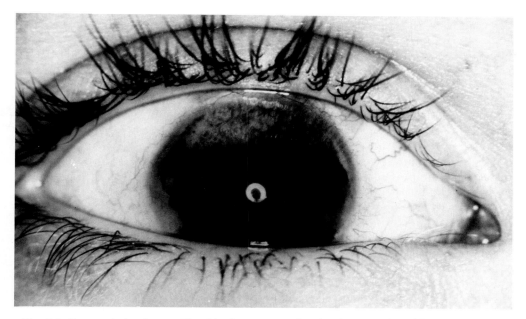

Fig. 7-3. Traumatic hyphema. Blood in the anterior chamber has not clotted but, during rest, forms a fluid meniscus.

in and out of the anterior chamber with a syringe. Attempts to remove clots by means of forceps are contraindicated because of the difficulty in distinguishing between the clots and the iris. A vitrectomy instrument (p. 362) may be inserted through the corneoscleral limbus into the anterior chamber. The clotted blood is then cut and aspirated from the eye. Extreme care must be taken not to touch the corneal endothelium, iris, or lens. General anesthesia is usually desirable because of the difficulty in anesthetizing the congested eye. If the intraocular pressure is increased, it is usually reduced by using intravenous mannitol before the incision into the anterior chamber is made.

Fracture-dislocations of orbital bones

Blunt trauma to the orbital region may give rise to fractures and dislocations affecting the bony margins or the walls of the orbit. Many of these injuries are associated with other facial fractures, head injury, and severe lacerations and cannot be treated until shock and life-threatening injuries have been managed. It is not necessary to make an emergency decision to remove an injured eye until adequate consultation has been obtained. Roentgenographic views of the skull and the orbit are essential, and laminography may indicate fractures not otherwise evident.

Examination should be particularly directed to asymmetry of the face and to the position of the canthal ligaments. Attention should be directed to possible brain injury associated with penetrating wounds of the walls of the orbit.

Fractures of the medial margin of the orbit are usually associated with nasal fractures. The nasolacrimal duct may be sheared as the nasolacrimal canal is displaced. A fracture causing a nasal accessory sinus to communicate with the orbit may permit air in the tissues (emphysema), which gives rise to a peculiar crepitation on palpation. Relatively minor trauma to the medial wall of the orbit may fracture the thin lamina papyracea of the ethmoid bone. This permits air to enter the orbit or the cutaneous tissue of the eyelid from the sinus. Violent blowing of the nose forces air into the tissues. The condition is self-limited and requires no treatment.

Fractures of the inferior orbital margin are often comminuted and associated with eyelid lacerations. The infraorbital nerve is severed in its canal, and there is anesthesia in its area of distribution. The bony fragments may often be placed in a better position, and depressed fractures may be elevated by forceps introduced through an existing laceration.

Fracture-dislocation of the zygomatic bone and arch occurs commonly. The lateral canthus is depressed, and the prominence of the cheekbone disappears. Relatively minor blows may be a cause. If the arch is fractured, it may be reduced through an incision at the posterior end of the arch and elevation by means of towel forceps or a periosteal elevator introduced into the temporalis muscle fossa. Much major cosmetic surgery may be avoided if such injuries are corrected within the first 24 hours.

Fractures of the superior rim of the orbit may involve the trochlea of the superior oblique muscle. This gives rise to the signs of paresis of this muscle and to a diplopia that is most marked when looking down and in, as in reading. The trochlea tends to reattach itself spontaneously, and treatment is not necessary.

Blowout fracture. Blunt trauma to the orbit may markedly increase intraorbital pressure, and the weak floor of the orbit gives way, causing a blowout fracture. The orbital contents prolapse into the maxillary sinus, and the entire globe may disappear from sight (Fig. 7-4). The palpebral fissure is narrowed. There is slight enophthalmos and inability to rotate the eye upward. In most cases roentgen-

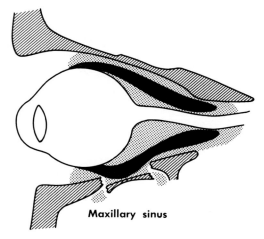

Fig. 7-4. Blowout fracture of the orbit with prolapse of the orbital tissue and the inferior rectus muscle into the maxillary sinus, where the muscle may become entrapped.

ograms show cloudiness of the maxillary sinus. There is anesthesia in the area of distribution of the infraorbital nerve, including the skin of the lower eyelid, side of the nose, and cheek. A blowout fracture of the orbit need be repaired only when there is diplopia and permanent restriction of ocular movement, indicating incarceration of orbital tissue in the fracture. The defect may be exposed through a skin incision of the inferior margin of the orbit, and the fracture opening may be bridged with bone or plastic.

BURNS
Chemical burns

Chemical burns of the conjunctiva and cornea are best treated by immediate dilution of the chemical with water. There should be no delay to learn the history, examine the eyes, measure vision, or seek the appropriate chemical neutralizer. The eye should be copiously irrigated with water. In most industries (Fig. 7-5), employees are routinely taught how to do this. The most effective method is to plunge the entire face into a container of

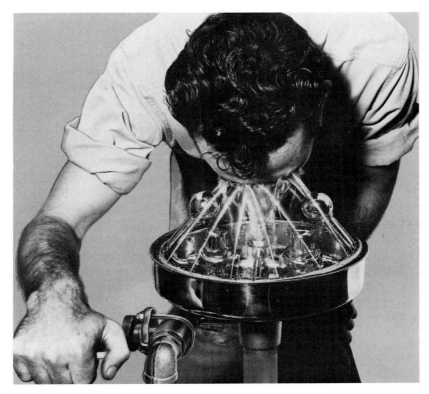

Fig. 7-5. Irrigation of a chemical burn of the eye with an eye-face wash fountain designed for industrial and school use. (Courtesy Haws Drinking Faucet Co., Berkeley, Calif.)

water and then open the eyes under water. Immediate dilution is the most important therapy. The fluid used need not be sterile, at body temperature, or even clean, provided the chemical is diluted promptly.

Acids are quickly buffered by the tissues, and the immediate injury is usually the full extent of the damage. Alkalis, however, continue to release hydroxyl ions into the tissue, and the injury is aggravated. Meticulous inspection of the conjunctiva is necessary, and all tissue containing alkali must be removed. Prolonged irrigation with saline solution is carried out, and as much of the chemical is removed as possible. Irrigation has been carried out for several days with good results. A scleral contact lens at-

tached to an irrigating system may provide continuous irrigation. Calcium hydroxide burns may be treated by means of chelation of the calcium ion using a chelating agent (p. 138) such as ethylenediaminetetraacetic acid. Infection is prevented by the use of systemic and local antibiotics. The pupils are dilated, and the ciliary muscle is paralyzed with topical atropine. The systemic use of corticosteroids in high doses after alkali burns appears to limit the amount of scarring. Symblepharon is prevented by the passage of a lubricated probe between the inner surface of the eyelids and the globe and by the use of a soft contact lens.

After alkaline burns, the corneal epithelial cells release collagenase enzymes, which lyse collagen gel and digest corneal stroma. Compounds such as acetylcysteine, penicillamine, and ethylenediaminetetraacetic acid, all of which inactivate collagenase by chelating the calcium needed for its activation, are used topically each hour. The failure of collagen synthesis in the alkali-burned cornea resembles that seen in scurvy. The systemic administration of ascorbate in experimental animals with alkali burns of the cornea has minimized corneal perforation. Medroxyprogesterone blocks collagenase formation and has been used topically and parenterally in experimental animals to limit alkali damage.

Chemical injuries of the eye may cause severe damage, and the prognosis must be guarded until the full extent of the burn is determined.

Thermal burns

Thermal burns of the eyelids usually do not involve the globe, since the blinking reflex provides natural protection. Additionally, tightly closed eyelids usually prevent involvement of the eyelid margins themselves.

Burns of the eyelids require prompt care to prevent severe ectropion (p. 203). First-aid measures consist of application of sterile dressings and systemic control of pain. Definitive treatment should be carried out within 12 hours of the injury. If dirty, the burned eyelids are cleaned gently with sterile saline solution and a sterile, bland soap. Fluid blebs are left intact. The most important step is suturing the upper to the lower eyelid with 4-0 black silk sutures or, if not available, with other suture material. A mattress suture is placed through the margin of the lower eyelid and through the margin of the upper eyelid, care being taken not to penetrate the globe. The sutures bring the two eyelids together in the closed position, preventing gross contracture and subsequent ectropion formation. Such sutures, if unnecessary, are easily removed. Early skin grafting in severe second- and third-degree burns may speed convalescence and prevent late deformities. Skin for this purpose may be obtained from behind the ear, the inner side of the forearm, or preferably, provided it is uninjured, from the opposite upper eyelid region.

Severe body burns are often associated with smoke inhalation and carbon monoxide poisoning. There are retinal hemorrhages, hyperemia of the optic disk, and venous and arterial congestion. The ocular changes resemble those seen in altitudinal hypoxemia (p. 197).

INJURIES CAUSED BY RADIANT ENERGY

Injury to the eye by radiant energy is related to absorption of the energy by the tissues of the eye (p. 98). Ultraviolet radiation is almost entirely absorbed by the cornea, and a small band causes ultraviolet keratitis. Infrared radiation is transmitted by the cornea and lens but comes to focus on the posterior ocular segment. If it increases the temperature of the tissues enough, it causes a chorioretinitis (p. 298) (the principle applied in photocoagulation of ocular disorders). Infrared radiation to the iris increases its temperature and that of the adjacent lens, causing an infrared type of cataract (p. 404).

Electromagnetic energy of long wavelength in the range of radar can cause cataract when focused on the eye for several minutes. The changes are presumably entirely caused by increased temperature of the lens and not specifically related to the type of energy. Electromagnetic energy of short wavelength (roentgen rays, gamma rays) may damage any part of the eye. Radiation cataract is produced through interferences with mitoses at the equator of the lens.

For the most part, industrial, warfare, and therapeutic sources of these energies are well known, and appropriate protective measures are undertaken. The majority of injuries are recognized quickly.

Ultraviolet burns of the cornea occur in arc welders, in mountain climbers and those exposed to snowfields (snow-blindness is ultraviolet keratitis), and in those who expose themselves unwisely to sun lamps. Like sunburn, ultraviolet radiation is cumulative; symptoms occur some time after exposure. A marked foreign body sensation in the eye, lacrimation, and photophobia are present. Symptoms are entirely relieved by a local anesthetic, which, however, delays epithelization of the cornea. The condition is entirely self-limited.

The use of fluorescent lighting to lower the bilirubin level in low birth weight infants who suffer from hyperbilirubinemia causes concern, because photoreceptors in lower animals show structural and functional changes after extended periods of exposure to illumination even at levels lower than those used to treat infants. In piglets, who have retinas similar to those of newborn infants, extensive retinal damage occurs after as little as 12 hours' exposure to light in the commercially produced infant phototherapy unit. Therefore, infants' eyes should be protected by intermittent patching during the phototherapy. In addition, some form of ultraviolet-absorbing material, such as a sheet of glass, should be placed between the infant and the fluorescent bulbs to protect the infants from ultraviolet radiation and to prevent injury from bulb breakage.

Another problem arises in infants who spend days and nights under the bright room lights of a nursery. It seems advisable that they should be protected from lights periodically to permit the visual cells to renew themselves.

THE BATTERED CHILD SYNDROME

The battered child syndrome includes nonaccidental trauma as well as other problems resulting from lack of reasonable care and protection of children by their parents, guardian, or other caretaker. Many cases are first suspected because of the implausible history offered in explanation of a child's injury, a discrepancy in the history provided by the two parents, or a delay in seeking medical care. Ocular injuries include acute hyphema, chemical burns of the eyes, dislocated lenses, and detached retina. Subdural hematomas are often the result of violent shaking and may cause coma and convulsions. Retinal hemorrhages are nearly always present.

Any child who is a victim of physical abuse requires the protection of admission to a hospital. Further management involves telling those involved the diagnosis, reporting the diagnosis to a protective agency, and seeking social service assistance. The child must not be returned to the caretakers until after adequate intervention.

ALTITUDINAL HYPOXEMIA

Acute mountain sickness occurs within 8 to 24 hours after rapid ascent to altitudes above 8,000 feet. Most individuals show symptoms at elevations of more than 15,000 feet. These symptoms occur within 8 to 24 hours after arrival and clear over a 4- to 8-day period. They include headache, lassitude, insomnia, and gastrointestinal upset. Ocular hemorrhages frequently occur in individuals who ascend to 17,500 feet. There is no association between the retinal hemorrhages and concomitant sickness. A prior history of migraine as well as rapid ascent and increased physical exertion places the climber at higher risk.

Other ocular changes include increase in the diameter, tortuosity, and cyanosis of the retinal arteries and veins together with cyanosis of the optic disk. There may be increased retinal blood flow and retinal blood volume while the mean retinal circulation time decreases. The concomitant hypoxia and Valsalva maneuvers required in physical exertion along with the hyperviscosity of the blood occurring at high altitudes may play a role. Similar changes occur in carbon monoxide poisoning in humans. Slow ascent to permit acclimatization as well as ingestion of acetazolamide for 48 hours before ascent to prevent cerebral edema appears to be beneficial.

BIBLIOGRAPHY

Crawford, J. S., Lewandowski, R. L., and Chan, W.: The effect of aspirin on rebleeding in traumatic hyphema, Am. J. Ophthalmol. **80:**543, 1975.

Dempsey, L. C., O'Donnell, J. J., and Hoff, J. T.: Carbon monoxide retinopathy, Am. J. Ophthalmol. **82:**692, 1976.

Edwards, W. C., and Layden, W. E.: Monocular versus binocular patching in traumatic hyphema, Am. J. Ophthalmol. **76:**359, 1973.

Grove, A. S., Jr., Radmor, R., New, P. F. J., and Momose, K. J.: Orbital fracture evaluation by coronal computed tomography, Am. J. Ophthalmol. **85:**679, 1978.

Newsome, D. A., and Gross, J.: Prevention by medroxyprogesterone of perforation in the alkali-burned rabbit cornea; inhibition of collagenolytic activity, Invest. Ophthalmol. **16:**21, 1977.

Paton, D., and Goldberg, M. F.: Management of ocular injuries, Philadelphia, 1976, W. B. Saunders Co.

Pfister, R. R., and Paterson, C. A.: Additional clinical and morphological observations on the favorable effect of ascorbate in experimental ocular alkali burns, Invest. Ophthalmol. **16:**478, 1977.

Robertson, D. M.: Safety glasses as protection against shotgun pellets, Am. J. Ophthalmol. **81:**671, 1976.

Rosenthal, A. R., Appleton, B., Zimmerman, R., and Hopkins, J. L.: Intraocular copper foreign bodies, Arch. Ophthalmol. **94:**1571, 1976.

Tseng, S. S., and Keys, M. P.: Battered child syndrome simulating congenital glaucoma, Arch. Ophthalmol. **94:**839, 1976.

Chapter 8

THE EYELIDS

The eyelids are thin, movable curtains composed of skin on their anterior surface and mucous membrane on their posterior surface. They contain striated and smooth muscle and the tarsus, a fibrous plate that contains meibomian glands. They protect the eye, distribute tears over its anterior surface, and limit the amount of light entering. The eyelids are divided by the orbitopalpebral sulcus into two portions: (1) the palpebral portion, adjacent to the eyelid margin, which ends at the margin of the tarsus and is involved in reflex blinking, and (2) the obital portion, the peripheral portion of which merges into the cheek below and the brow above.

The free margins of the eyelids contain the mucocutaneous junction of skin and conjunctiva (called the gray line), a triple line of eyelashes or cilia, the orifices of the meibomian glands, and the superior and inferior puncta, which are the openings of the superior and inferior canaliculus (Fig. 8-1). The margin is divided into two parts: (1) a lateral five sixths, the ciliary portion containing eyelashes, and (2) a medial one sixth, without eyelashes, containing the puncta. The lateral junction of the eyelid margins, the lateral canthus, forms a 60° angle located about 2 mm higher than the rounded medial margin, the medial canthus (p. 50).

The eyelids are covered by a thin, elastic, easily distensible skin that contains no subcutaneous fat. The skin is, of course, subject to the same diseases as skin elsewhere, but secondary involvement of the globe may overshadow the cutaneous disorder. The orbicularis oculi muscle (N VII) originates from the medial orbit and medial palpebral ligament, circles the orbit covering the orbital margin and the eyelids, and inserts into the lateral orbit and lateral palpebral ligament. The orbicularis oculi muscle is separated from orbital structures by the palpebral fascia, which limits the extension of inflammation, effusions, and fat from the orbit into the eyelids.

The upper eyelid is elevated by the levator palpebrae superioris muscle (N III). Müller smooth muscle (sympathetics) provides tone to the elevated eyelid. The eyelids are closed by the orbicularis oculi muscle (N VII). Only the palpebral portion is involved in reflex blinking, whereas both the orbital and palpebral portions are involved in forcible closure of the eyelids.

The eyelids contain numerous glands: sebaceous (Zeis) and sudoriferous (Moll) glands associated with the cilia, meibomian glands in the tarsal plates, and accessory lacrimal glands of Krause and Wolfring located in the conjunctival fornices (Fig. 1-40). Additionally, the skin of

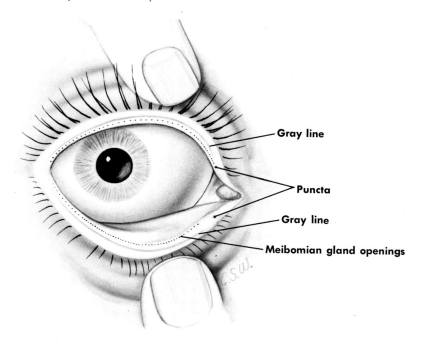

Fig. 8-1. The upper and lower puncta, the openings of the lacrimal canaliculi, divide the eyelids into ciliary and lacrimal portions. The openings of the meibomian glands are visible inside the gray lines.

the eyelids contains sweat and sebaceous glands subject to the same disorders as elsewhere.

SYMPTOMS AND SIGNS OF EYELID DISEASE

The variety of structures forming the eyelids, their importance in facial expression and appearance, and their function in the protection and health of the eye provide the basis for a wide variety of abnormalities.

The palpebral apertures are normally similar in size, shape, position, and movement, and the eyelids just conceal the corneoscleral limbus in the 12 and 6 o'clock meridians. The obliquity of the aperture varies in different races, being more slanted in Orientals. The upper eyelid is highest at the junction of the medial one third with the lateral two thirds, whereas the lower eyelid is lowest at the lateral one third. Retraction of the eyelids or forward protrusion of the globe exposes the sclera (scleral rim) above or below the corneoscleral limbus. When the eyelids are closed, the palpebral aperture becomes a fissure and the eye turns up and out (Bell phenomenon), providing protection to the cornea.

The eyelid margins are normally in close apposition to the globe, and the lashes are directed outward. The lashes are darker and more rigid than body hair, and they do not gray with aging. The inferior punctum turns slightly inward to dip into the lacrimal lake at the inner canthus. The lacrimal papillae, small prominences surrounding the punctum, become more obvious with aging.

The skin of the eyelids is thin and often translucent, so that a delicate tracery of

Table 8-1. Some abnormalities of the eyelids

Blepharochalasis	Loss of elasticity of skin of eyelids
Blepharoclonus	Excessive blinking
Blepharophimosis	Interpalpebral fissure congenitally short
Blepharoptosis	Upper eyelid not elevated properly
Blepharospasm	Persistent forcible closure of the eyelids
Distichiasis	Supernumerary row of lashes
Ectropion	Outturning of eyelid margin
Entropion	Inturning of eyelid margin
Epicanthus	Skin fold conceals medial canthus
Lagophthalmos	Eyelids do not close
Myokymia	Involuntary orbicularis oculi muscle contractions
Symblepharon	Adhesions between palpebral and bulbar conjunctivae
Trichiasis	Lashes directed toward the globe

blood vessels gives a slighty bluish cast to the eyelids. The skin is thrown into fine folds, and the superior and inferior palpebral furrows (p. 49) provide characteristic folds.

Periodic contraction of the tarsal portion of the orbicularis oculi muscle causes involuntary blinking. During attempts to squeeze both eyes closed, contracture is normally equal on both sides. The levator palpebrae superioris and Müller muscles elevate the eyelids to a similar height on the two sides.

The eyelids may be involved in many different abnormalities (Table 8-1). The symptoms vary widely. Inturning of the eyelid margins (entropion, p. 202) causes the lashes to irritate the cornea and bulbar conjunctiva. Failure of the eyelids to cover the globe, as in lagophthalmos (p. 206) or ectropion (p. 203), may expose the conjunctiva and cornea, causing inflammation. If the eyelids cover one or both pupils, there may be interference with vision. If one pupil is covered early in life, amblyopia (p. 426) may develop. If both eyelids cover the pupils, the patient often compensates by throwing his head back to expose the visual axis.

Pain, swelling, and redness of the eyelids occur with a variety of inflammations. Inflammatory or neoplastic disease may extend from the eyelids to involve the eye. Infection of the upper eyelid or the outer one third of the lower eyelid may cause enlargement of the preauricular (parotid) lymph nodes. Involvement of the medial two thirds of the lower eyelid may cause a submaxillary lymphadenopathy (p. 53 and Fig. 1-41).

Tearing may occur because of irritation of the eye or because the eyelids are not in apposition with the globe. Constant tearing may cause excoriation of the skin at the lateral and medial canthi.

CONGENITAL ABNORMALITIES

Failure of a eye to develop may result in ablepharon, which is absence of the eyelid. The eyelid may be imperfectly separated in ankyloblepharon. There may be failure of a portion of the eyelid to develop, causing a notching defect of its margin, a coloboma of the eyelid. Development of a supernumerary row of lashes, which are frequently directed backward to irritate the cornea, is known as distichiasis (p. 208). In blepharophimosis the interpalpebral fissure is congenitally narrowed.

Epicanthus is by far the most common congenital variation. A vertical skin fold occurs in the medial canthal region that conceals the medial angle and the caruncle. Such an epicanthal fold occurs normally in Orientals and is often combined

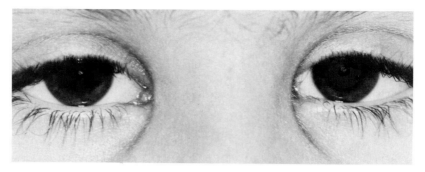

Fig. 8-2. A 5-year-old boy with bilateral epicanthus that is more marked on the left side. The concealment of the left sclera by the extra fold of skin simulates the appearance of an esotropia (pseudostrabismus, p. 425).

with a fold of skin overhanging the palpebral fissure (mongolian fold), giving it an almond shape (Fig. 8-2). It is present in many white infants until growth of the nose and face causes it to be obliterated. An epicanthal fold may conceal the medial sclera and may simulate the appearance of esotropia (pseudostrabismus). The presence or absence of esotropia is quickly determined by means of the cover-uncover test (p. 414).

ABNORMALITIES OF SHAPE AND POSITION

In entropion the eyelid margin is turned inward, and the eyelashes irritate the eye. In ectropion the eyelid margin is turned outward so that the conjunctival surface is exposed and becomes keratinized. In blepharoptosis the upper eyelid is not elevated properly so that the palpebral fissure is narrowed. Blepharoptosis and epicanthal folds may be associated. In lagophthalmos the eyelids fail to cover the globe.

Entropion

Entropion (Fig. 8-3) is a condition in which the eyelid margin is turned inward so that the lashes irritate the eye, causing corneal epithelial defects, conjunctival injection, tearing, and sometimes secondary infection of the cornea or the conjunc-

tiva. It occurs in three main forms: (1) spastic; (2) atonic, or senile; and (3) cicatricial. The spastic and atonic types affect only the lower eyelid, whereas the cicatricial form may affect either the upper or the lower eyelid.

The spastic form results from excessive contraction of the orbicularis oculi muscle (blepharospasm) and may complicate chronic conjunctivitis, keratitis, and ocular surgery. Primary treatment is directed toward removal of the cause. Surgical correction involves resection of a strip of skin and orbicularis oculi muscle parallel to the palpebral fissure in order to evert the eyelid margin.

The atonic type of entropion follows a loss of tone of the orbicularis oculi muscle combined with loss of elasticity of the skin. It occurs in the elderly. In the early stages the entropion is often intermittent but may be induced by having the patient forcibly squeeze the eyes closed. The irritation of the globe by the lashes causes a blepharospasm; therefore, both a spastic and an atonic entropion may be present. Surgery is usually required. Temporary relief in minor cases may be obtained by drawing the skin of the outer canthus down and out by means of an adhesive tape strip. The usual surgical procedure involves a resection or shortening of the orbicularis oculi muscle fibers ad-

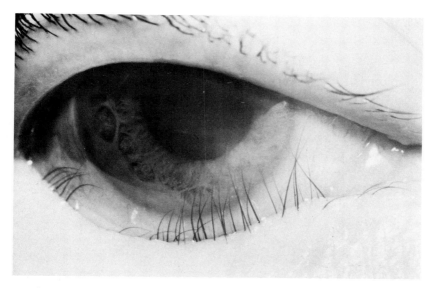

Fig. 8-3. Spastic entropion with irritation of the globe by the eyelashes.

jacent to the eyelid margin or a shortening of the inferior portion of the orbital septum.

Cicatricial entropion follows scarring of the palpebral conjunctiva, which may be caused by chemical injuries, lacerations, surgical procedures, radiant energy, trachoma, and erythema multiforme. Frequently the tarsus is deformed. The globe is usually irritated by the lashes; this results in a blepharospasm and spastic entropion. Primary treatment is directed toward removal of the cause. A number of surgical procedures have been devised to evert the eyelid margin and the lashes. It may be necessary to transplant mucous membrane from the mouth to replace scarred conjunctiva.

Ectropion

Ectropion (Fig. 8-4) is a condition in which the eyelid margin is turned away from the eye so that the bulbar and the palpebral conjunctivae are exposed. Symptoms result from exposure of the conjunctiva and the cornea. When the

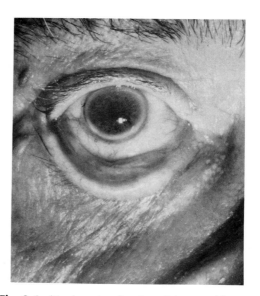

Fig. 8-4. Atonic ectropion in a 74-year-old man.

lower eyelid is involved, the inferior punctum is not adjacent to the lacrimal lake, and tearing may occur. Ectropion occurs in three main forms: (1) spastic, (2) atonic, and (3) cicatricial. Only the lower eyelid is involved in the spastic and atonic types, but the cicatricial type may affect either the upper or the lower eyelid.

Atonic ectropion is the most common type. It follows paralysis of the orbicularis oculi muscle (N VII). The lower eyelid sags outward, and there is marked tearing. Usually there is an associated paralysis of other facial muscles. Medical measures are ineffective. Any of a wide variety of surgical procedures can correct the condition. In diseases of the facial nerve, nerve grafting is the preferred procedure. If this is not practicable, a shortening operation on the eyelid is indicated. Surgery is not indicated if spontaneous recovery from the paralysis occurs.

Spastic ectropion usually follows conditions in which the eye is proptosed or the conjunctiva chronically thickened. In youth, the skin and muscle provide firm support of the eyelid, and the spasm of the orbicularis oculi muscle causes the eyelid margin to turn outward. Treatment is directed toward the cause.

Cicatricial ectropion follows burns, lacerations, and infections of the skin of the eyelids. With most thermal burns, the eyelids close tightly and the eyelid margins are uninvolved, there being an intact 1- or 2-mm margin present. Subsequent plastic surgery to correct contracture may be unnecessary if the eyelids are sutured together as early as possible. Early skin transplant is desirable in most instances of cicatricial ectropion. Skin of the opposite upper eyelid is ideal for this purpose, or skin may be obtained from over the mastoid region. The plastic surgery required for established cicatricial ectropion may be difficult and may necessitate skilled and prolonged care. Symptomatic treatment is usually not helpful.

Blepharoptosis

An abnormality in the innervation or musculature of the levator palpebrae superioris muscle gives rise to blepharoptosis (Fig. 8-5), in which the upper eyelid droops and the palpebral fissure is narrowed.

Blepharoptosis is often divided into

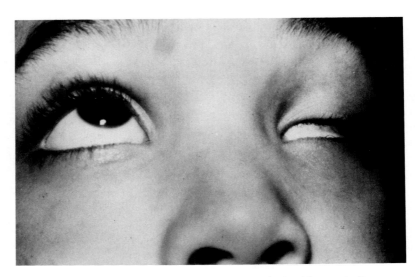

Fig. 8-5. Left blepharoptosis. The absence of a superior palpebral furrow indicates paralysis of the levator palpebrae superioris muscle.

congenital and acquired types. The congenital type, which is present at birth, is almost invariably the result of interference with the superior division of the oculomotor nerve (N III), which innervates only the levator palpebrae superioris muscle and the superior rectus muscle. There may also be weakness of the superior rectus muscle. The acquired type may be distinguished from the congenital type by the presence of a superior palpebral sulcus, which marks the insertion of the levator palpebrae superioris aponeurosis into the skin of the upper eyelid. If the muscle has never functioned, the sulcus is absent. Both the congenital and the acquired type may be hereditary or occur sporadically.

Congenital blepharoptosis. Congenital blepharoptosis may involve one or both eyelids. Most instances are caused by an abnormality of the superior branch of the oculomotor nerve (N III). The condition is apparent at birth or shortly thereafter, when it is evident that the palpebral fissure on one or both sides is narrower than normal and that the upper eyelid does not move upward with the eye. The degree of severity varies. If the visual axes of both eyes are covered by the drooping eyelids, the child acquires a characteristic posture with the head thrown back and forehead furrowed in a perpetual frown as he uses his frontalis muscle to elevate the eyelids. If only one eye is involved, the child may develop a sensory amblyopia (p. 426) that necessitates earlier surgical treatment than bilateral blepharoptosis.

Treatment is based on the degree of severity. If the pupils are not covered by the eyelids, treatment may be deferred for a long period. If only one eye is involved and the visual axis is covered, surgery should be carried out before the age of 1 year, and major attention should be directed toward the development of normal visual acuity in the affected eye. When the condition is bilateral, surgery is usually done between the ages of 3 and 5 years. Although myasthenia gravis does not usually affect children, it is customary to carry out a Tensilon test preoperatively to be certain that the condition is not caused by this muscle disorder.

Acquired blepharoptosis. Acquired blepharoptosis may result from any affection of the nerve supply of the upper eyelid musculature, from disease of the muscles themselves, or from mechanical interference in elevating the eyelid by the weight of a tumor. The most common acquired causes of oculomotor nerve involvement are ruptured intracranial aneurysms, head injuries, diabetes mellitus neuropathy, and toxic and inflammatory intracranial disease. Aneurysms of the internal carotid artery within the cavernous sinus may cause a complete ophthalmoplegia from involvement of nerves III, IV, and VI combined with anesthesia in the area of distribution of the maxillary (second) division of the trigeminal nerve (N V).

Interference with the sympathetic innervation of the smooth muscle (Müller), which provides tone to the upper eyelid, causes 1 to 2 mm of drooping, as is seen in Horner syndrome (p. 285). Blepharoptosis occurs in chronic progressive external ophthalmoplegia, myotonic dystrophy, and myasthenia gravis. It has also been observed in patients who have used topical corticosteroids for long periods. With aging, loss of tone of the levator palpebrae superioris muscle and Müller muscle together with loss of support caused by enophthalmos from atrophy of orbital fat may cause some eyelid sagging. Disinsertion or dehiscence, or both, of the aponeurosis of the levator palpebrae superioris muscle from the epitarsal tissues may cause a narrowed palpebral fissure in some patients, particularly those who have had akinesia of the eyelid muscles for ocular surgery.

Myasthenia gravis. Paresis of the levator palpebrae superioris muscle may be the initial sign of myasthenia gravis. Frequently the disease is limited to the upper eyelid and does not become more generalized. Most commonly only one side is affected. Inasmuch as the disease may be treated medically, it is most important to exclude myasthenia gravis (p. 568) before surgical correction of an acquired blepharoptosis.

Surgical correction of blepharoptosis. There are several surgical procedures used in the correction of blepharoptosis.

1. The levator palpebrae superioris muscle may be resected through either a skin or conjunctival incision. It is the procedure of choice when muscle function is present. Blepharoptosis after eyelid akinesia can be corrected by reattachment of the aponeurosis of the levator palpebrae superioris muscle to the tarsus.

2. Suspension of the upper eyelid from the frontalis muscle by means of fascia lata or other material provides mechanical elevation, but the cosmetic result may be less pleasing than with a levator palpebrae superioris muscle resection. If no muscle function is present, however, the procedure must be used.

Several ingenious devices, known as "ptosis crutches," attached to the frame of spectacles elevate the eyelid. They are not particularly well tolerated and, in individuals with unilateral ophthalmoplegia, a drooping eyelid may prevent diplopia.

Lagophthalmos

Lagophthalmos is an abnormality in which inadequate closure of the eyelids results in exposure of the eye. It may occur because of seventh cranial nerve weakness, proptosis, eyelid retraction, or enlargement of the globe. Exposure of the cornea occurs with drying and secondary infection (p. 266). Treatment is directed toward the cause. Surgery to pre-

vent exposure keratitis should be carried out as soon as it is evident that the cornea is threatened. Permanent or temporary adhesions may be created between the upper and the lower eyelids (tarsorrhaphy). These may be either lateral, medial, or central. In mild lagophthalmos only the central portion of the cornea may be exposed, and the instillation of an ointment base at bedtime may be all that is required to prevent corneal drying during sleep. Saran Wrap held in position with gummed cellophane tape may be used to cover the exposed eye and create a moist chamber. Alternatively, a soft contact lens and artificial tears may prevent corneal drying in a cosmetically more acceptable manner.

DISORDERS OF THE ORBICULARIS OCULI MUSCLE
Blinking

Blinking spreads tears over the surface of the eyeball and limits the amount of light entering the eye. It may be involuntary or voluntary. Involuntary blinking occurs as a periodic contraction of the tarsal portion of the orbicularis oculi muscle at a rate peculiar to each individual. It is absent in infants and is of low frequency in Parkinson disease and hyperthyroidism (Stellwag sign). A decreased rate of blinking or incomplete closure of the eyelids may aggravate the symptoms of keratoconjunctivitis sicca. Periodic blinking normally occurs once every 5 seconds and lasts about 0.3 second.

Reflex blinking may follow peripheral stimulation of the trigeminal, optic, or auditory nerves. Irritation of the cornea, conjunctiva, or eyelashes is following by eyelid closure. Bright lights or dazzling in the visual field may initiate blinking through a reflex arc that begins in the retina. A sudden loud noise may cause reflex closure of the eyelids.

Blepharoclonus

Blepharoclonus is an exaggerated form of reflex blinking in which either the rate of blinking is increased or the phase of closure is excessively long. There is often marked contraction of the orbital portion of the eyelids. Blepharoclonus may be initiated by irritation or inflammation of the conjunctiva or the cornea. Even after removal of the cause, blepharoclonus may continue as a tic, and other muscles of the face may be involved. When the stimulus cannot be found, effective treatment is difficult. A variety of surgical procedures have been described that aim at interrupting the facial nerve supply to the orbicularis oculi muscle or interrupting the muscle fibers themselves.

Children 5 to 10 years of age may develop episodes of rapid blinking. Apparently the child is unaware of blinking, but the parents may be distressed. Almost invariably, examination of the eyes indicates no ocular abnormality.

Orbicularis oculi muscle tremor

Involuntary contraction of a few fibers of the orbicularis oculi muscle (myokymia) causes the patient to sense an annoying twitching that feels conspicuous. Examination indicates a barely perceptible contraction of a few fibers of the orbicularis oculi muscle. The condition occurs most frequently with fatigue, but often no cause is found. Local instillation or systemic administration of anticholinesterase compounds, particularly the organophosphates, may cause myokymia. Quinine sulfate in doses of 200 to 400 mg increases the latent period of skeletal muscle contraction with relief of symptoms. If the entire muscle is involved, a search must be made for organic causes, particularly multiple sclerosis, Parkinson disease, tabes dorsalis, and hyperthyroidism.

Blepharospasm

Blepharospasm is an involuntary, tonic, spasmodic, bilateral contraction of the orbicularis oculi muscle that may last from several seconds to several minutes. It occurs mainly in individuals more than 60 years of age. It may involve other muscles of the face, and it causes a severe cosmetic deformity as well as failure to see because of persistence of the eyelid closure. It may occur in postencephalitic states, in hemiplegia from various causes, and after Bell palsy. In these patients the blepharospasm may not disappear during sleep. In another group the disease seems limited to the orbicularis oculi muscle. Careful dissection of the seventh nerve just anterior to the parotid gland with interruption of each nerve identified by a muscle stimulator as going to the orbicularis oculi muscle may be followed by relief. Some patients have been treated with psychotherapy and others with levodopa when this has been considered a form of Parkinson disease.

MISCELLANEOUS CONDITIONS
Blepharochalasis

Blepharochalasis is an abnormality in which there is atrophy and loss of elasticity of the skin of the eyelids. It occurs most commonly in aged persons. There is a loss of skin turgor, and a fold of skin may hang down over the eyelid margin. Treatment is usually not indicated. If the fold of skin interferes with vision by covering the pupillary area, the excess skin may be excised.

Baggy eyelids

Puffiness or swelling of the eyelids results from localized edema or protrusion of orbital fat through the orbital fascia. Systemic causes include hyperthyroidism, nephrosis, and angioneurotic edema. In premenstrual edema, fluid retention as well as vasodilation may be

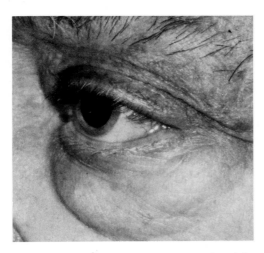

Fig. 8-6. Herniation of orbital fat through a dehiscence in the orbital septum.

conspicuous in this area, with the abundant vasculature of the eyelid evident through the nearly translucent skin.

Herniation of orbital fat through a dehiscence in the orbital fascia (Fig. 8-6) gives rise to a localized swelling in the eyelid that can sometimes be palpated as a small tumor. The inner portion of the upper eyelid and the middle portion of the lower eyelid are partially involved. Successful treatment requires surgical closure of the fascial defect, because excision of the fat only will be followed by replacement of more fat from the orbit.

Trichiasis

In this condition the lashes are directed toward the globe and irritate the cornea and the conjunctiva, causing secondary infection. The condition usually follows diseases that cause scarring of the eyelid margin. The cornea and conjunctiva may be protected by a soft contact lens, but usually treatment is directed toward destruction of the irritating lashes. The lash follicles may be destroyed by freezing the conjunctival surface of the eyelid margin with liquid nitrogen. If a number of lashes are involved, reconstruction of the margin of the eyelid may be necessary.

Distichiasis

Distichiasis is a congenital abnormality in which the meibomian glands atavistically revert to hair follicles to form an accessory line of lashes. Other congenital malformations may be present. If the lashes are numerous and cause irritation of the globe, the area must be excised and a graft substituted.

Hypertrophy of the eyelids

Immense overgrowth of the eyelids may occur in neurofibromatosis, hemangiomas (particularly in infancy), lymphangioma, and a variety of infections. Treatment is directed toward the cause.

INFLAMMATION

The glands in the eyelids may be involved in acute suppurative infections such as those occurring with sties that involve the glands of Zeis and Moll. The meibomian glands may be involved in an acute or chronic inflammation called chalazion.

The eyelid margins may be involved in inflammations (blepharitis), caused by bacteria, seborrheic dermatitis, or localized hypersensitivity reactions. The skin of the eyelids may be involved in a large variety of inflammations that may be more conspicuous than similar lesions elsewhere in the body bacause of the looseness of the skin, its exposed position, and secondary involvement of the eye. Contact dermatitis and reactions secondary to the application of drugs or cosmetics to the eyelids or conjunctival sac are common.

Hordeolum

Hordeolum, or sty (Fig. 8-7), is an acute suppurative inflammation of the follicle of an eyelash or the associated gland of Zeis (sebaceous) or Moll (special apo-

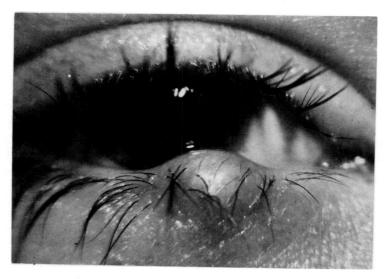

Fig. 8-7. Acute hordeolum of the lower eyelid.

crine sweat gland). Like pustules else-where, the usual cause is staphylococcal infection. The initial symptom is tender-ness of the eyelid that may become marked as the suppuration progresses. The initial sign is edema of the eyelid, which may be diffuse, followed by the development of a red, indurated area on the eyelid margin that may rupture. The main differential diagnosis involves an acute chalazion that tends to point on the conjunctival side of the eyelid and does not involve the eyelid margin unless the opening duct of the meibomian gland is involved. The chalazion is preceded and followed by a minute tumor in the sub-stance of the eyelid that feels like a small buckshot. Sties tend to occur in crops, be-cause the infecting organism spreads from one hair follicle to another, either directly or by the fingers. Treatment is the same as that of acute suppurative in-fection elsewhere in the body. Hot com-presses applied at frequent intervals hasten resolution of the lesion. When pointing occurs, incision and drainage are indicated. Frequently a topical sulfona-mide or an antibiotic prevents involve-ment of adjacent glands.

Chalazion

Chalazion is a chronic inflammatory lipogranuloma of one of the meibomian glands. It is characterized by a gradual painless swelling of the gland without gross inflammatory signs. Palpation indi-cates a small buckshotlike swelling in the substance of the eyelid, and this may be its only evidence. With increase in size, it may cause astigmatism by distortion of the globe or may be evident beneath the skin as a small mass (Fig. 8-8). It may be-come secondarily infected and give rise to an acute suppurative inflammation that usually points on the inside of the eyelid. The lesion is a lipogranuloma resembling that seen in sarcoidosis or tuberculosis with giant cells but without caseation.

Treatment is by excision, usually through a conjunctival incision. When small and asymptomatic, removal is not indicated, and the mass may disappear spontaneously. Many disappear after in-tralesional injection of 0.25 to 1.0 mg of

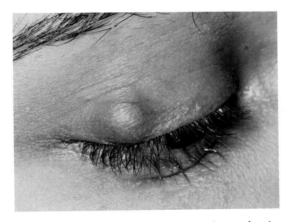

Fig. 8-8. Chronic chalazion (lipogranuloma of meibomian gland) of the upper eyelid.

triamcinolone suspended in 0.05 to 0.2 ml of normal saline solution. Some individuals tend to have a series of chalazia, apparently because of inspissation of the meibomian gland contents in the excretory ducts of Zeis or Moll. If pressure on the eyelid expresses a viscous secretion from the glands, massage of the eyelids, sometimes with a glass rod, may be helpful. Recurrence of what is believed to be a chalazion at the site where it has been excised should make one suspicious of a meibomian gland carcinoma.

Meibomianitis

In the middle years a passive retention of secretion by the meibomian glands may deposit a white, frothy secretion on the eyelid margins and at the canthi. The glands may be massaged to express an oily secretion, and eversion of the eyelids may show vertical yellowish streaks shining through the tarsal conjunctiva. Occasionally calcium is deposited in a gland. If this material penetrates the conjunctiva, it causes a foreign body sensation and must be removed.

Meibomianitis is often associated with blepharitis and chronic conjunctivitis and may give rise to recurrent chalazia. Treatment consists of tarsal massage and removal of the secretion with a moist cotton applicator.

Blepharitis

Blepharitis is a chronic inflammation of the eyelid margin that may be acute or chronic. It begins early in childhood and frequently continues throughout life. Staphylococcal infection and seborrheic dermatitis, often in combination, are its principal causes.

There are two forms of blepharitis: (1) simple squamous blepharitis and (2) ulcerated blepharitis. Both types are associated with dilated blood vessels on the eyelid margins, white lashes, loss of lashes, trichiasis, and scales around the cilia (collarettes). Almost invariably there is an associated chronic papillary conjunctivitis. Keratitis may occur, as may phlyctenulosis. *Pityrosporum ovale* and *Demodex folliculorum* mites may serve as vectors of staphylococci. It has been postulated that *Pityrosporum ovale* produces the disease by splitting lipids into irritating fatty acids.

Patients with rosacea have a greater than normal predisposition for blepharitis, and patients with atopic diseases also have a special predilection. If meibomian gland secretions are excessive, they should be expressed in the physician's office or at home by the patient or a relative. The eyelid margins should be cleaned by applying a mild baby shampoo or a $1/10\%$ selenium sulfide solution with a cotton-tipped applicator. Seborrhea should be treated by frequent shampoos with selenium sulfide. Depending on the sensitivity of the infecting organism, locally applied sulfacetamide, gentamicin, erythromycin, and bacitracin may be used. An ointment base is preferred.

Squamous blepharitis. Simple squamous blepharitis is characterized by a hyperemia usually limited to the eyelid margins. It is associated with scaling of the skin that may give rise to fine flakes and scales surrounding the lashes. In severe instances the eyelid margins may become thickened and everted. Most commonly, however, redness of the eyelid margins is the chief complaint. There may be burning and discomfort of the eyes and an associated chronic conjunctivitis (p. 225).

There is nearly always an associated seborrheic dermatitis of the scalp, which may also involve the eyebrows and give rise to an erythema of the cheeks. Irritation of the eyelid margins by chemical fumes, smoke, and smog may aggravate the hyperemia. Frequent rubbing of the eyelids may perpetuate the inflammation. In years past, uncorrected errors of refraction have been considered an important cause.

Treatment is directed mainly toward correction of the seborrheic dermatitis of the scalp by means of one of the specific shampoos available. Scales on the eyelid margin should be removed twice daily by means of a moistened cotton-tipped applicator. When indicated, refractive errors and imbalances of the ocular muscles should be corrected by means of lenses. Epinephrine is commonly used to cause vasoconstriction, but its action is evanescent and becomes less effective with repeated use. Numerous antibiotics, sulfonamides, and corticosteroids have been used locally and cause diminution of the inflammatory signs. For the most part, the condition tends to be arrested when the seborrheic dermatitis of the scalp is treated and to recur when treatment is stopped.

Ulcerative blepharitis. Ulcerative blepharitis arises from acute and chronic suppurative inflammation of the follicles of the lashes and the associated glands of Zeis and Moll. *Staphylococcus aureus* is usually the causative organism. The eyelid margins are red and inflamed. There are multiple suppurative lesions surrounded by yellow pus that crusts and is removed with difficulty, bringing with it eyelashes. Loss of lashes and the presence of necrotizing inflammation cause distortion of the eyelid margin, leading to ectropion, epiphora, and chronic conjunctivitis. Locally applied antibiotics such as neomycin and chloramphenicol or sulfonamides such as sulfacetamide and sulfisoxazole (Gantrisin) may be useful. Systemic antibiotics may be indicated in severe inflammation. In recent years ulcerative blepharitis has become uncommon.

Dermatitis

Infection of the skin of the eyelids may occur with a variety of microbial organisms, and it involves nearly the entire range of dermatitides. The thinness of the skin and its good blood supply allow enormous distension and injection, but more important, secondary infection of the conjunctiva, cornea, and intraocular contents may occur by direct extension from the skin. Conversely, inflammatory skin lesions may extend from the glands of the eyelid, conjunctiva, orbit, nasal accessory sinuses, or lacrimal apparatus.

Impetigo, erysipelas, anthrax malignant pustule, tuberculosis, chancre, leprosy, yaws, and tularemia may all involve the eyelid on occasion, often with enlargement of the parotid and submaxillary lymph glands.

Herpes zoster ophthalmicus causes a vesicular eruption of the eyelid that is less important than the frequent keratitis and uveitis. Verruca vulgaris and molluscum contagiosum infection of the eyelid margins are important because of the resulting conjunctivitis.

Fungus infections of the eyelid may occur either as a local infection or in the course of widespread systemic disease.

Infection of the eyelashes by lice may cause a blepharitis or secondary infection of the skin. Primary treatment is through delousing. The parasite attached to the lashes is poisoned by one of the anticholinesterase preparations used in the management of glaucoma and is easily removed.

Contact dermatitis. Contact dermatitis of the eyelids occurs commonly. It is characterized by a frequently recurrent, weeping, eczematous type of reaction of the skin. When chronic, the skin becomes indurated and brawny with moderate swelling and sometimes severe itching. Contact dermatitis may result from topical compounds applied locally to relieve inflammations and infections. Particular offenders are local antibiotics, anesthetics, antihistamines, atropine, and sulfonamides. Spectacle dermatitis may arise from the nickel in frames or from plastic frames. A variety of chemicals that are used in industry, detergents, nail polishes, cosmetics, and products dispensed in aerosol cans may be implicated. Often the agent is brought to the eye by the fingers and is most marked on the side of the dominant hand, although the hand is not inflamed.

Treatment is unsatisfactory unless the cause is removed. This may be difficult to determine, but it is sometimes aided by the patient's maintaining a diary in which he correlates his activities with the severity of the inflammation. The patient should be warned not to touch his eyelids with his fingers. In many instances it is a sound practice to discontinue all topical medications, to proscribe cosmetics and perfumes, and to advise the use of Basis soap. Sometimes a bland ointment such as Aquaphor will relieve symptoms. A systemic antihistamine may be useful, but removal of the cause and application of corticosteroid preparations are more reliable.

TUMORS

The eyelids are subject to the usual tumors of the skin. If the eyelid margin is not involved, excision is simple. Involvement of the eyelid margin necessitates skilled surgery to assure excision and satisfactory closure.

Cutaneous horns

Cutaneous horns are small, cylindric epidermoid growths of unknown origin. They occur near the eyelid margins or the outer canthus in middle-age or older people. They are excised easily.

Milia

Milia are small, white, round, slightly elevated cysts of the superficial dermis. They tend to occur in crops localized in a small area of the skin, sometimes on the eyelid. They may be derived from a hair follicle or its associated sebaceous gland. Excision may be desirable for cosmetic reasons.

Xanthelasma

Xanthelasma is a cutaneous deposition of lipid material that occurs most commonly at the inner portion of the upper or the lower eyelid. The lesion appears as a yellowish, slightly elevated area with sharply demarcated margins tending to be approximately parallel to the eyelid margin. The condition occurs with primary and secondary systemic lipid anomalies, but more commonly it occurs spontaneously without evident cause. It produces a cosmetic defect, and treatment is indicated only to remove the defect. The lesion may be excised surgically or destroyed by means of diathermy, photocoagulation, or chemicals. Recurrence is common.

Phakomatous choristomas

A choristoma, or aberrant rest, is a mass of tissue histologically normal for an organ or part of the body other than the site at which it is located. Small tumors located at the inner portion of the lower eyelid of infants appear to arise from the crystalline lens. These have been called phakomatous (lens) choristomas.

Carcinoma

Tumors of the eyelids may originate in the skin, mucous membranes, and glands. The tumors are relatively benign in that they are easily recognized and rarely metastasize.

Basal cell carcinoma is the most common neoplasm of the eyelids; squamous cell carcinoma is much less common. Both have a similar nodule appearance with elevated, irregular surfaces and sharply demarcated, pearly margins. The squamous cell tumor produces keratin and may appear more pearly white. The centers may be excavated, or ulceration occurs with enlargement (rodent ulcer). The basal cell tumor may be pigmented, although this may indicate nevus or malignant melanoma. Generally, the lower eyelid is involved (Fig. 8-9), particularly its outer portion. The patient may neglect the lesion for a long period inasmuch as it does not cause symptoms. There is a gradual increase in size of a typical tumor that has pearly margins and an excavated center (rodent ulcer). If the eyelid margin is not involved, treatment in the early stages is not particularly difficult; excision provides cure. When the eyelid margin is involved, surgical excision may necessitate a major plastic procedure.

Radiation therapy may cause keratinization of the conjunctiva and chronic irritation of the cornea and keratitis. This condition is most likely to follow treatment of lesions involving the middle portion of the upper eyelid. When the eyelid margin is involved, surgical excision is preferred to radiation inasmuch as inadequate radiation may be followed by metaplasia of the tumor to the squamous cell type, and removal is more nearly assured with excision. In tumors involving the inner canthus, radiation is frequently indicated, since damage to the

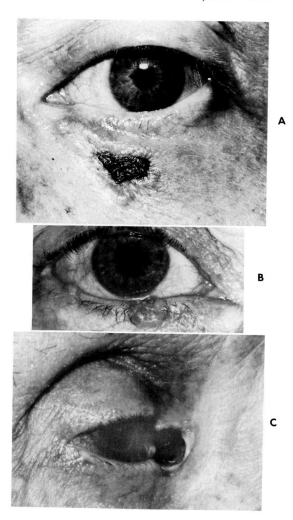

Fig. 8-9. **A** and **B**, Basal cell carcinomas of the lower eyelid. **C**, Extension of a basal cell carcinoma of the inner canthus into the nose in an 83-year-old man.

lacrimal drainage apparatus may be minimized. The globe is protected by means of a lead shield to prevent the formation of radiation cataract.

Neglected or mismanaged basal cell carcinoma may invade the orbit and the cranial cavity, causing a widespread destructive lesion.

The sweat glands (of Moll) of the eyelids are apocrine glands and, like such glands elsewhere (axilla, surrounding the nipples, and perianal and perigenital regions), may develop a special type of carcinoma, extramammary Paget disease. The diagnosis is usually based on the histologic appearance of the tissue, which is resected in the belief that the lesion is a basal cell carcinoma.

Adenocarcinoma may develop in the glandular portion of a meibomian gland. Most commonly, patients are treated for recurrent chalazion before the neoplastic nature of the lesion is evident. Such a delay may permit fatal metastasis. The tissue excised in all recurrent chalazia should be examined histologically.

BIBLIOGRAPHY

Beard, C.: Ptosis, ed. 2, St. Louis, 1976, The C. V. Mosby Co.

Fox, S. A.: Ophthalmic plastic surgery, ed. 5, New York, 1976, Grune & Stratton, Inc.

McMahon, R. T., Font, R. L., and McLean, I. W.: Phakomatous choristoma of eyelid, Arch. Ophthalmol. **94:**1778, 1976.

Pizzarello, L. D., Jacobiec, F. A., Hofeldt, A. J., and others: Intralesional corticosteroid therapy of chalazia, Am. J. Ophthalmol. **85:**818, 1978.

Reeh, M. J., Beyer, C. K., and Shannon, G. M.: Practical ophthalmic plastic and reconstructive surgery, Philadelphia, 1976, Lea & Febiger.

Smolin, G., and Okumoto, M.: Staphylococcal blepharitis, Arch. Ophthalmol. **95:**812, 1977.

Soll, D. B., editor: Management of complications in ophthalmic plastic surgery, Birmingham, 1976, Aesculapius Publishing Co.

Tenzel, R. R., Stewart, W. B., Boynton, J. R., and Zbar, M.: Sebaceous adenocarcinoma of eyelid, Arch. Ophthalmol. **95:**2203, 1977.

White, J. H.: Correction of distichiasis by tarsal resection and mucous membrane grafting, Am. J. Ophthalmol. **80:**507, 1975.

Chapter 9

THE CONJUNCTIVA

The conjunctiva is a thin, translucent mucous membrane that lines the posterior surfaces of the eyelids and covers the noncorneal portion of the anterior segment of the eye ("the white of the eye"). It is divided into the palpebral and bulbar portions and the regions connecting them, the superior and inferior fornices (p. 55). Its epithelium is continuous with that which covers the corneal stroma and lines the lacrimal passages and glands. It varies in thickness from two layers of nonstratified columnar epithelium at the tarsal plate to some 10 to 15 layers at the corneoscleral limbus. Goblet cells are scattered throughout with lymphocytes and melanocytes in the basal layers. The stroma is closely adherent to the tarsal plate but thrown into many folds in the fornices and loosely adherent to the globe. The stroma comprises loosely arranged bundles of coarse collagenous tissue containing numerous fibroblasts. Fibroblasts, macrophages, mast cells, and leukocytes are found extravascularly in the tissues. After the age of 3 or 4 months the superficial stroma in the fornices contains lymphoid tissue.

Because of its exposed position, the bulbar conjunctiva is the site of many degenerative changes. Inflammation may arise from exogenous microorganisms, chemical and mechanical foreign material, or radiant energy. Infection may extend from the areas adjacent to the conjunctiva or may be blood-borne, as in measles and chickenpox. Conjunctival allergic reactions may be conspicuous, as in hay fever or vernal conjunctivitis. Vascular abnormalities are readily apparent and may constitute an obvious part of systemic disease.

SYMPTOMS AND SIGNS OF CONJUNCTIVAL DISEASE

The main symptoms of conjunctival disorders are ocular discomfort or burning and sometimes exudation. Severe pain suggests corneal involvement rather than conjunctival disease. Itching is common in allergic conditions. Inflammatory exudates may excoriate the skin, particularly at the outer canthus, or agglutinate the eyelids together during sleep. Copious exudate may float across the cornea and blur vision or may even cause halos surrounding lights that disappear with rapid blinking.

The most serious symptoms of conjunctival disease arise from secondary corneal involvement. This may occur by extension of inflammation from the conjunctiva or by irritation of the cornea because of continued contact with keratinized epithelium of the tarsal conjunctiva. Corneal disease may be secondary to exposure in cicatricial conditions that limit eyelid mobility, or it may be caused by secretory failure of goblet cells or accessory lacrimal glands resulting in an abnormal tear film. Visual loss from corneal scarring is common, and indeed trachoma (p. 222), a chlamydial infection involving the conjunctiva initially, is probably the chief cause of blindness in the world.

The signs of conjunctival disease are mainly related to abnormalities of appearance, vascular changes, and edema (chemosis). The bulbar conjunctiva is easily inspected, but the tarsal conjunctiva can be seen only by eversion of the upper and lower eyelids (p. 169). Inspection of the superior fornix requires elevation of the upper eyelid by means of a retractor.

CONJUNCTIVAL BLOOD VESSELS
Injection

The normally inconspicuous posterior conjunctival arteries are dilated and engorged in conjunctival inflammations. Conjunctival injection is characterized by superficial bright red blood vessels, which are most conspicuous in the fornices and fade toward the corneoscleral limbus. These blood vessels move with the conjunctiva and are constricted by 1:1,000 epinephrine solution instilled in the conjunctival sac (see Table 6-1).

Both the conjunctival and ciliary vascular bed are usually injected in inflammations of the anterior segment, although one is more markedly involved than the other. To distinguish conjunctival diseases from deeper diseases of the eye, it is wiser to direct attention to signs of corneal and iris involvement, the pupillary reaction to light, and visual acuity (p. 158), rather than emphasize vascular engorgement.

Conjunctival hyperemia is a dilation of the conjunctival blood vessels that occurs without exudation or cellular infiltration. Symptoms may be absent, but often a gritty foreign body sensation is aggravated by prolonged close work. Many

patients are distressed by the conjunctival redness, which becomes more severe with wakefulness and is aggravated by fatigue.

Hyperemia is caused by the following: (1) irritation caused by tobacco smoke, smog, and chemical fumes; (2) exposure to wind and sun; (3) inadequate ocular protection from ultraviolet radiation; (4) uncorrected refractive errors and ocular muscle imbalance; (5) prolonged topical instillation of drugs, including vasoconstrictors; (6) acne rosacea; (7) blepharitis and excessive meibomian gland secretion; and (8) ganglionic blockage in the treatment of hypertension. Chronic conjunctivitis may be caused by many of the same entities (p. 225).

Treatment is directed toward removal of the cause. Temporary relief may be obtained by cold compresses or by local instillation of weak solutions of vasoconstrictors. Many commercial preparations containing epinephrine or phenylephrine are available and may provide temporary relief. Products containing corticosteroids should not be used because of the danger of inducing infection or glaucoma.

Subconjunctival hemorrhage

Rupture of a conjunctival blood vessel causes a bright red, sharply delineated area surrounded by normal-appearing conjunctiva. The hemorrhage is located beneath the bulbar conjunctiva and gradually fades in the course of 2 weeks. There are no symptoms, but many patients become alarmed by its appearance. A subconjunctival hemorrhage is caused by the same factors responsible for a black-and-blue spot elsewhere in the body: trauma, hypertension, blood dyscrasias, and the like. Usually no cause is found. Treatment is ineffective in hastening the absorption of the blood.

Subconjunctival hemorrhage involving the entire conjunctiva may follow fracture of one of the orbital bones or rupture of the posterior sclera. In 1978 several endemics of adenovirus conjunctivitis (p. 263) were associated with severe subconjunctival hemorrhage.

Systemic disease

Typical involvement of the conjunctival blood vessels has been described in (1) sickle cell disease (p. 562), (2) diabetes mellitus (p. 511), (3) riboflavin deficiency, and (4) cryoglobulinemia (p. 556). The changes are frequently evident only with biomicroscopic examination. Inasmuch as the conjunctival blood vessels often show dilation and tortuosity with advancing age and exposure to wind, the changes that accompany diabetes and riboflavin deficiency may be difficult to differentiate from aging changes.

Conjunctival vascular stasis may be present in hemoglobin SC disease and in blood hyperviscosity conditions. Biomicroscopic examination indicates isolated, sharply defined, twisted segments of capillaries with both the efferent and afferent connections empty of blood. The vessels are most involved in the bulbar conjunctiva adjacent to the inferior fornix. There are also nonspecific changes of microaneurysms, telangiectasis, and sausagelike dilation. The typical vascular stasis disappears with the local application of heat and is accentuated by cholinergic blockade and cold.

Cryoglobulinemia is associated with stasis of blood flow in conjunctival vessels that have a clumping of erythrocytes. Ice water irrigation of the conjunctival sac slows the bloodstream and causes an increase in segmentation of the blood column.

Venous congestion, microaneurysms, and venous dilation have been noted in the conjuctival vessels in diabetes mellitus. The changes are nonspecific and may be seen with aging, arteriosclerosis, and vascular hypertension.

Pigmentation

The dull, white sclera accentuates conjunctival pigmentation. A dull, grayish discoloration involving the conjunctiva in the lower fornix may follow repeated instillation of silver and mercury salts. The pigmentation arises from the deposition of the metallic ion and cannot be reversed. Prolonged instillation of epinephrine salts may cause deep black subconjunctival deposits of adrenochrome (oxidized epinephrine).

A yellowish discoloration of the conjunctiva may arise from an excess of plant pigment (carotene) in food faddists who eat many carrots. It must be distinguished from jaundice. Ochronosis and Addison disease also cause pigmentation of the conjunctiva. The conjunctiva and not the sclera is stained with bilirubin in jaundice.

CONJUNCTIVITIS

Conjunctivitis is an inflammation of the conjunctiva characterized by cellular infiltration and exudation. Classification is unsatisfactory but is often based on the cause (bacterial, viral, fungal, parasitic, toxic, chemical, mechanical, irritative, allergic, or lacrimal), the age of occurrence (ophthalmia neonatorum), the type of exudate (purulent, mucopurulent, membranous, pseudomembranous, or catarrhal), or course (acute, subacute, or chronic). There is often an associated corneal inflammation (keratoconjunctivitis).

Diagnosis

The diagnosis of conjunctivitis is based on (1) the history and clinical examination, (2) Gram and Wright stains of conjunctival scrapings, and (3) culture of conjunctival scrapings and identification of the cause.

The history of the inflammation may be helpful. Infectious disease is often bilateral and may involve other members of the family or community. Unilateral disease suggests a toxic, chemical, mechanical, or lacrimal origin. A copious exudate suggests a bacterial inflammation. A stringy, sparse exudate suggests an allergy or a viral infection. A preauricular adenopathy suggests an adenovirus infection.

Clinical examination requires good illumination and magnification. Attention should be directed to the presence or absence of preauricular adenopathy, involvement of the eyelid margins, patency of the lacrimal system, severity and nature of the conjunctival injection, occurrence of follicles or papillary hypertrophy (p. 219), and the nature of the secretion (Table 9-1).

Conjunctival scrapings are obtained with a platinum spatula, and the material is then placed on a clean glass slide. The smear is fixed by drying and is not heated.

Staining and culture. The gram-stained material is the basis for initial treatment based on gram-positive or gram-negative rods or cocci, mixed material, or none. Intraepithelial gram-negative diplococci of gonorrheal ophthalmia may be demon-

Table 9-1. Clinical findings in conjunctivitis

 I. Preauricular adenopathy
   A. Palpable and not tender: inclusion conjunctivitis, most APC viruses
   B. Visible and tender: adenovirus types 8 and 19, herpes simplex, sties, acute suppurative chalazion
   C. Gross enlargement with suppuration: Parinaud oculoglandular syndrome
 II. Blepharitis and meibomianitis: *Staphylococcus* sp.
 III. Excoriation of skin of medial and lateral canthus: diplobacillus of Morax-Axenfeld
 IV. Conjunctival injection
   A. Red: infectious disease
     1. Intense with petechial hemorrhages: *Streptococcus pneumoniae* or *Haemophilus aegyptius* (Koch-Weeks)
     2. Subconjunctival hemorrhage: adenovirus or acute hemorrhagic conjunctivitis (picornavirus)
   B. Pale whitish: allergy
 V. Chemosis: gonococcus, trichinosis, orbital infections
 VI. Exudate
   A. Stringy, white: allergy
   B. Purulent: gonococcus, meningococcus
   C. Mucopurulent: pyogenic bacteria
   D. Scanty: virus
   E. Foamy, whitish secretion: *Corynebacterium xerose*
   F. Pseudomembrane: *Corynebacterium diphtheriae, Streptococcus,* erythema multiforme, APC type 8, vernal conjunctivitis
 VII. Follicle formation (lymphatic hypertrophy)
   A. Lower eyelid: follicular conjunctivitis, APC viruses, adult inclusion blenorrhea, molluscum contagiosum, toxic effect of pilocarpine, eserine, and so on
   B. Upper eyelid: trachoma
 VIII. Papillary hyperplasia: vernal conjunctivitis (neovascularization with lymphocyte infiltration)
 IX. Conjunctival scarring
   A. Upper eyelid: trachoma
   B. Lower eyelid: erythema multiforme, alkali burns, radiation burns, ocular pemphigoid
   C. General: diphtheria
 X. Corneal involvement
   A. Purulent: gonococcus, *Pseudomonas aeruginosa*
   B. Marginal infiltrates: *Staphylococcus,* diplobacillus of Morax-Axenfeld
   C. Punctate epithelial defects: *Staphylococcus* (lower half), trachoma (upper half)
   D. Generalized epithelial defects: Sjögren syndrome
   E. Superior vascularization: pannus of trachoma, phlyctenular disease
 XI. Unilateral inflammation: Parinaud syndrome, adult gonococcus, contact allergy, lacrimal occlusion, viral infection

strated by Gram stain some 48 hours before their demonstration in bacterial culture.

The Wright-stained material is read for the predominant cell type present (Table 9-2). The Giemsa stain may be used to demonstrate inclusion bodies (chlamydial diseases), but the yield is low, and immunofluorescent staining is more useful.

The exudate for culture should be collected from the inferior cul-de-sac by using a moist swab without anesthetics. A transport medium should not be used; the media should not contain inhibitors and must be incubated immediately. Carbon dioxide must be provided for organisms such as *Neisseria* and certain strains of *Streptococcus pneumoniae*. Exudate is cultured on blood and chocolate agar, beef broth, or other media when diphtheria, gonorrhea, or fungi are suspected. Different parts of the same plate may be used to culture exudate from the eyelids and conjunctiva. Adequate material must be obtained from the site of active disease. Chance contamination can be distinguished from infection by the confluent or abundant colonies present on culture in infection. The chlamydia group may be cultured in the yolk sac of chicks or in tissue culture-irradiated–idoxuridine-treated McCoy cells.

Table 9-2. Cytologic findings in conjunctivitis

I. Polymorphonuclear leukocytes
  A. Neutrophils
    1. Bacterial and mycotic infections
    2. Erythema multiforme
    3. Chlamydial infections
  B. Basophils and eosinophils
    1. Allergies
      a. Vernal conjunctivitis (often fragmented)
      b. Hay fever
      c. Sensitivity to drugs, cosmetics, and so on
II. Monocytes
  A. Lymphocytes
    1. Virus infections
  B. Plasma cells
    1. Trachoma
  C. Phagocytes (Leber cells)
    1. Trachoma
III. Inclusion bodies
  A. Basophilic
    1. Upper tarsal: trachoma
    2. Lower tarsal: inclusion conjunctivitis
  B. Acidophilic
    1. Molluscum contagiosum
    2. Herpes simplex
IV. Epithelial cells
  A. Keratinized
    1. Sjögren syndrome
  B. Multinucleated
    1. Virus infection

Clinical types

The clinical manifestations of conjunctivitis vary with the cause. The onset is often insidious. The patient notices a fullness of the eyelids and a diffuse, gritty, foreign body sensation. Examination indicates diffuse conjunctival injection, a clear cornea, a distinct iris pattern, and normal pupillary reaction. Within several hours of the onset, there is exudation. There may be swelling of the eyelids and edema (chemosis) of the conjunctiva. The cornea should be stained with sterile fluorescein, and particular attention should be directed to the corneoscleral limbus and extension of the inflammation. The upper and lower eyelids should be everted and the tarsal conjunctiva studied.

Particular attention should be directed to the fornices to determine if papillary hypertrophy or follicle formation may be present. Papillary hypertrophy is characterized by folds or projections of hyperplastic epithelium that contain a core of blood vessels surrounded by edematous stroma infiltrated with lymphocytes and plasma cells. It is basically a vascular response with secondary monocytic infiltration and occurs characteristically in vernal conjunctivitis. Papillary hypertrophy occurs in vernal conjunctivitis and in exceptionally severe or prolonged conjunctival inflammation.

Follicular hypertrophy is characterized by small follicles that are smaller and paler than papillae and lack the central core of blood vessels. Basically it is a lymphoid hyperplasia and occurs in trachoma, drug sensitivities, and allergies.

Mucopurulent conjunctivitis. Bacterial organisms causing mucopurulent conjunctivitis in the United States include gram-positive cocci (*Staphylococcus aureus, Staphylococcus epidermidis, Streptococcus pyogenes,* and *Streptococcus pneumoniae*), gram-negative cocci (*Neisseria meningitidis, Moraxella lacunata* [of Morax-Axenfeld]), and gram-negative rods (genus *Haemophilus,* family Enterobacteriaceae [genera *Proteus* and *Klebsiella*]). (The tribe Mimeae sp. *polymorpha* is obsolete. It belongs to the family Neisseriaceae and is closely related to genus *Moraxella.*) Almost any bacteria may be involved. Additionally, the causative organism may be one of a number of bacteria or fungi intermediate between saprophytes and pathogens. They may be recovered in culture or found in epithelial scrapings stained with Gram iodine.

The onset is acute, and both eyes are involved with a mucopurulent exudate. Drying of inspissated pus during sleep may cause the eyelids to be agglutinated on awaking.

The physician must wash his hands thoroughly and use eye drops in individual containers to avoid transmitting infection. The patient should use only his own towels. Corticosteroids should not be used. The eye should not be patched.

Many bacterial inflammations of the conjunctiva are self-limited. However, treatment with topical sulfacetamide, sulfisoxazole, or antimicrobials may be helpful. Initial treatment should consist of hourly instillation of sulfonamides, topical bacitracin, or erythromycin. Baci-tracin-neomycin-polymyxin B (Neosporin) may cause local allergy. A poor clinical response after 48 to 72 hours indicates that an insensitive bacterium is the cause or that the cause is not bacterial. Further therapy should be based on the result of culture. Conjunctivitis caused by gonococci, *Chlamydia trachomatis,* or *Pseudomonas* organisms may require systemic as well as topical treatment.

Purulent conjunctivitis. This is a severe, acute, purulent conjunctivitis caused by *Neisseria gonorrhoeae.* It has an incubation period of 2 to 5 days. It occurs in newborn infants, who are infected during passage through the birth canal, and in adults as a result of self-contamination from acute urethritis.

The inflammation may have a relatively mild onset but progresses rapidly. Marked swelling and redness of the eyelids and severe chemosis of the conjunctiva occur. The exudate is first serous and then purulent. The disease is well established after 2 days, reaches its height in 4 or 5 days, and then regresses over a 4- to 6-week period. Involvement of the central cornea is common, and perforation may occur. The gram-negative intracellular organism may be demonstrated in conjunctival scrapings at the time of onset of the disease and in the exudate some 48 hours later.

Intramuscular and topical penicillin G is the treatment of choice. If penicillin sensitivity is present, tetracycline may be substituted. Care should be taken that a monocular infection does not spread to the fellow eye. Frequent irrigation of the eyes with normal saline solution will clear secretions.

Gonococcal urethritis is sometimes complicated by a bacteremia that causes an acute migratory polyarthritis or a tenosynovitis. A sterile catarrhal conjunctivitis occurs in about 10% of those affected. The condition must be differentiated from Reiter syndrome, which causes a sterile urethritis, arthritis, and iridocyclitis (p. 304).

Ophthalmia neonatorum. Ophthalmia neonatorum is a conjunctivitis that occurs within the first 10 days of life. In most states it is a reportable infectious disease. The most serious cause is *Neisseria gonorrhoeae.* More common causes today are inclusion body conjunctivitis (p. 454) and bacteria, mainly *Staphylococcus* and *Streptococcus pneumoniae.* Diagnosis is based on epithelial scrapings stained with Gram stain, on culture, and on cytology of the exudate. Treatment with systemic and local antibiotics is effective in bacterial disease. Inclusion conjunctivitis must be treated by means of systemic erythromycin and topical tetracycline.

Credé prophylaxis. Credé prophylaxis is the instillation of 1 drop of 1% silver nitrate into the lower conjunctival sac of each eye immediately after birth. Chemical conjunctivitis occurs in about 20% of the infants thus treated, but the treatment has eliminated gonorrheal ophthalmia as a cause of blindness. Credé prophylaxis does not prevent inclusion conjunctivitis.

Inasmuch as gonorrhea during pregnancy may be adequately treated by means of antibiotics, Credé prophylaxis is regarded by some to be outmoded. However, gonorrhea may be undetected and unsuspected during pregnancy, with resultant contamination of the eyes in the birth canal. In some hospitals the mother and infant may be discharged during the incubation period of the infection, and the inflammation may be well established before initiation of therapy. Although many of the antibiotics have proved as adequate as silver nitrate in prophylaxis of gonococcal conjunctivitis, none has been shown to be superior. Additionally, infants born of mothers who have gonor-

rhea should be given parenteral penicillin G immediately after birth.

Trachoma and inclusion conjunctivitis (TRIC). The genus *Chlamydia* (p. 454) contains two species, *Chlamydia trachomatis* and *Chlamydia psittaci. Chlamydia trachomatis* is parasitic principally in humans and causes a variety of oculourogenital diseases: trachoma, inclusion conjunctivitis, lymphogranuloma venereum, urethritis, and proctitis. Pneumonitis has recently been identified in neonates. *Chlamydia psittaci* is a parasite of vertebrates and causes a variety of nonocular disorders in birds and mammals.

Inclusion conjunctivitis. Inclusion conjunctivitis is an acute ocular inflammation caused by *Chlamydia trachomatis* in sexually active adults. Newborns are infected in the birth canal (inclusion blennorrhea) and develop an acute mucopurulent conjunctivitis after an incubation period of 5 to 14 days. Adult infection is transmitted venereally and by contaminated eye cosmetics. About 90% of the women who have chlamydial eye infection have an associated chlamydial genital infection.

Inclusion conjunctivitis is one cause of ophthalmia neonatorum. After a variable period of 5 to 14 days, an acute conjunctivitis occurs with profuse discharge. Inasmuch as the newborn does not have conjunctival lymphoid tissue until 4 to 6 weeks of age, there is no follicular reaction. Epithelial scrapings stained with Giemsa stain show many basophilic inclusion bodies combined with initial and elementary bodies. If not treated, the acute phase lasts 10 to 20 days and then subsides into a gradually diminishing chronic follicular conjunctivitis that persists 3 to 12 months. Infants should be treated daily for 21 days with both systemic erythromycin (30 mg/kg) and topical tetracycline ointment. Systemic tetracyclines are contraindicated in infants because of yellowing of future teeth. Both parents should be examined and treated.

Gonorrheal conjunctivitis may be differentiated by a shorter incubation period (1 to 3 days), by involvement of both the superior and inferior fornices, and by cytology and demonstration of the causative organism.

Inclusion conjunctivitis of the adult begins as an acute follicular conjunctivitis that becomes chronic. There may be an associated preauricular adenopathy and a punctate keratitis. The disease may be distinguished from adenovirus infections by the polymorphonuclear cytologic response and the basophilic intracytoplasmic inclusion bodies in contrast to the mononuclear response seen in adenoviral infections. Adults should be treated with both systemic and topical tetracyclines.

Trachoma. Trachoma is a chronic, bilateral, cicatrizing conjunctivitis caused by *Chlamydia trachomatis.* There are at least eight strains, and the disease varies considerably in severity. It is endemic, often associated with conjuncitivitis, and is likely the chief cause of blindness in the world. Basophilic inclusion bodies may be found, particularly in the acute stage, in epithelial scrapings stained with Giemsa stain. Antibodies to *Chlamydia* may be present both in eye secretions and in the serum. The severity of the disease varies markedly, and there are unexplained regional differences; in the United States, it is largely confined to American Indians in the Southwest. The disease occurs among the underprivileged and in regions with a warm, moist climate. Entire populations in regions of poor hygiene may be infected. There is corneal inflammation and vascularization with severe conjunctival scarring and deformity of the eyelids that may lead to blindness. The disease may be complicated by superimposed infection with

Neisseria gonorrhoeae or *Haemophilus aegyptius* (Koch-Weeks).

Chlamydia organisms are sensitive to sulfonamides and broad-spectrum antibiotics. The compounds must be administered systemically. In adults tetracycline or sulfadiazine (2 to 4 gm daily for 14 days) is the preferred agent. Entire communities may be treated prophylactically with sulfonamides, but attention must be directed to elimination of flies and improvement in hygiene, a major problem in regions without plumbing or running water. Active immunization by inoculation is complicated by the several strains, poor cross-immunity, and weak antigenicity. Surgery is commonly required for cicatricial distortion of the eyelids.

Virus inflammations. Invasions of the conjunctiva by a variety of viruses can cause conjunctivitis (p. 458). Many mild nonincapacitating conjunctival inflammations in which microorganisms are not demonstrated are probably caused by viruses. Conjunctival involvement may be part of a systemic infection, or the disease may be limited to the epithelium of the cornea and conjunctiva.

Adenovirus. This group of at least 31 human and 17 animal serotypes causes upper respiratory tract infection in infants, children, and military recruits. Some strains cause conjunctivitis and preauricular adenopathy together with fever and pharyngitis (acute pharyngoconjunctival fever), and others cause keratoconjunctivitis (p. 263).

ACUTE PHARYNGOCONJUNCTIVAL FEVER. This is one of a spectrum of infections caused by the adenoviruses and is characterized by fever, pharyngitis, cervical adenopathy, and conjunctivitis. The conjunctivitis is bilateral, often with intense hyperemia, particularly in the lower cul-de-sac, and a scanty secretion. Adenovirus types 3 and 7 are particularly implicated in infections in which conjunctival involvement is marked.

The parents of children with acute pharyngoconjunctival fever may develop a monocular conjunctivitis with follicle formation and preauricular adenopathy. Fever may occur in about one half.

Acute hemorrhagic conjunctivitis. This new disease, first seen in Africa in 1969 (and called Apollo conjunctivitis because it occurred at the time of the Apollo 11 moon landing), has appeared in west and north Africa, southeast Asia, Hong Kong, the Philippines, Taiwan, Japan, India, and Korea. There is an explosive onset of conjunctivitis with eyelid edema, tearing, serous discharge, and conjunctival hemorrhages. Conjunctival follicles and enlarged preauricular lymph nodes occur. Lumbosacral reticulomyelitis has been reported. Antigenically different strains of a new member of the picornavirus group have been implicated, but although acute and convalescent serums indicate increasing titers, the virus is seldom recovered from the eye. The spread seems to be by eye to eye or by hand to eye. The disease is highly contagious, having affected hundreds of thousands of patients. The differential diagnosis includes other diseases with acute follicular conjunctivitis, such as epidemic keratoconjunctivitis, pharyngoconjunctival fever, Newcastle disease of the conjunctiva, primary herpes simplex, inclusion conjunctivitis, and acute exacerbations of trachoma.

Acute bacterial conjunctivitis caused by *Streptococcus pneumoniae*, other bacterial pathogens, or adenovirus infections may produce conjunctival hemorrhages without follicular reaction. By contrast, acute hemorrhagic conjunctivitis is explosive at onset, bilateral, and characterized by eyelid edema, chemosis, follicles, and hemorrhages; the signs peak at 48 hours and clear rapidly thereafter.

Lacrimal conjunctivitis. Lacrimal conjunctivitis is a monocular conjunctivitis secondary to infections caused by microorganisms in an occluded lacrimal sac. The inflammation persists until drainage is established. Usually dacryocystitis does not involve the conjunctiva. Pneumococcus infection of the lacrimal sac is a common cause of serpiginous keratitis (p. 260). Fungus occlusion of the canaliculi is often recognized because of the scraping sound when the lacrimal system is probed.

Parinaud oculoglandular syndrome. This is an eponym traditional in ophthalmology, but the condition is rarely seen clinically. It consists of a monocular, granulomatous, necrotic conjunctival lesion associated with a suppurative preauricular adenopathy. Parinaud syndrome must be differentiated from Parinaud sign, which is the inability to rotate the eyes upward because of midbrain neoplasms, principally pinealoma. The chief causes of Parinaud oculoglandular syndrome include chancre, tuberculosis, lymphogranuloma venereum, leptotrichosis, and oculoglandular tularemia.

Mycotic inflammations. Fungus inflammations of the conjunctiva (p. 455) are uncommon. They may be primary in the conjunctival sac, secondary to mycotic obstructions of the lacrimal system, or contiguous to adjacent inflammation. Treatment is the same as that described for keratomycosis (p. 265).

Allergic conjunctivitis. A number of antigens may give rise to superficial conjunctival reactions. Because of the elasticity of the tissues, there may be considerable swelling. Most of the conditions are characterized by the presence of many eosinophils in the epithelial scrapings. A number of specific types are described.

Vernal conjunctivitis. Vernal conjunctivitis is a bilateral recurrent inflammation occurring during the warm months of the year, particularly in warm climates. Boys are affected more commonly than girls, usually during childhood. Two

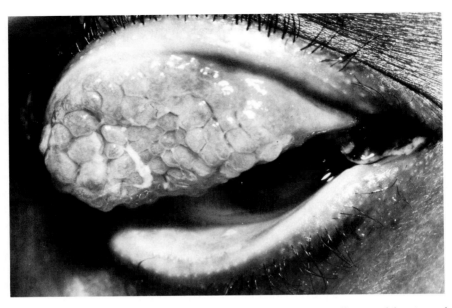

Fig. 9-1. Palpebral form of vernal conjunctivitis with marked papillary proliferation of the conjunctiva.

forms occur: (1) palpebral (Fig. 9-1), involving the tarsal conjunctiva of the upper eyelid with the formation of typical thickened gelatinous vegetations and sometimes a pseudomembrane, and (2) limbal, associated with inflammation of the circumference of the corneoscleral limbus with the formation of a gelatinous, elevated area about 4 mm wide. The chief symptom is itching, which may be nearly intolerable. Histologically there is hyperplasia and hyalinization of connective tissue, proliferation of epithelium, and cellular infiltration with numerous eosinophils. The serum and tear level of IgE is high, and many mast cells are present. The secretion is tenacious, stringy, and sticky. Moving to a cool climate is sometimes helpful. Treatment consists of local instillation of corticosteroids and weak solutions of epinephrine and application of epinephrine and application of cold compresses. Local application of cromolyn sodium may give relief. Radiation

therapy is contraindicated, but the excision of large palpebral vegetations may give symptomatic relief.

Atopic conjunctivitis. Atopic conjunctivitis is the conjunctival reaction to pollens in hypersensitive people who usually have hay fever. Atopic conjunctivitis may occur independent of pollen hypersensitivity, but there is usually a history of allergy. The onset is acute, and lacrimation, chemosis, and a watery discharge are present. The conjunctival secretion contains many eosinophils. The local instillation of the causative antigen causes similar symptoms. The condition responds to the local instillation of vasoconstrictors and to systemic antihistamines. Desensitization to the causative antigen may be unusually helpful. Locally applied antihistamines may cause a contact conjunctivitis.

Phlyctenular keratoconjunctivitis. Phlyctenular keratoconjunctivitis is a unilateral, localized hypersensitivity bulbar conjunctival nodule about 1 to 3 mm in size. It is considered a delayed hypersensitivity to bacterial protein, particularly tuberculoprotein. Classically it was believed to be a disease of undernourished children sensitive to tuberculoprotein. In the United States it is mainly an inflammation that affects adults. Staphylococci are considered the most common cause. The most serious complication is corneal vascularization. The phlyctenula progresses irregularly to the central cornea and is followed by a group of blood vessels; this causes corneal scarring and reduced vision. Topical instillation of corticosteroids usually suppresses the hypersensitivity, and healing follows.

Contact conjunctivitis. Contact conjunctivitis occurs in one of two forms: (1) allergic and (2) primary irritant. Allergic contact conjunctivitis is nearly always caused by the local instillation of medication used in the treatment of chronic ocular disease, such as pilocarpine and eserine in the treatment of glaucoma and atropine in the management of uveitis or retinal detachment. Local penicillin, streptomycin, sulfathiazole, topical anesthetics, and antihistamines are also common offenders. The condition is marked by itching, chemosis of the conjunctiva, and eosinophils in the scrapings.

Primary irritant contact conjunctivitis is a follicular type of conjunctivitis that is particularly marked in the lower cul-de-sac. Symptoms are minimal, and the disease is often listed as a chronic conjunctivitis. Eosinophils are not present in conjunctival scrapings. Almost any compound used in the treatment of ocular disease may be a source of such irritation. The conjunctivitis disappears when the compound is discontinued, and once it has improved, the drugs may be reinstituted without recurrence. The irritation may constitute an untoward reaction to the vehicle or a preservative rather than the active principle of the drug.

Chronic conjunctivitis. Chronic conjunctivitis is a generic term applied to persistent conjunctival inflammation. It may be caused by many agents. It is characterized by bilateral conjunctival injection, scanty exudation, and a tendency to periodic exacerbation and remission. Symptoms vary from mild grittiness or foreign body sensation, with heaviness of the eyelids, to burning, photophobia, and irritation. The symptoms may be severe enough to handicap the patient and are often disproportionately severe for the clinical signs of disease. Examination indicates hyperemia, microscopic papillae, thickening of the conjunctiva in the fornices, and a mucous secretion.

Causes include the following:

1. *Staphylococcus aureus* infection is usually associated with a chronic blepharitis and an epithelial keratitis involving the lower one half of the cornea.

2. A variety of microorganisms often considered nonpathogenic have been implicated. These organisms often reside on body surfaces but may be found in almost pure culture, and presumably when appropriate predisposing conditions are present, they may produce inflammation.

3. The significance of viruses is not established. Virus infections other than adenoviruses tend to involve the superior conjunctiva and to be associated with corneal filaments near the 12 o'clock meridian (see discussion on superficial punctate keratitis, p. 264).

4. Chemical and physical irritants and unsuspected foreign bodies may be a cause. The use of sun lamps without ocular protection may give rise to an actinic keratoconjunctivitis. Chemical irritation from the chlorine in swimming pools is an obvious cause. Drugs used to treat ocular disease may cause the inflammation.

5. Excessive meibomian secretion is characterized by a frothy secretion at the angles and may either cause or complicate chronic conjunctivitis.

6. Acne rosacea may have conjunctival involvement that precedes rosacea corneal vascularization.

Treatment of chronic conjunctivitis is difficult. Careful diagnosis is essential, and the cause must be eliminated if possible. Lesions of the eyelids and eyelid margins, such as cysts, verruca vulgaris, and molluscum contagiosum, must be eliminated. Keratoconjunctivitis sicca (p. 268) must be excluded, and the tear ducts must be tested for patency. Allergy and irritations caused by chemicals, smoke, and cosmetics must be minimized. Many of the same symptoms arise from abnormalities of the precorneal tear film (p. 83).

OTHER CONJUNCTIVAL DISORDERS
Ocular cicatricial pemphigoid

Ocular cicatricial pemphigoid (benign mucous membrane pemphigoid, essential shrinkage of the conjunctiva) is a chronic progressive disease characterized by marked scarring of the conjunctiva that results in trichiasis and drying of the eyes with eventual corneal opacification and reduced vision. This disorder begins with granulation tissue beneath the conjunctiva followed by fibrosis, causing conjunctival shrinkage. IgG, IgA, and complement are deposited in the conjunctival basement membrane, and antinuclear antibodies are present. Conjunctival scarring is also associated with radiation or chemical burns, erythema multiforme, epidermolysis bullosa, cutaneous pemphigus, bullous pemphigoid, and trachoma.

Symblepharon

Symblepharon is a condition in which there are adhesions between the palpebral and bulbar conjunctivae. It may obliterate conjunctival cul-de-sacs or form bands of scar tissue. Scarring follows conditions in which apposed areas of the conjunctiva lose their epithelial coverings. The chief causes are chemical burns (particularly caustics), trachoma, erythema multiforme (Stevens-Johnson syndrome), and benign mucous membrane pemphigus. The adhesions cause a mechanical defect, since the eyelids are adherent to the eyeball, and desiccation of the cornea and keratitis occur because of exposure. Treatment frequently is ineffective and disappointing. It is directed toward periodic lysis of the adhesions with a glass rod and protection of the corneas with a soft contact lens. Replacement of the scarred conjunctiva with a buccal mucous membrane graft may be necessary.

Pterygium

A pterygium is a triangular fold of bulbar conjunctivitis that advances progressively over the cornea in the interpalpebral fissure, usually from the nasal side (Fig. 9-2). It occurs in response to chronic recurrent dryness at the corneoscleral limbus and is often related to a corneal delle. A pinguecula often precedes its development, and elastotic degeneration of collagen is found in both pingueculae and pterygia. Most occur in individuals who spend much time outdoors in sunbaked lands. Initially there are signs of chronic conjunctivitis along with thickening of the conjunctiva. There may be

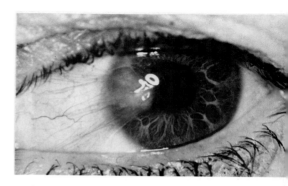

Fig. 9-2. Pterygium extending over the nasal portion of the cornea.

minor symptoms from the conjunctivitis, and the blood vessels in the peterygium may cause a cosmetic defect, but severe symptoms are absent unless the pterygium encroaches on the visual axis.

In the temperate zone of the United States pterygia seldom progress rapidly and usually require no treatment, but they respond well to any surgical procedure. In tropical areas pterygia progress rapidly, are commonly thick and vascular, and have a pronounced tendency to recur, irrespective of the type of surgery.

Every effort must be made to maintain a smooth corneal contour and avoid depressed areas of cornea that will create breaks in the precorneal tear film. Beta and grenz rays have been widely used to prevent recurrence. Beta-ray sources applied to the corneoscleral limbus may cause a sectorial radiation cataract caused by damage to cells in the replicative zone of the equatorial portion of the lens. Pre- and postoperatively, individuals with pterygia should be protected from ultraviolet light and irritation from wind or dust.

A secondary pterygium, or pseudopterygium, is a superficial fibrovascular overgrowth evoked by chronic superficial corneal disease near the corneoscleral limbus. Treatment must be directed to the exciting cause.

Pinguecula

A pinguecula is a benign degenerative tumor of the bulbar conjunctiva that appears as a yellowish white, slightly elevated, oval-shaped tissue mass on either side of the cornea in the palpebral fissure. The lesions are usually bilateral and located nasally. They become more common with advancing age. They cause a cosmetic defect and in some instances appear to precede a pterygium. Treatment is usually unnecessary, but excision is simple. Histologically, a pinguecula consists of a deposition of amorphous

hyaline substance in areas of degenerative elastic tissue. Rarely, a pinguecula becomes inflamed, causing a foreign body sensation and a surrounding conjunctival hyperemia. The apex of the pinguecula then stains with fluorescein. The inflammation responds quickly to local antibiotics.

Lymphangiectasis

The lymphatic channels of the conjunctiva may become dilated and give rise to clear, serous conjunctival cysts. These appear on the bulbar conjunctiva as minute tubules filled with clear fluid. Symptoms are minimal. There is no effective treatment.

Lithiasis

Degenerations of the conjunctival epithelium in the elderly or prolonged conjunctivitis may cause yellowish to white concretions in the epithelium. The deposits may be seen in the tarsal conjunctiva or the inferior fornix. Rarely, there is dehiscence of the overlying epithelium, causing exposure of the concretion along with foreign body symptoms. The area stains with fluorescein. Such concretions may be removed easily with a sharp needle-knife after the instillation of a conjunctival anesthetic.

Granulomas

Granulomas may follow faulty closure of a conjunctival incision. They occur particularly after retinal detachment and strabismus surgery. There is a formation of large, fungating, reddish masses, which bleed readily. Usually simple excision is all that is required. Retained foreign bodies may also cause a granuloma.

Tumors, cysts, and neoplasms

Choristomas. Choristomas are congenital tumors composed of tissues not normally found in the region. Dermoid cysts of the conjunctiva may be cystic or solid, containing stratified squamous epithelium, hair follicles, sebaceous glands, hair shafts, and debris. An epidermal cyst contains stratified squamous epithelium only. A dermatolipoma occurs usually at the superior temporal corneoscleral limbus and appears as a sharply circumscribed, round, slightly yellowish, elevated mass involving the cornea and the sclera. It occurs frequently in mandibulofacial dysostosis. Hamartomas are congenital tumors composed of tissues normally found in the region.

Lymphomas. Lymphomatous disease (benign lymphoma, lymphosarcoma, and reticulum cell sarcoma) may be manifest in the adenoid layer of the conjunctiva. A smooth, elevated tumor mass, which may be widespread, develops, and there is protrusion of the conjunctiva. Retrobulbar extension may cause proptosis. The condition may be localized to the conjunctiva or may be a manifestation of systemic disease. The conjunctival lesion is extremely sensitive to roentgen-ray therapy.

Telangiectasis. Telangiectasis of the conjunctiva occurs in all cases of ataxia telangiectasia (Louis-Bar syndrome). There is nystagmus (p. 536), progressive cerebellar ataxia, deficiency in IgA, and impaired lymphocyte transformation.

Carcinoma of the conjunctiva. This may appear as an exposure keratosis, as an inflammatory lesion, or as a leukoplakia with a white shining lesion caused by keratinization of the conjunctival epithelium.

Intraepithelial epitheliomas (Bowen disease). This is a slowly growing neoplasm usually associated with chronic conjunctival inflammation. It begins most commonly near the corneoscleral limbus. Usually men 60 years of age or older are affected. The tumor may give rise to an atypical squamous cell carcinoma or may metastasize without evidence of local invasion. Papanicolaou staining of scrapings may indicate carcinomatous cells. Complete excision often requires a lamellar corneal transplant. Recurrence is common.

Squamous cell carcinoma. Squamous cell carcinoma (Fig. 9-3) may be confined to the superficial tissues, or it may invade the adjacent tissues, such as the eye or orbit. The tumor is extremely sensitive to radiation, which should be used if excisional biopsy fails. Basal cell carcinoma rarely arises.

Pigmented lesions of the conjunctiva

Nevi. Nevi are extremely common on the conjunctiva and usually occur near the corneoscleral limbus. They appear as yellowish red areas or deeply pigmented masses, usually on the bulbar conjunctiva. Nevi are usually present before puberty but have junctional activity in adulthood.

Benign acquired melanosis (precancerous and cancerous melanosis). This is a benign acquired pigmented lesion that appears

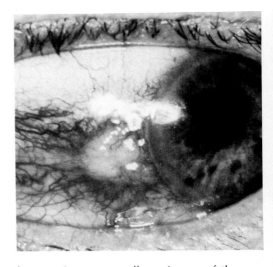

Fig. 9-3. Squamous cell carcinoma of the conjunctiva at the corneoscleral limbus. These tumors occur particularly in compromised hosts, and this 76-year-old patient had a pulmonary mass that could not be diagnosed.

at about the age of 40 to 50 years, unlike nevi, which are congenital or appear before puberty. The pigmentation is diffuse, flat, unilateral, and asymptomatic. Large areas of the conjunctiva may be involved over a period as long as 20 years. Sometimes after 5 or 10 years the lesion imperceptibly merges into a malignant melanoma. The lesion waxes and wanes, and clinical and histologic assessment of activity is difficult. The comparable lesion of the skin is called a senile melanotic freckle of Hutchinson. Treatment is difficult. In most individuals the tumor is benign, and periodic histologic study is indicated only when there is evidence of progression or activity. Exenteration of the orbit is indicated if frank malignant changes occur. Many regard the lesion as radiosensitive and believe radiation is indicated if metaplasia occurs.

BIBLIOGRAPHY

Allansmith, M. R., Hahn, G. S., and Simon, M. A.: Tissue, tear, and serum IgE concentrations in vernal conjunctivitis, Am. J. Ophthalmol. **81**:506, 1976.

Allansmith, M. R., Kajiyama, G., Abelson, M. B., and Simon, M. A.: Plasma cell content of main and accessory lacrimal glands and conjunctiva, Am. J. Ophthalmol. **82**:819, 1976.

Dawson, C. R.: How does the external eye resist infection, Invest. Ophthalmol. **15**:971, 1976.

Dawson, C. R., Hoshiwara, I., Daghfous, T., and others: Topical tetracycline and rifampicin therapy of endemic trachoma in Tunisia, Am. J. Ophthalmol. **79**:803, 1975.

Elsas, F. J., Green, W. R., and Ryan, S., Jr.: Benign pigmented tumors arising in acquired conjunctival melanosis, Am. J. Ophthalmol. **83**:718, 1977.

Furey, N., West, C., Andrews, T., and others: Immunofluorescent studies of ocular cicatricial pemphigoid, Am. J. Ophthalmol. **80**:825, 1975.

Greiner, J. V., Covington, H. I., and Allansmith, M. R.: Surface morphology of giant papillary conjunctivitis in contact lens wearers, Am. J. Ophthalmol. **85**:242, 1978.

Herron, B. E.: Immunologic aspects of cicatricial pemphigoid, Am. J. Ophthalmol. **79**:271, 1975.

Jampol, L. M., Marsh, J. C., Albert, D. M., and Zimmerman, L. E.: IgA associated lymphoplasmacytic tumor involving the conjunctiva, eyelid, and orbit, Am. J. Ophthalmol. **79**:279, 1975.

Markham, R. H. C., Richmond, S. J., Walshaw, N. W. D., and Easty, D. L.: Severe persistent inclusion conjunctivitis in a young child, Am. J. Ophthalmol. **83**:414, 1977.

Mondino, B. J., Ross, A. N., Rabin, B. S., and Brow, S. I.: Autoimmune phenomena in ocular cicatricial pemphigoid, Am. J. Ophthalmol. **83**:443, 1977.

Paton, D.: Pterygium management based upon a theory of pathogenesis, Trans. Am. Acad. Ophthalmol. Otolaryngol. **79**:603, 1975.

Tabbara, K. F., and Arafat, N. T.: Cromolyn effects on vernal keratoconjunctivitis in children, Arch. Ophthalmol. **95**:2184, 1977.

Waltman, S. R., and Yarian, D.: Circulating autoantibodies in ocular pemphigoid, Am. J. Ophthalmol. **77**:891, 1974.

Yang, Y. F., Hung, P. T., Lin, L. K., and others: Epidemic hemorrhagic keratoconjunctivitis, Am. J. Ophthalmol. **80**:192, 1975.

Chapter 10

THE LACRIMAL APPARATUS

The lacrimal apparatus consists of a secretory and a drainage portion. The secretory portion comprises the lacrimal gland, which is divided into palpebral and orbital lobes, and the accessory lacrimal glands of Wolfring and Krause scattered through the conjunctiva (p. 57). Additionally, goblet cells in the conjunctiva provide mucin to wet the hydrophobic epithelium, and the meibomian glands provide an oily secretion that minimizes tear evaporation. The drainage portion consists of epithelium-lined tubes leading from the two openings on the eyelid margins (the puncta) through the canaliculi to the lacrimal sac, which lies in the lacrimal fossa (p. 58). The lacrimal sac opens into the inferior nasal meatus by its inferior continuation, the nasolacrimal duct, which lies in the bony nasolacrimal canal.

The tears (p. 83) consist of a relatively stagnant layer overlying the cornea and a fluid layer that flows in the lower fornix to the inferior punctum. The corneal layer, the precorneal film, provides the smooth and regular anterior refracting surface of the eye. It has three layers: (1) a superficial oily layer derived from the meibomian glands that prevents evaporation, (2) a middle layer of fluid tears, and (3) an inner mucoid layer immediately adjacent to the corneal epithelium derived from the conjunctival goblet cells. The layer of

fluid tears is derived mainly from the accessory lacrimal glands, and the main lacrimal gland functions most conspicuously in psychic crying or when the eye is irritated.

SYMPTOMS AND SIGNS OF LACRIMAL APPARATUS DISEASE

Diseases of the lacrimal system are divided into those involving abnormalities of the lacrimal glands and those involving defects in the drainage system. Excessive tear secretion usually occurs because of reflex stimulation of the gland, whereas decreased tear formation arises because of either atrophy of glandular tissue or conjunctival scarring that occludes the orifices of the accessory and main lacrimal glands. Neoplasms and inflammatory diseases of the lacrimal gland give rise to a characteristic swelling that causes an S-shaped curve of the upper eyelid.

Diseases of the lacrimal drainage apparatus give rise to obstruction, which causes tearing. The obstructed lacrimal sac may become acutely or chronically inflamed. Acute inflammation causes a generalized cellulitis of the sac and surrounding structures. Chronic inflammation is associated with few signs other than painless swelling of the lacrimal sac region and pus flowing from the puncta when pressure is applied to the sac.

The main symptoms of diseases of the

lacrimal system are usually related to an excess or a deficiency of tears or to swelling of the lacrimal gland or lacrimal sac. Excessive tear formation or poor drainage is a nuisance, since vision is blurred by tears that overflow onto the face. Deficient tear secretion, however, may cause loss of the eye and may be associated with keratinization of the conjunctiva and cornea. It may cause nearly intolerable symptoms of burning and dryness of the eyes.

DISEASES OF THE LACRIMAL GLANDS

The lacrimal glands are tuburoracemose, similar in structure to the salivary glands. In general, they are subject to the same inflammations, diseases, and tumors. The two groups of glands are often involved in the same inflammatory and degenerative diseases.

Inflammation

Acute dacryoadenitis. Acute dacryoadenitis (Fig. 10-1) is a rare catarrhal inflammation of the lacrimal gland that usually accompanies systemic disease. Mumps and infectious mononucleosis are the usual systemic causes of an acute process. A purulent infection may be secondary to extension of inflammation from the eyelids or the conjunctiva.

Pain and discomfort in the upper outer portion of the orbit are the chief symptoms. Swelling and redness of the lacrimal gland cause a mechanical blepharoptosis of the upper eyelid and an S-shaped curve of the eyelid margin. Other causes of cellulitis of the skin and orbit must be considered in the differential diagnosis. Eversion of the upper eyelid indicates a swollen, reddened gland.

Treatment is directed to the cause. If a purulent infection is present, antibiotics and local hot compresses, possibly combined with incision and drainage, are indicated. Dacryoadenitis is usually self-limited, and therapy is directed toward preventing extension of the infection.

Chronic dacryoadenitis. Chronic dacryoadenitis is a proliferative inflammation of the lacrimal gland usually caused by specific granulomatous disease, particularly pseudotumor (p. 238), sarcoidosis, tuberculosis, and syphilis. Clinically, chronic dacryoadenitis is characterized by painless enlargement of the lacrimal glands, most evident when the upper eyelid is everted. Treatment must be directed toward the cause.

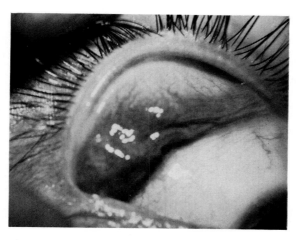

Fig. 10-1. Acute dacryoadenitis in an 18-year-old girl with infectious mononucleosis.

Mikulicz syndrome is the term applied to chronic bilateral swelling of the lacrimal and salivary glands. It may occur in the course of reticuloendothelial disease, leukemias, Hodgkin disease, sarcoid, and other granulomas. It is not a specific entity.

TEARING AND DRY EYES

Excessive tear formation (lacrimation) or defective drainage of tears (epiphora) (Table 10-1) is associated with blurring of vision and constant discomfort caused by tears running down the cheek. In all instances it is necessary to learn whether there is excessive production or defective drainage of tears.

Schirmer test

Tears are measured clinically by means of the Schirmer test using a 35 × 5 mm strip of Whatman No. 41 filter paper

Table 10-1. Tearing and dry eyes

I. Lacrimation (excessive tear production)
  A. Psychic stimulation
  B. Parasympathetic stimulation
    1. Cholinergic drugs
    2. Anticholinesterase drugs
  C. Lacrimal gland inflammations and neoplasms
  D. Trigeminal irritation
    1. Lesions of the eyelids, conjunctiva, cornea, iris
    2. Glaucoma
  E. Retinal stimulation by glare and excessive light
  F. Facial nerve
    1. Sphenopalatine ganglion stimulation by inflammation and neoplasms
    2. Misdirected regeneration following seventh nerve paralysis (crocodile tears)

II. Epiphora (defective tear drainage)
  A. Abnormalities of puncta
    1. Ectropion, orbicularis oculi muscle weakness, cicatrization, occlusion
  B. Lacrimal obstruction
    1. Canaliculi: inflammation, cicatrix, fungi impaction
    2. Lacrimal sac and duct
      a. Congenital abnormalities, inflammation, neoplasms
    3. Meatus
      a. Congenital or acquired stenosis, local nasal disease

III. Dry eyes
  A. Conjunctival cicatrization
    1. Erythema multiforme (Stevens-Johnson syndrome)
    2. Trachoma
    3. Ocular pemphigoid
    4. Thermal, chemical, and radiation burns
  B. Sjögren syndrome
  C. Lagophthalmos
  D. Riley-Day syndrome
  E. Absence of lacrimal gland
  F. Paralytic
    1. Facial nerve (between facial lacrimal nucleus and geniculate ganglion), greater superficial petrosal nerve, sphenopalatine ganglion
    2. Trigeminal nerve (decrease in reflex lacrimation)
  G. Toxic
    1. Cholinergic blockade (atropine)
    2. Deep anesthesia
    3. Debilitating disease

(available commercially as Iso-Sol strips). The filter strip is folded so that one end, 5 mm long, may be inserted at the mid-portion of the lower eyelid (Fig. 10-2). Generally, tear formation is considered normal if 10 mm or more of the paper from the point of the fold becomes wet in a 4-minute period. More than 25 mm of wetting indicates excessive tear formation. The eye and conjunctiva may be anesthetized and the same test carried out (basic secretion test) to measure secretion of the glands of Krause and Wolfring (wetting of first 8 to 15 mm is normal). The nasal mucosa may be irritated with a camel's-hair brush to excite reflex tearing from the lacrimal gland (Schirmer test II). Lacrimal gland secretion is stimulated only by irritation and emotion. The accessory lacrimal glands and the goblet cells in the conjunctiva are responsible for maintaining normal moistening of the eye.

Lacrimation

Lacrimation, or the overproduction of tears, results from emotional or reflex stimulation of the lacrimal gland, irritation of the cornea and conjunctiva, or stimulation of the retina by excess light.

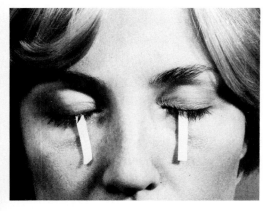

Fig. 10-2. Proper position of the filter paper to measure tear formation using the Schirmer test.

Local causes include allergy, infection, keratitis, trichinosis, or superficial foreign bodies. Extreme tearing may exhaust the lacrimal gland so that the Schirmer test shows normal or decreased tear formation. Abnormal regeneration of the seventh cranial nerve after facial nerve paralysis may result in concurrent tearing and salivation during eating (crocodile tears). Hyperthyroidism, tic douloureux, pseudobulbar palsy, cholinergic stimulation by either parasympathomimetic drugs or anticholinesterases may lead to a pharmacologic type of lacrimation. Often the cause of lacrimation can be easily identified and corrected.

Epiphora

Epiphora is that condition in which drainage of tears through the lacrimal passages is faulty. It arises from a variety of causes: faulty apposition of the lacrimal puncta in the lacrimal lake; scarring of the puncta; paresis or paralysis of the orbicularis oculi muscle, which eliminates the pumping action of the canaliculi; foreign bodies in the canaliculi; and obstructions in the lacrimal sac and the nasolacrimal duct. The accumulation of tears at the inner canthus causes irritation, which reflexly stimulates additional tear formation.

The adequacy and patency of the lacrimal system may be demonstrated in several ways (Table 10-2). Simple inspection indicates whether the puncta are in contact with the lacrimal lake. Normally, when the eye is rotated upward, the inferior punctum is not visible unless the eyelid is everted. Forcible closure of the eyelids indicates the adequacy of the function of the orbicularis oculi muscle.

Fluorescein tests. Fluorescein solution (2%) instilled in the conjunctival sac is diluted and normally disappears within 1 minute. If the fluorescein can then be demonstrated in the nose or pharynx, the lacrimal passages are patent (Jones test I).

Table 10-2. Tear formation and drainage tests

Type of test	Procedure
Schirmer I	Wetting of Whatman No. 41 filter paper
Schirmer II	Wetting of filter paper combined with trigeminal nerve stimulation
Basic secretion	Wetting of filter paper after topical anesthetization of conjunctiva
Dye disappearance	Fluorescein disappearance from cul-de-sac (normal 1 minute)
Norn	Fluorescein dilution in cul-de-sac
Jones I	Appearance of fluorescein* in the nose after conjunctival instillation
Jones II	Appearance of fluorescein* in the nose after lacrimal sac irrigation
Dacryocystography	Roentgenography after injection of radiopaque medium into lacrimal sac
Dacryoscintography	Gamma camera tracing of technetium Tc 99m instilled into cul-de-sac
Saccharine or quinine	Sweet or bitter taste after instillation of solution in conjunctival sac

*Use of cobalt light to excite fluorescence.

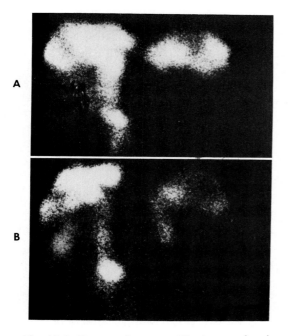

Fig. 10-3. Dacryoscintogram 15 minutes after the instillation of ⁹⁹ᵐTc in each cul-de-sac in a 72-year-old man who complained of tearing. **A,** Radioactive marker is seen to fill the entire nasal lacrimal excretory system on one side and to remain largely in the conjunctival sac and canaliculus on the opposite side. **B,** After 45 minutes, a complete obstruction is demonstrated at about the level of the entrance of the sac to the nasal lacrimal canal. (Courtesy Malcolm Cooper.)

A cobalt filter used to cause fluorescence of the fluorescein may enhance the accuracy. Sodium saccharide (10%) instilled in the conjunctival sac may be recognized by its sweet taste if it passes into the posterior pharynx.

If 2% fluorescein instilled in the conjunctival sac cannot be demonstrated in the nose or pharynx, the residual fluorescein is irrigated from the conjunctiva and the lacrimal system irrigated with normal saline solution. Fluorescein found in the nasopharynx is evidence that it has reached the lacrimal sac and that the obstruction is in the nasolacrimal duct (Jones test II). If fluorescein cannot be demonstrated in the nose or pharynx by irrigation, the functional block is most likely in the canaliculi.

Sodium pertechnetate (⁹⁹ᵐTc) in dilute solution may be instilled in each conjunctival sac; a scintigram taken with a gamma camera will indicate its passage through the lacrimal drainage system (Fig. 10-3). This is a physiologic method of demonstrating obstruction, particularly minor blockage by folds of mucous membrane. Injection of a radiopaque compound such as iophendylate (Pantopaque) through the punctum and canaliculus and subsequent roentgenographic study demonstrate the lacrimal system less physiologically than instillation of a radioactive isotope.

Irrigation of the lacrimal system through the punctum demonstrates severe obstructions. However, when a fold of mucous membrane obstructs, the force of irrigation may indicate a lacrimal sac to be patent.

The management of epiphora depends on its cause. Surgery of the eyelid is indicated when the punctum is not in contact with the lacrimal lake. Obstruction in the lacrimal sac may require anastomosis between the sac and the mucous membrane of the nose, a dacryocystorhinostomy. Atresia of the canaliculi may be difficult to correct. If the lacrimal sac has been obliterated, a glass tube extending from the conjunctival cul-de-sac into the nose or maxillary sinus will provide drainage.

Dry eye

Although a tearing eye may be a nuisance to the patient, it never causes loss of vision. Absence of tears causes keratinization of the corneal and conjunctival epithelium and possibly marked corneal scarring. Removal of the lacrimal gland is not associated with particular drying of the eye, although reflex and psychic tearing are lost. The accessory lacrimal glands seem to maintain normal moistening of the globe.

Decreased tear secretion is particularly associated with conjunctival cicatrization (trachoma, chemical burns, and erythema multiforme), which occludes the orifices of the lacrimal gland. Decreased tear secretion occurs prominantly in keratitis sicca (p. 268) and as an element of Sjögren syndrome, amyotrophic sclerosis, and some bulbar palsies. There is less than 10 mm of wetting of filter paper (Schirmer test) in a 4-minute period even after stimulation of the nasal mucosa. The eyes burn, feel dry, and have a constant foreign body sensation. Symptoms are aggravated by warmth and conditions that cause rapid evaporation of tears. There may be punctate epithelial erosions of the cornea and the conjunctiva.

Conditions associated with conjunctival scarring include (1) erythema multiforme in its various ocular manifestations of Stevens-Johnson syndrome and Reiter syndrome, (2) trachoma, (3) ocular pemphigoid, and (4) chemical and radiation burns of the conjunctiva. Sjögren syndrome is a systemic disease that has widespread manifestations, mainly of keratoconjunctivitis sicca and arthritis with laboratory signs of a severe infection. It occurs mainly in women near menopause (p. 563).

Deficiency of the mucin layer of tears adjacent to the corneal epithelium is measured by the tear film breakup time. A small amount of fluorescein covers the cornea, and the patient is instructed not to blink as the cornea is studied by using a cobalt blue filter with the biomicroscope. In normal eyes a dry spot appears within 15 to 34 seconds. In mucin-deficient eyes dry spots appear in less than 10 seconds.

The treatment of dry eyes is often unsatisfactory. Artificial tears are commercially available, and patients often experiment until they find one that provides relief. Frequent instillation may be required. Use of a soft contact lens requires careful evaluation inasmuch as the lens must be kept hydrated. A soft contact lens may lessen the frequency that artificial tears need to be used. Obstruction of the superior and inferior puncta to conserve tears cannot be effective if no tears are present. Avoidance of hot and dry atmospheres, which encourage tear evaporation, is helpful. Airtight covering of the eyes with diving goggles may help. If parotid gland secretion is not impaired, transplantation of the Stensen duct into the conjunctival sac may provide a generous salivary secretion.

DISEASES OF THE LACRIMAL PASSAGES
Canaliculitis

Canaliculitis is an inflammation of the canaliculi that occurs because of infection. Most attention has been directed to inflammation associated with obstruction by *Streptothrix (Actinomyces)*. Canaliculitis causes tearing and inflammation of the adjacent conjunctiva. Recovery of the organism from the canaliculus and a gritty foreign body sensation in the canaliculus establish the diagnosis.

Dacryocystitis

Dacryocystitis is an acute or chronic inflammation of the lacrimal sac. The cause is obstruction of the lacrimal sac or the nasolacrimal duct followed by bacterial infection.

Acute dacryocystitis. Acute dacryocystitis is a suppurative inflammation of the lacrimal sac with an associated cellulitis of the overlying tissues (Fig. 10-4, A). The onset is acute, and there are major symptoms of a suppurative infection at the inner canthus. Painful swelling occurs in the tissues overlying the lacrimal sac. Exquisite tenderness in the region is often combined with widespread cellulitis and associated constitutional symptoms. The main differential diagnosis involves other causes of acute suppurative inflammation in the area. Local hot compresses and systemic antibiotics are used in treatment. Incision and drainage are indicated if there is abscess formation.

Chronic dacryocystitis. Chronic dacryocystitis occurs because of obstruction of the nasolacrimal duct, and it is seen most frequently in the newborn period and in middle life (Fig. 10-4, B). The chief

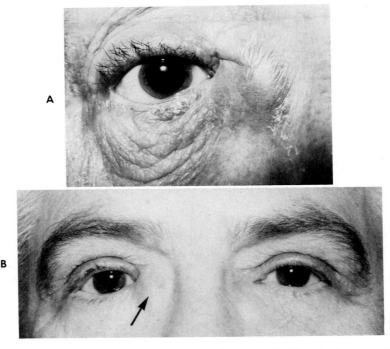

Fig. 10-4. A, Acute dacryocystitis in a 71-year-old woman. **B,** Chronic dacryocystitis with a mucocele of the lacrimal sac.

symptoms are epiphora and regurgitation of pus through the puncta when the lacrimal sac is massaged.

Infantile stenosis. Dacryocystitis in infants arises because of failure of the nasolacrimal duct to open into the inferior meatus, as normally occurs about the third week of life. The initial symptom is constant tearing of one eye. The tearing is distinguished from that in congenital glaucoma by the clear and transparent cornea and the absence of eye pain. Tearing is followed by regurgitation of pus through the puncta. Acute dacryocystitis is exceptional.

The treatment of stenosis is debated. There is a strong tendency toward spontaneous patency with spontaneous drainage and disappearance of the condition by the age of 6 months. Generally, a medication such as sulfacetamide is used locally to prevent lacrimal conjunctivitis. While awaiting spontaneous correction, the parents are instructed to massage the lacrimal sac daily to keep it empty of pus.

If the obstruction persists after the age of 6 months, lacrimal probing is indicated inasmuch as spontaneous patency is unlikely. The patient is mummified in a blanket, and a local anesthetic is instilled into the conjunctival sac. General anesthesia may be used. A lacrimal probe is inserted into the upper punctum, directed medially and into the lacrimal sac, and then turned at right angles into the nasolacrimal canal and the inferior meatus. The nose is inspected to be certain that the tip of the probe is not covered by mucous membrane. Rarely, more than one probing must be done. In exceptional instances the nasolacrimal duct fails to form, and a dacryocystorhinostomy is necessary. Such surgery is wisely deferred until the child is 3 or 4 years old. Because of the softness of the bone, it is an uncomplicated procedure in the very young.

Adult chronic dacryocystitis. Adult chronic dacryocystitis results from occlusion of the lacrimal sac, which may occur spontaneously or after injury or nasal disease in this region. Spontaneous atresia is more common in women in middle life. An annoying epiphora occurs initially, and as the occlusion continues, there is regurgitation of pus from the lacrimal sac. If neglected, extraordinary dilation and thinning of the lacrimal sac occur; this condition is known as mucocele or hydrops of the lacrimal sac. Acute suppuration is unusual. Differential diagnosis involves mainly the various causes of tearing and granulomatous infections of the lacrimal sac.

Surgery is the only satisfactory treatment. When not severe, instillation of zinc and epinephrine collyria may be helpful in the elderly. Probing of the lacrimal passages with probes of successively greater size may be useful, but for the most part relief is transient, and the procedure is painful. For a time, the threading of fine polyethylene tubes through the lacrimal passages was popular.

The surgical procedure of choice is a dacryocystorhinostomy, in which a communication is established between the lacrimal sac and the nose. Many procedures have been recommended. If the bony opening into the nose is large enough, the majority of patients improve. Preoperative dacryoscintography is helpful to outline the lacrimal sac and localize the obstruction and to rule out the rare neoplasm. Extirpation of the sac (dacryocystectomy) should not be carried out. In elderly patients who require intraocular surgery, the lacrimal sac is removed to eliminate the regurgitation of pus into the conjunctival sac.

Tumors

Three types of tumors involve the lacrimal gland: (1) lymphoma, 25%; (2) chronic granuloma arising from sarcoid or orbital pseudotumor (nonspecific granuloma), 25%; and (3) epithelial tumor, 50%. Pseudotumor is usually an inflammatory granuloma of unknown cause (p. 248). Lymphomatous disease may vary considerably in histologic type. It may be restricted to the lacrimal gland, or it may be only an incidental finding in the course of systemic disease. It is sensitive to radiation therapy. All are associated with a mass or fullness in the outer portion of the upper eyelid that may simulate the appearance of a blepharoptosis. There may be proptosis with displacement of the globe down and in. Granulomas and lymphomatous disease may be associated with intermittent inflammation. Eversion of the upper eyelid may indicate enlargement of the lacrimal gland. Pain is a prominent symptom of all tumors. The diagnosis can be made only by means of histologic study. Inasmuch as piecemeal removal of a malignant mixed tumor may be followed by seeding and dissemination of a malignancy, the capsule must be sutured after excision and complete removal carried out within 24 hours if the mass is malignant.

Tumors of the lacrimal gland are similar in both their histologic appearance and clinical course to neoplasms of the salivary glands, but mucoepidermoid carcinoma almost never affects the salivary gland. About one half are lymphoid tumors and inflammatory pseudotumors. The remainder are epithelial neoplasms. These may be classified as follows:

Benign
  Mixed tumor
  Adenoma
Malignant
  Mixed tumor
  Adenoid cystic carcinoma (cylindroma)
  Adenocarcinoma
    Squamous cell adenocarcinoma
  Mucinous carcinoma
  Undifferentiated

Mixed tumor is the most common epithelial tumor of the lacrimal gland. It originates from embryonic rests, and both epithelial and mesenchymal elements are present. It is slowly progressive, predominantly involves men (2:1), and occurs at a median age of 35 years. Both malignant and benign mixed tumors may erode the bone of the lacrimal fossa. Every effort must be made to excise the tumor within its capsule and to avoid seeding. If there is bony involvement, the bone should be resected. Both benign and malignant tumors recur if there is seeding, but only the malignant type metastasizes.

Malignant mixed tumor has no sex predilection and occurs at a median age of 51 years. It probably arises from a benign mixed cell tumor.

Adenoid cystic carcinoma occurs relatively more frequently in the lacrimal gland than in the salivary glands. It is invasive and metastasizes by way of the lymphatics and the blood vessels. Histologically it is composed of aggregates of small undifferentiated neoplastic cells separated by small and large cystoid spaces containing a mucinous material ("Swiss cheese"). Treatment is unsatisfactory, although the tumor is not rapidly fatal. The preferred treatment is exenteration of the orbit along with resection of the bone of the lacrimal fossa and any other involved tissues. The other types of malignant tumors listed have a similarly dismal prognosis, and radical surgery is indicated.

Tumors of the lacrimal sac are rare and involve its lining, the pseudostratified columnar epithelium. Most neoplasms are squamous cell carcinomas, transitional cell carcinomas, and adenocarcinomas. The initial symptom is tearing, which may be followed by the signs of chronic dacryocystitis with regurgitation of pus and mucus through the punctum.

Regurgitation of blood is nearly always caused by a malignant tumor of the lacrimal sac. A painless, nonreducible swelling then occurs in the region of the sac, and eventually there is extension of the tumor outside the lacrimal fossa. Tumors can be demonstrated roentgenographically after injection of contrast media into the lacrimal passages. Squamous cell tumors must be completely excised.

BIBLIOGRAPHY

Byers, R. M., Berkeley, R. G., Luna, M., and Jesse, R. H.: Combined therapeutic approach to malignant lacrimal gland tumors, Am. J. Ophthalmol. **79:**53, 1975.

Dohlman, C. H., Friend, J., Kalevar, V., and others: The glycoprotein (mucus) content of tears from normal and dry eye patients, Exp. Eye Res. **22:** 359, 1976.

Jones, L. T., and Wobig, J. L.: Surgery of the eyelids and lacrimal system, Birmingham, 1976, Aesculapius Publishing Co.

McClellan, B. H., Whitney, C. R., Newman, L. P., and Allansmith, M. R.: Immunoglobulins in tears, Am. J. Ophthalmol. **76:**89, 1973.

Murphy, M. B., and Rodrigues, M. M.: Benign mixed tumor of the (palpebral) lacrimal gland presenting as a nodular eyelid lesion, Am. J. Ophthalmol. **77:**108, 1974.

Ryan, S. J., and Font, R. L.: Primary epithelial neoplasms of the lacrimal sac, Am. J. Ophthalmol. **76:**73, 1973.

Taiara, C., and Smith, B.: Palpebral dacryoadenectomy, Am. J. Ophthalmol. **75:**461, 1973.

Chapter 11

THE ORBIT

The orbit is a pear-shaped cavity with a medial wall that extends directly anterior from its stem, or apex, and a lateral wall that diverges about 45°. The stem contains the annulus of Zinn, which is the circular fibrous origin of the recti muscles. It provides a passage for the blood vessels and nerves. The orbital apex is located about directly posterior to the medial canthus and not directly posterior to the fovea centralis. The middle portion is expanded to make room for the eye. The base forms the thick orbital margins for protection of the eye. Adjacent to the inferior wall of the orbit is the maxillary sinus. Adjacent to the medial wall is the ethmoid sinus. Laterally the temporalis muscle fossa is located anteriorly, whereas the temporal lobe of the brain is adjacent to the posterior part. Superiorly the frontal sinus is located anteriorly, and the frontal lobe of the brain is located posteriorly (Fig. 11-1). The junction of the anterior and middle cranial fossae is located at the apex of the orbits.

Affections of the orbit are a heterogeneous group of abnormalities (p. 243) that arise within a bony cavity that provides expansion only anteriorly. The orbit contains tissue of both ectodermal and mesodermal origin that may be primarily or secondarily affected. Tissues and tumors from the intracranial cavity or sinuses may herniate through bony defects into the orbit and cause displace-

ment of the eye and involvement of its motor nerves. The venous drainage of the orbit is into the cavernous sinus, and an increase in the intravascular pressure of the cavernous sinus from a carotid-cavernous sinus fistula may cause a pulsating protrusion of the globe (p. 533).

SYMPTOMS AND SIGNS OF ORBITAL DISEASE

Diseases of the orbit often manifest themselves by displacement of the globe sometimes associated with local pain, redness, and swelling. Proptosis usually refers to unilateral displacement and exophthalmos as well as to bilateral protrusion of the eyes. Abnormalities at the apex of the orbit may paralyze structures innervated by the motor nerves of the eyes, affect their sensory nerve supply, or cause optic atrophy.

In proptosis or exophthalmos, the palpebral fissure often widens, and a rim of sclera is visible above and below the cornea. In thyroid disease (p. 504), retraction of the upper eyelid accentuates the appearance. In enophthalmos, the palpebral aperture is more narrow, and a blepharoptosis may seem to be present.

Proptosis of an eye is best detected by viewing the eyes over the brow of the patient from above and behind (p. 168). Many devices are available to measure the distance between the anterior surface of the cornea and the zygomatic arch on

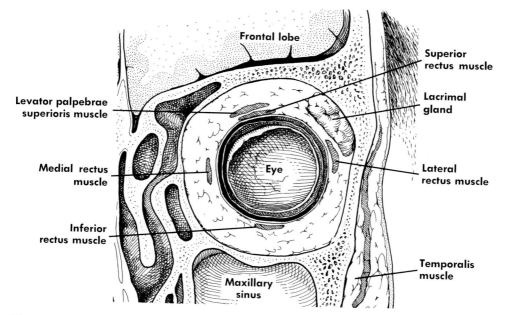

Fig. 11-1. Coronal section of the left orbit about 15 mm from the corneal apex. The frontal sinus is adjacent to the orbit in its anterior portion, whereas the frontal lobe is adjacent to the orbit posteriorly. Laterally the temporalis muscle is adjacent to the orbit anteriorly, whereas the temporal lobe of the brain is located posteriorly. The ethmoid sinus is located medially and the maxillary sinus inferiorly.

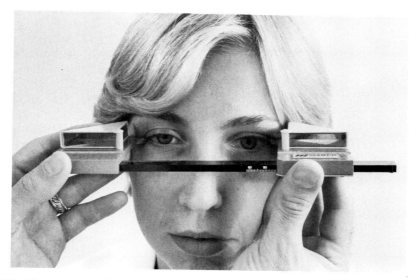

Fig. 11-2. Measurement of exophthalmos using a modified Hertel exophthalmometer. The observer views the position of the eyes in the mirrors. The numbers on the rule refer to the distance separating the two eyepieces and must be the same with repeated measurement.

the lateral margin of the orbit (Figs. 11-2 and 11-3). The measurements with the usual exophthalmometers are accurate to within 1 to 2 mm. An exophthalmometer may be improvised by viewing the front surface of the cornea over a ruler held against the zygoma or the maxilla.

Orbitonometry measures the backward displacement of the globe under different pressures. This may be estimated by means of palpation or measured by determining how much displacement of the globe occurs when a measured force is applied with a copper orbitotonometer.

The direction of displacement of the eye may suggest the most likely cause. Proptosis as a result of thyroid disease is usually equal bilaterally unless muscle contracture occurs. Tumors within the muscle cone cause a symmetric proptosis, whereas those outside of the muscle cone may cause the eye to be deviated up or down, in or out, in addition to forward.

Proptosis involves displacement of the globe, visual abnormalities, congestion and edema of the eyelids and conjunctiva,

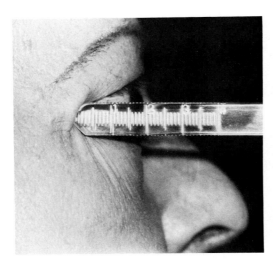

Fig. 11-3. Estimate of degree of proptosis using a transparent exophthalmometer (Luedde).

occasionally a bruit in the head, palpable tumors, choroidal folds, and other signs.

Displacement of the globe. A relatively small mass in the muscle cone causes early forward displacement of the globe. The nerve supply to the extraocular muscles may be affected, causing strabismus. Masses outside the muscle cone must be larger to displace the globe, and the proptosis is asymmetric. Tumors of the lacrimal gland may not cause proptosis, or they may displace the globe down and in. The lacrimal gland itself may be proptosed when there is a marked increase in the volume of the orbital contents.

Visual abnormalities. Diplopia is often an early sign of proptosis and may occur before development of gross displacement of the globe. Indentation of the posterior sclera by a tumor causes increased hyperopia often associated with decreasing vision and choroidal folds (p. 244).

Congestion and edema of the eyelids and conjunctiva. Marked congestion of the vessels of the globe is most suggestive of an inflammation, a thyroid abnormality with rapid progression of exophthalmos, or a carotid-cavernous sinus fistula.

Bruit in the head. An abnormal blowing sound heard on auscultation of the head is a classic sign of carotid-cavernous sinus fistula. The patient usually hears noises in the head, such as the sound of running water or the swishing of water. It may be most marked on the side of a carotid-cavernous sinus fistula (p. 530), but it has scant localizing value. The bruit is synchronous with the heart and may disappear when pressure is applied to the carotid artery in the neck. Bruits occur with some orbital and intracranial tumors, and they may be present in normal infants.

Palpable tumors. Tumors located in the anterior one half of the orbit may be palpated through the eyelids. Often a lateral canthotomy or a conjunctival incision in

Table 11-1. Diseases of the orbit (excluding the eye)

I. Developmental abnormalities of size, shape, and position
   A. Craniosynostosis
   B. Craniofacial dysostosis
   C. Mandibulofacial dysostosis
   D. Hypertelorism
   E. Failure of eye to develop or enucleation in infancy
II. Developmental anomalies of contents
   A. Hemangiomas
   B. Lymphangiomas
   C. Dermoid cysts
   D. Lipomas
   E. Choristomas
III. Herniation of adjacent structures through wall
   A. Mucocele
   B. Meningocele
   C. Encephalocele
IV. Inflammation of walls or contents
   A. Cellulitis
   B. Abscess
   C. Periostitis
   D. Chronic granuloma (pseudotumor)
   E. Gumma
   F. Tuberculoma
   G. Sarcoid granuloma
V. Vascular abnormalities
   A. Carotid-cavernous sinus fistula
   B. Cavernous sinus thrombosis
   C. Orbital aneurysm
   D. Hemorrhage
   E. Angioneurotic edema
VI. Tumors
   A. Primary
      1. Bone
         a. Chondrosarcoma
         b. Osteosarcoma
      2. Muscle
         a. Rhabdomyosarcoma
      3. Optic nerve
         a. Meningioma
         b. Glioma
      4. Lacrimal gland
         a. Benign: mixed, adenoma, cyst
         b. Malignant: mixed, adenocarcinoma, mucoepidermoid, squamous cell
      5. Connective tissue
         a. Fibroma
         b. Neurofibromatosis

VI. Tumors—cont'd
      6. Vascular
         a. Hemangioma
   B. Direct extension
      1. Eyelids
         a. Squamous cell
      2. Eye
         a. Malignant melanoma
         b. Retinoblastoma
      3. Intracranial cavity
         a. Meningioma
      4. Nasal accessory sinuses
         a. Osteoma
         b. Chondrosarcoma
         c. Malignancies
   C. Metastatic
      1. Sympathicoblastoma (neuroblastoma)
      2. Chloroma (in myeloblastic leukemia)
      3. Lymphoma (in lymphatic leukemia)
      4. Nephroblastoma
      5. Carcinoma: breast, uterus, thyroid, prostate, lung
VII. Systemic disorders
   A. Thyroid disease
   B. Osteitis deformans (Paget disease), osteosarcoma following osteitis deformans
   C. Histiocytosis
      1. Nevoxanthoendothelioma
      2. Eosinophilic granuloma
      3. Hand-Schüller-Christian disease
      4. Letterer-Siwe disease
   D. Hematopoietic system
      1. Lymphoma
         a. Malignant lymphoma, lymphocytic type (nodular or diffuse)
            (1) Well differentiated
            (2) Poorly differentiated
         b. Malignant lymphoma, histiocytic type (diffuse)
         c. Malignant lymphoma, mixed (nodular)
         d. Hodgkin type
      2. Plasma cell
         a. Primary
         b. Metastatic
      3. Granulocytic sarcoma (chloroma)
VIII. Injuries

the lower outer canthus will permit the surgeon to palpate deep in the orbit. Such as incision should never be used in the upper eyelid because of possible damage to the levator palpebrae superioris muscle (p. 52), causing blepharoptosis. The tendon of the superior oblique muscle, localized fat in the eyelids, and indurated orbital inflammatory tissue all simulate the tactile sensation of a tumor.

Choroidal folds. Orbital tumors, hyperopia, Graves disease, and hypotony may cause folds or striae in the posterior fundus. These appear as alternating bright and dark lines with the peaks bright and the valleys a darker shade of red. They are more common temporally than nasally and may be associated with congestion of the disk. Fluorescein angiography causes the peaks to fluoresce brightly, creating a pattern of alternate bright and dark lines. Vision is unaffected, although there may be a shift of refraction toward hyperopia because the posterior pole of the eye is displaced forward. With time, the slopes of the folds become pigmented.

Miscellaneous signs. Interference with the venous drainage of the optic nerve may cause a papilledema that may be followed by optic atrophy. Marked congestion of the orbit may severely restrict ocular movements. Prominence of the globe causes increased exposure of the cornea; lacrimation, photophobia, and exposure keratitis may develop.

DIAGNOSIS

An initial decision must be made as to whether ocular proptosis is actually present or whether the appearance is simulated by another condition. Retraction of the upper eyelid causes the eye to appear more prominent, although it is not displaced. Eyelid retraction is a common sign of thyroid disease (p. 504). A slight blepharoptosis, as occurs in Horner syndrome (p. 285), may simulate an ocular

proptosis of the opposite side. Abnormalities of orbital structure that cause a shallow orbit, as in Crouzon disease, simulate proptosis. Marked enlargement of the eye such as occurs in congenital glaucoma (p. 409) makes the eye more prominent without displacement.

Physical examination should be directed to possible neoplasms in areas adjacent to the orbit, notably the nasopharynx and the intracranial cavity. Thyroid disease, lymphomatous disease, and pseudotumor must always be excluded. A chest roentgenogram is desirable to exclude metastatic malignancy, although a normal chest film does not exclude this possibility. Blood tests should exclude hematopoietic disease and syphilis, and attention should be directed to the causes of chronic granulomas. Removal of a portion or all of a tumor may provide both cure and a diagnosis. It is essential that every precaution be taken to avoid seeding of a malignant neoplasm. Following excisional biopsy, it is desirable to base the decision concerning further therapy on the best possible histologic sections and not on frozen sections.

Roentgenography. Roentgen examination is essential in the diagnosis of orbital disease. Conventional roentgenography includes the standard frontal projection to permit a composite view of the bones forming the orbit. When both orbits are photographed on the same film, their dimensions and density can be compared. The Water technique is used for detailed study of the roof of the orbit. Separate oblique views are required for examination of the inner and outer walls. The Caldwell position is used for demonstration of the superior orbital (sphenoidal) fissure. Visualization of the inferior orbital (sphenomaxillary) fissure requires a special posteroanterior projection. This view demonstrates fractures of the floor of the orbit. Laminography is used to study details too small to be visible on conventional roentgen-ray examination and to visualize orbital structures without superimposition of surrounding structures.

In general, cerebral angiography and orbital phlebography are used in the diagnosis of vascular abnormalities but less frequently than previously.

Computed tomography (p. 179) is unusually helpful in the diagnosis of ocular disorders and has largely supplanted conventional roentgenography.

Ultrasonography. Sound waves with frequencies of more than 18,000 Hz are used in the diagnosis of both intraocular and orbital tumors. When the ultrasound encounters a change in elasticity or density of the medium, it is reflected toward its course. This reflected vibration (echo) is converted into an electric potential by piezoelectric crystal and displayed on a cathode ray oscillograph (p. 179).

Two types of ultrasonography are used. The A-scan measures the time or distance of changes in acoustic impedance from the transducer as well as acoustic density. The change is shown as a spike on the tracing. It is particularly useful in evaluating the density of tumors to suggest histologic type. The B-scan moves in a linear fashion across the eye, and any change in acoustic impedance is shown as an intensification on the line of the scan that builds up a picture of the eye and the orbit (Fig. 11-4). The B-scan is of particular value in examination of the orbit.

DEVELOPMENTAL ANOMALIES

The orbit and its contents may be affected by a number of congenital abnormalities involving the bones of the skull or the face. Frequently there is a characteristic shape of the head or facial appearance associated with exophthalmos, optic atrophy, papilledema, and strabismus.

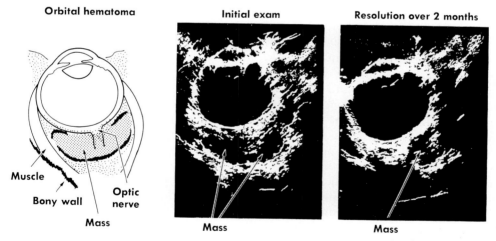

Fig. 11-4. Ultrasonograms of a compact orbital hematoma. By ultrasonic criteria the lesion appears to have many characteristics of a solid tumor. Repeat ultrasonography (right) two months after the original shows partial resolution of the lesion. Later it resolved completely without sequelae. More usual ultrasonic findings of orbital hemorrhage resemble those of orbital inflammation and are not confused with tumors. (From Dallow, R. L.: Ultrasonography in the diagnosis of orbital disease. In Brockhurst, R. J., Boruchoff, S. A., Hutchinson, B. T., and Lesse, S., editors: Controversy in ophthalmology, Philadelphia, 1977, W. B. Saunders Co.)

The common abnormalities may be classified as follows:

Craniosynostosis
    Scaphocephaly (boat skull): premature closure of sagittal suture
    Oxycephaly (tower skull): premature closure of coronal suture
    Trigonocephaly (egg-shaped skull): premature closure of frontal suture
    Brachycephaly (short skull, cloverleaf skull): premature closure of all sutures
Crouzon disease: brachycephaly with hypoplasia of maxillary bones
Mandibulofacial dysostosis (Franceschetti syndrome)
Apert syndrome (syndactyly)
Hypertelorism (Grieg syndrome)

Craniosynostosis. Craniosynostosis (Fig. 11-5) follows premature closure of one or more cranial sutures. The closure causes a complete arrest of bone growth perpendicular to the closed suture, and compensatory growth of the cranium in other diameters causes anomalies in the shape of the skull. The deformity progresses until the brain ceases to grow at about the age of 8 years.

Increased cerebrospinal fluid pressure is common and may be followed by secondary optic atrophy. Primary optic atrophy may occur because of traction on the optic nerve by downward displacement of the base of the brain or because of compression of the nerve in the optic foramen. The orbit may be unusually shallow because of an abnormality of the lesser wing of the sphenoid bone. Esotropia or exotropia may occur. The strabismus may be secondary to optic atrophy or may be the result of anatomic changes in the orbit.

Increased cerebrospinal fluid pressure, papilledema, and optic atrophy are indications for cranial surgery. Some physicians advocate craniectomy in the early months of life in all instances of craniosynostosis to prevent mental retardation and the cosmetic defect. Others believe

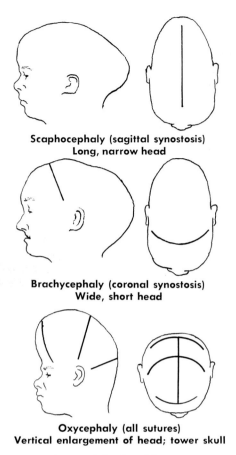

**Scaphocephaly (sagittal synostosis)
Long, narrow head**

**Brachycephaly (coronal synostosis)
Wide, short head**

**Oxycephaly (all sutures)
Vertical enlargement of head; tower skull**

Fig. 11-5. Shape of the head in some common types of premature fusion of a cranial suture.

that the procedure should be individualized, that a cosmetic defect is not constantly produced, and that mental retardation is not caused by the bony abnormality.

Orbital hypertelorism. The median cleft face syndrome consists of orbital hypertelorism (Grieg syndrome) with a V-shaped frontal hairline, primary telecanthus, cranium bifidum occultum, and median cleft upper lip, nose, and palate. There may be associated eyelid defects including epicanthal folds, accessory nasal tissue medially with displacement of the inferior puncti, colobomas of the eyelid, epibulbar dermoid tumors, unilateral microphthalmos, and hereditary vitreoretinal degeneration with retinal separation.

Craniofacial dysostosis. Craniofacial dysostosis (Crouzon disease) is an abnormality in which brachycephaly (short head) is combined with hypoplasia of the maxilla. The nose is broad and hooked. The palate is high, and the maxillary dentition is irregular. The earlobes are often large, and atresia of the external auditory canal is frequent.

The eyes are widely separated. A shallow orbit simulates an exophthalmos. Exotropia is common. The optic nerve may be involved, as in other forms of craniosynostoses. Exposure keratitis may necessitate a lateral blepharoplasty (p. 266).

Mandibulofacial dysostosis. Mandibulofacial dysostosis (Franceschetti syndrome) is a hereditary abnormality of the facial bone with hypoplasia of the zygoma and the mandible that causes a birdlike face. The inferior orbital margin is indistinct, and malformations of the lower eyelid are common. The palpebral fissure slants downward to the temporal side (antimongoloid), and there may be an ectropion. The external ear may be abnormally small (microtia), and there may be atresia of the external auditory canal. Atrophy of the mandible causes a prognathism of the upper jaw and an open bite. Associated skeletal anomalies are common, and dermolipomas of the conjunctiva occur.

Apert syndrome. In this abnormality the skull is tall; the occiput is flat with protuberant and widely placed eyes; and a flat and underdeveloped maxilla and nasal bridge are present. There are dilated cerebroventricles and mental retardation. In type I there is complete syndactyly of the fingers and toes ("mitten hands," "sock feet"), and in type II the syndactyly is incomplete.

ORBITAL INFLAMMATION
Acute inflammation

Acute orbital inflammation is most commonly caused by direct bacterial spread from the ethmoid or maxillary sinus, by pyogenic thrombophlebitis from a focus in the skin of the eyelids in regions drained by orbital veins, or by a penetrating orbital trauma. The orbital septum, which is the dense fascia that separates the anterior eyelids from the orbital contents, prevents anterior inflammations, mainly periorbital cellulitis, from extending into the orbit proper. Acute intraorbital inflammations are far more serious than anterior periorbital cellulitis and may involve both the anterior and posterior orbital contents.

Anterior periorbital cellulitis is characterized by severe edema of the eyelids, by injection and chemosis of the conjunctiva, and sometimes by pointing of the inflammation through the skin of the eyelid. Although there may be marked swelling of the eyelids, the globe moves freely and is not proptosed. Orally administered antibiotics are used.

Acute posterior orbital inflammation occurs with proptosis, ophthalmoplegia, and edema of the conjunctiva and eyelids. Pressure on the globe causes severe pain. The constitutional signs of infection occur: fever, malaise, and prostration. Exposure of the cornea may occur, and the orbit may be the source of metastatic infection or of a cavernous sinus thrombosis.

Posterior orbital inflammation before the age of 5 years is usually caused by ethmoid or maxillary sinusitis with infection by *Haemophilus influenzae* or *Streptococcus pneumoniae*. Initial management consists of immediate admission to the hospital, culture of the conjunctiva and posterior nasal pharynx, and broad-spectrum antibiotic treatment (often a combination such as methicillin and gentamicin), which is effective against both gram-positive and gram-negative bacteria. In children less than 2 years of age, in whom the causative organism is often *H. influenzae*, a combination of ampicillin and methicillin is used initially. Subsequent therapy is based on the results of culture. Orbital incision and drainage of an infected nasal sinus may be indicated if there is loss of vision with impairment of the pupillary reflex. Abscess formation is rare.

Cavernous sinus thrombosis. This is an acute thrombophlebitis that originates from a purulent infection of the face, sinus, ear, or other area that drains through veins to the cavernous sinus. Ophthalmoplegia occurs; the lateral rectus muscle is usually the first muscle involved. Involvement of the ophthalmic division of the trigeminal nerve causes severe pain. There may be papilledema, visual failure, and other signs of involvement of the nerves passing through the optic foramen and superior orbital fissure. The disease requires intensive antibiotic chemotherapy combined with anticoagulation.

Chronic (pseudotumor) inflammation

Chronic granulomas of the orbit are called pseudotumors and include a wide variety of torpid inflammations. A few are caused by specific granulomatous infections of the orbit: tuberculosis, syphilitic gumma, sarcoid (p. 471), and mycotic infections. The majority are nonspecific reactions and histologically are composed of fibroblasts combined with perivascular lymphocytic infiltration. Often there is a large eosinophilic component. The inflammation has no pathologic counterpart elsewhere in the body.

Middle-aged men are involved predominantly. The signs and symptoms are those of an orbital tumor. The onset is acute, and there is rapid development of proptosis and an associated diplopia. Often there is congestion of superficial orbital vessels along with redness of the eyelids. A tumor may be palpated. Extreme proptosis may develop rapidly with optic atrophy. Pain in the orbit is common.

The treatment is unsatisfactory, but often there is spontaneous remission. Excision is always incomplete and is usually followed by recurrence. A variety of surgical procedures may be used to protect the cornea from exposure, thus preventing keratitis e lagophthalmos. The chief treatment is systemic administration of corticosteroids often combined with retrobulbar corticosteroids. The fellow orbit becomes involved in about 25% of the cases.

INJURIES

Blunt trauma to the orbit may cause severe intraorbital hemorrhage that suffuses readily beneath the conjunctiva and under the eyelids and may limit ocular movements markedly. Severe hemorrhage may also be a sign of fracture of the wall of the orbit and may be associated with serious brain damage. Penetrating injuries of the orbit may perforate its thin posterior walls to enter the brain or the sinuses. The most common fracture of the orbit is the result of a marked increase in intraorbital pressure that causes a blowout of the floor (p. 194). The most common fracture of the orbital rim involves its medial margin and the nose and is particularly likely to occur in automobile accidents. Fractures of the superior margin of the orbit may damage the trochlea and may cause the symptoms of a superior oblique muscle paralysis. Fractures of the lateral margin are fairly common and result in loss of the cheekbone. Early elevation of the zygomatic arch can prevent the need for much corrective surgery. Fractures of the inferior margin are frequently comminuted and associated with fractures of other facial bones. The medial wall of the orbit may be ruptured, and emphysema of the orbital or eyelid tissues occurs. This may be recognized by the peculiar crepitation with palpation.

TUMORS AND RELATED CONDITIONS

A large variety of new growths, inflammations, congenital abnormalities, and systemic diseases may reflect themselves by orbital involvement. Diagnosis is complicated by the frequency with which the ocular manifestations of thyroid gland abnormalities (p. 504) and pseudotumors cause similar symptoms and signs. The medical history is helpful. A sudden onset and a rapid progression suggest a pseudotumor or other inflammatory process rather than a neoplasm. Orbital pain most commonly arises from inflammation, although tumors of the lacrimal gland are almost invariably painful. A history of hyperthyroidism suggests a thyroid abnormality even though the patient may be euthyroid or hypothyroid. A complaint of noise in the head is suggestive of a carotid-cavernous sinus fistula. Intermittent proptosis may be caused by varices of the orbit, and congestion is aggravated by increased venous pressure brought about by coughing or bending over.

The most common causes of proptosis of the adult orbit are thyroid disease, lymphomatous disease, pseudotumor, hemangioma, and mucocele of the frontal sinus. There is considerable variation in the orbital diseases encountered in different institutions; this most likely reflects the interests of the staff and the type of patient referred for care.

Meningioma of the sphenoidal region causes a slight proptosis, often combined with fullness of the temporal fossa. This is a brain tumor that is amenable to palliative surgery. Meningioma of the lateral one third of the sphenoidal region is particularly common in middle-aged women. It is readily diagnosed by roentgen-ray studies of the orbit.

Neuroblastomas in children and infants metastasize readily to the orbit. Gliomas of the optic nerve may be associated with signs of neurofibromatosis either in a child or in the parents. Rhabdomyosarcoma occurs more frequently in the orbit than elsewhere in the body and is the most common primary orbital malignancy in children.

Superior orbital fissure syndrome. The superior orbital fissure syndrome is characterized by local pain, proptosis, and paralysis of cranial nerves III, IV, and VI. There is loss of sensation in the area of distribution of usually only the ophthalmic division of the trigeminal nerve (N V). Proptosis and loss of corneal sensation distinguish the syndrome from cavernous sinus involvement (p. 530). Blepharoptosis is present, and the eye is usually turned down and out. The most common cause is a neoplasm that involves the apex of the orbit, but in many instances a pseudotumor may be responsible.

SURGERY OF THE ORBIT

Procedures involving the orbit include decompression to permit expansion of orbital contents that cannot be removed, excision of orbital tumors, exenteration of all orbital contents, enucleation of the eye, and correction of bony defects.

Orbital decompression is mainly indicated in thyroid disease in which expansion of the orbital contents causes so much proptosis that the cornea is no longer protected by the eyelids. Provision of an additional opening allows the orbital contents to expand without pushing the eye forward. The lateral approach with expansion into the temporalis fossa is favored by ophthalmologists; neurosurgeons often prefer a transtemporal approach with expansion into the frontal fossa; otolaryngologists prefer the maxillary antrum and the ethmoid sinus. Decompression is often combined with procedures designed to decrease the width of the palpebral fissure by suturing the upper eyelid to the lower eyelid (lateral blepharoplasty).

Tumors of the orbit may be approached from the orbit's anterior margin or its lateral or superior wall. The anterior approach is made by an incision through the eyebrow. Particular care must be taken to avoid injury to the levator palpebrae superioris muscle. This approach has relatively limited application and is used solely for palpable tumors.

The lateral approach to the orbit is usually combined with a lateral canthotomy and horizontal incision extending from the lateral canthus toward the tragus of the ear. The lateral bony margin of the orbit is incised with a Stryker saw that does not cut soft tissues, and the lateral wall is reflected backward by using the temporalis muscle as a hinge. There is good exposure of the lateral orbital contents, and this is the procedure of choice (among ophthalmologists) for the treatment of benign tumors of the posterior orbit. The anterior and the lateral approaches are combined for removal of benign lacrimal gland tumors, particularly the benign mixed cell type, which may recur or seed the operative area.

The superior orbital approach requires a craniotomy and retraction of the frontal lobe to expose the posterior portion of the orbit. Immediately beneath the periorbita of the superior wall is the levator palpebrae superioris muscle and the superior rectus muscle. This approach is mainly indicated in diseases involving both the cranial and orbital cavities, such as a meningioma. It is difficult to remove orbital tumors through a superior approach without damaging the ocular muscles.

The proptosed globe may be protected by adhesions created between the upper and lower eyelids (blepharoplasty). In a desperate situation in which the cornea is exposed and the eyelids cannot be drawn into position to protect it, the entire cornea may be covered with a conjunctival flap. A soft contact lens may also be used with good results.

Exenteration of the orbital contents is a mutilating procedure indicated mainly for malignancies of the lacrimal gland, for extension of eyelid malignancies into the orbit, for malignant melanoma of the conjunctiva, for a malignant melanoma or a retinoblastoma that has burst through the globe and caused marked orbital involvement, and for primary intraorbital malignancies such as rhabdomyosarcoma. The procedure may be lifesaving in lacrimal gland tumors in which areas of bony involvement must be removed. This usually necessitates exposing the dura mater. In malignancies that have extended into adjacent nasal sinuses and the intracranial cavity, the procedure is mainly palliative.

Removal of the eye. Enucleation of the eye is indicated in a blind and painful eye, in malignancies of the eye, in severe injuries of the globe when restoration of a functional eye is not possible, and in early sympathetic ophthalmia (p. 191). The conjunctiva is opened as close to the corneoscleral limbus as possible and each muscle separated from the globe at its insertion. The optic nerve is then severed as far behind the globe as possible.

A number of ingenious procedures have been proposed to provide motility to the ocular prosthesis after enucleation. In general, however, they do not work well. Nonetheless, with careful matching of the normal eye the cosmetic defect is minimal. The artificial eye should be removed only once or twice a month, and every precaution should be taken to prevent contamination.

Loss of an eye does not cause a 50% loss of visual efficiency (one may estimate the loss by covering one's own eye) but may be accompanied by severe emotional problems.

Bony defects of the orbit. These may be repaired by means of Silastic implants or bone taken from the iliac ridge. Commonly the surgery is indicated because of incarceration of an ocular muscle in an orbital fracture (p. 194), and considerable judgment is essential so as not to overcorrect the defect.

BIBLIOGRAPHY

Bleeker, G. M., Garston, J. B., Kronenberg, B., and Lyle, T. K., editors: Modern problems in ophthalmology. Vol. 14: Orbital disorders, Basel, Switzerland, 1975, S. Karger.

Blodi, F. C.: Pathology of orbital bones, Am. J. Ophthalmol. **81:**1, 1976.

Ellenbogen, E., and Lasky, M.: Rhabdomyosarcoma of the orbit, Am. J. Ophthalmol. **80:**1024, 1975.

Henderson, J. W., and Farrow, G. W.: Orbital tumors, Philadelphia, 1973, W. B. Saunders Co.

Jakobiec, F. A., Howard, G. M., Jones, I. S., and Tannenbaum, M.: Fibrous histiocytomas of the orbit, Am. J. Ophthalmol. **77:**333, 1974.

King, D. L., editor: Diagnostic ultrasound, St. Louis, 1974, The C. V. Mosby Co.

Kinsey, J. A., and Streeten, B. W.: Ocular abnormalities in the median cleft face syndrome, Am. J. Ophthalmol. **83:**261, 1977.

Knowles, D. M. II, and Jakobiec, F. A.: Rhabdomyoma of the orbit, Am. J. Ophthalmol. **80:**1011, 1975.

Newell, F. W.: Choroidal folds, Am. J. Ophthalmol. **75:**930, 1973.

Watters, E. D., Hiles, D. A., and Johnson, B. L.: Cloverleaf skull syndrome, Am. J. Ophthalmol. **76:**716, 1973.

Wolter, J. R.: Parallel horizontal choroidal folds secondary to an orbital tumor, Am. J. Ophthalmol. **77:**669, 1974.

Wolter, J. R., and Roosenberg, R. J.: Ectopic lymph node of the orbit simulating a lacrimal gland tumor, Am. J. Ophthalmol. **83:**908, 1977.

Zimmerman, L. E., and Font, R. L.: Ophthalmologic manifestations of granulocytic sarcoma (myeloid sarcoma or chloroma), Am. J. Ophthalmol. **80:**975, 1975.

Chapter 12

THE CORNEA

The cornea is the transparent, avascular structure that forms the anterior one sixth of the globe and through which the iris pattern and black pupil normally are clearly visible. Its most anterior layer, the precorneal tear film (p. 84), covers a constantly renewed epithelium whose basement membrane is attached to the corneal stroma. The stroma constitutes some 90% of the cornea; its anterior condensation, to which the basement membrane of the epithelium attaches, is the Bowman layer. The cornea is lined by a single endothelial cell layer adjacent to the aqueous humor of the anterior chamber. Descemet membrane, the basement membrane of the endothelium, separates it from the corneal stroma. The central cornea requires atmospheric oxygen for its aerobic metabolism, whereas the peripheral cornea is nurtured by the superficial and deep corneal plexuses derived from the anterior ciliary arteries. It is innervated by nonmedullated sensory fibers arising from the long and short ciliary nerves of the ophthalmic division of the trigeminal nerve.

The cornea, with its 40-diopter refractive power, is the principal refractive tissue of the eye because it separates air with an index of refraction of 1.0 and aqueous humor with an index of refraction of 1.34. The regular arrangement of the 200 corneal lamellae, the scarcity of keratocytes, the absence of blood vessels, and detumescence (dehydration) make the cornea transparent. Corneal transparency requires integrity of both the cornea and the endothelium.

The endothelium provides a mechanism (possibly a bicarbonate-activated ATPase [p. 81] system) that pumps fluid from the stroma to the aqueous humor. Failure of the endothelial pump causes a generalized corneal edema; the process is sometimes called endothelial decompensation. Damage to the corneal epithelium causes a subepithelial edema, and the anterior condensation of the corneal stroma (Bowman layer) prevents stromal swelling. When a contact lens that is not permeable to oxygen is worn for a long period, subepithelial corneal edema develops (Sattler veil). The edema disappears spontaneously when the cornea comes in contact with the atmosphere.

The corneal epithelium, which is five to six layers thick, is continuous with the outer layers of the conjunctival epithelium; thus, inflammatory diseases of the conjunctiva extend easily to the corneal epithelium. The basement membrane of the corneal epithelium must be adherent to the underlying condensation of the stroma (Bowman layer), or epithelial cells may be easily flicked away by blinking, which causes severe pain. Abnormalities of the eyelids or conjunctiva or a deficiency in the precorneal tear film results in localized areas of corneal drying.

SYMPTOMS AND SIGNS OF CORNEAL DISEASE

The three main symptoms of corneal disease are (1) iridescent vision (halos), (2) reduced visual acuity, and (3) pain. Iridescent vision results from epithelial and subepithelial edema, which divides white light into its component parts with blue in the center and red on the outside. Edema and the round pupil cause a halo sensation in which lights are surrounded by a shimmering rainbow (p. 151). Interference with the visual axis by scars, blood vessels, stromal edema, leukocytes, or other opacities reduces visual acuity.

The corneal epithelium is liberally innervated by delicate nerves without Schwann sheaths. Epithelial defects cause discomfort that may be described as a foreign body sensation, burning of the eyes, or pain so severe that it incapacitates the patient. Reflex lacrimation may occur.

The exposed position of the cornea and the anatomic lamination of the tissue allow easy observation and precise localization of corneal defects, which are enhanced by biomicroscopy. However, inspection through a +20 diopter condensing lens (p. 168) combined with penlight illumination often provides adequate magnification. Attention is directed to the diameter of the cornea, its shape, and the presence or absence of opacities in the normally transparent tissue. The normal cornea reflects a clear image of the examining light, whereas the light is distorted or dull in the area of disease. Corneal opacities or aqueous humor opacities may obscure the delicate pattern of the iris and prevent observation of the normally black pupil. Fluorescein strips or solutions (2% sterile) stain areas of absent corneal epithelium bright green. Corneal sensation is measured by touching the cornea with a wisp of cotton and observing the eyelid closure reflex. Many conjunctival abnormalities (p. 215), lacrimal disorders (p. 230), and eyelid disorders may result in corneal disease.

OPACITIES

Opacities in the cornea may be central or peripheral. When located in the visual axis they may impair vision; there may be a surprising degree of opacity with nearly normal vision. Conversely, a minor scar may severely distort vision because it disturbs the smooth curvature of the corneal refractive surface (irregular astigmatism).

Scars

Three degrees of scars involve the cornea:

1. Leukoma, in which the involved portion of the cornea is entirely opaque. Localized leukoma appears as a whitish scar surrounded by normal cornea. In generalized leukoma the entire cornea is white, often with conspicuous blood vessels coursing across its surface.
2. Macula, in which the involved cornea is translucent.
3. Nebula, which is a mild loss of corneal transparency.

Epithelial defects heal without scarring (p. 83), whereas the Bowman layer and the remaining stroma heal with permanent opacification. The human endothelium does not replicate, and if there are too few endothelial cells to flatten and cover a defect, stromal edema (p. 83) occurs. A corneal scar to which the iris is adherent is called an adherent leukoma.

Congenital leukomas. Infants born with central scarring of the cornea often have a severe intraocular abnormality that may be unilateral or bilateral. In the simplest type of scarring, the Descemet membrane is defective and bordered by iris adhesions. Glaucoma may occur. Avascular defects are often called Peters anomaly and, when vascularized, von Hippel internal corneal ulcer. When the iris and lens are adherent to a posterior corneal defect (also called Peters anomaly), vitreoretinal and systemic abnormalities are often present also. Most cases are sporadic. To prevent severe amblyopia (p. 426), keratoplasty is indicated within 3 months of birth.

Corneal vascularization

The central cornea has no blood vessels but depends on atmospheric oxygen for its aerobic metabolism. The peripheral cornea is nurtured by superficial and deep arteries at the corneoscleral limbus. Corneal vascularization follows corneal invasion by polymorphonuclear leukocytes. Lymphocytes do not cause neovascularization. The superficial corneal vascular plexus is the source of subepithelial neovascularization. Interstitial (anterior stromal) neovascularization arises from the deep corneal plexus; apposition of the major arterial circle of the iris or radial vessels of the iris to the cornea results in posterior stromal neovascularization. Blood vessels may extend from the entire corneal circumference or radially from a portion of the corneal margin (fascicular). Subepithelial neovascularization combined with fibroblastic proliferation is called *pannus;* it usually involves the superior portion of the cornea.

In the acute stage of corneal neovascularization new blood vessels are easily visible. They are associated with ciliary injection and a varying degree of corneal clouding. After the condition causing neovascularization subsides, these vessels may appear in a relatively clear cornea as a delicate bloodless network (ghost vessels). Corneal neovascularization is part of the normal inflammatory response. Many corneal inflammations and infections resolve quickly after vascularization.

The most serious consequence is the loss of corneal transparency combined with a biochemical modification of the corneal tissue that changes it from an avascular tissue not participating fully in the body's tissue immunity to one requiring a direct blood supply that partakes of antigen-antibody reactions.

Corneal edema

The integrity of both the epithelium and endothelium are necessary to maintain the cornea in its relatively dehydrated state. The zonula occludens of the epithelium provides a barrier to external aqueous fluids, and the endothelium removes fluid from the corneal stroma. Damage to either of these structures may result in corneal edema. (A drug must be lipid soluble to penetrate the epithelium and aqueous soluble to penetrate the stroma.)

If the corneal epithelium is deprived of atmospheric oxygen, as for example with a hard contact lens, or if the intraocular pressure rapidly increases to more than 50 mm Hg, an epithelial and a subepithelial edema develops. This is prevented from spreading deep into the stroma by the compactness of the Bowman membrane. The cornea appears dull, uneven, and hazy. The patient has decreased visual acuity and iridescent vision. The edema rapidly disappears when the cause is removed.

Stromal edema reflects the inability of the corneal endothelium to pump an adequate amount of fluid from the cornea into the aqueous humor. In minor cases of the disease, the cornea is thickened and has a dull appearance. In severe cases, even the epithelium may be disturbed; the condition is called bullous keratopathy. Vision is severely depressed.

Pigmentation

A delicate, brownish epithelial line occurs in normal eyes (Hudson-Stähli line:

horizontal), at the base of the cone in keratoconus (Fleischer ring: circular [p. 257]), at the head of a pterygium (Stocker line: vertical arc [p. 226]), and immediately anterior to a filtering bleb (Ferry line: horizontal). The lines are composed of ferritin deposited in widened intracellular spaces and within intracytoplasmic vacuoles of the corneal epithelium. Ferritin is composed of a protein shell (apoferritin) and a core of ferric hydroxide. How it is deposited in the corneal epithelium is not known.

In Wilson hepatolenticular degeneration (p. 488) deposition of a copper-containing material in the inner layers of the cornea extends into the trabecular meshwork of the anterior chamber recess (Kayser-Fleischer ring). It stops abruptly at the posterior edge of the meshwork. The ring is often incomplete—it may be concealed in its early stages by the corneoscleral limbus and can be seen only by using a gonioscope.

The Krukenberg spindle is a vertical pigment deposit on the endothelial surface of the cornea, probably derived from uveal pigment. It is deposited by convection currents in the anterior chamber and is usually arranged in an approximately triangular pattern with the apex near the center of the cornea and the base in the 6 o'clock meridian. In the pigment dispersion syndrome (p. 403) patchy areas of iris depigmentation appear as defects by iris transillumination combined with pigment accumulation in the anterior chamber angle recess. Glaucoma may occur.

Keratic precipitates, which are epithelioid inflammatory cells adherent to the endothelium in inflammations of the anterior segment, may occasionally become pigmented.

Blood staining of the cornea usually follows injuries in which there has been bleeding into the anterior chamber followed by an increase in intraocular pressure. The anterior layers of the cornea are transparent, but the endothelium becomes glazed with a brownish tan pigment, which may obscure the iris entirely. If the cornea is incised for a third or more of its circumference, as is done in cataract extraction, blood staining may occur without increased intraocular pressure, although blood must be present in the anterior chamber.

Heavy metals such as silver (argyria), iron (siderosis), gold (chrysiasis), copper (chalcosis), and mercury may be deposited in the stroma adjacent to the Descemet membrane. They are introduced by local medication (silver), intraocular foreign bodies (iron or copper), intraocular blood (iron), systemic therapy (gold), toxic vapors (mercury), or a disordered metabolism (copper in hepatolenticular degeneration).

ABNORMAL DEPOSITS IN SYSTEMIC DISEASE

The cornea is frequently the site of deposition of abnormal metabolic products circulating in the blood. Often the disorder is not particularly conspicuous and may be overlooked if special magnification is not used.

In corneal arcus (arcus senilis, gerontoxon) (see Fig. 24-6) there is a lipid infiltration (neutral fats, phospholipids, and steroids) at the corneal periphery. It consists of two concentric areas separated by a clear interval of about 1 mm and occurs almost universally after 60 years of age, although often involving only a sector of the cornea.

Corneal arcus tends to develop more commonly and earlier in life in blacks than in whites. Both races show a tendency to develop the lesion with increasing age. Myocardial infarction is twice as likely to occur in an individual aged 39 to 49 who has corneal arcus than in one who does not. Additionally, young patients with cornea arcus are more likely to have higher serum cholesterol levels and to be smokers. It does not occur invariably in familial hypercholesterolemia, and there is no relationship between corneal arcus and secondary types of hypercholesterolemia that occur in diabetes mellitus, lipoid nephrosis, and myxedema. Previous vascularization of the cornea leads to the deposition of lipid adjacent to the blood vessel in some patients with hypercholesterolemia and may occur in association with megalocornea. The optical zone of the cornea is not involved, there are no symptoms, and treatment is not indicated.

Jet-black patches of adrenochrome may be seen in the cornea and conjunctiva after long-term use of epinephrine salts in the treatment of glaucomas. In blacks an irregular melanosis is often present in the superficial layers of the peripheral cornea. These appear as extensions of conjunctival pigmentation and are irregularly arranged peninsulas of pigment.

Calcium is deposited in the cornea in two forms: (1) diffuse subepithelial deposition of crystals and (2) band keratopathy in which a horizontal grayish band is interspersed with round dark areas that appear as "holes." The first type of deposition is seen in the milk-alkali syndrome (ingestion of milk and calcium carbonate) and is associated with glasslike glistening crystals in the diffusely hyperemic conjunctiva. In hypophosphatemia, in which the tissues are unable to metabolize calcium because of a deficiency in the parathyroid hormone, the cornea, but not the conjunctiva, contains calcium crystals.

Band keratopathy arises from the deposition of noncrystalline phosphate and carbonate calcium salts in the epithelium, in the subepithelial tissue, and between the stromal lamellae. In juvenile rheumatoid arthritis (Still disease), band keratopathy may complicate the indolent chronic iridocyclitis. Other causes include hyperparathyroidism, vitamin D poison-

ing, sarcoidosis, multiple myeloma, renal disorders, and dry eyes. It occurs in diseases associated with hypercalcemia, in association with ocular inflammation, and with topical instillation of drugs that have calcium as a vehicle.

The calcium may be removed by first removing the corneal epithelium and then applying a chelating agent, usually EDTA (ethylenediaminetetraacetic acid). Visual improvement is often temporary inasmuch as additional calcium is deposited.

In some lysosomal storage diseases (p. 478), the cornea, among other tissues, accumulates an abnormal amount of the storage substances. The cornea is cloudy, not unlike its appearance in corneal edema, and the iris is seen with difficulty.

In cystine storage disease (p. 495), cystine crystals in the conjunctiva and cornea appear as tinsellike, fine refractile crystals uniformly scattered throughout the tissue.

In plasma cell dyscrasias (p. 555), particularly multiple myeloma, iridescent crystals may be scattered throughout the cornea and conjunctiva. Deep deposits giving rise to an appearance similar to that in corneal dystrophy may be present in cryoglobulinemia (p. 556).

Thickened corneal nerves occur in clear corneal stroma in two disorders: (1) commonly in multiple endocrine neoplasia type 2B and (2) occasionally in multiple endocrine neoplasia type 2A. Type 2B is characterized by the association of medullary thyroid carcinoma, one or more pheochromocytomas, and multiple mucosa neuromas in patients who usually have a marfanoid habitus and other developmental anomalies. In addition to the thickened corneal nerves, these patients have conjunctival and eyelid neuromas and keratoconjunctivitis sicca. Coexistence of medullary thyroid carcinoma and pheochromocytoma but absence of the marfanoid habitus, multiple mucosa neuromas, and other eye lesions characterize type 2A. Hyperparathyroidism often occurs.

Thickened corneal nerves may occasionally be seen as a consequence of corneal surgery or inflammation and in lattice dystrophy of the cornea. However, other associated disease is always present, and the cornea is not entirely clear, as in multiple endocrine neoplasia.

ABNORMALITIES OF SIZE AND SHAPE
Microcornea

In microcornea the cornea has a diameter of less than 10 mm together with a decreased radius of curvature. The majority of these eyes are hyperopic, and the development of glaucoma in later years is common. The term is reserved for eyes in which the small corneal diameter is the sole abnormality. When the entire eye is small, the condition is described as microphthalmia. Vision is reduced, and ocular nystagmus and strabismus may occur. Usually there are numerous associated developmental abnormalities, and sometimes only cystic remnants of the eye are present.

Megalocornea

Megalocornea (keratoglobus) is a bilateral abnormality in which each cornea has a diameter of more than 14 mm (Fig. 12-1). Glaucoma is not present, but many authorities believe that the corneal enlargement is secondary to an arrested congenital glaucoma. The anterior chamber is deep, the iris stroma atrophic, and the iris tremulous. Posterior subcapsular cataract occurs with aging. Megalocornea must be differentiated from congenital glaucoma (p. 409). Measurement of the intraocular pressure and study of the anterior chamber angle by means of a prism (gonioscopy) are essential in the differential diagnosis.

Keratoconus

Keratoconus (conical cornea) is an abnormality in which the symmetric curvature of the cornea is distorted by an abnormal thinning and forward bulging of

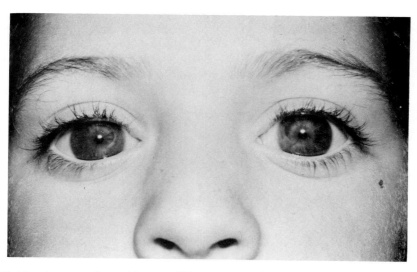

Fig. 12-1. Megalocornea in an 11-year-old boy. Despite the enlarged cornea, ocular tension and the optic nerves remain normal.

the central portion of the cornea (ectasia) (Fig. 12-2).

The condition is usually bilateral, but one eye may be involved long before its fellow. Its onset is usually at the time of puberty. Women are involved more frequently than men. Keratoconus progresses slowly over many years but may become stationary at any time. The chief symptom is decreased visual acuity for far and near combined with marked astigmatism, which as the disease progresses becomes irregular and cannot be improved with spectacles. Contact lenses provide a regular anterior curvature and usually provide visual improvement.

Diagnosis may be difficult in the early stages, although a contact lens may give normal vision. Viewing the cornea from above by looking down from behind the patient and over the brow, as is done in the diagnosis of proptosis (p. 168), may indicate the corneal cone. The corneal cone distorts the pattern of the Placido disk, a flat disk that has concentric black and white circles with a central opening to observe their corneal reflection. The

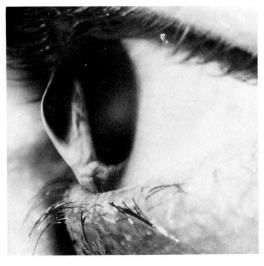

Fig. 12-2. Abnormal corneal profile in keratoconus.

epithelium at the base of the cone may be infiltrated with a ferritin pigment, causing Fleischer ring. Breaks in the Descemet membrane cause aqueous humor to enter the stroma and to produce a severe corneal edema, hydrops of the cornea, which is a common complication in Down syndrome.

Vision is usually maintained at a useful level by using contact lenses. If these cannot be used, a penetrating corneal transplant (p. 271) restores useful vision with a 95% success rate.

Staphyloma

An ectasia or bulging of the cornea that is lined with uveal tissue is an anterior staphyloma. It occurs, with iris prolapse, most commonly in degenerated eyes following perforation of a corneal ulcer. The anterior chamber is obliterated, and a secondary glaucoma is present. Often enucleation is required.

INFLAMMATION (KERATITIS)

Table 12-1 provides an etiologic classification of the various types of corneal inflammation. Although the same microbes often cause either keratitis or conjunctivitis, the corneal involvement is more serious because of the poorer defense response of the avascular cornea and impairment of vision caused by scarring, neovascularization, or disturbance of corneal curvature. Antigen-antibody reactions in the cornea may be particularly destructive. In addition to infectious causes, keratitis arises from deficiencies in the precorneal tear film, ischemia affecting the peripheral corneal arcade of blood vessels, nutritional deficiencies, exposure, anesthesia following interruption of the trigeminal nerve, and mechanical, radiational, or chemical trauma.

Because most inflammation interrupts the corneal epithelium, the defect stains with fluorescein. Discomfort varies from a foreign body sensation to severe pain.

Table 12-1. Corneal inflammation (keratitis)

Type	Etiology
Infection	
Bacterial	
Keratoconjunctivitis	Extension of conjunctivitis to cornea, staphylococci, streptococci
Keratitis	Enterobacteriaceae, fecal contamination
Necrotizing keratitis	*Pseudomonas aeruginosa* and trauma, contaminate and solutions
Acute hypopyon ulcer (pus in anterior chamber)	Trauma combined with *Streptococcus pneumoniae* or hemolytic streptococci
Indolent ulcer	*Haemophilus, Moraxella liquefaciens*
Pannus (vascularized scar)	*Chlamydia trachomatis*
Interstitial keratitis	Spirochaetaceae, *Treponema,* congenital syphilis (rare in acquired)
Fungal	
Keratomycosis	Injury by plant material, prolonged topical antibiotics and corticosteroids, compromised host
Viral	
Dendritic keratitis epitheliitis	Herpes simplex (*Herpesvirus hominis,* type 1)
Adenovirus keratitis	Any adenovirus
Epidemic keratoconjunctivitis	Adenovirus 8 and 19
Herpes zoster keratitis: epitheliitis (early), mucous plaques (late)	Varicella virus involving the ophthalmic branch of trigeminal nerve (N V)
Keratitis vaccinia or variola	Vaccination or smallpox
Hypersensitivity	
Marginal catarrhal ulcers	Staphylococcic conjunctivitis or blepharitis
Disciform keratitis, metaherpetic keratitis	*Herpesvirus hominis* hypersensitivity, T-cell reaction?
Phlyctenular keratitis	Cell-mediated to bacterial proteins, particularly *Mycobacterium tuberculosis*
Vascular disease	
Ring-type ulcer	Peripheral corneal ischemia
Cogan syndrome (interstitial keratitis, deafness), vertigo, and tinnitus (N VIII)	Arteritis?
Mooren ulcer	Elderly, peripheral corneal ischemia?
Nutritional deficiency	
Keratomalacia (xerophthalmia)	Vitamin A and protein deficiency
Acne rosacea	Nutritional?
Interruption of ophthalmic branch of trigeminal nerve (N V)	
Neurotrophic keratitis	Usually surgical section of N V and N VII
Exposure of cornea	
Keratitis e lagophthalmos	Failure of eyelids to cover eye: (1) proptosis, (2) facial nerve paralysis, (3) severe ectropion, and (4) absence of blinking
Defects in tear film	
Keratoconjunctivitis sicca	
Loss of aqueous portion	Sjögren syndrome
Loss of mucin	Erythema multiforme, ocular pemphigoid
Local drying (delle, *pl.* dellen)	Failure to wet epithelium, elevated conjunctival lesions
Superior limbic	Failure to wet epithelium
Trauma	
Radiational	
Ultraviolet	"Snow blindness," cumulative ultraviolet exposure as sunburn
Mechanical	
Chemical	
Climatic droplet keratopathy	Wind, particles of sand or snow

The grossly transparent cornea becomes infiltrated with inflammatory cells, and blood vessels may invade the avascular stroma. The anterior ciliary arteries become injected. Generally, peripheral involvement of the cornea is related to the same disorders affecting the conjunctiva, whereas central corneal involvement occurs without primary conjunctival inflammation.

Bacterial infections

Bacterial invasion of the cornea requires a break in the epithelium, either by trauma or by extension of an infection from the adjacent conjunctiva. The organism may be inoculated by a corneal foreign body; may be present in the lacrimal system, conjunctiva, or eyelids; or may be introduced into a damaged cornea by contamination.

The major bacterial families (p. 447) that cause keratitis are: (1) Micrococcaceae (*Staphylococcus aureus, Staphylococcus epidermidis,* and *Micrococcus),* (2) Streptococcaceae (hemolytic *Streptococcus* species and *Streptococcus pneumoniae),* (3) Pseudomonadaceae *(Pseudomonas aeruginosa),* and (4) Enterobacteriaceae.

Treatment must be initiated on the basis of the organism found in the Gram stain (Table 12-2). Bacitracin, erythromycin, and methicillin sodium are the preferred agents against gram-positive cocci. Gram-positive rods, which rarely cause keratitis, should be treated with bacitracin and cephalothin. Gram-negative rods are treated with gentamicin sulfate and carbenicillin disodium. If no organisms are demonstrated by Gram stain, a combination of bacitracin and gentamicin may be used. After isolation of the organism, its antibiotic sensitivity will indicate the specific therapy.

Acute hypopyon ulcer. An acute hypopyon ulcer (serpiginous) is a severe bacterial inflammation of the cornea associated with pus in the anterior chamber (hypopyon) and a severe iridocyclitis (Fig. 12-3). *Streptococcus pneumoniae* (pneumococcus) is the usual cause, and the organism often has a focus in the lacrimal system. Frequently the keratitis is preceded by mild trauma and removal of corneal epithelium, which allows entry of the organism. The ulcer is a dirty gray color with overhanging margins, and it causes marked thinning of the cornea. The conjunctiva is violently inflamed. If

Table 12-2. Treatment of bacterial keratitis

Size of ulcer		
Less than 2-mm size, anterior ⅓ cornea	Ointment every hour (every 2 hours at night)	
2-5 mm, anterior ⅔ cornea	Concentrated antibiotic drops every 15 minutes, subconjunctival antibiotic daily	
6 mm or larger, inner ⅓ cornea	Concentrated antibiotic drops, subconjunctival antibiotic 2 times daily, intravenous antibiotics	
Unknown organism	**Topical**	**Subconjunctival or intravenous**
Gram-positive cocci	Bacitracin	Methicillin
Gram-negative cocci	Bacitracin*	Penicillin G†
Gram-negative rods	Gentamicin and carbenicillin	Same
Mixed or none	Bacitracin and gentamicin	Methicillin and gentamicin

Modified from Jones, D. B.: A plan for antimicrobial therapy in bacterial keratitis, Trans. Am. Acad. Ophthalmol. Otolaryngol. **79:**95, 1975.
*Not recommended for *Neisseria* gonococcus keratitis; use penicillin systemically and locally.
†Penicillin hypersensitive patients: vancomycin or cephalothin derivative.

untreated, the cornea may perforate, and the eye may be lost because of purulent inflammation.

The bacteria are sensitive to many antibiotics or sulfonamides, and the ulcer responds quickly to treatment. A concurrent pneumococcal dacryocystitis may necessitate dacryocystorhinostomy or temporary occlusion of the canaliculi.

Pseudomonas aeruginosa ulcer. *Pseudomonas aeruginosa* ulcer is caused by a gram-negative aerobic bacillus found on the normal skin and in the intestinal tract of humans. It is a common cause of corneal ulceration. Rapid liquefaction progresses to perforation if not treated intensively. The bacteria produce an extracellular protease that enzymatically degrades corneal proteoglycans. Additionally, the invading polymorphonuclear leukocytes and the cornea itself produce collagenases and proteases that contribute to corneal degradation. The lesion usually begins centrally, spreads quickly, and may cause perforation and loss of the eye within 48 hours. Treatment is by means of frequent instillation of polymyxin B or E (colistin), gentamicin, or tobramycin, sometimes combined with subconjunctival injection.

Viral infections

Viral infections of the human cornea arise mainly from *Herpesvirus hominis* (herpes simplex), various adenoviruses, and zoster and in association with many systemic viral disorders (p. 458). Conjunctival scrapings generally show a mononuclear leukocyte response in ocular involvement, or the virus may be isolated in tissue culture. Fluorescent antibody staining of scrapings may indicate the virus. A fourfold increase in adenovirus antibody titer between acute and convalescent serum suggests the diagnosis of adenoidal-pharyngeal-conjunctival (APC) infection.

Herpesvirus hominis infection. The two types of *Herpesvirus hominis* are type 1, the cause of facial, oral, or ocular lesions,

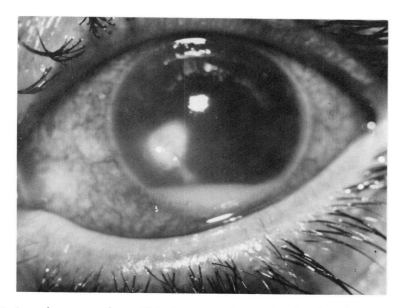

Fig. 12-3. Acute hypopyon ulcer with leukocytes in the anterior chamber. The ulcer is spreading toward the center of the cornea, and a tract of leukocytes extends through the entire corneal thickness.

and type 2, associated mainly with genital vesiculation. Primary ocular infection is rare, and nearly all corneal infection occurs in patients previously infected.

Primary infection occurs in childhood after the first 6 months of life and involves some 90% of the population. Less than 10% of those infected have clinical signs, but all become carriers and are subject to recurrent infection. Primary infection is usually transmitted by an individual with an acute herpes infection of the lips or mouth. If the primary infected individual has clinical signs, there may be vesiculation of the lips, mouth, or skin or a severe systemic disorder (0.1%). Primary herpes infection of the eye is exceptional. It is usually initiated by herpes vesicles on the lips followed by a unilateral ulcerative blepharitis with preauricular adenopathy. Follicular, or pseudomembranous, conjunctivitis may occur with regional lymphadenopathy. The rare corneal involvement resembles small phlyctenular spicules. Infection by type 2 herpesvirus in the birth canal may cause keratitis, conjunctivitis, cataract, chorioretinitis, optic atrophy, and a necrotizing retinitis.

After primary infection with type 1, recurrent inflammation occurs throughout life in an infected individual. Most individuals have no specific initiating factor; but in some, fever, ultraviolet light, trauma, emotional upset, menstruation, or corticosteroid therapy may trigger replication of the virus. The most common clinical signs are vesiculation of the lips or mouth. A much smaller group may have recurrent keratitis.

Dendritic keratitis. Dendritic keratitis (Gr. *dendron*, tree) is an acute and chronic corneal inflammation that occurs in an individual who has had a primary infection with *Herpesvirus hominis* type 1. The latent virus may reside in the trigeminal ganglion; it may be chronically shed in the tears; or it may remain in corneal

nerves. Thereafter, the same factors that cause recurrent inflammation elsewhere may trigger keratitis (p. 460).

Epithelial keratitis (Fig. 12-4) begins as delicate punctate epithelial opacities that become vesicular and coalesce in a branching linear pattern that stains with fluorescein. Corneal sensitivity is markedly diminished. If not arrested, the epithelium between the branches is lost; the result is a sharply demarcated, irregularly shaped geographic ulcer. Both eyes are infected in less than 10% of patients and rarely simultaneously. Symptoms include foreign body sensation, lacrimation, and reduction of vision if the optical area of the cornea is involved. After frequent attacks, the patient is aware of recurrence even before signs of inflammation are present.

Initial treatment consists of instillation of idoxuridine (IDU) ointment (p. 136) every 2 hours during waking hours and at bedtime. This may be combined with mechanical removal of the virus-laden epithelial cells by means of a cotton-tipped applicator or gentle scraping with a scalpel blade; damage to the basement membrane should be carefully avoided.

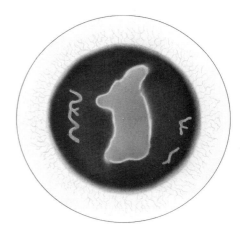

Fig. 12-4. Herpes simplex keratitis with central disciform lesion and peripheral dendritic lesions.

If the lesion has progressed to the geographic ulcer stage, medication should be used every hour and atropine instilled topically. Treatment should be continued for at least 1 week after the lesion heals. Resistant lesions may be treated with a soft contact lens. In individuals who are sensitive to IDU or who have an apparent IDU-resistant virus, one may substitute vidarabine (adenine arabinoside) ophthalmic ointment (p. 136). Clinical trials suggest that 1% trifluorothymidine (F_3T) (p. 136) eye drops are significantly superior to either IDU or vidarabine preparations. Corticosteroid preparations should not be used.

Stromal involvement occurs in several forms. The most common, disciform keratitis (Fig. 12-4), forms beneath an epithelial ulcer 5 to 10 days after the attack begins. It appears as a disk-shaped gray area that may involve the full thickness of the cornea or merely the stroma adjacent to the epithelium. This disciform lesion is presumably a hypersensitivity reaction, possibly of the delayed type, to the virus. It may heal without residue or may cause severe scarring and vascularization of the cornea. Treatment usually consists of antiviral agents to prevent replication of the virus combined with cautious topical administration of corticosteroids to combat the hypersensitivity reaction.

Stromal disease may occur in previously affected eyes without involvement of the epithelium. The eyes appear similar to those with severe bacterial or mycotic infection.

Recurrent inflammation of the stroma and epithelium with corneal vascularization, redness, discomfort, and a prolonged course is usually classified as keratitis metaherpetica. The inflammation is presumably the result of previous damage to the cornea caused by the virus and not the result of active virus replication. The inflammation commonly recurs until the abnormal tissue is excised and re-

placed with normal cornea in a penetrating transplant.

Adenokeratoconjunctivitis. Adenokeratoconjunctivitis is responsible for many sporadic cases of keratoconjunctivitis. Epidemic keratoconjunctivitis (EKC) is caused by adenovirus types 8 and 19, and outbreaks occur commonly in factories and hospitals.

Upper respiratory tract infection caused by adenovirus (pharyngoconjunctival fever) is a common disease, especially among children. Transmission from the respiratory tract to the eye is responsible for most instances of sporadic keratoconjunctivitis. Eye to eye transmission is the common cause of epidemic keratoconjunctivitis (p. 465).

Adults between the ages of 20 to 40 years are most commonly affected, and the disease is more common in men than women (2:1). The incubation period ranges between 2 and 14 days, usually 7 to 9 days. The infection starts unilaterally as conjunctivitis with preauricular adenopathy. In most cases, keratitis develops 2 to 7 days later.

The initial symptoms are foreign body sensation, photophobia, lacrimation, discharge, and swelling. As revealed by examination, the bulbar conjunctiva is hyperemic, sometimes with severe chemosis. Conjunctival hemorrhages may occur with adenovirus types 8 and 19. Hyperemia is moderately severe, and diffuse infiltration and papillary and follicular hypertrophy are present. Papillary hypertrophy is more severe in the upper tarsal conjunctiva and may persist for 2 to 4 weeks. Follicular hypertrophy is moderately severe and present mainly in the upper and lower fornices. Pseudomembranes may occur in severe cases of adenoconjunctivitis 8 and 19. Preauricular adenopathy is present.

Mild to moderate epithelial punctate keratitis with small corneal infiltrations may develop in the early stages. The duration of sporadic keratoconjunctivitis is less than 3 weeks, but epidemic keratoconjunctivitis lasts much longer. Subepithelial punctate keratitis with large, dense, well-marked corneal opacities in the subepithelial area of the cornea may develop in association with adenoviruses in both types of conjunctivitis. Generally, these opacities resolve within 3 months in all cases. Those caused by adenoviruses 8 and 19 may persist for several years.

Epidemic keratoconjunctivitis may occur in hospitals, outpatient departments, schools, and swimming pools. Institutional transmission may result from contaminated eye solutions, instruments, and contaminated fingers of doctors and nurses.

The differential diagnosis involves herpetic keratoconjunctivitis and chlamydial and bacterial conjunctivitis. Although the adenovirus has some in vitro sensitivity to idoxuridine and trifluorothymidine, no effective treatment is available. Frequent topical applications of antibiotic drops may soothe the eye and prevent secondary bacterial infection.

Superficial punctate keratitis. Superficial punctate keratitis is probably a specific viral infection of both eyes characterized by a punctate epithelial keratitis that persists from 6 months to 4 years. There are numerous remissions and exacerbations and eventual healing without corneal scars. Patients complain of intermittent burning, irritation, tearing, and blurred vision. Magnification is required to see from 1 to 50 (usually about 20) minute, oval, corneal opacities composed of a conglomeration of minute dots. New lesions appear as old ones heal, so that their distribution varies from examination to examination. There is hyperemia of the conjunctiva in the 12 o'clock meridian. Topical corticosteroids have a dramatic suppressive effect, and other medications are of no particular value.

A recurrent punctate erosion of the corneal epithelium may follow inadvertent injury to the eyes with aerosol products. The patient is usually unaware of the injury, but the cornea is studded with minute epithelial defects that stain with fluorescein solution. Once the cause is learned, more cautious use of aerosols prevents recurrence.

Systemic virus diseases. Corneal inflammation occurs in a large number of virus diseases (p. 458) and may or may not be associated with systemic abnormalities that dominate the clinical picture. Many of the adenoviruses (p. 222) cause ocular signs with corneal inflammation. Zoster ophthalmicus (p. 461) caused by *Herpesvirus varicellae* may cause severe anterior uveitis and keratitis. The photophobia observed in measles (p. 464) is caused by a frequently undiagnosed keratoconjunctivitis, whereas mumps (p. 464) may cause a transient corneal edema. Smallpox was previously a common cause of blindness, and accidental inoculation of the cornea was seen after vaccination.

Other infections

Keratomycosis. Since the introduction of topical administration of corticosteroids and antibiotics, infection of the cornea by fungi has increased some fifteenfold. The filaments of a fungus are usually introduced by injury, frequently by a foreign body contaminated with vegetable matter, such as a tree or shrub. Keratomycosis, especially that caused by *Candida,* may also complicate prolonged therapy with corticosteroids and antibiotics, and a fungus should be considered in every persistent corneal ulceration.

The fungus ulcer (Fig. 12-5) appears as a fluffy, white, elevated protuberance surrounded by a shallow crater that in turn is surrounded by a grayish, sharply demarcated halo that persists for months. The central lesion may have satellite lesions of pseudopods. Vascularization is minimal, and hypopyon is frequent. The conjunctival injection may be disproportionately severe for the amount of keratitis present. A specimen obtained by scraping the base and edges of the ulcer rather than culturing the exudate is essential to the diagnosis. Careful culture of the material at room temperature in Sabouraud media containing chloramphenicol, but no other inhibitors such as chlorhexidine, is required for identification of the fungus.

Many "nonpathogenic" fungi have been recognized as causes of keratitis, particularly in eyes treated with corticosteroids and antibiotics. The three most common fungi that cause corneal ulcers are (1) *Aspergillus fumigatus,* (2) *Candida albicans,* and (3) *Fusarium solanae.* The relative sensitivities of these fungi to treatment are shown in Table 12-3.

Many eyes do not heal until a conjunctival flap is drawn over the cornea surgically. Mechanical removal of the fungi by curettage may have a beneficial effect. Rapidly progressive deep ulcers with descemetocele or perforation require a penetrating transplant of a diameter that encompasses all of the pseudopods to remove as much of the fungi as possible. A lamellar corneal transplant is not satisfactory because of the many fungi remaining in the host cornea.

Interstitial keratitis. Interstitial keratitis is a corneal inflammation characterized by deep vascularization of the cornea often associated with a severe iridocyclitis. Congenital syphilis (p. 449) was formerly the most common cause. A severe bilateral anterior uveitis was followed by interstitial corneal vascularization between the ages of 5 and 20 years. The disease is entirely prevented by adequate treatment of congenital syphilis, but once the inflammation has developed, antisyphilitic therapy is of no value.

Interstitial keratitis with deafness (Cogan syndrome) is a rare disease affecting young adults. Either the eye or the ear may be affected initially, but involvement of the other organ follows within 2 months.

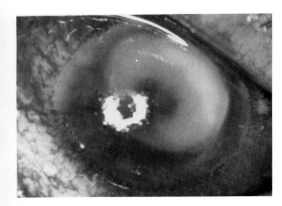

Fig. 12-5. Fungus ulcer of cornea with deep infiltrate and severe ciliary injection. There is no corneal vascularization.

Table 12-3. Treatment of mycotic corneal ulcer

Fungus	Polyenes (from Streptomyces)			Pyrimidines		
	Nystatin 3.3% ung	Amphotericin B 0.1-0.3%	Natamycin (pimaricin) 5% suspension	Flucystosine (5-fluorocytosine) 1-1.5%	Clotrimazole 1%	Miconazole 1%
Aspergillus	±	+	++	±	+++	++
Candida	+	++	++	+++	++	++
Fusarium	±	+	++	0	±	±

Modified from Jones, B. R.: Principles in the management of oculomycosis, Am. J. Ophthalmol. **79:**719, 1975.

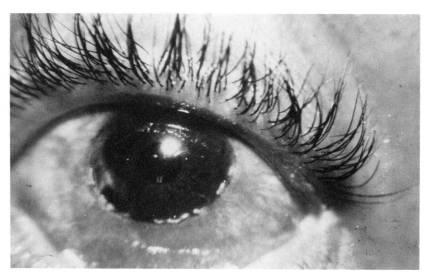

Fig. 12-6. Acute *Staphylococcus aureus* conjunctivitis with marginal corneal infiltrates caused by sensitivity to the exotoxin of the bacteria.

The ocular involvement consists of patchy, deep, peripheral corneal infiltrates that fluctuate in intensity and distribution and are accompanied by interstitial corneal vascularization. Vestibuloauditory symptoms consist of the simultaneous onset of vertigo, tinnitus, and deafness. Complete nerve deafness and nonresponsive labyrinths usually result. Treatment is symptomatic. Systemic corticosteroids seem useful.

Hypersensitivity

Marginal catarrhal ulcers. Marginal catarrhal ulcers are attributed to a hypersensitivity to the exotoxin of *Staphylococcus aureus* and other substances. They may be associated with conjunctivitis or blepharitis (Fig. 12-6), in which the staphylococci can be isolated. The inflammation responds to the topical instillation of corticosteroids.

Phlyctenular keratoconjunctivitis. Phlyctenular keratoconjunctivitis (p. 224) is a cell-mediated immune response of the cornea and conjunctiva. It is a common cause of decreased vision among Eskimos, presumably because of their sensitivity to tuberculosis.

Other disorders

Neurotrophic keratitis. Neurotrophic keratitis is a corneal inflammation that arises from anesthesia of the cornea, which permits trauma and desiccation of the corneal epithelium without reflex protection. In addition, the trigeminal nerve may play a role in the metabolism of the cornea. Inasmuch as the cornea is anesthetic, there is no pain, but the conjunctiva is injected, and there may be marked loss of vision. The lesion begins inferiorly with exfoliation and ulceration, and it may progress until there is loss of the globe. Suturing the upper to the lower eyelid (tarsorrhaphy, Fig. 12-7) is the usual method of treatment. If it is probable that both the trigeminal and facial nerves will be sacrificed in a neurosurgical procedure, as in a cerebellar angle tumor, the keratitis should be anticipated, and tarsorrhaphy should be performed before the cornea ulcerates.

Exposure keratitis. Exposure keratitis,

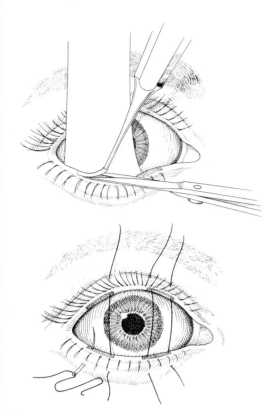

Fig. 12-7. Temporary tarsorrhaphy in which posterior portions of the upper and lower eyelid margin are denuded and brought together with sutures to prevent exposure of the cornea.

sometimes called keratitis e lagophthalmos, is an inflammation caused by the failure of the eyelids to cover the globe (p. 206). There is exfoliation of the corneal epithelium followed by secondary infection. The condition is most commonly associated with facial nerve disorders in which the orbicularis oculi muscle is paralyzed. The cornea may be similarly exposed following blepharoptosis surgery or in severe proptosis.

Keratitis e lagophthalmos causes pain and ciliary injection. It is evident on examination that the cornea is not protected by closure of the eyelids. Treatment is directed toward prevention of corneal drying. In mild cases the instillation of an ointment at bedtime and protection of the globe are all that is required. In facial nerve paralysis a temporary blepharoplasty may be carried out. Soft contact lenses may be useful. If the paralysis is permanent and there is no likelihood of restoration of the facial nerve function, a permanent type of blepharoplasty is carried out. Proptosis with exposure keratitis requires a central tarsorrhaphy.

Keratomalacia. Softening of the cornea arises from vitamin A deficiency, which causes desiccation and necrosis of the cornea and the conjunctiva. Vitamin A is a fat-soluble vitamin derived either from conversion of carotene or from preformed vitamin in the diet. Carotene occurs in many plants, particularly leafy greens and yellow vegetables. Preformed vitamin A is derived from butterfat, cheese, and liver. Failure to ingest adequate vitamin A or its precursor is commonly associated with other dietary deficiencies, notably inadequate protein. Secondary deficiency occurs because of inadequate saponification of vitamin A in the gut and is observed in sprue, celiac disease, and cystic fibrosis of the pancreas. In cirrhosis of the liver, there is a failure to store vitamin A.

Vitamin A deficiency in the retina has been studied carefully, particularly in animals in whom nutrition can be supported by administration of vitamin A acid, which is not converted to retinal (p. 93). In humans, vitamin A deficiency causes blindness by the following: (1) destruction of the cornea in xerophthalmia (dry eye) and keratomalacia (corneal softening), (2) loss of retinal in the photopigments of the retina, (3) faulty growth of bone causing optic nerve compression in the optic canal, and (4) faulty fetal development in a vitamin-deficient mother.

In children with acute but not chronic deficiency, dryness of the conjunctiva (xerosis conjunctivae) is the initial external sign of the deficiency. It is paralleled by night-blindness, which may not be noticed. Bitot spot is seen, particularly in male children, and occurs on the exposed bulbar conjunctiva, usually in the palpebral fissure on the temporal side. It appears as a highly refractile mass with a silvery gray hue and a foamy surface. It is extremely superficial, and the foam may be rubbed off, leaving a roughened conjunctival surface that fills with foam in several days.

The keratomalacia, or softening of the cornea, may be generalized or localized. It may lead to destruction of the eye if infection occurs. It is particularly common with an associated protein deficiency. Generally, it occurs in infants and not in adults.

Mild vitamin A deficiency caused by improper nutrition may be reversed by food rich in protein and carotene. Severe disease requires supplemental vitamin A.

Climatic droplet keratopathy (Labrador keratopathy). This acquired degenerative corneal disease occurs mainly in elderly patients as subepithelial, spherical, golden, dropletlike opacities of various sizes in the superficial stroma. It arises from exposure to extreme heat or cold, dust, snow, ice particles, and ultraviolet radiation. The material is deposited in a horizontal manner in the exposed portion of the cornea in a way similar to band keratopathy.

Keratoconjunctivitis sicca. Keratoconjunctivitis sicca is a common symptom complex arising secondary to an abnormal precorneal tear film. Patients complain of gritty, sandy, foreign body sensations in the eye or irritation and itching, all of which are worsened by hot, dry atmosphere and tobacco smoke. Symptoms may be aggravated by reading or by infrequent or incomplete blinking. The cornea loses its usual glossy appearance, and mucus floats as strands, sheets, or blobs in the tear film. Filamentary strands of epithelium may adhere to the cornea. The conjunctiva and corneal epithelium stain with a 1% rose bengal solution (also see dry eye, p. 235).

The precorneal tear film is composed of an external lipid layer rising from the meibomian glands and a much thicker aqueous layer derived from conjunctival goblet cells absorbed on the microvilli of the corneal epithelium. When the eye is open some of the tear film evaporates, but in the normal eye blinking causes an exchange in the tear film spread over the exposed cornea and conjunctiva. In keratoconjunctivitis the stability of this tear film is disturbed, and dry spots form on the corneal epithelium. Mucous plaque may adhere to the corneal epithelium, and filaments may be present. *Staphylococcus* conjunctivitis and blepharitis are common. Four types occur.

1. In the fluid deficiency type there has been atrophy of the main or accessory lacrimal glands, and the aqueous portion of the tear film is thinned and deficient. This is the classical type seen in Sjögren syndrome (p. 563). A decreased lacrimal gland system occurs in collagen diseases, neurologically in the Riley-Day syndrome (p. 539), and may be pharmacologically induced by ganglionic blockade.

2. Mucin deficiency occurs in conjunctival diseases such as ocular erythema multiforme (Stevens-Johnson syndrome) (p. 568) and ocular pemphigoid (p. 226). These diseases also cause an eventual loss of the lacrimal aqueous phase as a result of scarring of the secretory duct. Vitamin A deficiency and chemical burns also cause a loss of mucus. The mucus is necessary to wet the hydrophobic corneal epithelium.

3. Elevated lesions of the cornea or conjunctiva (uncommon) may cause the tear film to break up at the apex of the lesion. This may occur in trachoma, herpes simplex, or other diseases in

which the corneal surface is irregular. A similar mechanism may cause the relatively depressed area adjacent to the elevated area to become dry with failure of corneal stroma renewal and the creation of a pit (Ger. *dellen,* pits or depressions).

4. Failure of blinking or infrequent or incomplete blinking may cause inadequate spread of tears with normal components. This occurs in neuroparalytic keratitis, dellen, and pterygium.

Any of a variety of artificial tears may be used, and their viscosity may be increased to lengthen the time of contact. Occasionally, soft contact lenses are helpful. Occlusion of the lacrimal puncta may be beneficial. Diving goggles may prevent evaporation of tears. Membrane release systems placed in the lower cul-de-sac that gradually melt and provide a tear film stabilizer are being studied.

Superior limbic keratoconjunctivitis. This bilateral, chronic keratinization of the superior bulbar conjunctiva results in a papillary reaction in the tarsal conjunctiva and fine, punctate staining of the superior cornea. It occurs most often in women, about 25% of whom have signs of current or previous hyperthyroidism. The symptoms appear to originate from inadequate wetting of the superior cornea and may be treated with artificial tears, a soft contact lens, and, if necessary, resection of the superior conjunctiva so the cornea will be moistened by the tears.

CORNEAL DYSTROPHIES

Corneal dystrophies are hereditary disorders affecting both corneas that are occasionally present at birth but more frequently develop during adolescence and progress slowly throughout life. They are often described on the basis of their appearance or the level of the cornea involved. Many do not interfere with vision but create interesting patterns in the normally transparent cornea. Most are transmitted as autosomal dominant dis-

orders, but central macular dystrophy (Groenouw type II) is transmitted as an autosomal recessive defect.

The juvenile epithelial dystrophy (of Meesmann) is a rare disorder with clear dots or cysts in the corneal epithelium that occasionally rupture and stain. They are aggregates of an amorphous electron-dense material and marked irregularities in the architecture of the epithelium. Treatment is solely symptomatic.

Granular dystrophy (Groenouw type I) appears as irregularly shaped white spots surrounded by clear cornea in stroma underlying the Bowman membrane. The disease begins in childhood and slowly progresses by late middle age, rarely resulting in loss of useful vision. Corneal transplantation may be performed, if necessary, to restore useful vision.

Central macular dystrophy of the cornea (Groenouw type II) begins in childhood as a diffuse clouding and progresses until, by middle age, the entire thickness of the cornea contains gray confluent spots. It constitutes a local accumulation of mucopolysaccharides with keratocytes.

Lattice dystrophy becomes evident in young adults; their anterior corneal stroma contains lines in irregular patterns made up of amyloid that has been locally synthesized by the cornea. Painful epithelial erosions occur in early life, and early lamellar keratoplasty may be indicated.

Endothelial dystrophy

Human corneal endothelium does not regenerate, but when cells are lost, the adjoining cells spread out to cover the defect. If the defect is not covered, the Descemet membrane develops round, wartlike excrescences that dip into the anterior chamber. These normally occur as a degenerative change with aging, are located at the periphery of the cornea, and are called Hassall-Henle bodies. They are of no clinical significance except as an indication of aging.

A similar loss of endothelium of the central cornea causes an endothelial dystrophy (Fuchs dystrophy, or cornea guttata). The condition is bilateral, and one eye is more extensively involved than the other. Biomicroscopically, minute spheres appear imbedded on the posterior cornea. There may be few or so many as to impair vision. The deposits may act as a diffraction grating and may cause iridescent vision.

When extensive, the deturgescent action of the endothelium (p. 81) is lost, and the cornea becomes edematous. This may occur spontaneously or may follow cataract surgery, corneal trauma, prolonged wearing of contact lenses, or tonography. The substantia propria is thickened and opaque, and epithelial edema is followed by erosion and bullae (bullous keratopathy or combined epithelial-endothelial dystrophy). Vision is markedly reduced. The bullae may rupture and expose corneal nerve endings, resulting in severe pain. Soft contact lenses relieve discomfort. Hypertonic saline or glucose solutions dehydrate the edematous cornea and may improve vision. Early endothelial and epithelial dystrophy responds well to penetrating transplant, provided all of the diseased tissue is removed.

Superficial corneal lines

Microscopically thin parallel lines arranged in whorls and other concentric patterns originate in the epithelium and subepithelial tissue. The most common type, called fingerprint lines, may be associated with recurrent corneal erosion (below). Inasmuch as they are often bilateral, these may constitute a type of superficial corneal dystrophy.

Recurrent corneal erosion

Occasionally, following an uncomplicated corneal abrasion, the regenerated epithelium does not appear to adhere to the underlying basement membrane. In such an instance the patient, on awakening in the morning and opening or rubbing his eyes, will remove the epithelium. There is sudden onset of a foreign body sensation and lacrimation. Examination with high magnification between attacks shows a minute opacification in the subepithelial area. This area stains with fluorescein when the epithelium is removed. The disorder is disabling because of recurrent pain, but it causes no visual disability. Treatment is difficult. Some cases are caused by the subepithelial inclusion of ointment in the treatment of corneal abrasion. Once recurrent corneal erosion has occurred, it is treated by removal of the abnormal epithelium and pressure dressing in the hope that the epithelium will attach itself normally to the underlying tissue. In some cases corticosteroids are used locally following removal of the epithelium. Often several treatments are required. The instillation of an ointment at bedtime may prevent the eyelid from adhering to the loose epithelium and may prevent flicking the epithelium off when the eyes are opened. A soft contact lens is sometimes successful in preventing loss of epithelium.

The disorder may occur familialy and may constitute a corneal dystrophy.

Therapeutic soft contact lenses

Soft contact lenses are hemispherical shells that cover the cornea and a portion of the adjacent sclera. When hydrated the lens is soft and pliable, and when dry it is hard and brittle. A dry lens requires about 2 hours of soaking in normal saline solution to become completely hydrated. Soft contact lenses are usually better tolerated than hard contact lenses, although visual improvement may not be as good. Soft contact lenses have been useful in the treatment of bullous keratopathy, recurrent corneal erosion, and corneal ulcerations. They may protect the cornea in trichiasis.

In dry eye syndromes (such as Sjögren disease, ocular pemphigoid, erythema multiforme, and other conditions in which there is inadequate tearing), the lens is often not effective.

KERATOPLASTY

Corneal transplant, or keratoplasty, is the excision of corneal tissue and its replacement by a cornea from a human donor. One of two techniques is used: (1) the penetrating graft (Fig. 12-8), in which the entire thickness of cornea is removed and replaced by transparent corneal tissue, and (2) the nonpenetrating, or lamellar, keratoplasty, in which a superficial layer is removed and replaced without entry into the anterior chamber. The graft may vary in size from replacement of the entire cornea (total keratoplasty) to one in which a portion of the cornea is excised (partial). A diameter of 5 mm is the minimal size that will remain transparent in humans.

Because of improved surgery and better selection of donor material, the indications for transplant have been defined more in terms of the ocular disease necessitating the procedure rather than the preoperative visual acuity. Nonetheless, some corneal surgeons will not recommend keratoplasty unless vision is reduced to 6/60 (20/200) or less in both eyes. In diseases such as keratoconus, in which there is no corneal vascularization, the likelihood for marked improvement in vision is excellent. In corneal scars, particularly those following alkali burns, in which vascularization is superficial

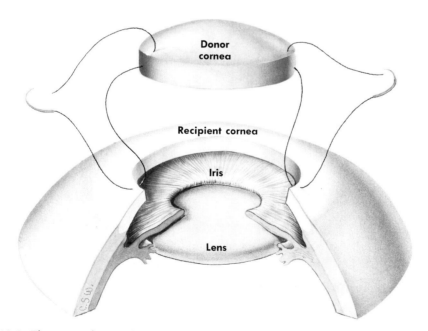

Fig. 12-8. The excised central portion of the cornea is being replaced with a clear donor cornea.

and deep, the graft is less likely to remain transparent. In every case, light perception and projection must be normal before surgery is considered. The prognosis in corneal dystrophy (p. 269) varies with the type and extent of the corneal abnormality.

Donor material is obtained from a non-infected adult, preferably between 25 and 35 years of age, who has died from an acute disease or from injury. Eyes from stillborn infants are less desirable, as are those of patients who were ill for a long period before death. Eyes should not be used from patients who had terminal septicemia, Creutzfeldt-Jakob disease or other possible slow-virus disorders, hepatitis, tumors of the anterior ocular segment, or leukemia. Eyes from individuals more than 60 years of age are undesirable.

The donor eye should be enucleated within an hour after death using sterile instruments and a sterile technique. If the eyelids are closed and a small icebag is placed over each eye, delays up to 5 hours are permissible. Many eye banks store donor corneal tissues as whole eyes in refrigerated, moist chambers for periods of 24 to 48 hours. Corneas may be stored for longer periods by carefully removing the cornea with a 3-mm rim of scleral tissue attached. The corneas must not be folded, because this damages the endothelium. The cornea is stored in a modified tissue-culture medium (M-K medium) and stored at a temperature of 4° C.

Persons who wish to donate their eyes for use in keratoplasty should write to an eye bank that is a member of the Eye Bank Association of America.*

Penetrating keratoplasty

The excision of all layers of a central portion of the cornea (partial penetrating) and replacement with a clear donor cornea is the traditional type of keratoplasty. A penetrating transplant is complete when the entire cornea is excised and partial when it is not.

The operation is usually performed using topical and retrobulbar anesthesia and akinesia. The graft is removed from the donor eye with a trephine. The same trephine is used to remove the diseased area from the recipient eye. The donor cornea is then sutured into position.

To align the graft, preplaced sutures may be inserted equidistantly in the four principal meridians of the donor button. Monofilament nylon (10-0) is used as either a continuous or an interrupted suture.

Lamellar keratoplasty

Since all layers of the cornea are not removed in nonpenetrating, or lamellar, keratoplasty, it has a more limited application than the penetrating type. Conversely, the procedure is associated with fewer postoperative complications than penetrating keratoplasty, may be repeated with a good likelihood of success even after earlier failures, and does not complicate a subsequent penetrating graft.

Keratoprosthesis

Corneal implants (keratoprostheses) made of nonreactive plastic are used in individuals in whom corneal transplantation was previously contraindicated or foredoomed to failure because of excessive scarring or neovascularization. In densely scarred corneas, a central optical cylinder of plastic supported by a cuff of plastic or dentin from a tooth extracted from the patient may provide a marked improvement in vision.

INJURIES

Foreign bodies of the cornea (p. 185) constitute about 25% of all significant eye injuries.

---

*Eye Bank Association of America, 2401 Queen Street, Winston-Salem, N.C. 27103, telephone (919) 724-5621.

Abrasions

Removal of the corneal epithelium by an abrasion or ultraviolet light causes considerable pain and lacrimation, but the lesion heals quickly and is of little clinical importance unless infection occurs. The abraded area stains with fluorescein. The eye is usually more comfortable if tightly patched, and the majority of corneal abrasions heal with no treatment other than patching. Local anesthetics are contraindicated because they may delay epithelization. If infection is feared, it is probably better to use sulfacetamide solution locally than to use a broad-spectrum antibiotic.

Lacerations

Corneal lacerations (p. 190) are particularly serious, because the interior of the eye is opened to infection and there is the likelihood of additional injury to intraocular structures. Treatment is directed toward prevention of infection by administration of an antibiotic, avoidance of prolapse of intraocular contents that may occur with repeated examinations, and closure of the laceration with sutures after excision of prolapsed intraocular tissue. If the lens is lacerated, it is removed at the time the corneal laceration is repaired.

BIBLIOGRAPHY

Allansmith, M. R., and McClellan, B. H.: Immunoglobulins in the human cornea, Am. J. Ophthalmol. **80**:123, 1975.

Aquavella, J. V., Buxton, J. N., and Shaw, E. L.: Thermokeratoplasty in treatment of persistent corneal hydrops, Arch. Ophthalmol. **95**:81, 1977.

Aquavella, J. V., Van Horn, D. L., and Haggerty, C. J.: Corneal preservation using M-K medium, Am. J. Ophthalmol. **80**:791, 1975.

Bigar, F., Kaufman, H. E., McCarey, B. E., and Binder, P. S.: Improved corneal storage for penetrating keratoplasties in man, Am. J. Ophthalmol. **79**:115, 1975.

Biglan, A. W., Brown, S. I., and Johnson, B. L.: Keratoglobus and blue sclera, Am. J. Ophthalmol. **83**:225, 1977.

Binder, P. S.: Review; herpes simplex keratitis, Surv. Ophthalmol. **21**:313, 1977.

Bloomfield, S. E., Gasset, A. R., Forstot, S. L., and Brown, S. I.: Treatment of filamentary keratitis with the soft contact lens, Am. J. Ophthalmol. **76**:978, 1973.

Bourne, W. M., and Kaufman, H. E.: Specular microscopy of human corneal endothelium in vivo, Am. J. Ophthalmol. **81**:319, 1976.

Brinser, J. H., and Torczynski, E.: Unusual *Pseudomonas* corneal ulcers, Am. J. Ophthalmol. **84**:462, 1977.

Brown, N. A., and Bron, A. J.: Superficial lines and associated disorders of the cornea, Am. J. Ophthalmol. **81**:34, 1976.

Capella, J. A., Edelhauser, H. F., and Van Horn, D. L., editors: Corneal preservation; clinical evaluation of current methods, Springfield, Ill., 1973, Charles C Thomas, Publisher.

Chin, G. N., Nyndiuk, R. A., Kwasny, G. P., and Schultz, R. O.: Keratomycosis in Wisconsin, Am. J. Ophthalmol. **79**:121, 1975.

DeVoe, A. G.: Complications of keratoplasty, Am. J. Ophthalmol. **79**:907, 1975.

Fine, M., and Cignetti, F. E.: Penetrating keratoplasty in herpes simplex keratitis, Arch. Ophthalmol. **95**:613, 1977.

Fraunfelder, F. T., and Hanna, C.: Spheroidal degeneration of cornea and conjunctiva. 3. Incidences, classification, and etiology, Am. J. Ophthalmol. **76**:41, 1973.

Gasset, A. R., and Kaufman, H. E.: Thermokeratoplasty in the treatment of keratoconus, Am. J. Ophthalmol. **79**:226, 1975.

Gasset, A. R., and Lobo, L.: Simplified soft contact lens treatment in corneal disease, Ann. Ophthalmol. **9**:843, 1977.

Iwamoto, T., and DeVoe, A. G.: Electron microscopical study of Fleischer ring, Arch. Ophthalmol. **94**:1579, 1976.

Jones, B. R.: Principles in the management of oculomycosis, Am. J. Ophthalmol. **79**:719, 1975.

Kaufman, H. E.: Contamination of donor eyes, Am. J. Ophthalmol. **84**:746, 1977.

Keates, R. H., Mishler, K. E., and Riedinger, D.: Bacterial contamination of donor eyes, Am. J. Ophthalmol. **84**:617, 1977.

Kessler, E., Mondino, B. J., and Brown, S. I.: The corneal response to *Pseudomonas aeruginosa*; histopathological and enzymatic characterization, Invest. Ophthalmol. **16**:116, 1977.

Kim, H-B., and Ostler, H. B.: Marginal corneal ulcer due to B-streptococcus, Arch. Ophthalmol. **95**:454, 1977.

Lemp, M. A., and Ralph, R. A.: Rapid development of band keratopathy in dry eyes, Am. J. Ophthalmol. **83**:657, 1977.

Marsh, R. J., Fraunfelder, F. T., and McGill, J. I.:

Herpetic corneal epithelial disease, Arch. Ophthalmol. **94**:1899, 1976.

Mondino, B. J., Shahinian, L. R., Johnson, B. L., and Brown, S. I.: Peters' anomaly with the fetal transfusion syndrome, Am. J. Ophthalmol. **82**:55, 1976.

O'Day, D. M., Gyer, B., Hierholzer, J. C., and others: Clinical and laboratory evaluation of epidemic keratoconjunctivitis due to adenovirus types 8 and 19, Am. J. Ophthalmol. **81**:207, 1976.

O'Day, D. M., Poirier, R. H., Jones, D. B., and Elliott, J. H.: Vidarabine therapy of complicated herpes simplex keratitis, Am. J. Ophthalmol. **81**: 642, 1976.

Okumoto, M., and Smolin, G.: Pneumococcal infections of the eye, Am. J. Ophthalmol. **77**:346, 1974.

Ostler, H. B., and Okumoto, M.: Anaerobic streptococcal corneal ulcer, Am. J. Ophthalmol. **81**: 518, 1976.

Pavan-Langston, D., Buchanan, R. A., and Alford, C. A., Jr., editors: Adenine arabinoside; an antiviral agent, New York, 1975, Raven Press.

Polack, F. M.: The endothelium of failed corneal graft, Am. J. Ophthalmol. **79**:251, 1975.

Robertson, D. M., Sizemore, G. W., and Gordon, H.: Thickened corneal nerves as a manifestation of multiple endocrine neoplasia, Trans. Am. Acad. Ophthalmol. Otolaryngol. **79**:772, 1975.

Townsend, W. M., Font, R. L., and Zimmerman, L. E.: Congenital corneal leukomas. 2. Histopathologic findings in 19 eyes with central defect in Descemet's membrane, Am. J. Ophthalmol. **77**:192, 1974.

Townsend, W. M., Font, R. L., and Zimmerman, L. E.: Congenital corneal leukomas. 3. Histopathologic findings in 13 eyes with noncentral defect in Descemet's membrane, Am. J. Ophthalmol. **77**: 400, 1974.

Van Horn, D. L., Schultz, R. O., and DeBruin, J.: Endothelial survival in corneal tissue stored in M-K medium, Am. J. Ophthalmol. **80**:642, 1975.

Vanley, G. T., Leopold, I. H., and Gregg, T. H.: Interpretation of tear film breakup, Arch. Ophthalmol. **95**:445, 1977.

Wilensky, J. T., Buerk, K. M., and Podos, S. M.: Krukenberg's spindles, Am. J. Ophthalmol. **79**: 220, 1975.

Wilson, L. A., and Ahearn, D. G.: *Pseudomonas*-induced corneal ulcers associated with contaminated eye mascaras, Am. J. Ophthalmol. **84**: 112, 1977.

Young, J. D. H., and Finlay, R. D.: Primary spheroidal degeneration of the cornea in Labrador and northern Newfoundland, Am. J. Ophthalmol. **79**:129, 1975.

Chapter 13

THE SCLERA

The sclera is a dense, connective tissue structure composed of collagen bundles of varying diameters. It constitutes the posterior five sixths of the globe. Its anterior portion is visible beneath the transparent conjunctiva as the white of the eye, but careful examination will show the delicate plexus of blood vessels that make up the richly vascularized episclera located mainly in the anterior segment of the globe. Inflammations, often associated with connective tissue disorders, are the main disorders of the sclera. The tissue, however, undergoes changes in shape, size, and translucency that play an important role in the pathogenesis of other ocular disorders.

SYMPTOMS AND SIGNS OF SCLERAL DISEASE

Because of its rich sensory nerve innervation, inflammations of the sclera may cause severe or dull pain that is aggravated by contraction of an ocular muscle if the sclera is inflamed near its insertion. No signs may be apparent in inflammations of the posterior sclera, but pain on ocular movement suggests the cause. There is no loss of vision, which distinguishes the pain from that occurring in retrobulbar neuritis.

Inflammation of the anterior portion of the sclera causes generalized or localized areas of deep reddish injection of the episcleral tissues. These areas may be painful on palpation. In thinning or necrosis of the sclera, the bluish-black choroidal pigment may be exposed.

INTRASCLERAL NERVE LOOP

An intrascleral nerve loop is an anatomic variation in which an anomalous loop of the long ciliary nerve partially or completely perforates the sclera and then returns to the inner surface of the sclera, often accompanied by a blood vessel. It appears as a 1- to 2-mm black dot on the sclera, mainly in the lower half of the eye, some 2 to 4 mm from the corneoscleral limbus. Its unchanging appearance and location indicate its nature. Treatment is not indicated.

PIGMENTATION OF THE SCLERA

Pigmentation of the sclera mainly involves underlying lesions of the uveal tract. Thus, a blue nevus may be associated with an underlying choroidal nevus or a melanocytoma with an underlying melanocytosis. The most serious abnormality is extension of a choroidal malignant melanoma through the sclera, often at the site of one of the small openings for the transmission of nerves or blood vessels. The differential diagnosis of a black elevated mass in the sclera includes staphyloma with an extremely thin sclera or extraocular extension of an intraocular malignant melanoma.

The sclera is not pigmented in jaundice; the yellowish appearance of the globe arises from bilirubin in the conjunctiva.

STAPHYLOMA AND ECTASIA

Staphylomas and ectasias are bulgings or enlargements of the sclera secondary to embryologic defects of the sclera, localized areas of degeneration, or increased intraocular pressure. If only the sclera stretches, the condition is called an ectasia, whereas if the uvea lines the bulging sclera it is called a staphyloma.

Ectasias are usually associated with abnormalities in closure of the optic vesicle; thus, concurrent colobomas of the uveal tract and retina are common. Failure of the scleral mesoderm to form the lamina cribrosa has the appearance of an enormous but normal disk at the bottom of a deep pit. In myopia a localized bulging of sclera may develop between the insertions of the recti muscles, and it may be associated with a retinal separation. In adult glaucoma, the sclera propria (and cornea) is resistant to the increased intraocular pressure, but a partial ectasia forms at the lamina cribrosa along with the characteristic glaucomatous excavation (cupping) of the optic disk.

Staphylomas may be total or partial. In congenital glaucoma, uniform stretching of the sclera occurs before the scleral and corneal collagen fibers have matured. The result is the total staphyloma of buphthalmos.

Localized staphylomas are divided into anterior and posterior types. Anterior staphylomas occur anterior to the equator, calary or ciliary staphylomas over the ciliary body, and intracalary staphylomas between the ciliary body and the corneoscleral limbus. These bulgings most often follow inflammation of the anterior uveal tract or laceration of the sclera combined with constantly increased intraocular pressure. The involved area appears as a region of scleral thinning lined with the dark pigment of the uveal tract.

Posterior staphylomas occur in pathologic myopia in which there is thinning and stretching of the posterior pole as the axial length of the globe increases (p. 434). Vision is decreased. Ophthalmoscopic examination shows central retinal degeneration. Indirect ophthalmoscopic examination shows a sharp, well-defined edge of posterior scleral outpouching.

Equatorial staphylomas and ectasias involve the areas near the points of exit of the four vortex veins from the eye. The localized bulging of the sclera may be a factor in retinal separation (p. 349), though often not detected until the area is exposed surgically.

SCLERAL THINNING

In long-standing scleral or uveal inflammation, in Marfan syndrome, and in osteogenesis imperfecta, the underlying uveal pigment is visible because of scleral thinning. The sclera appears more blue than white. This coloration may be vivid in osteogenesis imperfecta.

INFLAMMATIONS

The sclera proper has a poor blood supply and an inactive metabolism, but the episclera has a rich vascular network. Inflammations (Table 13-1) tend to be torpid. Most instances of scleritis are associated with connective tissue disorders or suggest an antigen-induced immune response or an autoimmunity.

Episcleritis

Episcleritis (Fig. 13-1) is an inflammation of the episcleral tissue in the region between the insertion of the recti muscles and the corneoscleral limbus. It affects women twice as frequently as men and has its peak incidence between the

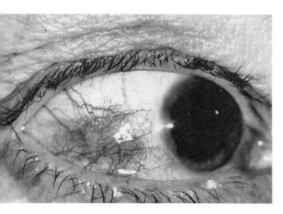

Fig. 13-1. Localized area of acute episcleritis on the temporal side of the sclera in a 35-year-old woman.

Table 13-1. Inflammation of the sclera

Episcleritis
   Simple
   Nodular
Anterior scleritis
   Diffuse
   Nodular
   Necrotizing
      With inflammation
      Without inflammation (scleromalacia perforans)
Posterior scleritis

Modified from Watson, P. G., and Hazleman, B. L.: Major problems in ophthalmology. Vol. 2: The sclera and systemic disorders, Philadelphia, 1976, W. B. Saunders Co.

ages of 30 and 40 years. The onset is sudden with intense redness, usually involving only one quadrant of the globe but sometimes all, and a sharpness or pricking discomfort. The affected episclera is edematous, and the blood vessels are engorged. The condition tends to spontaneous remission, sometimes within a few hours or days. There is a marked tendency for recurrence, sometimes cyclic, over a period of years.

Nodular episcleritis is similar to simple episcleritis but is associated with a tender nodule some 2 to 3 mm in size. There may be deep, boring pain, most severe at night, but the inflammation generally disappears spontaneously after 4 to 5 weeks, sometimes leaving a residue of a faintly pigmented patch to which the conjunctiva is adherent.

Scleritis

Scleritis is a more serious disease than episcleritis and is associated with more intense pain. Scleritis is more likely to be bilateral than episcleritis. Like episcleritis, it tends to recur.

Diffuse anterior scleritis has an insidious onset with generalized orbital aching. The blood vessels are intensely injected and appear as deep-seated, small, numerous radial vessels surrounded by numerous capillaries.

Nodular scleritis is intensely painful with an extremely tender, firm, immobile nodule completely separated from the overlying congested episcleral tissues. The nodules may be multiple. Avascularity or progressive increase in size of the nodule indicates scleral necrosis.

Necrotizing anterior scleritis occurs in two forms. In one, the inflammatory reaction is severe with much discomfort and pain and multiple ocular complications. In the other, inflammatory reaction is minimal (scleromalacia perforans). The disease may progress from earlier anterior scleritis, or it may have a dramatic onset with avascular patches that may perforate. The noninflammatory type may cause painless, large scleral defects through which the choroid bulges, usually without perforation, a disaster that may be precipitated by subconjunctival injections.

Diagnosis of posterior scleritis is difficult, but there is deep-seated pain in the eye with reduction of visual acuity and changes in the fundus caused by the scleral inflammation. Connective tissue disease is not usually present.

Treatment is difficult. Episcleritis improves spontaneously, although recov-

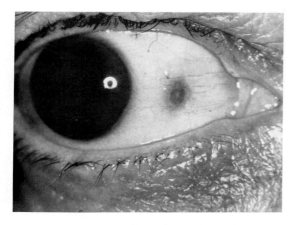

Fig. 13-2. Senile hyaline plaque located immediately in front of the insertion of the lateral rectus muscle in a 65-year-old man. The plaque shells out of the sclera easily and contains calcium sulfate (gypsum).

ery may be hastened by administration of noncorticosteroidal anti-inflammatory drugs. Large doses of corticosteroids may be used, but the dangers of cataract and glaucoma must be appreciated. However, in severe necrotizing disease corticosteroids as well as immunosuppressive therapy and other compounds used in the treatment of connective tissue disease may be necessary.

DEGENERATIONS: SENILE HYALINE PLAQUE

Senile hyaline plaque (Fig. 13-2) is the term mistakenly applied to a darkish deposition located immediately anterior to the insertion of the medial or lateral rectus muscle in the sclera. It occurs only in individuals more than 50 years of age. It appears as an area of translucency in the sclera. It was formerly thought to be caused by thinning of the sclera because of traction of the recti muscles. The plaque may be easily shelled out of the slightly thinned sclera and histologically may contain calcium sulfate (gypsum).

INJURIES

Laceration of the sclera invariably involves the underlying uveal coat and is unusually serious. Blunt trauma to the globe may rupture the posterior sclera as the result of contrecoup phenomenon. The history of blunt trauma associated with severe subconjunctival hemorrhage and a persistently soft globe suggests a posterior rupture of the globe. Usually an associated rupture of the retina and choroid occurs along with vitreous hemorrhage obscuring the tissues.

BIBLIOGRAPHY

Crandall, A. S., Yanoff, M., and Schaffer, D. B.: Intrascleral nerve loop mistakenly identified as foreign body, Arch. Ophthalmol. **95**:497, 1977.

Feldon, S. E., Sigelman, J., Albert, D. M., and Taylor, R. S.: Clinical manifestations of brawny scleritis, Am. J. Ophthalmol. **85**:781, 1978.

Watson, P. G., and Hazleman, B. L.: Major problems in ophthalmology. Vol. 2: The sclera and systemic disorders, Philadelphia, 1976, W. B. Saunders Co.

Chapter 14

THE PUPIL

The pupil is the central aperture of the iris. It controls the amount of light entering the eye by constricting in bright illumination and dilating in the dark. Pupillary size is controlled by the opposed actions of two nonstriated muscles, both derived from the neuroectoderm of the secondary optic vesicle: the sphincter pupillae (N III parasympathetics) and the dilatator pupillae (sympathetics). The two layers of secondary optic vesicle fuse to form the pigment layer of the iris, and its most anterior portion at the pupillary margin may form a pigmented pupillary frill, conspicuous in ectropion uveae.

Normal pupils are round, regular in shape, and nearly equal in size. There may rarely be a physiologic difference in pupil size (physiologic anisocoria). Each pupil is located with its center a little below and slightly to the nasal side of the cornea. The pupils are constricted in infancy and in old age and are at their maximal size during childhood and adolescence. In bright illumination the pupils are constricted (miosis), and in dim illumination the pupils are dilated (mydriasis). Pupils are considered miotic if less than 2 mm in diameter and mydriatic if more than 6 mm in diameter. Unequal size of the pupils is called anisocoria.

The sphincter pupillae muscle (p. 22) is a typical annular sphincter muscle located next to the pupillary margin deep in the iris stroma. It is innervated by efferent visceral fibers that originate in the Edinger-Westphal portion of the oculomotor nucleus (N III). These fibers enter the orbit with the inferior branch of the oculomotor nerve. A short motor branch is sent to the ciliary ganglion, where synapse is made with postganglionic fibers. Three to six postganglionic nerves extend forward from the ganglion to divide into 6 to 20 short ciliary nerves that penetrate the sclera around the optic nerve and pass forward in the suprachoroidal space; about 97% of the fibers are distributed to the ciliary muscle (accommodation) and the remainder to the sphincter pupillae muscle (miosis).

The dilatator pupillae muscle (p. 22) is arranged radially in the iris stroma. It extends from the outer edge of the sphincter muscle to the root of the iris and contains pigment. It is innervated by sympathetic fibers that probably originate in the hypothalamus. From here the fibers descend in the lateral columns of the cervical cord and emerge with the eighth cervical and first thoracic ventral nerve roots. The fibers then ascend the sympathetic chain to the superior cervical ganglion, where they synapse. Postganglionic fibers extend cranially along the internal carotid artery and reach the dilatator pupillae muscle mainly with the two long ciliary nerve branches of the nasciliary branch of the fifth (trigeminal) cranial nerve. The sympathetic fibers that pass through and do not synapse in the ciliary ganglion are mainly vasomotor and do not innervate the dilatator pupillae muscle.

Inasmuch as the sphincter pupillae muscle and the dilatator muscle are an integral part of the iris (p. 20), their function may be altered in iris inflammations, degenerations, and congenital abnormalities. Additionally, the pupil provides the pathway between the posterior and anterior chambers for passage of aqueous humor. If aqueous humor is prevented from passing through the pupil (pupillary block or iris bombé), glaucoma occurs (p. 406).

PUPILLARY REFLEXES

When light is directed into one eye, the pupil constricts (direct light reflex) and, with rare exceptions (in cases of consensual deficit), the opposite pupil simultaneously constricts a similar amount (consensual light reflex). The receptors for the light reflex are the retinal rods and cones. The afferent axons responsible for conduction of the impulse are separate from the visual fibers but follow the same course in the optic nerve and chiasm; they separate from visual fibers at the level of the lateral geniculate body and do not synapse but pass through the brachium of the superior colliculus and synapse in the pretectal region. Here fibers pass with partial decussation to the Edinger-Westphal portion of the oculomotor nucleus (N III). Visceral motor efferent fibers pass from the nucleus in the oculomotor nerve to synapse in the ciliary ganglion (p. 63). Postganglionic fibers reach the sphincter pupillae muscle by the short ciliary nerves.

In an eye blind from disease of the retina or the optic nerve, the direct light reflex is abolished, and there is no consensual reflex in the opposite eye. However, the blind eye has an intact consensual reflex so that its pupil constricts when the normal fellow eye is stimulated with light. In an eye with hemianopia arising from an optic tract lesion (thus, anterior to the lateral geniculate body), light stimulation of the portion of the retina corresponding to the field defect causes a diminished or absent direct light reflex. This is called the hemianopic pupillary reflex. Detection requires a small bundle of light rays so that the uninvolved side is not stimulated by scattered light within the eye. In hemianopia caused by involvement of the nerve fibers posterior to the lateral geniculate body, the pupillary reaction to light is intact, since the afferent pupillary fibers have already separated from the visual fibers.

Synkinetic, or associated, constriction of the pupil occurs with convergence and is not a true reflex but an associated reaction involving the common innervation of the medial rectus muscle involved in convergence and the sphincter pupillae muscle (p. 111). A less commonly observed synkinetic reaction is the pupillary constriction that may follow contraction of the orbicularis oculi muscle innervated by nerve VII.

Hippus, a rhythmic dilation and contraction of the pupils (physiologic pupillary unrest), cannot be reliably associated with any nervous disorder.

SYMPTOMS AND SIGNS OF PUPILLARY ABNORMALITIES

The chief symptoms arising from abnormalities of the pupil relate to its function as a diaphragm in controlling the amount of light that enters the eye. When the pupil is dilated, approximately 50 times as much energy enters as when it is constricted. Dilation and constriction occur constantly in the normal eye (p. 110) in response to the amount of light stimulating the retina.

A convex lens (p. 168) provides magnification to observe minimal pupillary reflexes, which may be difficult to evaluate when the pupils are constricted.

A dilated pupil causes more chromatic and spherical aberration and less depth of focus, as is true of a camera with the diaphragm opened widely. (The normal eye is about f 5.6.)

A marked constriction of the pupil interferes with vision in dim illumination because of failure of the pupil to dilate in response to the reduced lighting. Visual loss arising from minor opacities of the lens may be severely aggravated by pupillary constriction, which is often a serious problem in the treatment of glaucoma (p. 401).

Openings in the iris in addition to the pupil may cause monocular double vision (diplopia). Surgical iridectomies are usually located near the 12 o'clock meridian; they are covered by the upper eyelid and cause no symptoms. In conditions such as polycoria (multiple pupils) or iridodialysis, which is a separation of the base of the iris from the ciliary body (Fig. 14-1), diplopia may be an annoying symptom.

The signs of pupillary abnormalities arise from the pupil's shape, position, and response to stimulation. The pupils of the two eyes are usually of about equal size and respond similarly to stimulation. Distortion and irregularity of the pupil may arise from disease or injury of the iris. In abnormalities reflected in differences in size of the two pupils (anisocoria, p. 284) or in disturbances of pupillary reflexes (p. 111), one must determine if the condition arises from a localized iris abnormality, inequality, or an interruption of the sympathetic or parasympathetic efferent innervation.

CONGENITAL ABNORMALITIES

Inasmuch as the pupil is an opening in the iris, it is evident that developmental pupillary abnormalities arise because of abnormalities of the iris or the innervation of its muscles. However, the most striking change may be the alteration in the appearance of the pupil. In aniridia (p. 290) the iris is rudimentary, and the eye appears to be jet black with no iris present. A coloboma of the iris (Figs. 14-1 and 15-3) may be associated with faulty closure of the retinal fissure and typical defects in the optic nerve and choroid.

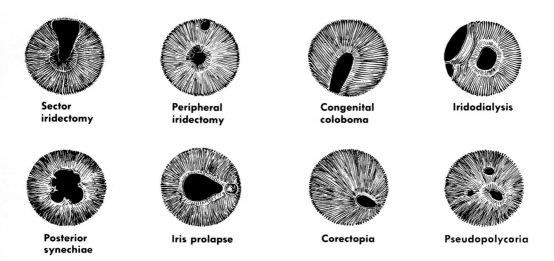

Sector iridectomy   Peripheral iridectomy   Congenital coloboma   Iridodialysis

Posterior synechiae   Iris prolapse   Corectopia   Pseudopolycoria

Fig. 14-1. Irregularity of the pupil in various disorders.

More common is simple coloboma of the iris, in which a single or all layers of the iris are absent in a localized area, either extending as far as the ciliary body (total) or involving only a portion of a sector (partial). The pupil is pear shaped (Fig. 14-1) because of the absence of iris, but the usual layers are retained in the normal sector, and thus the iris shows normal reflexes. Colobomas may be completely surrounded by iris tissue (Fig. 14-1) and appear as additional pupils (pseudopolycoria). True polycoria, with multiple pupils each having a sphincter muscle, is extremely rare. The condition of multiple pupils without sphincters is called pseudopolycoria. Conspicuous displacement of the pupil from its normal position is corectopia, or ectopic pupil. Except for the cosmetic blemish, it causes no symptoms.

MIOSIS AND MYDRIASIS
Miosis

Constriction of the pupil to less than 2.0 mm is called miosis. The pupil is abnormal if it does not dilate in darkness. The most common cause of the condition is the instillation of cholinergic-stimulating drugs, which contract the sphincter pupillae muscle, in the treatment of glaucoma. Accidental or systemic administration of these compounds may cause miosis, depending on the dose. Morphine causes extreme constriction of the pupil. During sleep the pupils constrict, and the miosis may distinguish true sleep from simulated sleep (as does involuntary fluttering of the eyelids in simulated sleep). With aging, the pupils normally become smaller (senile miosis), but normal reflexes are retained. Bilateral adhesion of the iris to the lens (posterior synechiae, p. 301) may cause small, irregular pupils. Congenital absence of the dilatator pupillae muscle results in miosis because of unopposed action of the sphincter pupillae muscle.

Constriction of the pupil after blinking is caused by dark adaptation. It does not occur in darkness. The pupil dilates on closure because of dark adaptation but is miotic in sleep. Irritation of the conjunctiva or the cornea may cause miosis.

Mydriasis

Dilation of both pupils to more than 6.0 mm combined with failure to constrict when stimulated with light follows local instillation of drugs that paralyze the sphincter pupillae muscle (Table 14-1). Pupils dilated with drugs such as atropine do not constrict promptly when 1% pilocarpine solution is instilled. Pupils that are dilated as a result of interference with the nerves involved in the reflex arc constrict promptly after instillation of pilocarpine. Usually, systemic administration of compounds has a minimal pupillary effect, and its chief action involves the ciliary muscle in decreased accommodation. In bilateral blindness caused by lesions anterior to the lateral geniculate body, the pupils are dilated and, of course, fail to constrict when stimulated with light.

During general anesthesia the pupils are usually dilated in stages I and II because of excitement, alarm, or adrenergic stimuli. During stage III the pupils reflect the miosis of coma. In stage IV, hypoxia of the midbrain and the Edinger-Westphal nuclei causes pupillary dilation. Surprise, fear, and pain cause dilation of the pupil, as does any strong emotion, pleasant or unpleasant, or vestibular stimulation.

The pupil may be dilated in carotid artery aneurysm and in orbital or intracranial trauma caused by injury to pupillary fibers in the oculomotor nerve (N III). In acute angle-closure glaucoma the pupil may be middilated because of sphincter hypoxia and may be fixed (p. 404). In Adie syndrome, the pupil reacts

Table 14-1. Possible causes of a dilated pupil that does not constrict to light

---

  I. Iris involvement*
   A. Inflammatory disease, posterior synechiae
   B. Ischemia sphincter with acute increase in intraocular pressure
   C. Contusion injury to sphincter (traumatic iridoplegia)
   D. Cholinergic blockage of sphincter (atropine and so on)
 II. Ciliary ganglion or short ciliary nerves†
   A. Adie syndrome
   B. Ciliary ganglion inflammation (zoster, viral ganglionitis)
   C. Orbital or choroidal trauma or tumor
III. Preganglionic N III†
   A. Aneurysm of circle of Willis
   B. Herniation of the uncus of the temporal lobe
   C. Parasellar tumors (pituitary adenoma, meningioma, craniopharyngioma, nasopharyngeal carcinoma)
   D. Parasellar inflammation (Tolosa-Hunt syndrome, zoster, giant cell arteritis)
IV. Edinger-Westphal nucleus†
   A. Dorsal: uncommon, bilateral, near-vision reaction retained, supranuclear vertical gaze palsy present
   B. Ventral: associated neurologic defects (Nothnagel, Benedikt, Weber syndromes) and paralysis of ocular
      muscles, innervated N III

---

*Pupil does not constrict with topical 1% pilocarpine.
†Pupil constricts with topical 1% pilocarpine.

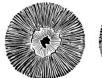

Argyll Robertson pupil
Miotic, irregular, unreactive to light,
reacts to convergence

Oculomotor paralysis with fixed
dilated pupil likely with lost accommodation

Horner syndrome
Miosis, ptosis, anhidrosis on side of
sympathetic innervation interruption

Adie syndrome
Pupil larger or smaller than fellow,
reacts slowly to light and accommodation

Fig. 14-2. Some neurologic causes of unequal pupils.

slowly to light and is larger initially than the fellow pupil.

Anisocoria

Anisocoria (Fig. 14-2), or unequal size of the pupils, is a relatively common normal variation. The normal difference in diameter, however, is slight, and often it is not noted. About 2% of apparently normal individuals have a 0.5- to 2.0-mm difference in the size of the pupils with normal pupillary reflexes. The cause is unknown but may be hereditary.

Inequality in size of the pupils or a difference in their reflex reactions or responses to locally instilled drugs may indicate serious ocular or neurologic disease, which demands careful study. If the afferent pupillary fibers in one eye and the optic nerve are intact, the pupils of both eyes will remain equal in size even if there is a lesion of the optic nerve of the fellow eye. This is because of the decussation of the efferent outflow so that the iris muscles of the involved eye are innervated normally (p. 111). Anisocoria thus mainly reflects an abnormality involving the iris musculature of one eye, the eye itself, or the efferent parasympathetic or sympathetic motor innervation. The involved pupil may be either smaller or larger than the fellow. Irritative lesions of the parasympathetic pathway cause constriction, whereas paralytic lesions cause dilation. Irritative lesions of the sympathetic pathway cause dilation, whereas paralytic lesions cause constriction.

Table 14-2. Some causes of inequality of pupil size (anisocoria)

I. Local ocular causes
  A. Drugs topically instilled: mydriasis or miosis
  B. Injury
    1. Rupture of iris sphincter with contusion (traumatic iridoplegia)
    2. Adhesions between iris and cornea following laceration (adherent leukoma or anterior synechiae)
  C. Inflammation
    1. Keratitis (miosis)
    2. Acute iridocyclitis (middilation)
    3. Adhesions between iris and lens (posterior synechiae)
  D. Angle-closure glaucoma (middilation)
  E. Ischemia of iris
    1. Retinal separation surgery
    2. Internal carotid artery insufficiency (dilation)
  F. Diseases of iris
    1. Essential atrophy
    2. Aniridia
    3. Congenital variation
II. Paralysis of sphincter pupillae muscle (pupil dilated)
  A. Intracranial disease
    1. Neoplasm, aneurysm, degeneration
    2. Infection: syphilis, herpes zoster ophthalmicus, meningitis, encephalitis, botulism, diphtheria, tuberculous meningitis (pupil dilated, fixed)
    3. Vascular disease: cavernous sinus thrombosis, hemorrhage
  B. Toxic polyneuritis (alcohol, lead, arsenic, carbon dioxide)
  C. Diabetes mellitus (pupil spared in 75% of cases of diabetic ophthalmoplegia)
III. Paralysis of dilatator pupillae muscle (pupil constricted)
  A. Horner syndrome
IV. Lesion of intercalated neuron
  A. Argyll Robertson pupil (tabes dorsalis, pupil constricted)

Tonic pupil (Adie syndrome)

Tonic pupil (Fig. 14-2) is an abnormality in which disturbances of pupillary reaction are associated with abnormalities of tendon reflexes in patients who do not have syphilis. The shape of the pupil is slightly irregular, and one pupil may be larger than the other. Although the condition is mainly limited to one side, it can be bilateral. In the complete form of Adie syndrome the pupil reacts barely, if at all, to light. Initially the tonic pupil is large but becomes smaller with time. When the patient makes an attempt to fix a near point, a slow and delayed pupillary constriction appears. This response may be marked and may exceed that of the normal pupil. After the pupil constricts for near vision, it slowly redilates and may remain smaller than the normal pupil for some time. There is an associated diminution or absence of tendon reflexes; however, the pupillary signs may occur without involvement of the deep tendons.

There is supersensitivity to cholinergic stimulation, and the pupil constricts after instillation of 0.10% pilocarpine, a concentration that does not affect the normal eye. This suggests the supersensitivity of denervation and indicates that the lesion is located either at the level of the ciliary ganglion or its postganglionic outflow. The disease is entirely benign, and no treatment is indicated.

Horner syndrome

Interruption of the sympathetic nerve supply to the dilatator pupillae muscle results in a constricted pupil. The miosis is not marked and is often not noticed. Interruption of the sympathetic nerves anywhere in their course from the hypothalamus to the orbit results in Horner syndrome. In addition to the miosis, there is blepharoptosis, anhidrosis, and, in experimental animals but not in humans, an enophthalmos.

The blepharoptosis is the result of loss of sympathetic nerve supply to the Müller smooth muscle of the upper eyelid, which provides its "tone" (p. 54). The eyelid droops only 1 or 2 mm. The anhidrosis follows loss of the sympathetic nerve fibers to the face and neck. The sweating fibers follow the external carotid artery, and in lesions occurring between the bifurcation of the common carotid artery and the orbit, they are not affected. The enophthalmos is not present in humans but is simulated by the slight blepharoptosis. It is marked in animals that have much smooth muscle in the orbit.

Horner syndrome is usually caused by interruption of the cervical sympathetic trunk or the lower cervical and upper thoracic anterior spinal roots. The most common causes are mediastinal tumors, particularly bronchogenic carcinoma, Hodgkin disease, and metastatic tumors.

Table 14-3. Pharmacologic response of unequal pupils

Compound	Normal pupil	Horner syndrome		Oculomotor nerve	
		Pre-ganglionic lesion	Post-ganglionic lesion	Pre-ganglionic	Post-ganglionic*
Epinephrine (0.1%)	0	0	Dilation	0	0
Hydroxyamphetamine (1%)	Dilation	Dilation	0	Dilation	Dilation
Cocaine (4%)	Dilation	0	0	Dilation	Dilation
Pilocarpine (0.1%)	0	0	0	0	Miosis
Pilocarpine (1%)	Constriction	Constriction	Constriction	Constriction	Constriction

*Excludes absent response in sphincter pupillae involvement in inflammation, posterior synechiae, cholinergic blockade (atropine).

Large adenomas of the thyroid gland and neurofibromatosis may be causes. Surgical and accidental traumas to the neck are the next most common causes. Diseases within the central nervous system that may cause this syndrome include occlusion of the posterior inferior cerebellar artery, multiple sclerosis or syringomyelia involving the reticular substance of the pons, and tumors of the cervical cord. Congenital Horner syndrome may be associated with less pigment in the iris on the affected side than in the fellow eye (heterochromia iridis) (p. 293).

The affected pupil does not dilate after instillation of cocaine solution, but the normal pupil does. If the lesion causing Horner syndrome involves the sympathetic nerves between the synapse in the superior cervical ganglion and the eye, the pupil is supersensitive to epinephrine and dilates after instillation of 1: 1,000 epinephrine hydrochloride, a concentration that does not affect the normal pupil. This reaction helps to distinguish between pre- and postganglionic lesions causing Horner syndrome. In preganglionic Horner syndrome, the pupil dilates after instillation of the indirect-acting mydriatic hydroxyamphetamine (1%), a drug that does not affect the postganglionic Horner lesion.

Argyll Robertson pupil

The Douglas M. C. L. Argyll Robertson pupil (Fig. 14-2) is a bilateral abnormality characterized by failure of the pupils to constrict with light but retention of pupillary constriction with convergence and accommodation. The entire syndrome includes miotic, irregular, and unequal pupils, the presence of some vision in each eye, failure of the pupils to dilate after local scopolamine instillation, and further miosis after eserine instillation. When all signs are present, they characterize tabes dorsalis of central nervous system syphilis. The lesion is thought to be in the pretectal region, where the afferent pupillary fibers synapse. Hemorrhage and tumors involving the pretectal region may be associated with failure of the pupils to react to light and retention of the reaction to convergence; however, the pupils are not miotic, unequal, or irregular and are not typical of those described by Robertson.

Afferent pupillary defect

The afferent pupillary defect (Robert Marcus Gunn), or pupillary escape phenomenon, occurs in defects of the visual pathway anterior to the chiasm. It consists of a diminished amplitude of pupillary light reaction, a lengthened latent period, and pupillary dilation (escape) with continuous light stimulus. Patients with this disorder note a decreased light sensitivity on the affected side indicative of a conduction interference. The pupils are of equal size.

The test for its detection has been called the swinging flashlight test. There is dilation of both pupils when the light stimulus is moved from the unaffected eye to the affected eye. Normally, if penlight illumination is alternately directed to each eye, the pupils constrict and do not vary as the light alternates between the eyes. In the afferent pupillary defect, both pupils dilate when light is directed into the affected eye and constrict when light is directed into the normal eye.

The pupillary sign occurs most conspicuously in optic neuritis and serves to distinguish the reduction of visual acuity caused by optic neuritis from that occurring in central retinal edema. However, it is present in a variety of conditions affecting the conduction of light impulses. Thus it may occur in extensive retinal disease in which there is failure of a nerve signal to be propagated to the optic nerve, in compression of the optic nerve secondary to mass lesions, and in unilateral optic atrophy.

The normally slow dilation of the pupil because of retinal adaptation as light continues to be directed into the eye must be distinguished from the more rapid dilation that occurs in afferent pupillary defects. Patients with strabismic and related types of amblyopia have nearly normal pupillary reflexes; patients with conversion reactions or simulated loss of vision have normal pupillary reflexes.

Irregularity

The pupils may be of irregular shape in a variety of disorders (Fig. 14-1). Following a corneal laceration, the iris prolapses into the wound, causing a tear-shaped pupil. Following blunt trauma to the eye, the iris may be torn from its insertion at the scleral spur, causing an iridodialysis. The sector of the pupil corresponding to the iridodialysis is flattened and becomes a chord of the circular pupil.

In uveitis the iris may be bound to the lens by posterior synechiae. These may be evident only when the pupil is dilated, but if they formed when the pupil was miotic, the irregularity of the pupillary margin will be marked.

Surgical excisions of part of the iris may be recognized by their usual location near the 12 o'clock meridian and by the deficiency of the iris pigment frill at the edges of the incision. A congenital coloboma involves the inferior nasal iris, and the frill of pupillary pigment lines the margins.

Persistent pupillary fibers. The anterior portion of the tunica vasculosa lentis, which nourishes the lens during embryonic life, is derived from anterior ciliary vessels. These ordinarily undergo atrophy about the eighth month and recede to the collarette of the pupil. Occasionally, delicate strands of fibers remain extended from the collarette to the anterior lens capsule. Sometimes they may be sturdy and covered with pigment, but they do not interfere with vision.

Ectopia lentis et pupillae. This is a rare autosomal recessive disorder characterized by oval or slit-shaped pupils displaced temporally, whereas the lens is displaced nasally.

BIBLIOGRAPHY

Bourgon, P., Pilley, S. F. J., and Thompson, H. S.: Cholinergic supersensitivity of the iris sphincter in Adie's tonic pupil, Am. J. Ophthalmol. **85:**373, 1978.

Kaback, M. B., Burde, R. M., and Becker, B.: Relative afferent pupillary defect in glaucoma, Am. J. Ophthalmol. **81:**462, 1976.

Miller, S. D., and Thompson, H. S.: Pupil cycle time in optic neuritis, Am. J. Ophthalmol. **85:**635, 1978.

Purcell, J. J., Jr., Krachmer, J. H., and Thompson, H. S.: Corneal sensation in Adie's syndrome, Am. J. Ophthalmol. **84:**496, 1977.

Sharpe, J. A., and Glaser, J. S.: Tournay's phenomenon; a reappraisal of anisocoria in lateral gaze, Am. J. Ophthalmol. **77:**250, 1974.

Chapter 15

THE MIDDLE COAT: THE UVEA

The middle coat of the eye, the uvea (L. *uva*, grape), consists of the choroid, the ciliary body, and the iris. The choroid is the vascular layer of the posterior three fifths of the eye that nurtures the adjacent retinal pigment epithelium and the outer portion of the sensory retina. The ciliary body secretes aqueous humor and contains the smooth muscle (N III) that governs accommodation (p. 105). The iris, a diaphragm that rests upon the lens, separates the anterior and posterior chambers of the eye. It contains a central opening, the pupil (Chapter 14), through which aqueous humor passes from the posterior to the anterior chamber; it also contains two muscles, the sphincter pupillae (N III, parasympathetics) and the dilatator pupillae (sympathetics), which regulate the amount of light entering the eye.

The choroid extends from the edge of the optic nerve posteriorly to the ciliary body anteriorly. It consists of the choriocapillaris, an inner layer of specialized, large-diameter (21μ), fenestrated capillaries (Fig. 15-1), which is separated from the retinal pigment epithelium by the lamina basalis choroideae (Bruch membrane, lamina vitrea of light microscopy [obsolete], p. 15). The outer layer of the choroid, which is closest to the sclera, consists of arteries and veins of successively larger diameter that empty into

four vortex veins. The blood supply of the posterior one half of the choroid is derived from 10 to 20 short posterior ciliary arteries, and that of the anterior one half is derived from the long posterior and anterior ciliary arteries. The iris and ciliary body have the same blood supply as the anterior choroid.

The ciliary body (p. 17) is composed of (1) a corona ciliaris, which contains ciliary processes, and (2) an orbicularis ciliaris, or pars plana, a transitional area with the choroid. The ciliary processes secrete the aqueous humor into the posterior chamber.

Located within the ciliary body is the ciliary muscle, divided into well-defined longitudinal and circular muscle fibers and poorly defined radial muscle fibers. Zonular fibers, which do not have contractile properties, connect the equatorial area of the lens with the ciliary muscles. Contraction of the ciliary muscles relaxes the zonule so that the lens becomes more spherical (accommodation).

The iris (p. 20) contains a variable amount of pigment in its anterior stroma. The anterior stroma is absent in some areas, forming iris crypts. The stroma rests upon a layer of pigment epithelium continuous with the retina. It contains the dilatator pupillae muscle on its anterior surface. The sphincter pupillae muscle is located near the pupil in the posterior iris

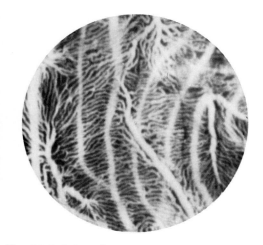

Fig. 15-1. Injected specimen of human choroid showing choriocapillaris and large collecting veins. The choriocapillaris is composed of such large vessels that it resembles vascular sinuses rather than the usual capillaries.

stroma. Both muscles arise from neural ectoderm. The iris is divided into a central pupillary zone (concentric with the pupil) and a peripheral ciliary zone by the collarette, the remnant of the minor vascular circle of the iris. The blood vessels of the iris are arranged in a radial pattern and have a thick adventitia. The blood vessels of the iris and ciliary body (and retina) are not permeable to large molecules (blood-aqueous barrier, p. 113). Additionally, some organic acids are actively transported by the ciliary body epithelium.

SYMPTOMS AND SIGNS OF UVEAL DISEASE

The symptoms and signs vary considerably with the portion of the uvea affected. Abnormalities of the iris may distort the shape of the pupil or may interfere with its dilation and constriction (p. 281). Inflammations of the iris and the ciliary body cause a ciliary type of injection (p. 173). Diseases of the ciliary body and the iris may be associated with se-

vere, deep, boring, dull, aching pain within the eye. Inflammation of the posterior choroid occurs without ciliary injection or pain.

Most local diseases of the ciliary body cause contraction of the ciliary muscle along with disturbed accommodation. Diseases affecting the oculomotor nerve supply result in pupillary dilation and loss of accommodation. Diseases of the choroid often affect the overlying retina and interfere with vision. If choroidal nutrition of the fovea centralis is impaired, abnormalities of visual acuity occur. Peripheral visual field changes follow interference with the extracentral retina. Inflammations of the choroid often extend into the overlying retina, and there is exudation of inflammatory cells and protein into the vitreous cavity along with decreased vision. Ciliary body inflammations release cells and protein into both the vitreous cavity and anterior chamber, whereas iris inflammatory signs are confined to the anterior chamber.

The iris may be examined directly, and the cornea provides magnification for study. The ciliary body can be seen only with a gonioscope (p. 397) after maximal pupillary dilation.

Ophthalmoscopic visualization of choroidal details is usually impaired by the pigment epithelium of the retina, causing the fundus to appear reddish brown. Often a portion of the choroid is visible at the temporal side of the optic disk as a choroidal crescent. In blonde individuals the large veins may be seen. A whitish sclera may be observed between blood vessels that usually belong to the outer vessel layer of the choroid (Haller), which consists of veins that have a considerably larger diameter than the corresponding retinal arteries. Details of the choriocapillaris may be seen with fluorescein angiography, but ophthalmoscopically it consists of a thin sheet of blood that results in the red fundus reflex.

In atrophy of the choriocapillaris, the choroidal veins may be seen as a dense network of whitish vessels (Fig. 15-4).

The pigment of the choroid is more brownish than the jet-black retinal pigment. The choroidal pigment cells do not proliferate in inflammatory irritation as does the retinal pigment epithelium.

The lamina basalis choroideae (Bruch membrane) is composed of the basement membrane of the choriocapillaris, endothelium, an elastic tissue layer sandwiched between two collagen layers, and the basement membrane of the retinal pigment epithelium (p. 15). Deficiencies in the elastic layer cause a variety of fundus abnormalities, such as angioid streaks (p. 345) and rare hereditary diseases (p. 562), and likely precede subretinal neovascularization (p. 345), which underlies a variety of retinal disorders.

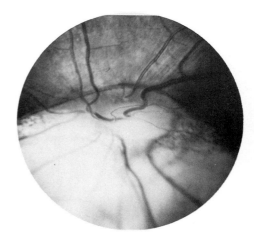

Fig. 15-2. Large coloboma of the inferior choroid. The retinal arteries and veins are present, but the large white area is sclera photographed through the transparent sensory retina, which lacks its normal blood supply for its outer layers.

CONGENITAL AND DEVELOPMENTAL ANOMALIES
Coloboma

Failure of the optic cup (p. 75) to close in the region of the retinal fissure results in a coloboma, absence of uveal tissue in the region. Colobomas involve the inferior nasal quadrant and may extend from the optic nerve to the pupil. The retinal pigment epithelium is missing; the sensory retina is usually present but is transparent, and only its blood vessels can be seen with the ophthalmoscope.

The white sclera is seen ophthalmoscopically at the base of choroidal colobomas (Fig. 15-2). A scleral ectasia may be present. A coloboma of the ciliary body may be associated with a notching defect of the lens corresponding to the deficient zonule in the area. The appearance of a coloboma may be simulated by prenatal retinochoroiditis caused by toxoplasmosis (p. 466). These inflammatory lesions, however, are usually not present in the inferior nasal quadrant, and there is proliferation of the retinal pigment epithelium.

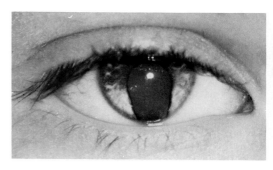

Fig. 15-3. Congenital coloboma of the iris in the characteristic down and slightly nasal position in the region of the site of closure of the fetal fissure.

Typical congenital colobomas of the iris involve the inferior nasal portion and give rise to a defect in the shape of the pupil (Fig. 15-3). The margins of the coloboma show the pupillary frill with pigment epithelium, unlike surgical iridectomies.

Aniridia

Aniridia is a congenital abnormality in which the anterior growth and differentiation of the optic cup fail. It occurs in a hereditary, usually autosomal dominant form and in a sporadic, nonhereditary form. This growth failure results in a rudimentary iris concealed behind the corneoscleral limbus and visible only by gonioscopy. Involvement is usually bilateral but unequal. The corneal region appears black with no iris visible. Photophobia may be present. In the usual phenotype the aniridia is associated with foveal hypoplasia, nystagmus, corneal pannus, and secondary glaucoma. Visual acuity is about 6/60 (20/200) and deteriorates further with corneal opacification and glaucomatous optic atrophy. In a rare phenotype, the iris defect predominates, and visual acuity may be normal. In the third type mental retardation and congenital cataract may be present.

Nonhereditary aniridia may be associated with a variety of systemic disorders: mental retardation, microcephaly, hemihypertrophy, horseshoe kidney, and genital abnormalities (cryptorchidism, hypospadias, and pseudohermaphrodism). A Wilms tumor may develop by the age of 3 years (one in 200 cases of nonhereditary aniridia). Rhabdomyosarcoma, nephroblastoma, adrenal tumors, hepatoblastoma, and gonadoblastoma have also been described, although less often than Wilms tumor.

Provision of an artificial pupil by means of an iris painted on a contact lens reduces photophobia but does not improve vision. Glaucoma often develops in adolescence. The glaucoma responds poorly to surgery and medical treatment.

Choroidal sclerosis (vascular atrophy of the choroid)

These terms describe the fundus changes in which the choroidal vessels are more visible ophthalmoscopically than usual and are combined with abnormalities in caliber and color. Two forms of the disorder are seen: (1) a benign form in myopia and aging (depigmentation in situ), in which there is no functional impairment, and (2) a degenerative form, which may be either generalized or focal, in which functional impairment is severe. In the benign type the sole pathologic change is attenuated pigment in the retinal pigment epithelium. In the degenerative type the choriocapillaris is absent, as are the retinal pigment epithelium and the outer layers of the sensory retina in the affected areas. Actual sclerosis of the choroidal vessels does not occur in either condition.

Benign choroidal sclerosis is seen commonly in simple myopia and less frequently as a change with aging. The choroidal vasculature is conspicuous in the fundus. As in partial albinism, vision and fluorescein angiography are normal.

Degenerative choriocapillary atrophy occurs in a generalized or diffuse form or in a focal form confined to the posterior pole of the eye. The generalized form occurs sporadically (Fig. 15-4) in X chromosome–linked choroideremia (p. 292), in gyrate atrophy, and in hereditary and toxic retinal pigmentary degeneration (p. 353). The focal type (also known as central areolar choroidal sclerosis, central progressive areolar choroidal dystrophy, central choroidal sclerosis) occurs mainly as an autosomal disorder. Central vision is reduced in both types. In the generalized type there is night blindness, loss of the electroretinographic response to light, and a reduced electro-oculography light-dark ratio.

Degenerative choroidal sclerosis begins in the pigment epithelium and is followed shortly thereafter by impaired filling of the lobules of the choriocapillaris and then atrophy. With atrophy, the retinal pigment epithelium together with the adjacent outer retina degenerates, and the major arteries and veins of the choroid become visible. The precapillary arterioles and branches of the short posterior ciliary arteries also atrophy, but to a lesser extent than the choriocapillaris, and, additionally, shunt blood to choroi-

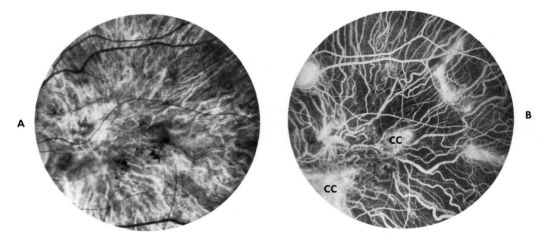

Fig. 15-4. A, Light ophthalmoscopy of choriocapillaris atrophy. The choroidal vessels appear as white lines through the decreased pigment epithelium. **B,** Choroidal circulation in the late phase of fluorescein angiography. There is atrophy of the choriocapillaris, and the choroidal arteries and veins are clearly seen. Some islands of choriocapillaris *(CC)* remain.

dal veins. Loss of retinal capillaries in affected areas is a curious, unexplained abnormality.

Focal choroidal atrophy. The most common type of hereditary atrophy involves the choriocapillaris of the posterior pole and is transmitted as an autosomal dominant or recessive characteristic. This abnormality causes patches of atrophy in the posterior fundus with exposure of the sclera. The time of onset varies with the pedigree. The symptoms may be minimal when the atrophy is confined to the nasal portion of the posterior fundus, or there may be loss of central and color vision when the central retinal region is affected. There is no effective treatment. A similar atrophy occurs in myopia in excess of 6 diopters (pathologic myopia, p. 435).

Choroideremia. Choroideremia is an X chromosome–linked choroidal atrophy with secondary atrophy of the retina, causing night blindness.

In the female carrier, the condition is asymptomatic and is associated with pigmentation and depigmentation of the fundus that is most marked in the equatorial region. The pigment granules have an irregular, square appearance like chunks of coal, and their size is about the diameter of the central retinal artery. Under or adjacent to the clumps of pigment are depigmented areas up to 0.5 disk diameter in size. They may appear paler than the rest of the fundus or have a bright yellow color.

Choroideremia in the homozygous male usually has its onset between the ages of 10 and 13 years. Night blindness, which becomes complete in about 10 years, is the initial symptom. The peripheral field then begins to contract, and finally, after about 35 years, all vision is lost. The earliest fundus lesions resemble the pigmentary changes of the female carriers. Eventually atrophic changes dominate, and the white sclera becomes exposed in the equatorial region. At this time, night blindness occurs and an annular scotoma is present. The atrophy then spreads centrally and peripherally until all vision is lost. The retinal vessels are normal.

Gyrate atrophy of the choroid. This is a progressive, autosomal recessive, diffuse atrophy of the choroid, pigment epithelium, and sensory retina that begins in childhood. There is associated night blindness, myopia, and complicated cataract. The disorder begins at the fundus equator with sharply punched-out oval areas of atrophy that progress until the sclera is seen. The disease progresses toward the central retina, which is preserved until late. Clinically the disorder resembles choroideremia in appearance but involves women as well as men. In the late stages of gyrate atrophy there is fine, velvetlike pigmentation with glittering crystals not seen in choroideremia. Additionally, the central retinal pigmentation conceals the choroid, which is exposed in choroideremia.

The plasma nonprotein amino acid ornithine, an intermediate in the synthesis of arginine, is increased some ten- to twentyfold. As revealed by enzyme studies, skin fibroblasts in patients with gyrate atrophy are deficient in the enzyme ornithine ketoacid aminotransferase. Heterozygotes for the defect have intermediate levels of the enzyme. The ornithine, lysine, and taurine levels are normal in other choroidal atrophies and in pigmentary degenerations of the retina.

Congenital ectropion uveae

The pigmented margin of the pupil marks the anterior border of the secondary optic cup. Rarely, flocculi or cystic dilations of the marginal sinus of the pupillary margin develop into dark brown bodies that may extend on the surface of the iris. They may occasionally break free to appear as movable pigment masses on the iris surface. They have no harmful effects.

Heterochromia iridis

In heterochromia iridis the two irises differ in color. In simple heterochromia iridis there is a relative hypoplasia of the lighter-colored iris combined with a relative hyperplasia of the iris architecture on the side of the darker-colored iris. The abnormality may be transmitted as an autosomal dominant trait or may be associated with displacement of the medial canthi, hypertrophy of the nasal bridge, white forelock, and deafness (Waardenburg-Klein syndrome).

In hypochromic heterochromia the eye with the lighter-colored iris is abnormal. The difference between the two eyes may be extremely slight when both irises are blue. The condition occurs in many different disorders. In Horner syndrome there is paralysis of the sympathetic nerves to the dilatator muscle of the iris (p. 285). In Fuchs heterochromic cyclitis there is a mild inflammation of the iris as well as the ciliary body, often complicated with cataract and sometimes with glaucoma (p. 403). In glaucomatocyclitic crises there is diffuse iris atrophy secondary to inflammation, trauma, and ischemia of the iris. Infiltration of the iris by any nonpigmented tumor causes a hypochromic iridis.

In hyperchromic iridis, the iris on the side of the anomaly or disease is darker than its fellow. The condition occurs with retention of an iron foreign body in the eye (siderosis), with malignant melanoma of the iris, in monocular melanosis in which there are excess chromatophores in the iris stroma, following anterior chamber hemorrhage from any cause, following perforating injuries or contusion of the globe before the age of 10 years, and in association with microcornea.

Iris atrophy

Normally the pupillary zone of the iris is relatively flat because of an absence of the anterior leaf of the stroma (p. 20). The delicate gossamer appearance of the ciliary zone may be lost in conditions in which the blood vessels and fine collagen fibers undergo atrophy and are replaced by a sclerosed network. Hypochromia iridis causes such an atrophy combined

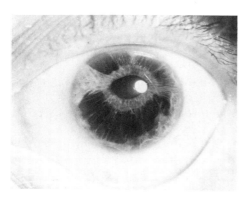

Fig. 15-5. Essential atrophy of the iris with loss of iris stroma below and an opening through the full iris above in a 33-year-old woman. Intraocular pressure is easily controlled by instillation of 2% pilocarpine, but pressure rises precipitously with corneal edema and loss of vision when treatment is omitted.

with a loss of chromatophores; if chromatophores are not lost, the iris appears dull and patternless with the same color as its fellow. Such atrophy may be diffuse or localized. Minor degrees of iris atrophy occur with aging, and the atrophy may be severe after ocular inflammation, trauma, ischemia, and glaucoma. It may follow interruption of the ciliary ganglion and may occur in tabes dorsalis without pupillary abnormalities.

Essential iris atrophy. Essential iris atrophy (Fig. 15-5) is a rare, progressive, usually unilateral disease predominantly affecting women (38.6 years). It is characterized by a distorted, displaced pupil, corneal endothelial degeneration, patchy atrophy of the iris with partial or complete hole formation, peripheral anterior synechiae, and secondary glaucoma. The onset is gradual, and the patient is aware only of a change in shape or position of the pupil. During the next several years holes develop in the iris. Secondary glaucoma then ensues from peripheral anterior synechiae and damage to the trabecular meshwork from a cuticular membrane.

Direct inspection of the iris indicates the loss of iris tissue and migration of the pupil. Treatment is directed toward the secondary glaucoma and is often not effective. Visual loss arises either from corneal edema or secondary glaucoma.

A less severe form of iris atrophy (Chandler syndrome) is associated with an endothelial disturbance and corneal edema combined with multiple small nodules and an ectopic Descemet membrane on the iris surface. Glaucoma eventually may occur secondary to obstruction of outflow by peripheral anterior synechiae. Corneal edema (p. 254) occurs with minor increases in intraocular pressure. Iris nodules appear in the iris stroma as little spheres of tissue. They vary in color from dark brown to yellowish white. Such nodules may be seen in neurofibromatosis, melanomas, iridocorneal dysgenesis, flocculus of the iris, and essential iris atrophy and as inflammatory granuloma. Mesodermal dysgenesis of the cornea and iris (Rieger anomaly) may be associated with dark, wartlike iris nodules located near the pupillary margin.

Secondary iris atrophy. Secondary iris atrophy does not cause the frank holes seen in the essential type. The atrophy may result from anterior uveitis (p. 300), ocular trauma, or herpes zoster. The iris sphincter muscle may atrophy after an attack of angle-closure glaucoma (p. 404). Iris atrophy may be caused by ischemia of the iris secondary to closure of the anterior ciliary arteries or long ciliary arteries that may follow carotid artery insufficiency and lupus erythematosus. Local interference with blood supply may follow retinal detachment operations, freezing or cauterizing of the corneoscleral limbus region, or detachment of three or four recti muscles.

Rubeosis of the iris (rubeosis iridis)

Neovascularization of the iris (Fig. 15-6) occurs as a coarse and irregularly

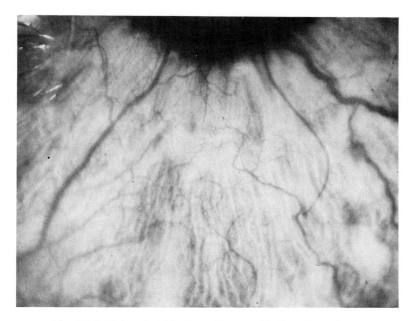

Fig. 15-6. Rubeosis iridis in a 48-year-old diabetic patient.

distributed network of new vessels on the iris surface and stroma or as a fine, markedly tortuous, anastomosed, tightly meshed network on the surface and stroma of the entire iris. The new blood vessels may cover the trabecular meshwork, cause peripheral anterior synechiae, and give rise to an intractable angle-closure type of glaucoma. Hemorrhage into the anterior chamber occurs.

Diabetes mellitus is a frequent cause of rubeosis iridis. The disorder follows central vein closure and, more rarely, central retinal artery closure. It occurs in many abnormalities, such as aortic arch syndrome, carotid artery occlusive disease, carotid artery fistula, giant cell arteritis, anterior ocular segment ischemia, and intraocular tumors, and after ocular radiation and intraocular inflammation presumably because of an iris hypoxia. The neovascularization occurs commonly in eyes blind from the primary disorder.

Relief of the secondary glaucoma by surgical methods may be difficult, and in recent years a number of photocoagulation procedures have been described. Retrobulbar alcohol will relieve pain. Enucleation may be deferred if the eye is not too unsightly and one is assured by ultrasonography that no intraocular tumor is present.

Panphotocoagulation (ablation) of the retina may be followed by involution of rubeosis iridis.

INFLAMMATORY DISORDERS

Inflammation of the uveal tract includes conditions that vary in severity from abscess formation caused by pyogenic bacteria to the evanescent asymptomatic iritis in mumps. Because of their common blood supply, the iris, ciliary body, and anterior choroid tend to be involved to a greater or lesser extent in the same inflammatory process. Inflammations of the posterior choroid, however, unless exceptionally severe, do not involve the anterior uveal tract. Inflammatory reactions are frequently designated as acute, subacute, or chronic. They may also be designated according to the site of the most severe reaction: iritis, cyclitis, iridocyclitis, choroiditis, anterior uveitis, or posterior uveitis.

Inflammations of the choroid often affect the overlying retina, resulting in a loss of vision. Inflammatory cells from the ciliary body may cloud the vitreous, enter the aqueous, and adhere to the cornea (keratic precipitates, KPs). There may be retinal edema with elevation of the central retina. Adhesions between the iris and lens (synechiae) may cause a pupillary block glaucoma (iris bombé). Inflammatory debris in the trabecular meshwork that prevents the outflow of aqueous humor causes an open-angle secondary glaucoma.

Three types of uveal inflammation are seen (Table 15-1): (1) acute suppurative inflammation with a polymorphonuclear leukocyte reaction; (2) acute, subacute, and chronic nonsuppurative inflammation with a predominantly lymphocytic and plasma cell reaction; and (3) chronic nonsuppurative inflammation with an epithelioid cell reaction. After long periods of uveitis the second type may merge into the third. The acute suppura-

tive type involves one or more walls and chambers of the eye and follows an acute fulminating course. The nonsuppurative inflammations with plasma cells and lymphocytes tend to involve the anterior uveal tract, whereas those with an epithelioid cell response may involve the anterior or posterior uvea.

The inflammations may occur because of endogenous or exogenous causes. In exogenous disease the causative agent is introduced from the outside directly into the eye through an opening in the cornea or sclera. Endogenous inflammations arise from systemic disease, from intraocular abnormalities such as hypermature cataract or uveal tissue necrosis, or because of an immunologic response of a previously sensitized area.

In the past, acute inflammation of the iris and ciliary body (iridocyclitis) was classed as a nongranulomatous type of uveitis and chronic inflammation as a granulomatous type of uveitis. Nongranulomatous inflammations were considered to be the result of humoral antigen-antibody reactions. Granulomatous inflammations were thought to be caused by cell-mediated immunity reactions. However, granulomas do not occur in all

Table 15-1. Classification of uveitis

I. Acute suppurative uveitis (polymorphonuclear leukocyte reaction)
  A. Exogenous
  B. Endogenous
II. Acute, subacute, and chronic uveitis with lymphocytic and plasma cell reaction (nongranulomatous)
  A. Exogenous
  B. Endogenous
    1. Without evident systemic disorder
    2. With noninfectious systemic disorder
    3. With infectious systemic disease
    4. Ocular syndromes
III. Chronic uveitis with epithelioid cell reaction (sometimes granulomatous)
  A. Exogenous
  B. Endogenous
    1. Without evident systemic disorder
    2. With noninfectious systemic disorder
    3. With infectious systemic disease
    4. Ocular syndromes

chronic inflammations, even those that have a prominent epithelioid cell reaction. The use of these terms, associated with definite histologic lesions, to describe clinical disease is protested by those who believe they are cumbrous expressions for acute (nongranulomatous) and chronic (granulomatous) uveal inflammation. The present tendency is toward a more precise description of the inflammatory involvement that emphasizes the morphology of the lesion without attempting to classify or to suggest the underlying mechanism of the inflammation.

Suppurative uveitis

Suppurative uveitis is caused mainly by pyogenic (pus-producing) bacteria and rarely by fungi (Table 15-2). In exogenous infection the organisms are introduced into the eye after an accidental or surgical penetrating wound, after rupture of a corneal ulcer, or through a cystic filtering bleb following glaucoma surgery. Endogenous septic emboli may infect the eye in bacterial endocarditis or during the bacteremic stage of meningococcic meningitis. Septicemia may follow surgical procedures performed elsewhere in the body, particularly genitourinary tract operations in the elderly. Common organisms include *Staphylococcus aureus, Bacillus subtilis, Pseudomonas aeruginosa, Proteus,* coliform bacilli, and fungi. The purulent inflammation is classified as either a panophthalmitis involving the vitreous cavity and all coats of the eye including the sclera or an endophthalmitis limited to the intraocular contents.

Panophthalmitis. Panophthalmitis is an acute suppurative inflammation of the inner eye with necrosis of the sclera, and sometimes the cornea, and extension of the inflammation into the orbit. The causes are mainly bacterial. The incubation period is only a few hours, and the disease follows a fulminating course. The eyelids are red and swollen, and there is severe chemosis of the conjunctiva. Extension to the orbit may cause proptosis. The cornea is often a whitish mass of necrotic tissue, and if there has been a laceration or surgical incision, pus exudes from the wound. There may be severe ocular pain, and the globe may rupture. The signs gradually subside, and the eye becomes a shrunken mass of fibrous tissue (phthisis bulbi).

Although it is often not successful, treatment must be prompt and vigorous. Inasmuch as the causative organism and its antibiotic sensitivity are not known until culture, broad-spectrum antibiotics to which penicillinase-producing staphylococci and gram-negative bacteria are sensitive are used systemically, topically, subconjunctivally, and intraocularly. The pus from the wound, the aqueous humor, and the vitreous humor are stained and cultured. Initial treatment is based on the findings of the Gram stain, but in about half of the patients no organism is found. A vitrectomy to remove microbes and leukocytes and passage through a Milli-

---

Table 15-2. Suppurative uveitis

I. Exogenous
   A. Intraocular infection with pus-producing bacteria after accidental or surgical penetrating wound, rupture of corneal ulcer, or microbial invasion of intraocular filtering bleb after glaucoma surgery
II. Endogenous
   A. Septic emboli in bacterial endocarditis, meningococcemia, bacteremia, viremia, and fungemia; septic emboli after urologic surgery
   B. Spread from adjacent structure: orbital abscess, pharyngeal phycomycosis

pore filter may concentrate the organism for staining and culture. Initial antibiotic therapy is modified as necessary on the basis of the cultured characteristics and antibiotic sensitivity of the organism. Systemic corticosteroids may minimize the fibroblastic response to inflammation. Once it is evident that a useful eye will not result, the entire intraocular contents are removed (evisceration).

Endophthalmitis. Endophthalmitis is a suppurative inflammation of the intraocular contents in which not all layers of the globe are affected and in which the eye does not rupture. It follows penetrating wounds of the eye (either surgical or accidental), metastatic infections, or intraocular foreign bodies. The onset is less violent than that of panophthalmitis; the inflammation gradually increases in se-

verity. Fungi, necrosis of intraocular tumors, and retained intraocular foreign bodies often cause a purulent endophthalmitis. Leukocytes may accumulate in the anterior chamber (hypopyon), and the vitreous body may be filled with inflammatory cells. Treatment is the same as for panophthalmitis.

Acute, subacute, or chronic uveitis with lymphocytic and plasma cell reaction

This nonsuppurative, self-limited, often recurrent inflammation of the uveal tract is characterized by edema, capillary dilation, and an exudation of polymorphonuclear leukocytes, which are quickly replaced by lymphocytes and plasma cells. Inflammation of the anterior segment is characterized by acute and severe inflammatory signs with a sudden onset,

Table 15-3. Characteristics of acute and chronic uveitis

	Chronic	Acute
Anterior uvea		
Pain, photophobia	Minimal or absent	Severe
Vision	Gradual reduction	Abrupt reduction
Course	Protracted, remissions, and exacerbations	Self-limited (1-6 weeks), often recurrent
Keratic deposits	Heavy, coalescent, often "mutton fat," crenated margins, macrophages, phagocytized pigment	Pinpoint
Aqueous humor	Few cells, often large, little aqueous flare	Many cells, intense aqueous flare, sometimes protein coagulation
Iris nodules and precipitates	Frequent	None
Posterior uvea		
Retinal and subretinal edema	Usually slight or moderate and localized around exudates	Marked and generalized, with blurring of neuroretinal margins and retinal vascular bed
Choroidal exudates	Heavy massive exudates with edges blurred by surrounding retinal and subretinal edema	No heavy massive exudates, occasionally localized areas of deeper infiltration
Secondary retinal involvement	Almost invariable, with retinal destruction	None or limited to pigment epithelium and rods and cones
Residual organic damage	Heavy glial scars with massive pigment surrounding the lesion	None or fine granular changes in pigment epithelium with damage to neuroepithelium and superficial gliosis
Anterior segment changes	Sometimes mutton-fat keratic deposits	Usually none
Vitreous changes	Usually heavy vitreous blurring; heavy, veillike opacities frequent	Slight to intense general blurring, fine, stringlike, fibrinous opacities

severe symptoms, and a tendency to spontaneous remission. The disease may recur or continue chronically (Table 15-3). Lesions in the choroid are rare and are associated with fine cells in the vitreous body and retinal edema without exudation.

The inflammation may be exogenous or endogenous (Table 15-4). Exogenous causes include ocular contusion, which often produces a transient anterior uveitis or traumatic iridocyclitis, alkali burns of the external eye, noninfected foreign bodies, blood and its degradation products, and necrotic intraocular tissue.

There are numerous endogenous causes. In most instances there is no obvious ocular or systemic cause. Chronic idiopathic uveitis constitutes the most prevalent type of inflammation. Noninfectious systemic disorders ranging from arthritis to atrophic diseases may be associated with uveitis of varying degree of severity. Uveitis with rubella, rubeola, and mumps is usually not diagnosed. Uveitis secondary to ocular syndromes is easily recognized.

Chronic uveitis with epithelioid cell reaction

Chronic uveitis with epithelioid cell reaction (sometimes granulomatous) is a chronic, usually progressive inflammation of the uveal tract in which there is cellular infiltration, chiefly by mononuclear cells, macrophages, and epithe-

Table 15-4. Acute, subacute, or chronic uveitis with lymphocytic and plasma cell reaction

I. Exogenous
  A. Ocular contusion (traumatic iridocyclitis)
  B. Alkali burns
  C. Accidental and surgical penetrating injuries with noncontaminated foreign bodies, blood and its degradation products, necrotic intraocular tissue
II. Endogenous
  A. Without evident systemic disease: chronic idiopathic uveitis (the common type)
  B. With noninfectious systemic disease: rheumatoid arthritis, ankylosing spondylitis, Still disease, Reiter syndrome, Behçet disease, collagen disorders, regional enteritis, atopic disorders
  C. With infectious systemic disease: rubella, rubeola, mumps, herpes simplex, subacute sclerosing panencephalitis
  D. Ocular syndromes: uveal effusion, glaucoma-cyclitis crisis, heterochromic iridocyclitis, pars planitis

Table 15-5. Chronic uveitis with epithelioid cell reaction

I. Exogenous
  A. Foreign body granuloma
II. Endogenous
  A. With infectious systemic or local disease
    1. Bacterial: *Mycobacterium tuberculosis, M. leprae, Treponema, Francisella tularensis*
    2. Fungal: *Blastomyces dermatitidis, Cryptococcus neoformans, Coccidioides immitis,* rhinosporidiosis
    3. Viral: herpes zoster, cytomegalic inclusion disease
    4. Parasitic: *Cysticercus cellulosae, Toxocara canis, Toxoplasma gondii, Trichinella spiralis, Echinococcus granulosus,* schistosomiasis
  B. With noninfectious systemic disease: sarcoidosis, Vogt-Koyanagi-Harada syndrome, familial chronic granulomatous disease of childhood, Chédiak-Higashi syndrome, juvenile xanthogranuloma, relapsing febrile nodular nonsuppurative panniculitis
  C. Ocular syndromes: sympathetic ophthalmia, phacoanaphylactica, granulomatous scleritis, granulomatous reaction to degeneration of Descemet membrane

lioid cells, with tissue necrosis and repair by fibrosis. Involvement of the anterior uvea in granulomatous inflammation is characterized by a torpid, chronic course and minimal signs of infection. "Mutton fat" KPs form, and there is a mild aqueous flare with few cells in the aqueous humor. There is a marked tendency to the formation of posterior synechiae and interference with ocular function.

Chronic uveitis of the posterior eye clouds the vitreous with heavy, veillike opacities. One or more choroidal exudative areas that involve the overlying pigment epithelium of the retina may be present.

Rarely, a retained intraocular foreign body stimulates an epithelioid cell reaction, but mainly only endogenous disease occurs (Table 15-5). The inflammation may be caused by microbes or parasites, or it may occur with a wide variety of noninfectious systemic diseases. There are a number of purely ocular causes.

Symptoms and signs of uveitis

The symptoms of nonsuppurative uveitis vary with the portion of the uveal tract involved. Visual loss is the main symptom of posterior inflammations, whereas anterior uveitis may initially cause pain, photophobia, and lacrimation. Pain is more common in acute iridocyclitis than in chronic iridocyclitis and is particularly severe when associated with keratitis. It centers in the periorbital and ocular region and is aggravated by exposure to light and by pressure on the eye. Photophobia varies in severity and may be so marked that the eyelids cannot be opened to examine the eye. Lacrimation is usually proportionate to the degree of photophobia. Decreased vision arises because of exudation of cells and protein-rich fluid and fibrin into either the anterior chamber or vitreous body or because of involvement of the

overlying retina in posterior uveitis. Inflammation of the choroid beneath the fovea centralis causes an early loss of visual acuity that is often disproportionately severe in comparison with the amount of choroidal involvement. Uveitis adjacent to the disk (Jensen choroiditis juxtapapillaris) may cause a nerve fiber bundle defect (p. 397). Choroidal inflammation that is distant from the posterior pole, although damaging to the overlying retina, may cause only minimal changes in the peripheral visual field. Toxic edema of the posterior pole of the eye along with swelling of the optic disk (papillitis) and central cystoid edema (p. 307) occurs with severe inflammations of both the anterior and posterior uvea and causes decreased vision.

Anterior uveitis. The signs of anterior uveitis include ciliary injection, exudation into the anterior chamber, iris changes, and adhesions between the iris and lens (posterior synechiae).

Ciliary injection. Dilation and congestion of the anterior ciliary arteries that nurture the iris and ciliary body are referred to as ciliary injection. This must be distinguished from conjunctival injection seen in conjunctivitis (see Table 6-2). The severity varies with the degree of inflammation. Little or none occurs in chronic iridocyclitis, whereas in severe acute inflammation there may be associated episcleral and conjunctival injection and conjunctival edema. In less acute inflammation there is a deep circumcorneal injection with a violet hue. The injection fades in the conjunctival fornix and does not bleach when 1:1,000 epinephrine is instilled.

Exudation into the anterior chamber. Inflammation of the iris and ciliary body releases prostaglandins, particularly from the anterior ciliary body, and breaks down the blood-aqueous barrier, so there are increased protein, fibrin, and inflammatory cells in the aqueous humor. The protein gives rise to a translucence of the aqueous humor, called aqueous flare, which can be seen with the biomicroscope. The cells are suspended in the aqueous humor and, because of thermal convection currents, rise when close to the iris and descend at the cooler cornea. Inflammatory cells adhere to the endothelial surface of the cornea, giving rise to keratic precipitates (KPs). Two main types of KPs occur: (1) large, heavy, greasy, fat KPs (mutton-fat KPs) composed of macrophages and phagocytized pigment and (2) small, white, punctate accumulations composed of lymphocytes and plasma cells. Similar cellular accumulations may occur at the pupillary margin (Koeppe nodules), on the surface of the iris (floccules of Busacca), on the lens surface, and in the anterior chamber angle. Occasionally in severe acute iridocyclitis so many cells are present that a hypopyon forms, or rarely diapedesis of erythrocytes causes a hyphema.

Iris changes. In acute iridocyclitis the pupil may be constricted or in middilation. The iris may be edematous with its pattern blurred ("muddy") and the capillaries engorged. In chronic iridocyclitis, nodules may arise from proliferation of the iris pigment epithelium or infiltration of the iris with round cells and macrophages. Rarely, typical granulomatous nodules such as tubercles or sarcoid nodules may be found. These may be followed by a patchy area of iris atrophy. Diffuse iris atrophy with loss of iris pattern follows prolonged iridocyclitis and may involve both the stroma (mesodermal) and pigment (ectodermal) layers.

Posterior synechiae. These adhesions bind the iris to the lens. They cause a small, irregular pupil that does not constrict to light in the area of the adhesions. Sometimes a large clump of iris pigment remains on the anterior lens capsule, a sign pathognomonic of past or present iris inflammation. If posterior synechiae involve the entire pupillary margin, aqueous humor cannot flow from the posterior chamber into the anterior chamber, and the resultant iris bombé causes a secondary pupillary block glaucoma.

Posterior uveitis. The two most important signs of posterior uveitis are vitreous opacities and chorioretinitis (choroiditis).

Vitreous opacities. A variable degree of cloudiness of the vitreous arises in posterior uveitis because of exudation of inflammatory cells and a protein-rich fluid combined with erythrocytes and tissue cells. Vitreous opacities consist of aggregates of cells, coagulated exudate and fibrin, and strands of degenerated vitreous body that are visible with the ophthalmoscope. They appear as black dots against the red background of the fundus or may be so numerous as to make all fundus details indistinct. They are best studied by means of the biomicroscope combined with a concave lens to neutralize the refractive power of the cornea.

Choroiditis. In the acute stage, choroiditis appears ophthalmoscopically as an ill-defined grayish yellow or grayish white area surrounded by the normal colored fundus. The lesions may be single or multiple. The adjacent sensory retina becomes edematous and opaque and is so commonly inflamed that the lesion is described as chorioretinitis. Inflammatory cells and exudate may burst through the Bruch membrane and cause vitreous clouding, which further obscures the ophthalmoscopic details of the lesion.

With healing, the margins of the lesion become more sharply defined and the vitreous clouding clears. If the choroid has been the main site of the lesion, it appears as a whitish yellow area delicately stippled with pigment. When the retina has been destroyed, a whitish patch of scar appears that consists of either a fibrous replacement of retina and choroid or stark, white sclera over which both the retina and choroid have been destroyed. The retinal pigment epithelium proliferates, particularly at the margins of the lesions, and the final ophthalmoscopic appearance is often one of white sclera surrounded by black pigment. Pigment proliferation does not always occur following severe inflammation, presumably because of destruction of the retinal pigment epithelium.

In presumed ocular histoplasmosis (p. 304), subretinal neovascularization beneath the central retina minutely hemorrhages between the Bruch membrane and the retinal pigment epithelium. Ophthalmoscopically there is a deep, dark, grayish, well-defined exudate surrounded by a greenish deposit of subretinal blood. Occasionally the hemorrhage breaks into the sensory retina to form an arc of bright red blood adjacent to the primary lesion.

Diagnosis and etiology

The diagnosis of suppurative uveitis presents no marked difficulties. Acute iridocyclitis presents the signs and symptoms of the red eye (p. 173), and angle-closure glaucoma, keratitis, or conjunctivitis is usually easily excluded. The diagnosis is confirmed by biomicroscopic examination and observation of keratic precipitates, aqueous flare, and cells. Clouding of the vitreous and ophthalmoscopic observation of a chorioretinal inflammatory lesion are diagnostic of posterior uveitis.

The exogenous cause of uveitis is usually evident. The endogenous etiologic factor may be immediately evident when associated with systemic disease, but in many instances it is impossible to demonstrate. The problem of diagnosis is complicated by the inability to secure uveal tissue for study, so that even after effective specific therapy, the cause remains presumptive. In many patients the etiologic factor is diagnosed only by exclusion of other possible causes; in other patients, such as those with arthritis or genitourinary tract disease, one knows only that the uveal tissue is inflamed, as are other portions of the body. Moreover, the uveal inflammation may not be caused by a systemic disease that is present, even if the disease is often associated with uveal inflammation.

Many patients in whom the cause of uveitis is not found have only a single attack; others are seen with chorioretinal scars or anterior segment lesions from asymptomatic inflammations that have occurred previously. In conditions such as heterochromic cyclitis (p. 293) and glaucomatocyclitic crises, no systemic abnormality has ever been found and etiologic studies are usually not emphasized. Virtually every systemic infection may cause uveitis. However, unless there is visual disturbance, attention is often not directed to the eyes.

Local ocular disease with uveitis. A variety of inflammations and diseases primarily involving the eye or its adnexa may be associated with uveitis:

1. Inflammation of adjacent tissues.
    a. Severe infection of the conjunctiva or cornea, which may involve the uvea by direct extension or by entry of the exotoxin into the eye (the infection may be bacterial, viral [often herpes simplex], or fungal). Herpes zoster ophthalmicus (p. 461) is associated with both uveitis and keratitis.
    b. Orbital abscess extending along the vortex veins.
    c. Meningitis extending along the sheaths of the optic nerve.
2. Disease of the lens.
    a. Hypermature cataract with release of toxic polypeptides within the eye.
    b. Endophthalmitis phacoanaphylactica, an autoimmune process in which the eye has become sensitive to its own lens protein. Usually

the sensitization occurs when one lens is removed extracapsularly so that lens protein is retained in the eye and gives rise to antibody production. With extracapsular extraction of the lens in the fellow eye, an antigen-antibody reaction occurs.

   c. Retention of the lens nucleus or particles after extracapsular lens extraction.

3. Trauma.

   a. Sympathetic ophthalmia (p. 191), a rare bilateral granulomatous inflammation that follows a laceration of one eye and possibly constitutes an autosensitization to uveal pigment.

   b. Retained intraocular foreign body.

   c. Contusion damage from blunt trauma.

   d. Chemical injury.

   e. Blood within the eye following trauma or hemorrhagic intraocular disease.

   f. Perforation of the lens.

4. Heterochromic cyclitis (p. 293), a nongranulomatous iridocyclitis occurring in an eye lighter in color than the fellow eye.

5. Blind eyes with degenerative changes. Often these eyes have a chronic uveitis, and a decision must be made as to whether it is worthwhile to retain or enucleate the eye.

6. Necrosis of intraocular tumor. In most instances the cause of the uveitis is obvious. Ultrasonography may be valuable in demonstrating a tumor if the fundus cannot be seen.

The etiologic diagnosis of uveitis is often based on the following:

1. A uveitis of a type associated with a particular systemic disease.

2. A positive focal reaction occurring after the diagnostic or therapeutic administration of an antigen when there is a marked aggravation of the inflammation—a dangerous test that is usually observed inadvertently and is sometimes inaccurate.

3. Exclusion of all other likely causes of the uveitis.

4. Therapeutic improvement with specific medication. Many inflammations are self-limited, and a diagnosis based on improvement with specific medication may be erroneous.

The major conditions considered in the diagnosis of uveitis without obvious cause vary with time and locality. In the United States, tuberculosis and syphilis are no longer major causes. Rather, attention is directed to sarcoidosis, arthritis, genitourinary tract disease, toxoplasmosis, histoplasmosis, and delineation of specific syndromes such as pars planitis.

Sarcoidosis. Sarcoid (p. 471) involves the uveal tract in about 25% of the cases. The disease may excite a minimal inflammatory reaction, and attention is not directed to the eyes. Anterior inflammation is associated with a granulomatous type of inflammation with numerous mutton-fat KPs and a few cells evident by means of biomicroscopy of the anterior chamber. Periphlebitis of veins in the peripheral fundus may occur with neovascularization. The choroidal lesion causes destruction of the overlying retina, and there may be a severe inflammatory reaction with exudation of cells into the vitreous body and the formation of veils and membranes. The lesion shows little tendency to heal, and pigment proliferation is minimal.

Arthritis (p. 464). Patients with ankylosing spondylitis (Marie-Strümpell disease) develop an intermittent nongranulomatous anterior uveitis in 15% of the cases. The ocular disease is never particularly severe and responds readily to local medication. Ocular inflammation may precede joint disease. Young men are mainly affected; often there is a family history of ankylosing spondylitis or rheumatoid arthritis. The involvement of cervical vertebrae often makes it difficult for such a patient to place his head in position for biomicroscopy. However, the lumbosacral spine is initially involved, and the disease may easily escape diagnosis.

Uveitis may occur with juvenile rheumatoid arthritis (Still disease), although band keratopathy is more common. The initial sign of the disease may be uveitis with minimal inflammatory signs that lead, however, to many complications.

Genitourinary tract disease. In the period when focal infection was considered a source of many ocular infections, the genitourinary tract was second in importance to the nasal accessory sinuses and nasopharynx. An occasional patient is seen in whom a chronic prostatitis appears to play a role in uveitis, but such instances are so uncommon that a causal relationship is unlikely. Uveitis may complicate a metastatic gonorrhea (p. 451) in which there is an acute or chronic urethritis followed by arthralgia and ocular inflammation. Even before specific treatment for gonorrhea, such instances were uncommon.

Two uncommon syndromes are related to genitourinary tract disease: (1) Behçet disease and (2) Reiter syndrome.

Behçet disease is a widespread systemic disorder classically associated with aphthous ulceration of the mouth (canker sores) and genital region combined with as iridocyclitis and leukocytes in the anterior chamber (hypopyon). Arthropathy, erythema nodosum with high fever, meningoencephalitis, pyoderma, colitis, and venous thrombosis may occur.

The iridocyclitis may be associated with optic nerve atrophy, decrease in caliber and sheathing of retinal blood vessels, retinal hemorrhages, episcleritis, conjunctivitis, and central serous retinopathy. Blindness occurs about 3 years after the onset of ocular symptoms. Immune suppression with chlorambucil for a period of at least 1 year with treatment continuing for at least 6 months after arrest of the disease has proved helpful.

Reiter syndrome consists of a sterile urethritis, polyarthritis, and ocular involvement of conjunctivitis or iritis. Arthritis may be the earliest sign of the disease. Cutaneous lesions may occur in about 25% of the patients. The cause of the disease is not known, but the histocompatibility antigen, HLA-W27, is found in most patients with the syndrome. The iritis or iridocyclitis may not be diagnosed, and undoubtedly many instances of conjunctivitis reported are examples of ciliary injection secondary to iridocyclitis. The urethritis may be erroneously diagnosed as gonorrheal in origin. The arthritis varies in severity and is migratory. The uveitis is often mild, and diagnosis requires biomicroscopy. The disease is characterized by remissions and recurrences and is refractory to therapy.

Histoplasmosis (p. 457). Histoplasmosis is a fungus infection caused by *Histoplasma capsulatum* endemic in the Mississippi Valley, and it occurs mainly as a subclinical disease demonstrable only by skin hypersensitivity and positive complement fixation. The organism has not been found in the eye except in endophthalmitis, and its role in causing chorioretinal disease is speculative.

Presumed ocular histoplasmosis is initially diagnosed because of loss of vision caused by an elevated central retinal lesion. Recurrent hemorrhage beneath the retinal pigment epithelium is common. Blood sometimes seeps into the sensory retina, giving rise to a dark lesion caused by the deeper blood and a bright red lesion caused by blood in the sensory retina. There are multiple, small, discrete, atrophic areas ("histo spots") of healed chorioretinitis at the equator and a healed chorioretinal inflammation at the disk margin resembling a choroidal crescent. The cellular reaction is minimal.

Peripheral uveitis. Peripheral uveitis (chronic cyclitis, pars planitis) is a chorioretinitis that involves the peripheral fundus with cellular exudation into the vitreous body. It is often bilateral and occurs in the first two decades of life. Periodic exacerbation and remission occur with chronic progression, and there is cystoid central retinal degeneration with loss of vision. Treatment is difficult. In unilateral cases sub-Tenon injections of corticosteroids are used. In cases that do not respond to treatment cryotherapy of the inflamed retina may be helpful.

Immunologic processes and the uvea

An infectious agent is rarely found in nonsuppurative types of uveitis. In many instances it seems likely that either microorganisms or other antigens in the uvea stimulate the accumulation of immunologically competent lymphocytes within the tissue. Further exposure to the same antigen then results in reactivation of these lymphocytes within the eye, causing uveitis. In other instances the eye appears to demonstrate an autoimmune reaction.

The cornea and lens, because of their avascularity, and the retina, because of the blood-retinal barrier, partake minimally in antigen-antibody reactions. However, the choroid, with its fenestrated capillaries, and the highly vascular perilimbal conjunctiva are susceptible to deposition of immune complexes, so that once stimulated, these tissues are able to form antibody in a manner analogous to a regional lymph node. The type of subsequent inflammation depends on whether humoral (B lymphocytes) or cell-mediated (T lymphocytes) lymphocytes are involved.

An ocular antigen-antibody reaction is easily produced in the laboratory and is described as immunogenic uveitis.

It may be produced by inducing either a systemic or an ocular hypersensitivity to an antigen. The antigen selected is usually an animal serum albumin, whole blood, egg albumin, antitoxin, or a similarly well-defined protein. If the animal is sensitized by means of a systemically administered antigen, subsequent injection of the same antigen into the vitreous body causes a severe self-limited uveitis.

If the antigen is injected initially into the vitreous body, there is an immediate inflammatory response, presumably to the trauma of injection, which persists several days and then subsides. A uveitis of several days' duration occurs 7 to 14 days later. This delayed inflammation can be prevented by whole-body x-radiation, but it is not prevented by x-radiation of the eye only. The uveitis is likely caused by the reaction of antibody to antigen that is still retained within the eye. Once the eye is sensitized, ocular or systemic administration of the same protein elicits a violent uveitis.

Diagnostic measures

Previously, an elaborate battery of diagnostic tests was applied to each patient with uveitis not obviously of ocular origin or complicating a readily evident systemic disease. Often such surveys revealed no cause or alternatively so many causes that the findings were not helpful.

Frequently the etiologic factor is not actively sought in self-limited acute inflammations, because they respond readily to corticosteroids. When such inflammations are recurrent, as they often are, attention is usually directed to a possible complement-dependent hypersensitivity and to systemic diseases such as rheumatoid arthritis or infections of the genitourinary tract.

In chronic inflammations the etiologic diagnosis is based on the ophthalmoscopic appearance of the lesions in the diagnosis of toxoplasmosis and histoplasmosis. Sarcoid is sought in black patients. If the inflammation is unusually severe and requires systemic corticosteroids for suppression, the drugs are not discontinued to determine bacterial hypersensitivity by means of skin testing.

In many patients the following diagnostic steps are carried out: (1) the serum fluorescent treponemal antibody absorption test for syphilis is performed; (2) chest roentgenograms are studied, and particular attention is directed to healed primary tuberculosis, sarcoid, and histoplasmosis; (3) leukocyte and eosinophil count and sedimentation rate are determined; (4) tests for immunologic abnormalities occurring in connective tissue disorders are performed; (5) skin testing with tuberculin is done to detect delayed hypersensitivity; (6) indirect fluorescent antibody test for toxoplasmosis is performed; and (7) the complement-fixation test for histoplasmosis is done (prior histoplasmin skin testing may increase the complement-fixation titer).

The medical history and systemic physical examination are often noncontributory. History of exposure to puppies and kittens is important in *Toxocara* infections (p. 468). Physical examination is directed particularly to evidence of infection in the teeth, pharynx, nasal accessory sinuses, and genitourinary tract. In patients with uveitis, elimination of any infection is desirable on a general hygienic basis. Cutaneous and mucous membrane lesions should be sought. Involvement of joints in arthritic lesions should be excluded.

Treatment

If possible, specific treatment is carried out. For inflammation of unknown cause that is confined to the iris and the ciliary body, the pupil is dilated and accommodation paralyzed by topical instillation of 1% atropine solution. Maximal pupillary dilation is desired to prevent posterior synechiae. Corticosteroid preparations are instilled at frequent intervals. Subconjunctival injections may be used. Care must be taken not to induce corticosteroid glaucoma in genetically sensitive individuals (p. 399).

Systemic corticosteroids are the main treatment for posterior uveitis. Retrobulbar or sub-Tenon injection of corticosteroids and, rarely, systemic cytotoxic anti-inflammatory agents may be used. Specific therapy is usually not possible. Early syphilitic inflammations respond readily to antibiotics. Tuberculosis responds to ethambutol and similar agents, but there are few cases in which they are indicated. Antibiotics are not administered empirically.

Complications

The tendency for inflammation of the uveal tract to extend to adjacent tissues leads to many complications. Often the complications dominate the disease picture and may lead to marked loss of vision.

Keratitis and keratopathy. Corneal involvement may occur in several ways. The corneal and anterior uvea may be nearly simultaneously inflamed in herpes zoster ophthalmicus and syphilitic interstitial keratitis. Iridocyclitis, sometimes with hemorrhage, is a late complication of severe herpes simplex keratitis.

Prolonged iridocyclitis damages the corneal endothelium, causing folds, haziness, and stromal and subepithelial edema. Continued edema is followed by vascularization of the cornea.

Band keratopathy (p. 256), in which there is a progressive, superficial deposition of calcium in a horizontal band across the cornea, often complicates uveitis in young persons. It has been described principally in juvenile rheumatoid arthritis (Still disease, p. 565), but it also occurs in older individuals after severe ocular damage. The calcium may be removed with chelating agents (p. 138), but if the cause is not removed, it recurs.

Intraocular pressure. Uveitis causes a hyposecretion of aqueous humor, and the intraocular pressure is usually low. Glaucoma may occur by one of several mechanisms. Topical instillation of corticosteroids in genetically susceptible individuals (p. 399) increases resistance to outflow from the anterior chamber in a manner identical to that in open-angle glaucoma. The trabecular meshwork may be occluded with inflammatory cells and protein in severe acute iridocyclitis or may itself be inflamed. Repeated or prolonged inflammation may damage the trabecular meshwork and lead to a permanent glaucoma similar to open-angle glaucoma.

Pupillary occlusion by posterior synechiae causes an angle-closure glaucoma by preventing the aqueous humor from passing from the posterior to the anterior chamber (iris bombé). Peripheral anterior synechiae may form between the iris and the cornea because of a shallow anterior chamber, exudate between the two structures, or edema of the root of the iris or ciliary body.

The treatment of glaucoma complicating uveitis necessitates a delicate balance between measures directed against the increased intraocular pressure and those used to treat the inflammation. The use of corticosteroids is minimized. The pupil is not constricted. Carbonic anhydrase inhibitors (p. 126) are used systemically and often combined with the local instillation of epinephrine drops. Removal of the anterior aqueous humor by means of keratocentesis provides material for microscopy and microbial culture and temporarily reduces ocular pressure. Sometimes keratocentesis is followed by a decrease in inflammation. In iris bombé, the iris ballooning forward is opened with a knife passed from the corneoscleral limbus (iris transfixation).

Ocular surgical procedures required because of peripheral anterior synechiae or damage to the trabecular meshwork should be postponed as long as possible after cessation of the inflammation.

Cataract. Systemic corticosteroid administration for a long period, particularly in patients with rheumatoid arthritis, may cause posterior subcapsular cataracts identical to those caused by uveitis. The typical cataract in uveitis (complicated cataract) occurs in long-standing cyclitis and involves the posterior subcapsular region in a lens opacity that has many colors (polychromatic). In particularly severe cyclitis the cataract may involve both the anterior and posterior subcapsular regions. Cataract commonly develops when there is an inflammation with a depigmentation of the iris, leading many to believe that this constitutes a specific entity of cyclitis, heterochromia iridis, cataract, and glaucoma.

Cystoid central retinal edema. In this abnormality the capillaries of the central retina become abnormally permeable with edema of the posterior pole. Vision is markedly reduced. A uveitis in the region of the ora serrata (peripheral uveitis, pars planitis, or cyclitis) is only one of the numerous causes (p. 336) of this abnormality. The inflammation can be seen only by means of indirect ophthalmoscopy or biomicroscopy combined with a contact lens. It is therefore not readily diagnosed, and attention is directed to the retinal periphery when unexplained central retinal edema occurs.

Optic nerve edema. Severe choroiditis may cause a papillitis as a toxic phenomenon. In Jensen choroiditis juxtapapillaris (adjacent to the disk), the optic nerve involvement is so marked that the choroiditis may be unrecognized.

Retinal separation. Fibrovascular proliferation after exudation into the vitreous may create vitreous traction bands that detach the sensory retina. Severe effusion from the uveal tract may elevate the retina. Often a similar secondary retinal separation may occur in soft eyes with shallow anterior chambers. This may be called choroidal detachment, although the choroid is firmly attached to the sclera and does not detach.

Two syndromes with chronic bilateral exudative uveitis that occur mainly in middle-aged Orientals are associated with retinal separation. In Vogt-Koyanagi syndrome, predominantly anterior uveitis is associated with vitiligo, alopecia, localized whiteness of the hair (poliosis), and deafness. The prognosis is poor. In Harada syndrome the uveitis is posterior, retinal separation is more common, and meningeal irritation with increased cerebrospinal fluid protein level and pleocytosis occurs. Hearing defects are common, but skin and hair changes are rare. Prognosis is better than in Vogt-Koyanagi syndrome, but the two diseases may be combined.

Chorioretinitis may cause a periphlebitis or localized venous sclerosis in adjacent veins. Peripheral neovascularization similar to that seen in sickle cell disease (p. 552) may occur with secondary retinal separation.

CENTRAL SEROUS CHOROIDOPATHY

The choriocapillaris of the choroid provides the nutrition of the Bruch membrane, the retinal pigment epithelium, and the portion of the sensory retina adjacent. The numerous plasma infoldings at the bases of the pigment epithelium cells suggest an extremely active fluid exchange. The cell junctions suggest a local permeability barrier that limits or prevents fluid from passing between cells.

Fluid accumulates in three main situations: (1) retinal separation (p. 348) or serous detachment of the retina, when there is a massive collection of fluid between the pigment epithelium and sensory retina; (2) inflammations of the

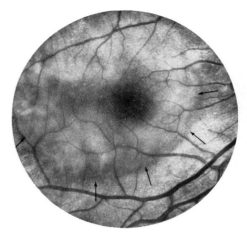

Fig. 15-7. Central serous choroidopathy with elevation of sensory retina in the region of the central retina. Arrows indicate lower border of the elevation. A fluid level is visible just above the foveal region. Small white dots adjacent to the superior blood vessel are residues of chronic edema.

choroid, particularly presumed histoplasmosis (p. 304), in which subretinal neovascularization occurs and serum or blood collects beneath either the pigment epithelium or the sensory retina (hemorrhagic detachment of the central retina); and (3) central serous choroidopathy.

When central serous choroidopathy affects the central retina, vision is disturbed (Fig. 15-7). Many terms are used to describe the condition: central serous retinopathy, central serous choroidosis, serous or hemorrhagic disciform detachment of the central retina, and central angiospastic retinopathy. A similar choroidopathy may affect the peripheral retina, but vision is not affected. As revealed by fluorescein angiography (Fig. 15-8), peripheral choroidopathy often accompanies central serous choroidopathy.

Ophthalmoscopically the fundus lesion is characterized by a circumscribed elevation of the retina or pigment epithelium in the central retinal region. There may be a serous or hemorrhagic extrava-

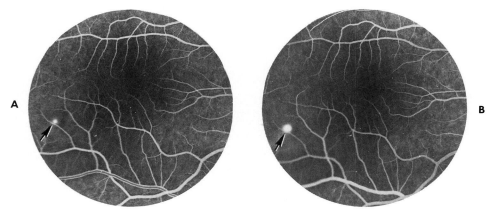

Fig. 15-8. Fluorescein angiograms of peripheral serous choroidopathy. **A,** Early phase with leakage of fluorescein from the choriocapillaris through the retinal pigment epithelium and under the sensory retina *(arrow).* **B,** Late venous phase showing an increased accumulation of fluorescein between the retinal pigment epithelium and the sensory retina.

sation. The lesions tend to remain unchanged for long periods. Histologically there is dilation and stasis in the orbital and vortex veins and their tributaries, and the lesion is suggestive of a widespread hemodynamic disturbance. The lesion may involve the retina only or the choroid only; more commonly, both are involved. There may be active proliferation of the pigment epithelium, producing elevated, pigmented lesions that suggest chorioretinitis. The lesions tend to disappear, leaving a residue of whitish-yellowish deposits deep to the sensory retina or mounds of pigment proliferation. A tumor may be suspected, although hemorrhage and involvement of the posterior pole are both unusual with tumor.

The cause of the reduced vision may be difficult to establish. If a small penlight is directed into the eye for 10 seconds, vision may be reduced one line or more in eyes with serous choroidopathy, whereas eyes with optic nerve disease recover within 30 seconds. Pupillary constriction to light stimulation is prompt in choroidopathy, whereas in optic nerve inflammation an afferent pupillary lesion occurs, and there is slow or absent constriction (p. 286).

An area of leakage in the choriocapillaris may be demonstrated with fluorescein angiography. Prompt photocoagulation of this area may be followed by resolution of the lesion. Usually vision tends to return to normal levels without treatment, but recurrent attacks are often treated.

INJURIES
Contusions

In persons more than 30 years of age blunt trauma is often followed by a severe nonabsorbing intraocular hemorrhage.

Contusion to the eye may cause a variety of injuries: (1) rupture of the sphincter pupillae muscle, with a dilated, unresponsive pupil (iridoplegia); (2) iridodialysis, in which the root of the iris is torn from its insertion, causing an additional opening at the periphery of the iris and the pupil in the sector of the defect to become a chord rather than an arc; (3) hemorrhage into the anterior chamber (hyphema, p. 192); and (4) glaucoma (p. 399).

The ciliary body is seldom visibly involved. However, many hyphemas probably originate from a tearing of the ciliary body from the scleral spur with bleeding from the major arterial circle of the iris. Previous injury to the ciliary body may well be the chief cause of a unilateral glaucoma that appears to be of the open-angle type. Gonioscopy indicates a localized deepening (recession) of the anterior chamber angle.

Hemorrhage into the choroid varies from a small intrachoroidal hemorrhage to a massive expulsive hemorrhage of the type that may occur with intraocular surgery. Bleeding occurring secondary to trauma gives rise to no particular problems of differential diagnosis. When located in the choroid, the hemorrhagic area is dark brown with pinkish to red edges evident in retroillumination. Hemorrhagic areas frequently absorb very slowly over a long period of time and disappear, leaving a residue of marked pigment disturbance.

Choroidal tears (Fig. 15-9) are a common result of severe contusions to the an-terior segment of the eyeball. They occur most frequently on the temporal side of the eye and are concentric with the disk, usually located between the disk and the central retina or temporal to the central retina. They may be single or multiple. They probably result from stretching of the posterior choroid caused by compression of the eye, the temporal side being more vulnerable because of its greater extent and the blow being more commonly directed from the less protected temporal side.

The tears are crescentic, vertical, and of variable length. Hemorrhage into the choroid, the subretinal area, or the retina frequently accompanies a disruption of the tissue. As hemorrhage and edema absorb, the yellowish gray lesions become well defined. When the tear is between the disk and the central retina, vision is usually reduced, and disruption of the overlying sensory retina causes a nerve fiber bundle defect. Tears of the choroid lateral to the fovea may affect vision minimally. Treatment is complete bed rest, instillation of a cycloplegic, and binocular patching of the eyes.

Serous choroidal detachment

Serous choroidal detachment occurs frequently as a complication of intraocular surgery. The disorder occurs after an uncomplicated cataract extraction in which there has been prompt re-formation of the anterior chamber and apparent uncomplicated convalescence. In 5 to 15 days after the procedure the anterior chamber becomes shallow, and there are many folds in the Descemet membrane. The ocular pressure is low, and occasionally aqueous humor leaks from the corneoscleral wound. Through a widely dilated pupil, the detachment of the choroid, visible by oblique illumination, appears as a dark gray-brown mass. As revealed by ophthalmoscopy, the detachment is a smooth, rounded swelling,

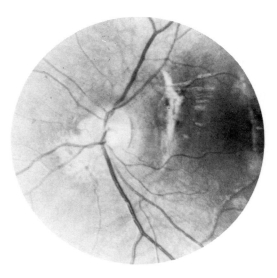

Fig. 15-9. Choroidal tears following blunt trauma to the anterior portion of the eye.

extending hemispherically into the vitreous cavity. The detachment may be single or multiple and usually rises anterior to the equator inferiorly. The borders are dark and well defined. The retinal vessels appear normal as they course over the elevated lesion.

Trauma combined with decreased intraocular pressure (hypotony) is required to produce choroidal detachment. The normal pressure relationships within the choroid are disturbed, producing a transudation of fluid in the suprachoroidal space and resulting in choroidal detachment. The serous choroidal detachment recedes once the wound heals, and the injury from the surgical manipulation subsides. This may occur within several days or, occasionally, weeks. One of the most common reasons for a serous choroidal detachment not receding rapidly is persistence of a small fistula that permits loss of aqueous humor. If this cause can be excluded, the persistence may be caused by hemorrhage. The latter complication may take months to resorb or may persist, owing to organization of blood in the suprachoroidal space.

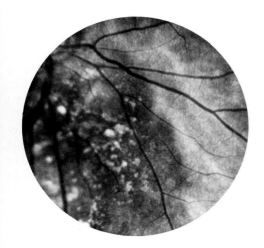

Fig. 15-10. Malignant melanoma of the choroid causing a solid retinal detachment. Numerous drusen are evident over the surface of the tumor.

Lacerations

A laceration of the cornea is followed immediately by prolapse of the iris into the wound. If the wound is small, the pupil is distorted and has a teardrop shape. If extensive, the entire iris may be prolapsed (p. 190).

Prolapse of the ciliary body through a scleral or corneal laceration is particularly serious inasmuch as vitreous humor is lost and the zonule (p. 191) is damaged. Neglected prolapse of the ciliary body is more likely to cause a sympathetic ophthalmia (p. 191) than prolapse of other portions of the uveal tract.

TUMORS OF THE CHOROID
Malignant melanoma

The most common intraocular tumors are malignant melanomas of the choroid (Fig. 15-10). They usually occur after puberty and increase in incidence with advancing age. Rare in blacks, they are slightly more common in men than women. Most malignant melanomas of the uveal tract result from a preexisting benign melanoma, commonly designated as a nevus. (All melanin-bearing tumors primarily arise from cells of the neural crest and have the potential of forming a variety of neuroectodermal and peripheral end organs.) Most benign melanomas never undergo malignant transformation; however, most eyes removed with malignant melanomas contain benign nevi along the edges or within the tumor. Malignant melanomas are found in approximately 10% of eyes blind from injury or inflammation, a finding that suggests that irritation may play a role in malignant transformation.

Malignant melanomas originate most frequently in the outer layers of the choroid and may spread carpetlike between the sclera and lamina basalis choroideae. Tumors may remain quiescent for long periods and then without apparent reason suddenly begin rapid

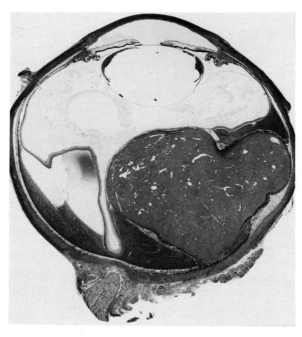

Fig. 15-11. Malignant melanoma of the choroid that has ruptured through the Bruch membrane into the eye. (Hematoxylin and eosin stain; ×5.)

growth. With increase in size (Fig. 15-11), there may be globular growth inward. Eventually the lamina basalis choroideae is perforated, and there is sudden growth of a mushroom or collar-button shape.

Symptoms and signs. The chief symptoms of malignant melanoma result from the secondary retinal detachment caused by the increase in choroidal volume. Early metamorphopsia may be associated with macropsia or micropsia (p. 152). This may be followed by a loss of visual field in the area corresponding to the tumor. The visual field loss characteristically is larger than would be anticipated from the size of the tumor. Glaucoma occurs late in the course of the disease, but in the early stages decreased pressure occurs because of decreased aqueous humor secretion. Intraocular inflammation occurs, and this must be considered in the diagnosis of the cause of any obscure intraocular in-

flammation, particularly when corneal scarring or cataract makes it impossible to inspect the fundus. Ultrasonography and computed tomography aid in the diagnosis of such eyes.

Sudden loss of vision or sudden increase in the size of a mass over several days' time suggests that a lesion is not a malignant melanoma. A drawing of the tumor, with emphasis on its relationship to blood vessels, and photography with fluorescein angiography of the lesion may be helpful in making an exact diagnosis and in following slight increases in size of the tumor. Physical examination should be done to exclude metastatic disease, although the presence of another malignancy does not exclude a primary ocular malignant melanoma. Neovascularization or vasodilation of episcleral vessels in the quadrant of involvement suggests a neoplasm, as does melanosis oculi. A vascularized mass on the sclera suggests an extraocular extension. Anesthesia of the cornea, partial paralysis of the iris, or dilated iris vessels occurring in the sector of tumor involvement have been noted uncommonly.

Ophthalmoscopy indicates a retinal detachment of grayish brown color. The pigmentation is distinctly lighter than the jet-black color seen in inflammatory retinal pigment proliferation. Discrete spots of light orange pigmentation may occur over the detachment. The retina is smoothly elevated, usually without a break, and has little tendency to form traction folds. There may be two areas of detachment, seemingly not connected. With increase in size a malignant melanoma becomes more distinct, but with inflammation the lesion becomes less distinct. Bed rest does not reduce the extent of the detachment in malignant melanoma.

Vessels on the retinal surface not associated with the retinal vasculature are suggestive of tumor. Hemorrhage is uncommon in malignant melanoma. The only exception is in large necrotic tumors that have broken through the Bruch membrane.

Biomicroscopy of the fundus by using a Goldmann or Hruby lens with the pupil fully dilated provides retinal details. Increased retinal thickness suggests a hemangioma. Cystoid degeneration of the overlying retina suggests a malignant melanoma. Conversely, a fine sprinkling of lipidlike deposits in the retina (edema residues) is never present immediately overlying the melanoma. Cells in the vitreous body and an indistinct retina suggest an inflammatory lesion, unless a necrotic tumor has broken through the Bruch membrane. Ophthalmoscopic study of the border of an elevated lesion may show a reddish or pink halo, indicating a hemorrhage rather than a tumor.

Transscleral illumination is of doubtful diagnostic value. It is done by placing a source point of light on the scleral surface behind the lesion and observing the general illumination of the widely dilated pupil. Alternatively, the fundus may be observed with the unilluminated ophthalmoscope. If the lesion is far posterior, it is necessary to incise the conjunctiva to place the light source behind the lesion. Patients may be unable to observe the light when it is at the site of a malignant melanoma because of failure of the rods and cones in a small area overlying the tumor. Marked pigmentation of a normal eye, hemorrhage, and dense inflammatory areas may give rise to faulty interpretation of decreased transillumination. Similarly, small tumors and lightly pigmented neoplasms will not interfere with light transmission.

Visual field studies are valuable in differentiating between a benign and malignant melanoma. Usually the choriocapillaris is intact when a benign melanoma is present; either there is no field defect or the defect is proportionate to the size of the lesion. In malignant melanoma the defect is larger and progressive. Careful visual field testing with a convex lens in front of the patient's eye to compensate for the detachment may demonstrate little, if any, visual field defect. A hemangioma causes a sector-shaped field defect associated with thickening of the retina.

After intravenous injection of sodium fluorescein, most malignant melanomas of the choroid begin to fluoresce slightly before or during the retinal arterial phase. Their fluorescence increases in intensity, and staining of the tumor may persist for 45 to 60 minutes after injection. Metastatic tumors of the choroid and hemangiomas may have a similar hyperfluorescence. Sometimes hemorrhage or pigment overlying a malignant melanoma will prevent visualization of the fluorescence.

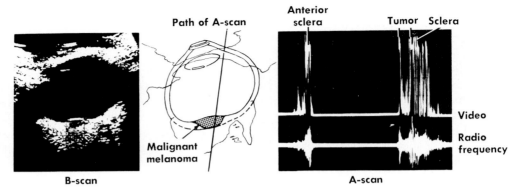

Fig. 15-12. Comparison of the B- and A-scan patterns through a malignant melanoma of the uvea. A malignant melanoma usually provides a high initial echo followed by echoes that are 10% to 40% of the sclera echo. The percentage echo trace is best judged from the radio-frequency trace. (From Coleman, D. J., Lizzi, F. L., and Jack, R. L.: Ultrasonography of the eye and orbit, Philadelphia, 1977, Lea & Febiger.)

Ultrasonography (p. 179) is unusually valuable in the diagnosis of uveal tumors, particularly when an opaque media makes ophthalmoscopic visualization difficult. Generally, the A-scan (Fig. 15-12) suggests the histologic type and the B-scan the size.

Measurement of the uptake of radioactive phosphorus is helpful in the differential diagnosis. Usually measurements are made 48 hours after the administration of the isotope. The lesion is accurately localized and the probe placed directly over it by using a conjunctival incision if necessary. A difference of more than 100% in the number of counts over the tumor and over a normal area of the same eye is considered positive.

Biopsy of an intraocular tumor is rarely indicated and may cause seeding of tumor cells along the needle tract.

The single most important prognostic factor is the size of the tumor. If the largest tumor diameter in contact with the sclera is 10 mm or less (⅔ disk diameters), the mortality is 13%, but if the size exceeds 12 mm, the mortality is 70%.

Thus, in small tumors in which the diagnosis is unclear, procrastination is permissible until the clinical diagnosis is clear.

Treatment. Once the clinical diagnosis has been clearly established, the treatment of malignant melanoma of the choroid is enucleation. If the eye is blind and painful, particularly if the media are opaque, early enucleation is indicated. In eyes with good vision and small tumors, enucleation is not an emergency procedure.

The treatment of a malignant melanoma in the only useful eye is a particular problem. There is obviously no effective therapy for a large, rapidly growing tumor except enucleation. In the case of small, flat, slowly progressive growths, excision is sometimes possible; irradiation by means of radioactive cobalt attached to the sclera, diathermy, or photocoagulation may arrest the growth. For successful results the tumor must be small, and inasmuch as histologic diagnosis is impossible, there is no certainty that the tumor is malignant. Additionally, like malignant melanomas elsewhere in the body, the tumor cells may remain quiescent for long periods and then show renewed activity without known cause.

Chemotherapy with dimethyltriazeno-imidazole (DTIC) is more useful than with other chemotherapeutic agents. The addition of a nonspecific immunopotentiating agent, such as bacillus Calmette-Guérin (BCG), increases the duration of remission and survival.

Benign melanoma

Benign melanomas of the choroid are oval or circular in outline, vary from 0.5 to 4 disk diameters in size, and occur most commonly at the posterior half of the fundus. The lesion is sharply demarcated from the surrounding fundus, but the contrast between the melanoma and the adjacent choroid may be so slight that careful ophthalmoscopic examination is necessary for detection. The lesion usually becomes pigmented between the sixth and tenth years of life.

The tumor varies in color from "slate gray" to "blue ointment." There is no overlying retinal abnormality, and the choroidal pattern can easily be seen surrounding, but not over, the tumor. There may be single or multiple lesions. Since a benign melanoma does not involve the choriocapillaris layer, there is usually no field defect, which is an important distinction from malignant melanoma.

Benign melanomas may become malignant, a change that is recognizable by stippling or irregular pigmentation over the tumor. Increase in size suggests malignancy, and for this reason benign melanomas should be followed by means of serial photographs.

Hemangioma

Hemangiomas (angiomas) of the choroid are a rare condition associated in about half of the cases with skin nevi elsewhere on the body, frequently in the area innervated by the first or second branch of the trigeminal nerve. Secondary open-angle glaucoma may occur. A monocular buphthalmos is associated with either choroidal or retinal hemangiomas. Neurologic signs may occur occasionally; the hemangiomas are then a manifestation of the Sturge-Weber syndrome.

Choroidal hemangiomas may vary in size from 2 to 17 mm in diameter and from 1 to 9 mm in thickness. They may increase slowly in thickness, giving rise to a progressive hyperopia when the hemangioma involves the posterior pole. Rarely, both eyes may be involved in a similar process.

Metastatic carcinoma

The breast is the most common primary site of malignant disease that metastasizes to the choroid. Other structures that may be involved include the lung, kidney, and stomach, and there are reports citing nearly every area and type of malignancy. The complication is fairly common in the terminal stages of a malignant disease; however, patients are often so ill that the diagnosis is not made. The left eye is affected more frequently than the right eye, probably because the left carotid artery is a direct branch of the aorta, whereas the right carotid artery is a branch of the innominate artery. In many cases the disease is bilateral, although further advanced in one eye. Involvement of the choroid in preference to the retina probably reflects the greater number of blood vessels going to the choroid from the ophthalmic artery.

Metastasis to the choroid leads to retinal detachment with loss of vision in the area of involvement. The posterior segment is involved, and early loss of central vision occurs. The ophthalmoscopic appearance is characteristic. There is a sharply circumscribed detachment with abrupt delineation and no retinal breaks. There may be rapid growth of the tumor anteriorly, but usually there is a rim of undetached retina between the tumor and the periphery. The color of the detachment is much lighter than that seen in malignant melanoma.

The diagnosis depends to a large extent on accurate history and physical examination. The primary malignancy may have been removed from months to years before the onset of symptoms. There may be no evidence of metastasis elsewhere in the body, but commonly osteolytic or pulmonary lesions can be demonstrated.

Treatment of a metastatic malignancy to the choroid must be directed to the primary disease. In tumors that are not hormonal dependent, the ocular treatment is related to the life expectancy and whether both eyes are involved. Enucleation is generally not indicated. Radiotherapy with a tumor dose of 2,500 to 3,500 r may be used, with appropriate precautions to protect the lens. However, the adult lens is resistant enough to radiation that cataract formation will probably not be a problem in view of the limited life expectancy of the patient. If the metastasis is binocular and the patient is not within the final weeks of life, radiotherapy may be carried out on both eyes.

CILIARY BODY TUMORS

Tumors of the ciliary body may involve the pigmented or nonpigmented epithelium or the stroma. The epithelium may be involved in a variety of uncommon types of hyperplasia or in a neoplastic process, medulloblastoma. The stromal tumors are essentially the same as those of the choroid, and malignant melanoma is the predominating type. A leiomyoma may arise from muscle cells.

Malignant melanoma

These tumors occur less frequently in the ciliary body than in the choroid. They

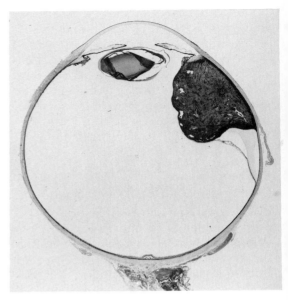

Fig. 15-13. Malignant melanoma of the ciliary body that has detached the peripheral retina. (Hematoxylin and eosin stain; ×4.)

tend to extend to involve either the choroid, the iris, or both. They may spread ringlike around the ciliary body, following the course of the major arterial circle of the iris. Because of their location, symptoms are minimal, and diagnosis may be delayed until the tumor has caused a retinal detachment or has become visible in the anterior chamber (Fig. 15-13). The mass may be demonstrated by transillumination, and by using maximal pupillary dilation, one may observe it directly.

Treatment is often based on the size: large tumors require enucleation, and small tumors are resected. Inasmuch as melanomas of the ciliary body are often benign and have a low degree of malignancy, resection is often good treatment.

Medulloepithelioma (diktyoma)

The nonpigmented epithelium of the ciliary body (pars ciliaris retinae) is derived from the optic vesicle, and the rare

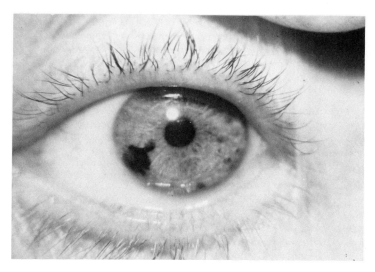

Fig. 15-14. Benign melanoma of the iris. There are freckles in the temporal portion of the iris. Gonioscopy indicates that the benign melanoma does not extend to the insertion of the iris.

tumors that arise in it resemble embryonic retina. Symptoms arise between the third and sixth year secondary to glaucoma, staphyloma, or uveitis. Enucleation is necessary.

Acquired adenocarcinoma of the nonpigmented epithelium was formerly viewed as arising from undifferentiated medullary epithelium. However, these tumors, often an unanticipated finding in eyes removed because of pain or inflammation, are now recognized as arising from fully differentiated ciliary epithelium that has undergone neoplastic changes.

TUMORS OF THE IRIS

There is considerable variation in the amount of pigment in the anterior stroma of the iris. About one half of all whites have pigment flecks on the surface of the iris that are of no pathologic significance. Histologically they belong to the group of benign melanomas. The term *benign melanoma* is preferable but should be limited to slightly elevated, localized pigmented areas extending deep into the stroma. These benign melanomas are not progressive and do not cause pupillary distortion (Fig. 15-14).

Malignant melanoma of the iris often originates from benign melanoma. There are usually no symptoms, and the tumor is "diagnosed" by the patient or a friend who notices the brownish mass on the iris surface. A malignant melanoma is progressive and extends into the anterior chamber angle. It has blood vessels growing in it, and there may be associated seeding of the remaining iris. The pupil is distorted, and this defect is accentuated when the pupil is dilated. In some patients the malignant melanoma is diffuse and causes an increasing pigmentation of the iris with an associated glaucoma. If the tumor is localized and confined to the iris, it may be treated by iridectomy. The tumors rarely metastasize and may be managed with careful observation and local resection; if the tumor is too diffuse, enucleation may be deferred until there is obvious progression.

BIBLIOGRAPHY

Colvard, D. M., Robertson, D. M., and O'Duffy, J. D.: Ocular manifestations of Behçet's disease, Arch. Ophthalmol. **95**:1813, 1977.

Cotlier, E., Rose, M., and Moel, S. A.: Aniridia, cataracts, and Wilms' tumor in monozygous twins, Am. J. Ophthalmol. **86**:129, 1978.

Elsas, F. J., Maumenee, I. H., Kenyon, K. R., and Yoder, F.: Familial aniridia with preserved ocular function, Am. J. Ophthalmol. **83**:718, 1977.

Fraunfelder, F. T., Boozman, F. W. III, Wilson, R. S., and Thomas, A. H.: No-touch technique for intraocular malignant melanomas, Arch. Ophthalmol. **95**:1616, 1977.

Ganley, J. P., and Comstock, G. W.: Benign nevi and malignant melanomas of the choroid, Am. J. Ophthalmol. **76**:19, 1973.

Gass, J. D. M.: Differential diagnosis of intraocular tumors; a stereoscopic presentation, St. Louis, 1974, The C. V. Mosby Co.

Godfrey, W. A., Epstein, W. V., O'Connor, G. R., and others: The use of chlorambucil in intractable idiopathic uveitis, Am. J. Ophthalmol. **78**:415, 1974.

Grant, W. M., and Walton, D. S.: Progressive changes in the angle in congenital aniridia, with development of glaucoma, Am. J. Ophthalmol. **78**:842, 1974.

Hamming, N., and Wilensky, J.: Persistent pupillary membrane associated with aniridia, Am. J. Ophthalmol. **86**:118, 1978.

Henkind, P.: Ocular neovascularization, Am. J. Ophthalmol. **85**:287, 1978.

Hodes, B. L., and Chromokos, E.: Standardized A-scan echographic diagnosis of choroidal malignant melanomas, Arch. Ophthalmol. **95**:593, 1977.

Jampol, L. M., Rosser, M. J., and Sears, M. L.: Unusual aspects of progressive essential iris atrophy, Am. J. Ophthalmol. **77**:353, 1974.

Jocson, V. L.: Microvascular injection studies in rubeosis iridis and neovascular glaucoma, Am. J. Ophthalmol. **83**:508, 1977.

Kaiser-Kupfer, M., Kuwabara, T., and Kupfer, C.: Progressive bilateral essential iris atrophy, Am. J. Ophthalmol. **83**:340, 1977.

Kaiser-Kupfer, M., Valle, D., and Del Valle, L. A.: A specific enzyme defect in gyrate atrophy, Am. J. Ophthalmol. **85**:192, 1978.

L'Esperance, F. A., Jr.: Current diagnosis and management of chorioretinal diseases, St. Louis, 1977, The C. V. Mosby Co.

Little, H. L., Rosenthal, A. R., Dellaporta, A., and Jacobson, D. R.: The effect of pan-retinal photocoagulation on rubeosis iridis, Am. J. Ophthalmol. **81**:804, 1976.

Mamo, J. G.: Treatment of Behçet disease with chlorambucil, Arch. Ophthalmol. **94**:580, 1976.

Ohno, S., Char, D. H., Kimura, S. J., and O'Connor, G. R.: Vogt-Koyanagi-Harada syndrome, Am. J. Ophthalmol. **83**:735, 1977.

O'Rourke, J.: Nuclear ophthalmology; dynamic function studies in intraocular disease, Philadelphia, 1976, W. B. Saunders Co.

Perry, H. D., and Font, R. L.: Clinical and histopathological observations in severe Vogt-Koyanagi-Harada syndrome, Am. J. Ophthalmol. **83**:242, 1977.

Ruiz, R. S., and Howerton, E. E., Jr.: Choroidal melanoma size and accuracy with the radioactive phosphorus test, Am. J. Ophthalmol. **78**:794, 1974.

Scheie, H. G., Yanoff, M., and Kellogg, W. T.: Essential iris atrophy, Arch. Ophthalmol. **94**:1315, 1976.

Schlaegel, T. F., Jr.: Ocular histoplasmosis, New York, 1977, Grune & Stratton, Inc.

Shabo, A. L., and Maxwell, D. S.: Experimental immunogenic proliferative retinopathy in monkeys, Am. J. Ophthalmol. **83**:471, 1977.

Shammas, H. F., and Blodi, F. C.: Prognostic factors in choroidal and ciliary body melanomas, Arch. Ophthalmol. **95**:63, 1977.

Shields, J. A., McDonald, P. R., Leonard, B. C., and Canny, C. L. B.: The diagnosis of uveal malignant melanomas in eyes with opaque media, Am. J. Ophthalmol. **83**:95, 1977.

Shields, M. B., Campbell, D. G., and Simmons, R. J.: The essential iris atrophies, Am. J. Ophthalmol. **85**:749, 1978.

Shields, M. B., Campbell, D. G., Simmons, R. J., and Hutchinson, B. T.: Iris nodules in essential iris atrophy, Arch. Ophthalmol. **94**:406, 1976.

Smith, L. T., and Irvine, A. R.: Diagnostic significance of orange pigment accumulation over choroidal tumors, Am. J. Ophthalmol. **76**:212, 1973.

Smith, R. E., Godfrey, W. A., and Kimura, S. J.: Complications of chronic cyclitis, Am. J. Ophthalmol. **82**:283, 1976.

Chapter 16

THE RETINA

The invagination of the lateral optic vesicles in embryonic life forms the double-walled secondary optic vesicles, or optic cups (p. 71). The inner wall differentiates to form the light-sensitive sensory retina. The outer wall thins to a single layer, the retinal pigment epithelium. The photosensitive pigment molecules located in the disks of the rod and cone outer segments (p. 24) absorb light that passes through the transparent inner portion of the sensory retina (*inner*, nearer the vitreous cavity; *outer*, nearer the choriocapillaris). The light converts 11-*cis*-retinal of the pigment molecule to an all-*trans* configuration. This process initiates a graded potential that is modulated and amplified in the retina and transmitted to the brain as spike discharges (p. 97). Axons of the rods and cones synapse with bipolar and horizontal cells that have their cell bodies in the inner nuclear layer. Bipolar and amacrine cells synapse with each other and with ganglion cells. The axons of ganglion cells are the nerve fiber layer of the sensory retina and pass in the optic nerve to synapse in the lateral geniculate body (visual) or the pretectal region (pupil).

The retinal pigment epithelium lines the outer sensory retina in intimate apposition, with the outer segments enmeshed in the pigment epithelium microvilli. The disks of the outer segments are continuously renewed by their cell bodies, and clumps of the oldest disks are phagocytized by the retinal pigment epithelium. If this phagocytosis stops, the sensory retina degenerates.

The sensory retina may be divided into a central portion (macula) containing the fovea centralis and concerned mainly with form vision and into four peripheral quadrants serving mainly spacial orientation. The central retina, located between the superior and inferior temporal vessels, extends temporally from the optic disk to about 2 disk diameters lateral to the fovea centralis (p. 177). It contains the fovea centralis, a pit in the retina in which the innermost layers of the sensory retina are displaced so that light falls directly upon the cone photoreceptors without transversing the inner retinal layers. This region functions in bright illumination (photopic vision), form vision, and color vision. Rod photoreceptors are most common in the peripheral quadrants and function in dim illumination (scotopic vision).

The blood supply to the retina (p. 58) in humans is derived from two sources: (1) the choriocapillaris, which nurtures the retinal pigment epithelium and the outer portion of the sensory retina adjacent to the choroid, and (2) the branches of the central retinal artery, which supply the innermost half of the retina. Both systems are necessary for retinal function.

The central retinal artery is a medium-sized artery that branches from the ophthalmic artery immediately after its entry into the orbit; consequently, its intravascular pressure is high. The central retinal artery within the optic nerve has the usual three layers of intima, media, and adventitia, with well-developed elastic and muscular components. As the artery passes through the lamina cribrosa, the internal elastic lamina is reduced to a single layer and is entirely lost after the first or second bifurcation. Within the eye the muscle of the medial coat of the arterioles is markedly decreased, although contractile elements persist to the precapillary arterioles.

The retinal arteriovenous crossings share a common adventitial sheath. A similar anatomic arrangement is seen elsewhere only in the afferent and efferent arteries of the glomerulus. The common adventitial sheath is the anatomic cause of some branch retinal vein occlusions and the basis for arteriolar sclerosis at arteriovenous crossings.

SYMPTOMS

The main symptom of retinal abnormalities is visual disturbance without pain. Disorders that predominantly affect peripheral (rod) function are associated with night blindness, impaired vision in reduced illumination, or impaired peripheral vision. Disorders of central (cone) function result in reduced visual acuity and impaired color vision. (Optic nerve disorders that cause symptoms similar to those of cone disease are associated with an impaired pupillary constriction to light.) Opacities of the ocular media that interfere with image formation at the fovea cause a generalized depression of vision. Localized disturbance in the fovea centralis area, such as hemorrhage, edema, deposits, or tumors, may cause micropsia (small images) or macropsia (large images).

Traction upon the retina gives rise to photopsia, which consists of sparks, rings, lightning flashes, or luminous bodies observed when the eyes are closed. Unlike visual hallucinations arising from lesions in the temporal or occipital lobes, photopsia does not involve both eyes simultaneously. Frequently the patient is unaware of retinal disease, and the abnormality is detected by means of functional testing or ophthalmoscopic examination.

FUNCTION

Five main factors determine the function of the sensory retina: (1) visual acuity (the form sense, p. 158), (2) dark adaptation (p. 99), (3) color vision (p. 165), (4) central and peripheral visual fields (p. 161), and (5) electroretinography. The function of the retinal pigment epithelium is inferred from electro-oculography (p. 102).

To exclude refractive errors as a cause of decreased vision, visual acuity must be measured while the patient is wearing corrective lenses suitable for the distance of vision being tested. Measurement of dark adaptation is a sensitive index of the synthesis of photopigments, particularly rhodopsin, in the rods. Color vision testing requires careful interpretation. The common types of hereditary defects in color perception are transmitted as X chromosome–linked recessive defects, and affected individuals have good visual acuity. In most patients with acquired central retinal lesions, such as central retinal degeneration, the defect in color perception parallels the reduction in visual acuity. Some individuals may have marked impairment of color vision, decreased visual acuity, and nystagmus transmitted as an autosomal recessive condition (achromatopsia); others may be born with normal color vision but develop hereditary types of cone degenerations heralded by characteristic impairment in color perception and in the photopic electroretinogram. Parietal lobe disorders may impair color-naming ability and sometimes color perception.

Measurement of the central visual field tests the retinal function with an area of 30° from the fixation point. Measurement of the peripheral field is less sensitive and determines the function of the entire retina. Inasmuch as the optic nerve is composed of axons of the ganglion cell layer that form the nerve fiber layer of the retina, optic nerve disease may cause many of the same symptoms as retinal disease.

Electroretinography measures the action potential evoked by light stimulation of the retina. Because this is a mass response, it may be normal when retinal lesions are focal.

Electro-oculography measures the standing potential between the cornea and the retina. A decrease in the ratio between the response in the light- and dark-adapted retina indicates a disorder of the retinal pigment epithelium.

OPHTHALMOSCOPIC FINDINGS

The retina is examined with a direct or indirect ophthalmoscope or with a biomicroscope and a concave lens to neutralize corneal refraction (p. 174).

The main ophthalmoscopic abnormalities of the retina include the following: (1) disturbances of the blood vessels (p. 543); (2) opacities of the sensory retina varying from hemorrhage to exudates to edema residues, cotton-wool patches, and glial and fibrous tissue proliferation; (3) disturbances in the position of the sensory retina in primary and secondary retinal separation; (4) derangements of the retinal pigment epithelium; and (5) abnormalities of the Bruch membrane.

Disturbances of blood vessels

The skilled observer constantly changes the focus of the direct ophthalmoscope to better define the size, shape, and depth of lesions. One knows that the major retinal vessels are located in the nerve fiber layer and that capillary plexuses are in this layer and the inner nuclear layer. Occlusive disease of the blood vessels affects mainly the inner layers of the retina. New blood vessel formation arises on the inner (vitreal) surface of the retina and the surface of the optic nerve. Other disorders arise from neovascularization of the choriocapillaris, spreading a fibrovascular network beneath the retinal pigment epithelium or between the retinal pigment epithelium and the sensory retina.

The retinal blood vessels are normally transparent tubes through which the contained blood is visible with an ophthalmoscope. The oxygenated blood in the artery is brighter red than in the veins, and the medial coat of the artery reflects light and causes a white reflex paralleling the axis of the vessel. Inasmuch as retinal vessels lack direct nervous innervation, their constriction and dilation are based on autoregulation (intravascular resistance-pressure and P_{CO_2}). The endothelial cells lining the retinal vessels are non-fenestrated and tightly joined, so that such vessels provide a blood-retinal barrier similar to the blood-brain barrier. The retinal blood vessels are susceptible to the same diseases as blood vessels elsewhere in the body; but because their intravascular pressure must exceed the intraocular pressure to prevent collapse, they form a highly specialized vascular bed without counterpart elsewhere. Thus, changes observed ophthalmoscopically (p. 174) must be extrapolated with considerable caution from similar changes in blood vessels of comparable size elsewhere in the vascular tree.

Vascular pulsation. Visible pulsation of arteries or veins occurs when the intraocular pressure equals the pressure within the vessel. The normal pulsation of the central retinal vein is best seen on the surface of the optic disk. It is synchronous with the heart, and it arises from transmitted central retinal artery pulsation. If the venous pulsation cannot be detected, gentle pressure upon the globe will elicit it. Venous pulsation is absent and cannot be elicited in impending central vein closure, and it usually cannot be elicited in papilledema.

Spontaneous arterial pulsation is always pathologic. It occurs when the intraocular pressure is equal to the diastolic blood pressure and in aortic regurgitation, in which there is a high pulse pressure. It may be elicited by pressure on the globe as is done diagnostically in ophthalmo-dynamometry (p. 530).

Venous dilation. Increased venous pressure or markedly decreased intraocular pressure causes dilated veins. Tortuosity increases, because the vessel wall widens in three dimensions. Thus, dilated veins are visible in diabetes mellitus at any stage, in papilledema, in impending closure of the central retinal vein, in vascular tumors of the retinal blood vessels, and in hyperviscosity blood syndromes.

Neovascularization. New blood vessels arise on the inner surface of the retina, on the surface of the optic disk, between the choriocapillaris and the retinal pigment epithelium, or between the retinal pigment epithelium and the sensory retina.

Neovascularization of the retina is seen in a variety of conditions in which the circulation is impaired; stasis is caused by hyperviscosity of the blood or decreased blood flow, vascular occlusion (particularly venous closure), sickle cell trait, inflammation, sarcoidosis, diabetes mellitus, and retinopathy of prematurity. The first arteriovenous crossing in the superior temporal quadrant is the most vulnerable area, followed in turn by the inferior temporal quadrant, the superior nasal quadrant, and the inferior nasal quadrant. In conditions associated with retinal neovascularization, preexisting vascular channels located within the sensory retina may dilate, with far more vascular channels evident than is usual (microangiopathy). New blood vessels may creep along the inner surface of the retina. They may grow into the vitreous as delicate, weblike, endothelial channels (rete mirabile) or with supporting fibrous tissue (proliferative retinopathy, see Fig. 25-7).

Subretinal neovascularization affects the central retinal region particularly and is a common denominator in presumed ocular histoplasmosis (p. 304), Kuhnt-Junius disease (p. 346), degenerative myopia, and other central retinal degenerations. The vessels originate from the choriocapillaris and may lie between the lamina vitrea and the retinal pigment epithelium or between the retinal pigment epithelium and the sensory retina. Occasionally, large subretinal vessels surrounded by hyperpigmentation may be seen on ophthalmoscopy. Hemorrhage occurs in about two thirds of the instances of subretinal neovascularization and is often crescent shaped at the outer edge of the neovascularization. The stimulus to new blood vessel formation is uncertain. Presumably, defects in the Bruch membrane permit blood vessels to grow beneath the retinal pigment epithelium. Loss of adhesion between retinal epithelial cells permits new blood vessels to grow between these cells and the photoreceptors. Serous detachment of the pigment epithelium may precede the neovascularization.

Retinal neovascularization requires a diseased retina combined with a disturbed vascular bed; new vessels form predominantly from veins. The stimulus is presumably a diffusable factor, because new vessels may be stimulated to form on the optic disk and iris. The vitreous humor also contains a factor that normally inhibits neovascularization. The vessels consist of fenestrated endothelial tubes that leak protein and tend to bleed. Some neovascularization is reversible and may disappear when the stimulus disappears or after retinal photocoagulation.

Hemorrhage. Hemorrhages within the retina assume different shapes, depending on the layer in which they occur. Preretinal hemorrhages (Fig. 16-1) occur between the retina and the vitreous body. They are characteristically large with a tendency to meniscus formation because the blood is not clotted and is only loosely restricted. Flame-shaped hemorrhages occur at the level of the nerve fiber layer and tend to parallel the course of the nerve fibers in the region of the retina where they occur. Round hemorrhages originate from the deep capillaries of the retina, and they are confined by Müller cells and the axons of the inner and outer plexiform layers (p. 29). Hemorrhages in the sensory layer of the retina have a bright red color and tend to absorb slowly. Hemorrhage between the pigment epithelium and the Bruch membrane is dark colored, well circumscribed, elevated, and may simulate a neoplasm.

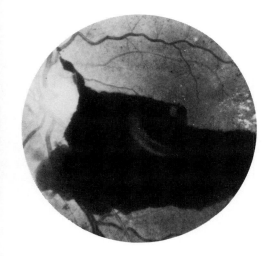

Fig. 16-1. Preretinal hemorrhages surrounding the optic disk in diabetes mellitus. Additionally, the veins are dilated.

Retinal and subhyaloid (preretinal) hemorrhages occur in 20% to 40% of the adults and almost 70% of the young children with subarachnoid hemorrhage. The mortality in individuals with intraocular hemorrhages exceeds 50%, as contrasted with a mortality of about 20% in those without such hemorrhages. Mortality is higher in those with bilateral intraocular hemorrhages (58%) as contrasted with those with uniocular hemorrhage (48%). Usually the hemorrhages absorb without sequelae. However, when they break into the vitreous, they result in the same complications as other intravitreal bleeding.

Retinal hemorrhages occur because of an abnormality between the blood pressure within a vessel and the ocular pressure surrounding it, because of abnormalities of the blood vessel wall, or because of diseases of the blood. Ocular causes include trauma, vascular obstruction, and vasculitis. Systemic causes include diabetes mellitus, arteriosclerosis, hypertension, and blood dyscrasias. A preretinal hemorrhage adjacent to the optic disk may be a sign of subarachnoid hemorrhage.

Microaneurysms. Microaneurysms constitute a common retinal abnormality. Large numbers form in diabetes mellitus (see Fig. 25-5), and these are characteristically on the venous side of the capillary network. Microaneurysms may be seen in most of the conditions associated with retinal venous stasis—central or branch vein obstruction, Coats disease, periphlebitis, and hyperviscosity of the blood. Microaneurysms can be identified with certainty by fluorescein angiography or histologic examination. Ophthalmoscopically they appear as minute red dots of unchanging appearance that are unrelated to visible blood vessels. They seem to remain for months but are eventually converted to minute white dots. Small, deep, round hemorrhages with similar appearance absorb more rapidly and disappear without leaving a residue. Although microaneurysms occur in many conditions, it is only in diabetes mellitus that large numbers occur predominantly at the posterior pole.

The resolving power of the direct ophthalmoscope is about 75μ. The majority of retinal microaneurysms are smaller than this and are invisible ophthalmoscopically, but they may be demonstrated by fluorescein angiography or histologically in flat preparations of the retina.

Capillary perfusion. Fluorescein angiography indicates that poor retinal function in vascular closure and diabetic retinopathy is secondary to inadequate perfusion of the retinal capillaries (see Fig. 25-5). Although with light ophthalmoscopy the areas appear no different than that surrounding, fluorescein angiography indicates patchy areas in which the capillaries do not fill with fluorescein.

The various abnormalities causing decreased capillary perfusion are discussed in several different sections: carotid artery occlusive disease (p. 529); ophthalmic artery occlusive disease; ischemic neuropathy of the optic nerve (p. 372); vascular stasis in glaucoma (p. 397); blood disorders such as leukemia (p. 556), polycythemia (p. 555), hemoglobinopathies (p. 552), hemorrhage, and plasma cell dyscrasias (p. 555); vascular inflammations (p. 336); diabetes (p. 511); and vascular hypertension (p. 549).

Opacities of the sensory retina

The sensory retina is ophthalmoscopically transparent with a red background caused by blood in the choriocapillaris more or less obscured by the pigment in the retinal pigment epithelium. Hemorrhages, exudates, cotton-wool patches, edema, microaneurysms, and tissue proliferation in the sensory retina cause generalized or localized loss of transparency and disappearance of the normal reddish fundus reflex.

Exudates in the retina are opacities resulting from inflammation. Such areas may be obscured by inflammatory cells in the vitreous. They are usually dirty white with ill-defined margins. The underlying retinal pigment epithelium and choroid are often destroyed, and the cells of the retinal pigment epithelium eventually proliferate.

Deposit is the term usually applied to opacities arising from localized areas of retinal edema. In chronic edema, these deposits are sharply defined (hard) and may be the site of lipid deposition, which gives them a bright yellow color (Fig. 16-2). In acute edema caused by acute focal ischemia, the opacities appear whitish or silvery with ill-defined margins (cotton-wool patches, p. 325), and these constitute intracellular accumulation of cellular organelles. Microscopically, they are termed cytoid bodies.

Chronic edema that involves the outer plexiform layer of the retina in the posterior pole surrounding the fovea centralis may cause deposits of a more or less complete arcuate or circular shape that sur-

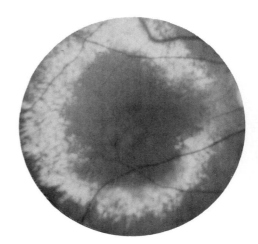

Fig. 16-2. Circinate pattern of chronic edema residues in a 59-year-old woman.

rounds the pathologic region (Fig. 16-2). This ring probably marks the location at which normal retinal capillaries collect serous fluid that leaks from abnormal capillaries. Such a circinate figure may be seen in diabetes mellitus, vascular hypertension, and other retinopathies. Chronic edema residues in the outer plexiform layer of the fovea centralis (Henle layer) form broken lines radiating from the uninvolved fovea centralis. Such a star-shaped figure is seen in severe vascular hypertension, papilledema, and papillitis.

Cystoid central retinal edema (p. 336) arises from a variety of conditions that cause abnormal permeability of the capillaries surrounding the fovea centralis. The retina appears slightly raised and white; the loss of vision directs most attention to the condition. However, fluorescein angiography provides a typical picture with spokes radiating from the fovea centralis.

Cotton-wool patches (cytoid bodies). Cotton-wool patches appear ophthalmoscopically as indistinct, white retinal

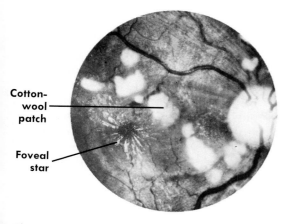

opacities with a hazy, irregular outline ("soft" exudates) (Fig. 16-3). They are usually ovoid in shape, about one third of a disk diameter in size, few in number, and are mainly seen in the posterior segment. They arise in the nerve fiber layer of the retina as a result of capillary infarction. Cotton-wool patches occur in the retina during the course of severe arterial hypertension, following retinal trauma, and in severe anemia, papilledema, diabetic retinopathy, generalized carcinomatosis, acute systemic lupus erythematosus, and dermatomyositis.

Microscopically, cotton-wool patches occur in ganglion cell axons. They consist of an accumulation of cell organelles and may reflect failure of axonal transport. Similar change in the central nervous system is known as wallerian degeneration.

Scarring. Retinal scarring results from proliferation of three retinal elements: (1) glia from Müller cells, (2) mesodermal tissue from blood vessel walls, and (3) retinal pigment epithelium. Glial proliferation causes a diffuse, white, usually well-defined retinal opacity that may become so extensive as to resemble a neoplasm. Connective tissue is usually diffuse and coarse. The retinal pigment epithelium causes a jet-black pigmented area that surrounds areas of retinal destruction (see Fig. 16-11).

Disturbances in the position of the sensory retina

The sensory retina normally lines the globe smoothly without elevation or distortion. In retinoschisis, cleavage of the sensory retina into two layers separates the layer of rods and cones and the outer nuclear and plexiform layers from the inner layers of the retina and the internal limiting membrane.

In retinal detachment or separation serous fluid or blood accumulates between the sensory retina and the retinal

Cotton-wool patch

Foveal star

Fig. 16-3. Foveal star of edema in the plexiform layer of the retina (Henle layer), which delimits the foveola. The cotton-wool patches are in the nerve fiber layer. These changes occurred in a 39-year-old man with accelerated vascular hypertension.

pigment epithelium. Inasmuch as the outer retinal layers no longer receive adequate nutrition from the choriocapillaris, vision is impaired in the region of the abnormality. The entire sensory retina or a localized portion may be involved. The involved retina has a diminished red reflex, and the arteries and veins appear to have similar oxygenation.

In detachments of the retinal pigment epithelium there is serous fluid or blood between the pigment epithelium and the Bruch membrane along with local elevation of the retina in the area.

Derangements of the retinal pigment epithelium

The retinal pigment epithelium obscures the view of the choriocapillaris, and the amount of melanin in its cells largely determines the degree of redness of the normal ocular fundus (p. 175). A decrease in pigmentation occurs in aging and myopia and in atrophy of the choriocapillaris (see Fig. 15-4). The choroidal blood vessels are seen with striking clarity, and if the choroid is lightly pigmented, the white sclera may be seen. In destructive inflammatory lesions involving both the choroid and the retina, all retinal and choroidal layers may be destroyed so that the dead-white sclera is visible. Proliferation of the retinal pigment epithelium is stimulated in inflammatory processes, with resultant deep black pigmentation that commonly surrounds an area of chorioretinitis. In tapetoretinal degenerations the pigment often has a central nucleus with dendrites and is most marked at the equator. Degenerative disease at the fovea may also be associated with pigment proliferation.

Abnormalities of the Bruch membrane (lamina basalis choroideae)

The Bruch membrane (p. 15) separates the choriocapillaris from the retinal pigment epithelium. It is derived from both.

The main abnormality recognized ophthalmoscopically is angioid streaks (p. 345) in which breaks occur in its elastic tissue portion. Disciform degeneration of the central retina (Kuhnt-Junius disease, p. 346) arises because of abnormalities in the Bruch membrane permitting new blood vessels to invade the sensory retina from the choriocapillaris layer of the choroid.

CONGENITAL AND DEVELOPMENTAL ABNORMALITIES

Myelinated nerve fibers. Myelination of the optic nerve is completed shortly after birth. Sometimes the process does not stop at the lamina cribrosa but extends a short distance over the retinal surface (see Fig. 18-3).

Additionally, the nerve fiber layer in the peripheral retina may be myelinated (Fig. 16-4). The involved area is translucent, with the blood vessels visible beneath a thin, stark white opacity that is more dense nearer the disk and follows the distribution of the nerve fiber layer. The visual field is normal; once formed, there is no progression.

Melanosis of the retina. Melanosis of the retina, or grouped pigmentation, is a rare nonfamilial, nonprogressive retinal abnormality characterized by small grayish to black spots scattered throughout the fundus or limited to a single quadrant. They vary in size and sometimes are grouped aggregations that resemble animal footprints ("bear tracks") on the surface of the retina. They are composed of densely pigmented accumulations of cells from the retinal pigment epithelium that have migrated to the region normally occupied by photoreceptors that have failed to develop. There are no symptoms, although minute visual field defects may be demonstrated in these areas.

Retinal dysplasia. Retinal dysplasia is a congenital, sometimes hereditary, often bilateral retinal abnormality character-

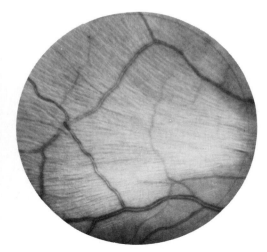

Fig. 16-4. Medullation of the nerve fiber layer of the peripheral retina.

ized by outer nuclear retinal cells at various stages of differentiation, arranged in a palisading or radiating pattern surrounding a central ocular space. The eye is often microphthalmic with a shallow anterior chamber. The retina forms tubes, and one-, two-, or three-layer rosettes form that are suggestive of a detached mature retina that has been thrown into folds.

The condition may occur because of separation of the sensory retina from the adjacent retinal pigment epithelium during a critical stage of its differentiation. Retinal dysplasia is associated with a variety of disorders: trisomy 13-15 and other chromosomal abnormalities, congenital retinal folds, Norrie disease, colobomas or cysts, and cyclopia. A small blind eye with a white mass in the pupil characterizes the condition.

Pseudoglioma (pseudoretinoblastoma) and leukocoria are obsolete terms used to describe eyes with a white pupil not resulting from a cataract. The causes include retinal dysplasia, persistent hyperplastic primary vitreous (p. 360), retinopathy of prematurity (p. 328), Coats disease (p. 328), retinoblastoma (p. 353), toxocaral endophthal-mitis (p. 469), and Norrie disease (p. 490).

Phakomatoses. This is a group of conditions in which there are congenital, disseminated, usually benign tumors of blood vessels or neural tissues (disseminated hamartomas). There are often ocular, cutaneous, and intracranial tumors. A variety of conditions are included: (1) neurofibromatosis (von Recklinghausen), (2) tuberous sclerosis (Bourneville-Pringle), (3) encephalofacial angiomatosis (Sturge-Weber-Dimitri), (4) angiomatosis retinae (von Hippel), (5) angiomatosis retinae with cerebellar hemangioblastoma (von Hippel-Lindau), (6) ataxia telangiectasia (Louis-Bar), and (7) encephalo-ocular arteriovenous shunts (Wyburn-Mason).

Neurofibromatosis is an irregular autosomal disorder with multiple tumors derived from glial cells of the central nervous system and Schwann cells of peripheral nerves. Cutaneous neurofibromatosis gives rise to widespread café au lait spots. Orbital tumors occur, sometimes with glaucoma, and about 10% of the patients with gliomas of the optic nerve have neurofibromatosis. Glial hamartomas may involve the brain, meninges, or spinal cord. Glial hamartomas (astrocytomas) of the retina and optic disk appear as hemispheres placed against a refractile, white, slightly uneven base.

Tuberous sclerosis is a heredofamilial disorder with the diagnostic triad of mental retardation (about one half), adenoma sebaceum (angiofibroma), and seizures. Retina glial hamartomas are smooth, translucent or semitransparent, flat lesions that develop into elevated, nodular, calcified masses with a tapioca-like appearance. Computed tomography demonstrates more intracranial lesions than does conventional roentgenography. Giant drusen (astrocytic hamartomas) of the optic nerve may occur.

Encephalofacial angiomatosis is a congenital, nonhereditary disorder in which there is a nevus flammeus (port-wine stain) along the distribution of the trigeminal nerve, a cavernous hemangioma of the choroid causing glaucoma, and hemangioma of the meninges on the same side often associated with intracranial calcification. Focal seizures and mental retardation are common.

Angiomatosis retinae is an autosomal dominant disorder with retinal hemangioblastoma involving one or both eyes. Similar tumors may occur in the cerebellum and spinal cord, and cysts of the kidney and pancreas may occur. Ophthalmoscopic examination reveals a reddish, slightly elevated tumor about the size of the optic disk or smaller that is nourished by a large artery and vein. Coagulation of the tumor by means of photocoagulation or transscleral diathermy prevents formation of hemorrhages and deposits and a secondary glaucoma.

Ataxia telangiectasia is an autosomal recessive disorder with cerebellar ataxia, nystagmus, and conjunctival and skin telangiectasis. There is reduced or absent IgA and IgE, and there is IgM in the serum. The alpha-fetoprotein of the serum, which usually reaches a peak concentration at about the thirteenth week of gestation, is elevated. There are widespread immunologic defects related mainly to T-lymphocyte functions. The conjunctival telangiectasia appears as a group of dilated blood vessels on the bulbar conjunctiva.

Encephalo-ocular arteriovenous shunts are a familial abnormality with an absence of capillaries between arteries and veins giving rise to aneurysms and angiomas in the retina, midbrain, and face. There may be ocular muscle paralysis, pulsating exophthalmos, and intracranial calcification.

Coats disease. Coats disease is a chronic, progressive retinal abnormality characterized by retinal exudates and usually associated with malformation of retinal blood vessels. It begins in youth (average age is 16 years), involves boys predominantly, and is usually unilateral, but when both eyes are involved one is affected more severely than the other.

The main symptom is decrease in central or peripheral vision. In the very young, attention may be directed to the abnormality because of a white mass behind the lens, suggesting a retinoblastoma, which may lead to enucleation. Pathologic examination indicates initial rod and cone degeneration followed by exudates, extensive detachment, and neofibrovascularization.

Ophthalmoscopic examination reveals yellowish white exudative patches beneath retinal blood vessels. These wax and wane and may disappear in one area while occurring in another. Subretinal hemorrhages are frequent and are usually associated with numerous glistening cholesterol deposits. The retinal vessels may have a tortuous course, aneurysms, fusiform dilatations, loops, and glomerulus-like formations. Hemorrhage into the vitreous body may occur with subsequent development of proliferative retinopathy. Eventually there may be detachment of the entire retina, iritis, cataract, and glaucoma.

Treatment is frequently ineffective, but early photocoagulation appears to be of limited usefulness.

Retinopathy of prematurity. The retinopathy of prematurity, or retrolental fibroplasia, is a bilateral, primary abnormality of retinal vascularization. It occurs almost exclusively in premature infants who have a birth weight of less than 1,500 grams and who have been subjected to a high oxygen environment during the first 10 days of life.

The human retina is avascular until the fourth gestational month, when vessels begin at the optic nerve and extend toward the ora serrata. The nasal periphery is vascularized by the eighth month, but the process is completed in the temporal periphery only after full-term birth. During the period of incomplete vascularization, the retinal vessels respond to excess oxygen (and to other factors) by vasoconstriction and obliteration, leading to suppression of the normal retinal vascularization. Thereafter, even though exposed to normal oxygen levels, the vessels dilate and become tortuous, and there is proliferation of the remaining capillaries with new blood vessels growing into the vitreous. The sensory retina detaches with retinal and vitreous hemorrhages. In the most severe form, the retrolental space is filled with fibrous tissues and the eye is blind.

The ocular fundi of premature infants may be studied with the indirect ophthalmoscope after topical application of 2½% phenylephrine and 0.5% cyclopentolate. The eyelids are separated with an infant speculum, and particular attention is directed to the retinal periphery, using scleral depression if necessary.

The normal premature retina has arteries and veins that branch at 30° to 60° and decrease in caliber as the retina passes from vascular to avascular regions. In the earliest stage of retinopathy there is a proliferation of primitive vascular tissue and an abundance of small, dilated venules with branches for the most part at the junction of the vascular and avascular retina. The condition may gradually involve arborization of both arterioles and venules with an abrupt, rather than gradual, junction between the vascular and avascular retina, especially in the temporal fundus. Usually during the next 11 to 16 weeks, spontaneous resolution permits normal retinal vascularization, and the vessels form their normal 30° to 60° branches.

If the condition progresses, a ridge forms between the two retinal zones, the terminal arborization becomes engorged, and new capillaries extend into the vitreous as polyps or plaques. The arterioles and venules of the posterior retina become dilated and tortuous. This usually recovers by 20 to 23 weeks or may progress.

In the fully developed condition the diagnosis is evident. The eyes are small and sunken, with faded, fetal, grayish blue irises. A white mass presses against the lens, and frequently glaucoma develops accompanied by tearing and corneal edema but without ocular enlargement. The infant will often sit, rocking back and forth and grinding his eyes with his fists.

Incomplete retrolental fibroplasia may be associated with gradual ocular deterioration in adolescence. Visual acuity may be reduced, and macular pigmentation and esotropia occur. Myopia is common. The minimal scarring in the peripheral retina may give rise to retinal separation requiring surgical correction.

The idiopathic respiratory distress syndrome affects some 10% of all infants weighing less than 2,500 grams at birth. High concentrations of oxygen are required for several days after birth. The cardiac and pulmonary deficiencies may disappear at any time, but the high oxygen concentration of the arterial blood causes retinal damage.

The retinopathy of prematurity does not reflect poor, dangerous, or inept medical care. Rather, it reflects essential care for an often fatal condition. Pediatricians and parents must weigh the risk of treatment and ocular involvement.

The ocular status of the premature infant should be evaluated when oxygen treatment is no longer required. The purpose of the ocular examination is to learn the presence or absence of ocular disease and to advise the parents. If there are signs of retinopathy, the infant should be reexamined at 3 months to learn if it has progressed. Thereafter, the child should be examined every 3 months for the first 2 years, every 4 months for the next 2 years, every 6 months for the next 3 years, and then annually. In all infants, oxygen must be administered only when hypoxia necessitates it, and the oxygen should be terminated, reduced, or used intermittently as early as the general condition permits. Photocoagulation of the ridge between the avascular and vascular retina may be beneficial.

VASCULAR DISORDERS

In humans, capillaries derived from branches of the central retinal artery nurture the inner layers of the sensory retina. There are capillaries at the level of the nerve fiber layer and in the inner nuclear layer. Interference with blood flow through these capillaries results in decrease or failure of retinal perfusion and loss of function in the affected portion of the retina. Normal perfusion necessitates a blood pressure in the central retinal artery in excess of the intraocular pressure and patency of the retinal vessels and capillaries.

Retinal vein occlusion

Occlusive disease of the retinal veins is a local circulatory disturbance characterized by retinal edema, hemorrhage, and engorgement of the venous tree. It may involve the central retinal vein (Fig. 16-5) or its branches. Branch retinal vein occlusion may occur near the optic disk and involve a major quadrant of the retina, or it may occur at peripheral crossing of the artery and vein. The rapidity of onset and the severity of symptoms vary with the portion of the retina affected. Occlusion of the central retinal vein may cause complete loss of vision, whereas occlusion of a nasal branch (rare) of the central retinal vein may be asymptomatic, as may be an occlusion of the portion of the temporal vein lateral to the fovea centralis. The pathogenesis is complex. If capillary perfusion is not impaired, vision often returns to normal. If arteriolar perfusion is

impaired or if there is actual arteriolar insufficiency and retinal ischemia, permanent retinal changes occur. Ophthalmoscopically, retinal hemorrhages, retinal edema, and sometimes cotton-wool patches are seen. The involved vein is dilated and tortuous and may appear segmented. Fluorescein angiography may show diffuse staining and leakage from the involved venous and arterial trees. As the hemorrhage clears, one may see areas of nonperfusion surrounded by microaneurysms, intraretinal microvascular abnormalities, and new blood vessel formation. Cystoid central retinal edema may be seen (p. 336).

Three basic occlusive mechanisms are usually described. First, external compression of the vein arises (1) from an atherosclerotic process affecting the central retinal artery adjacent to the central vein, (2) from a connective tissue strand within the floor of the physiologic excavation, or (3) from the cribriform plate. On

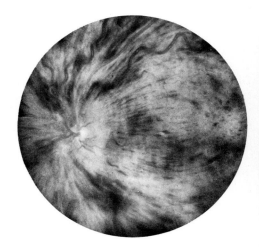

Fig. 16-5. Occlusion of the central vein of the retina. The old term "retinal apoplexy" is highly descriptive. Disk margins and arteries are blurred by retinal edema. Veins are dilated. There are retinal hemorrhages that parallel the distribution of the nerve fiber layer of the retina in the central retinal area.

the retinal surface, occlusion is favored by multiple crossings of the same artery or vein or congenital loops or twists of the vein in some patients. The initial event may be a transient occlusion of the retinal artery with the vein being involved because of the surrounding retinal edema combined with a low intravenous perfusion pressure. Second, occlusion from venous stasis reduces vascular perfusion pressure, causing collapse of the vein. Causes of stasis include glaucoma, spasm in the corresponding retinal artery arteriole, blood dyscrasias, increased viscosity of the blood, sudden reduction of systemic blood pressure, cardiac decompensation, surgical or traumatic shock, therapy for arterial hypertension, and carotid occlusive disease. Glaucoma must be excluded as a cause of venous occlusion in every patient. Retinal phlebitis causes stasis with venous occlusion, particularly in youthful patients. Third, degenerative disease of the venous endothelium causes intravascular detachment, proliferation, and hydrops. This occurs in severe systemic disease, such as arterial hypertension, cardiac decompensation, and diabetes mellitus. A similar mechanism may result from inflammation of the optic nerve or from systemic granulomatous disease.

The pathologic changes are dominated by hemorrhage, retinal edema, neovascularization, and glaucoma. There is secondary destruction of the retina, which is replaced with fibrous tissue. Some affected eyes ultimately require removal because of neovascularization of the iris (rubeosis iridis, p. 294), which causes a painful, hemorrhagic glaucoma.

The main symptom is painless loss of vision, which either involves all function or corresponds to the affected retinal sector. Transient decrease of vision occurs frequently before complete occlusion. This decrease is never as complete as that in carotid-basilar occlusive disease. Visu-

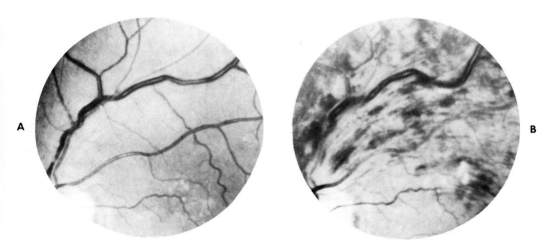

Fig. 16-6. Retinal branch vein closure in a 70-year-old woman. **A,** When the woman was 66 years old the superior temporal vein was found to have multiple arteriovenous crossings with notching and peripheral dilation. There were a few drusen inferiorly. **B,** Four years later a branch vein occlusion occurred with flame-shaped hemorrhages and deposits; vision was reduced to 6/18 (20/60).

al loss with frank venous occlusion does not occur suddenly, as in retinal artery closure, but develops over a period of several hours. Vision tends to remain poor or to deteriorate after occlusion.

Ophthalmoscopic examination indicates engorgement of the venous tree (Fig. 16-6), or portions of it, associated with edema of the corresponding sector of the optic disk and the retina along involved tributaries. Physiologic pulsation of the involved vein is absent and cannot be elicited by pressure upon the eye.

When complete occlusion takes place, the involved retina is splashed with numerous superficial and deep hemorrhages. The disk may be covered with hemorrhages, which may break into the vitreous body. The veins are enlarged, engorged, tortuous, and dark blue. Segments may be hidden beneath edematous retina. Cotton-wool patches are numerous. Fluorescein angiography shows marked leakage of the dye at the site of the occlusion.

In branch vein closure the superior temporal quadrant is the most common site, and the next most common site is the inferior temporal quadrant. The closure is often at an arteriovenous crossing.

After branch vein closure, hemorrhages and exudates tend to reabsorb, and most visual improvement may occur within 6 to 7 months of the initial episode. Improvement of vision depends on the adequacy of the circulation, and the prognosis is poorest when perfusion through the accompanying artery is impaired. In branch vein closures that do not affect the venous tributaries of the central retina there is a fairly good prospect of improved vision. Inasmuch as the causative mechanism is difficult to influence, the long-term prognosis for vision and life must be guarded. Often there is neovascularization on the surface of the optic disk, and the veins are narrowed and obscured by white streaks (parallel sheathing [Fig. 16-7]).

In branch vein occlusion, dilated and tortuous collateral vessels may course across the central retina and the median raphe from normal to abnormal retina. The capillaries are dilated, and they leak plasma. Surface neovascularization occurs, and there may be proliferative retinopathy and vitreous bleeding. The leakage of plasma from capillaries causes central retinal edema with reduced vision even after the absorption of the hemorrhage.

The main differential diagnosis includes those conditions causing dilation and tortuosity of retinal veins in the prodromal stage and the same vascular signs associated with hemorrhage after frank occlusion has occurred. The best diagnostic sign is the absence of spontaneous or induced venous pulsation in occlusion. Those conditions that may cause venous dilation include diabetes mellitus, blood dyscrasias (particularly those with associated increased blood viscosity), congenital tortuosity of retinal vessels, arteriovenous aneurysms of the retina, angiomas of the retina, papille-

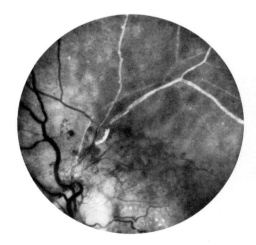

Fig. 16-7. Parallel sheathing of superior temporal vessels of the left eye after combined artery and vein occlusion. There is neovascularization on the surface of the optic disk together with hemorrhages and chronic edema residues.

dema, and congenital heart disease. Retinal hemorrhages are rarely as marked in any other condition as in vein closure.

Treatment is directed toward (1) removal of the underlying cause if possible, (2) use of anticoagulant drugs to permit collateral venous channels to develop, (3) recognition and treatment of preexisting glaucoma, and (4) photocoagulation of the retina.

The main causes of retinal vein occlusion that can be specifically treated include granulomatous infection, particularly tuberculosis and syphilis. Sudden reduction of blood pressure in individuals with advanced arterial disease should be avoided as much as possible.

Anticoagulation is usually carried out with bishydroxycoumarin (Dicumarol) or a related drug combined with careful observation of the prothrombin level, which is usually maintained at about the 10% to 20% level. Anticoagulation is generally contraindicated in occlusion secondary to venous inflammation. Best results are obtained when therapy is carried out in patients who are in good health, have only a mild degree of retinal atherosclerosis, and have had a sudden onset of occlusion suggestive of a stagnation factor. Impending occlusion is the chief indication for anticoagulation. Patients and physicians must be on the alert for transient diminution of vision and signs of venous engorgement, particularly if one eye has been lost from a venous occlusion. Anticoagulation may have to be continued indefinitely. Venous occlusion during therapy suggests failure to maintain the prothrombin level in a therapeutic range. Primary glaucoma must always be excluded as the cause.

In branch vein closure in which vision is reduced because of central retinal edema, destruction of hypoxic retina by means of xenon photocoagulation causes atrophy of the collateral supplying the hypoxic retina and decreased capillary leakage with absorption of the central retinal edema and improvement of vision. Photocoagulation in central retinal vein occlusion may prevent the development of rubeosis iridis but does not benefit vision. A problem in all therapy is the inability to correct the underlying vascular defect. Recurrence of the closure or involvement of other veins is a constant threat.

I sometimes empirically prescribe 300 mg of aspirin daily to reduce platelet adhesiveness. Glaucoma must be vigorously treated when present. Even when glaucoma is not present, I sometimes prescribe instillation of 2% pilocarpine twice daily in the affected eye or systemic acetazolamide (Diamox). Controlled studies have not been done.

Hyperviscosity syndromes. Extreme hyperviscosity of the blood gives rise to an ophthalmoscopic picture of venous dilation and tortuosity, hemorrhages, microaneurysms, exudates, and papilledema. The condition resembles an impending venous closure and may cause frank occlusion. The blood serum causes include macroglobulinemia, hyperglobulinemia, and cryoglobulinemia, whereas the blood cell causes are leukemia and polycythemia. A similar picture occurs in stasis retinopathy (p. 530) secondary to carotid artery occlusive disease.

Retinal artery occlusion

Occlusion of the central retinal artery (Fig. 16-8) causes sudden, painless loss of vision. Occlusion of a branch causes a defect in the field of vision corresponding to the branch affected. The main causes of central retinal artery occlusion are emboli from atherosclerotic plaques in older patients or from valvular heart disease in younger individuals and thrombosis with arteriosclerotic heart disease (Table 16-1). Branch artery occlusions are usually caused by emboli. Other conditions that cause arterial occlusion include atheroma formation complicated by subintimal hemorrhage, vascular spasm, and

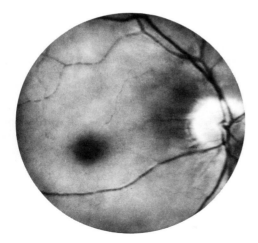

Fig. 16-8. Central retinal artery occlusion in a 19-year-old woman with mitral heart disease. Vision was suddenly lost 24 hours earlier. The sensory retina is edematous, and the choroidal circulation is visible at the foveola, causing a cherry-red spot. The blood column is segmented ("box cars") in the superior temporal artery.

Table 16-1. Causes of central retinal artery occlusion

   I. Cardiac disease
     A. Valvular
       1. Mitral stenosis or regurgitation
       2. Aortic stenosis
     B. Atrial myxoma
  II. Carotid artery disease
     A. Atherosclerosis
 III. Systemic vascular disease
     A. Hypertension
     B. Atherosclerosis
     C. Giant cell arteritis
 IV. Increased blood coagulation
  V. Systemic disease
     A. Sickle cell
     B. Syphilis
     C. Diabetes

---

a dissecting aneurysm of the central retinal artery. Arterial emboli may develop in patients with chronic rheumatic valvulitis (particularly mitral stenosis) and in myocardial infarction with mural thrombi. Vasospasm is secondary to arteritis in the

elderly or to vasomotor instability in younger individuals.

Embolic disease causes a sudden, complete loss of vision without premonitory symptoms. Vasospastic disease is usually preceded by repeated transient episodes of decreased vision or blindness in the affected eye (amaurosis fugax), and finally there is an attack in which vision does not return. The symptom of unilateral periodic blindness must be differentiated from the vascular spasm in internal carotid-basilar occlusive disease (p. 530), in which ophthalmodynamometry indicates a decreased pressure. Visual loss in carotid occlusive disease is seldom permanent or complete, even though the carotid artery is completely occluded, provided the central retinal artery is patent.

In central retinal artery occlusion, on ophthalmoscopic examination the inner layers of the sensory retina are opaque and white because of edema. Inasmuch as the inner layers are absent at the fovea, it stands out conspicuously as a cherry-red spot. The retinal arteries appear as thin red threads. The blood column may be segmented so that there are segments with blood interspersed with empty segments. On fluorescein angiography, the artery fills with the dye after a delay, but the dye does not perfuse the retinal capillaries (p. 324). After a week, the retina resumes its normal ophthalmoscopic appearance. The arteries, however, may remain as thin lines that, in time, develop parallel sheathing and appear as white threads. The optic nerve becomes atrophic and appears dead-white against the normally red fundus background.

Occlusion of the arterial blood supply causes an ischemia with cloudy swelling of the inner layers of the retina supplied by the artery or its branches. This is followed by autolysis and macrophages loaded with fat granules. In the final stages the inner retinal layers are replaced with glial tissue, which rests upon the outer nuclear layer.

The prognosis is related to the cause, the degree of obstruction, and the length of time the occlusion has persisted. Relief within 1 hour may restore all vision, whereas relief within 3 or 4 hours may restore peripheral vision with a persistent defect of central vision. After this period has elapsed, the visual defect is likely to be permanent.

Treatment is directed toward relief of vasospasm or an attempt to dislodge an embolus to a more peripheral and smaller vessel. Immediate intermittent massage of the globe is indicated. Moderate pressure is applied to the globe for a period of 5 seconds, then suddenly released for 5 seconds, and then repeated. Respiration of 5% carbon dioxide and 95% oxygen for 10 minutes each hour may be helpful. Stellate ganglion block with procaine or lidocaine (Xylocaine) may be helpful, as may retrobulbar injection with the same drugs or with acetylcholine, tolazoline, or papaverine. Anticoagulants may be helpful in the early stage of occlusion, and intravenous heparin is the drug of choice.

Transient emboli of the retinal arteries may arise from atherosclerotic occlusive disease of the carotid arteries (p. 529) or from diseased heart valves. The emboli are of two main types: cholesterol ester flakes from atheromatous ulcers in the carotid artery (see Fig. 27-1) or platelet-fibrin aggregates from thrombi in the carotid artery or the heart. The embolus causes a transient loss of vision corresponding to the branch in which it lodges. Attacks caused by platelet emboli are brief and frequent and often involve the same vessel. There is no residual abnormality in the retinal blood vessel. Those caused by cholesterol emboli are more variable both in severity and frequence. They may be associated with a lasting field defect and visible emboli in the retinal blood vessels.

Patients with retinal artery occlusion require careful evaluation of the cardiovascular system, especially the carotid arteries (auscultation for bruits, palpation of facial pulses, ophthalmoscopy for emboli, ophthalmodynamometry, and angiography when suggested by previous findings). Systemic diseases include those associated with atherosclerotic cardiovascular disease and with hypertension. In addition to hematologic and systemic disease studies, patients less than 40 years of age require echocardiogram or cardiac catheterization, or both, to screen for atrial myxoma.

Retinal vasculitis

Retinal vasculitis is primarily limited to veins. The most frequent cause is extension of an adjacent chorioretinitis. Other causes include necrotizing angiitis (p. 339), multiple sclerosis (p. 538), tuberculosis, sarcoidosis, syphilis, Behçet disease, and cytomegalic inclusion disease. The capillaries of the central retina may be inflamed in a number of conditions and cause a cystoid central retinal edema with the reduced vision.

Retinal arteriolitis may occur spontaneously or in cases of necrotizing angiitis. Inflammation of both arteries and veins leads to localized thrombus formation followed by neovascularization.

Retinal phlebitis. Phlebitis may rarely involve the central vein. It has the appearance of a papillitis. If it occurs in a major branch, the appearance is that of a branch vein closure, which clears spontaneously. Vaso-obliterative vasculitis may occur in peripheral retinal veins.

Eales disease is a nonspecific peripheral periphlebitis that mainly affects men between the ages of 15 and 30 years. It is characterized by recurrent retinal hemorrhage adjacent to the involved veins and by vitreous hemorrhage. Both eyes are involved in about one half of the cases. The cause is not known, but the condition may result from a nonspecific reaction to various antigens. The chief symptom is loss of vision caused by vitreous hemorrhage. Although this hemorrhage tends to absorb rapidly, repeated hemorrhages result in vascularization of the vitreous body, chronic uveitis, and glaucoma.

Ophthalmoscopic examination indicates segmental, dilated, beaded, occluded veins, with sheathing or exudation, and blood in the vitreous body and the retina.

Occlusion of the affected vessels by means of photocoagulation is remarkably effective in preventing progression. Photocoagulation may have to be repeated.

Retinal arteriolitis. Arteriolitis is less common than phlebitis. In segmental retinal periarteritis, discrete white plaques are deposited along the walls of retinal arterioles. The retinal arteries in retinal arteriolitis become dilated and tortuous. The dark blood column in the vessel indicates a slow flow, which in turn is followed by retinal neovascularization.

Cystoid central retinal edema

This is a condition of the sensory retina in which the capillary bed in and surrounding the fovea centralis becomes abnormally permeable and leaks fluid into the retina. The fluid accumulates in the outer plexiform layer, which in this region courses tangentially to the retinal surface, and gives rise to swelling and cystlike spaces. Vision is reduced often to 6/60 (20/200), but ophthalmoscopic signs are minimal, although flame-shaped hemorrhages may be present. However, fluorescein angiography demonstrates leakage of the dye from the perifoveal capillaries and accumulation within the retina. In the late stages this causes a wheellike pattern with the fluorescein in

Table 16-2. Cystoid central retinal edema caused by leakage from the perifoveal capillary bed of the retina*

Retinal vascular disorders
Diabetic retinopathy
Hypertensive retinopathy, severe
Central retinal vein obstruction
Retinal branch vein obstruction
Retinal telangiectasis
Radiation retinopathy
Intraocular inflammation
Pars planitis
Behçet disease
Acute nongranulomatous iridocyclitis
Acute recurrent (nodular) cyclitis
Sarcoidosis
Nematode endophthalmitis
Degenerations
Preretinal fibrosis
Retinitis pigmentosa
Senile "vitreitis"
After ocular surgery
Cataract extraction
Penetrating keratoplasty
Retinal reattachment
Glaucoma filtering procedure
Pars plana vitrectomy

*A partial list of ocular conditions. (Modified from Michels, R. F., and Maumenee, A. E.: Am. J. Ophthalmol. **80:**379, 1975.)

a circle surrounding a fluorescein-free area that marks the floor of the foveola where the plexiform layer is absent.

There are many causes. Originally the disorder was described as following cataract extraction (40% to 60%), particularly with vitreous adherent to the wound edges (Irvine-Gass syndrome). However, the lesion is nonspecific and occurs with a variety of retinal vascular abnormalities, degeneration, and intraocular inflammations as well as ocular surgery (Table 16-2).

Treatment is not effective, but the condition is often self-limited with spontaneous improvement. Topical epinephrine in aphakic eyes may cause the edema, which is reversible with discontinuation of the medication.

Shunt vessels between choroidal and vascular circulation

Anastomoses between the retinal and choroidal vascular beds are relatively common and consist mainly of capillaries. Large, anomalous shunt vessels that cause retinal blood to be drained into the choroidal circulation on the surface of the disk occur fairly commonly in occlusive retinal venous disease, in glaucomatous optic atrophy, in retinal proliferative vascular syndromes, and, occasionally, congenitally. When there is interference with the venous outflow in the optic nerve just behind the globe, convoluted dilated channels of preexisting capillaries develop on the surface of the disk. These occur with optic nerve gliomas, chronic atrophic papilledema, orbital cysts, and orbital meningiomas. The triad of shunt vessels, disk pallor, and loss of vision occurring in women is highly suggestive of an intraobital meningioma. The outlook for retained vision is poor.

RETINAL INFLAMMATIONS

The retina may be inflamed in exogenous and endogenous inflammations of the vitreous body, choroid, or retinal vessels. The main cause is an inflammatory lesion in the adjacent choroid causing a chorioretinitis (p. 298). Inflammation of the sensory retina leads to an exudation of cells into the vitreous body, and if marked, this may cause diffraction of light and interference with vision. Inflammations affecting the posterior pole disturb the fovea centralis and visual acuity. Ophthalmoscopically, in the acute stage the inflamed area appears yellowish white with ill-defined borders. With healing, a purely retinal inflammation may expose the underlying choroidal vascular bed, and ophthalmoscopically there are regions of brighter red than the surrounding fundus crossed by relatively large choroidal veins.

The retinal pigment epithelium proliferates in chorioretinitis, and on destruction of the choroid and retina the exposed white sclera is surrounded by deep black pigment. The choroidal pigment does not proliferate.

Retinal infection occurs in the compromised host because of protozoa, viruses, and fungi not recognized previously as infecting the retina. The inflammatory response varies with the degree of immunosuppression, and the disease may terminate spontaneously with healing and pigment proliferation. Often death from septicemia occurs in the course of the retinitis.

Rubella. Fetal rubella (p. 464) involves predominantly the retinal pigment epithelium and causes a slight disturbance in the melanin distribution. Ophthalmoscopically, there are discrete areas of pigmentation and depigmentation (Fig. 16-9). The electroretinogram (p. 103) is of limited value, since it may be normal, subnormal, or extinguished. The retinopathy does not progress, in contrast to primary retinal degenerations.

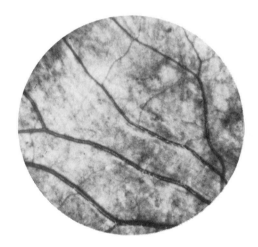

Fig. 16-9. Areas of pigmentation and depigmentation of the peripheral retina in fetal rubella.

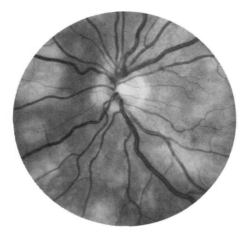

Fig. 16-10. Acute posterior multifocal placoid pigment epitheliopathy with multiple lesions deep to the sensory retina.

Acute posterior multifocal placoid pigment epitheliopathy. This is an inflammatory disease characterized by the acute onset of multiple, flat, yellow-white lesions of the posterior pole at the level of the retinal pigment epithelium (Fig. 16-10). These resolve spontaneously, leaving extensive derangement of the pigment epithelium, as shown on fluorescein angiography, but with minimal alteration of the choroid or retina. Lesions located in the central retinal area rapidly reduce visual acuity, which may improve spontaneously over several weeks. In the early stages the disease blocks the transmission of choroidal fluorescence, and the lesions gradually stain and fluoresce in the later stage. This appearance may be the result of a vasculitis of the choriocapillaris causing a transient occlusion. After the disease has healed, there are extensive transmission defects in the pigment epithelium without late staining or leakage of dye.

The disease particularly affects young adults, who often give a history of an upper respiratory tract illness some 1 or 2 weeks before onset. There may be an associated mild uveitis with keratic precipitates and aqueous humor flare and cells in the vitreous. Rarely, the presence of headache and cells in the cerebrospinal fluid suggests a mild cerebral vasculitis. The severity of involvement of the pigment epithelium suggests that the disease selects this level, but the involvement of the uveal tract elsewhere suggests that the lesion is in the choriocapillaris layer of the choroid. Serologic tests of the serum for a variety of viruses and other microbes have not implicated any group.

Acute retinal pigment epitheliitis. This is a self-limited, benign condition in which tiny black spots surrounded by a yellow, halolike zone occur in the pigment epithelium. The lesion may be single, but it more commonly occurs in grapelike clusters in the posterior pole. Vision may be blurred, but symptoms may not occur. Fluorescein angiography of the black dots at the posterior pole shows transmission defects in the retinal pigment epithelium that do not leak or change in size and shape. Men are affected predominantly (75%). The median age is 45 years, and there is bilateral involvement in 38% of the cases.

Uveal effusion. In this abnormality, a large quantity of fluid between the retinal pigment epithelium and the sensory retina causes a shifting retinal separation, depending on the position of the head. It occurs primarily in males who do not have retinal holes. The spinal fluid protein is increased. Ophthalmoscopically, the retina has a large bullous detachment that changes position. The eyes frequently become blind, or the fluid absorbs and the sensory retina returns to its normal position, but visual function is not restored. The condition seems to be a variant of idiopathic central serous chorioretinopathy, acute placoid pigment cell epitheliopathy, and acute epitheliitis.

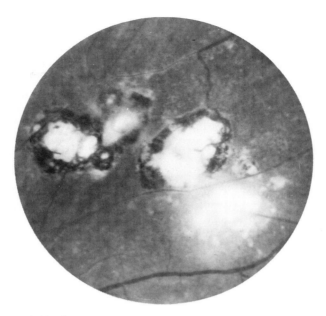

Fig. 16-11. Active retinitis *(lower right)* with inactive lesions above. Destruction of the retina and choroid has made the sclera visible. The retinal pigment epithelium proliferated with healing to give the black margins. The multiple lesions, their appearance, and the occurrence of an active satellite inflammation adjacent to an apparently healed area are characteristics of the retinochoroiditis of toxoplasmosis.

Toxoplasmosis. Toxoplasmosis (p. 466) is likely the main infectious cause of retinitis and occurs in both a congenital and an acquired form. There tends to be secondary involvement of the choroid with destruction of both the retina and the choroid, producing the ophthalmoscopic appearance of a sharply defined area of dull white sclera surrounded by irregular areas of pigment proliferation (Fig. 16-11). The congenital form of the disease is associated with cerebral calcification and internal hydrocephalus. The topic is fully discussed on p. 466.

Cytomegalovirus disease. Infection (p. 462) (as indicated by antibodies) is common with this DNA virus, but manifest disease is rare except in patients receiving immunosuppressants. Cytomegalovirus retinitis shows grayish patches

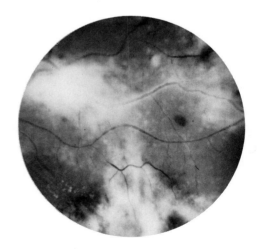

Fig. 16-12. Necrotizing cytomegalovirus retinopathy in a 25-year-old woman treated with chemotherapy for fulminating Hodgkin disease.

or scattered white dots with irregular sheathing of adjacent blood vessels and vitreous clouding (Fig. 16-12). There are superimposed hemorrhages followed by healing along with retinal atrophy. The inflammation is aggravated by systemic corticosteroid administration.

Toxocariasis. The larva of the common roundworm of the dog or cat (p. 468) may cause an eosinophilic granuloma of the central retina. It appears as a whitish, slightly elevated area approximately the size of the optic disk. The dark-colored larva, which excites little cellular or pigmentary reaction, may sometimes be seen in the mass. Less common is a chronic endophthalmitis, which may lead to enucleation because of a diagnosis of retinoblastoma (p. 353). Treatment is ineffective, but the disease may be prevented by regular deworming of dogs likely to come in contact with children.

RETINAL DEGENERATIONS

Genetic defects, inflammation, trauma, vascular disease, or aging causes either local or widespread retinal degeneration. An accurate diagnosis may necessitate psychophysical and ophthalmic studies combined with fluorescein angiography of the patient and family members. Unfortunately, many of these disorders have not been studied histologically or they have been studied only in their end stages, when nonspecific changes predominated. Histologic and biochemical studies of human eyes in the early stages of disease are essential to provide more precise information.

Previously the retinal pigment epithelium was called the tapetum (Gr., rug). The term *tapetoretinal degeneration* describes hereditary disorders of the layer, although the primary site is not always in this layer. Sometimes the retinal pigment epithelium fails in phagocytosis of rod outer segments. In other individuals, atrophy of the choriocapillaris reduces the blood supply to the overlying pigment epithelium and outer portion of the retina. Some disorders seem to affect the longevity of rods and cones, whereas others cause defects in lipid transport, defects in synthesis of rod membranes, or faulty or absent visual pigments. New blood vessel formation beneath the retinal pigment epithelium or between the retinal pigment epithelium and the sensory retina is the basis of a variety of central retinal degenerations, some of which are genetically determined, such as degenerative myopia. Many disorders once thought to involve the central retina predominantly are now recognized as involving the entire retina, with attention directed to the fovea centralis because of defective visual acuity.

Retinal pigment epithelium. Most pigmentary degenerations of the retina involve predominantly the photoreceptors and the retinal pigment epithelium. All nutrition for the photoreceptor layer must pass through the pigment epithelial layer, and the pigment epithelial layer is intimately involved in the phagocytosis and renewal of the rod outer segments. Failure of the lysosomal system of the pigment epithelium results in a failure to digest rod outer segments or in accumulation of cellular debris, which distorts the overlying receptors.

Primary pigmentary dystrophy of the retina ("retinitis pigmentosa"). This group of hereditary diseases is caused by different genes primarily affecting retinal rods but eventually resulting in impairment of all visual cells. X chromosome–linked forms of the disease (mainly recessive) are the most severe, and autosomal dominant forms are the mildest; autosomal recessive forms are intermediate. The disease begins in adolescence with night blindness followed by a ring scotoma that extends peripherally and centrally until only a small, contracted central field remains (tubular vision). The scotopic electroretinographic response is abolished, and dark adaptation is impaired. All vision may be lost by the age of 50 or 60 years.

Ophthalmoscopic examination (Fig. 16-13) reveals a waxy, yellowish atrophy of the optic nerve, severe arterial attenuation, patchy areas of choriocapillaris atrophy with prominent underlying veins, and usually conspicuous pigment proliferation with deposits that have a dense center and irregular processes, often referred to as bone corpuscle in shape. The appearance of the optic disks and retinal vessels aids in the diagnosis, even when pigment is sparse or absent. Pigment proliferation often begins in the equatorial region with fine areas of pigmentation and depigmentation; the pigment becomes more dense centrally.

The course of the disease is variable. Central retinal involvement with loss of central vision may occur early, or alternatively, central vision may be preserved until middle life, although loss of the peripheral field limits motility. Posterior subcapsular cataract may reduce vision and require extraction. Most instances of primary pigmentary dystrophy occur in individuals without other evident genetic defects. However, in many patients an apparently identical pigmentary degeneration occurs with widespread motor and visceral defects, mental retardation, cerebellar ataxia, ophthalmoplegia, and convulsions. The disorder is progressive with periods of remission. Evaluation of the effects of therapy requires long-term observation and double-masked clinical trials.

There have been a number of different treatments suggested: vitamin A in high doses, cataract extraction, various subconjunctival injections, and the like. In 1916 Leber suggested that exposure to light accelerated the process and the degeneration of the retina. Animals deficient in vitamin A develop retinal degeneration only when they are exposed to light. Thus, the most recent trials aim to preserve vision in one eye by excluding it from light by means of an opaque shell. Evaluation of treatment requires exact diagnosis of the type of disease, knowledge of its hereditary pattern, and long-term observation. Inability to provide effective treatment has made the victims of the disease and their families easy prey for many nostrums.

I suggest the following regimen for patients afflicted with any form of retinitis pigmentosa:

1. Examination of the eyes annually to determine the progression of the disease.
2. Complete family history and examination to classify the disorder accurately. The possibility of affected children in the future may be estimated through known family inheritance patterns.
3. Small doses of vitamins A and E, which may be helpful. The standard vitamin dosage should not be exceeded.

I believe it unwise for individuals with pigmentary degeneration to be exposed

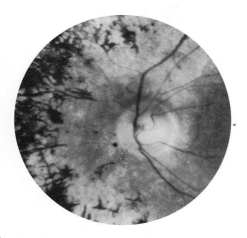

Fig. 16-13. Bone-corpuscle pigment proliferation and attenuated arterioles of primary pigmentary dystrophy of the retina (retinitis pigmentosa).

to bright sunlight. If such exposure is necessary, extremely dark sunglasses should be worn (lenses with less than 15% transmission). Additionally, pupillary constriction markedly limits the amount of light that can enter the eye. However, cautious consideration should be given to the use of drugs that constrict the pupil, because these drugs may also cause minor opacities in the lens.

Secondary pigmentary degeneration of the retina occurs in choroiditis, particularly that caused by syphilis; this makes it difficult to distinguish from primary pigmentary dystrophy. Secondary degeneration, however, has a less regular pigment, is distributed beneath blood vessels, is associated with areas of chorioretinitis, and produces an incomplete ring scotoma.

Leber congenital amaurosis. This is a recessively inherited, often consanguineous disorder in which there is either no light perception or near blindness from birth. The pupillary constriction to light is sluggish or absent. Pendular nystagmus and photophobia may be present. Initially the fundus may seem normal, but it subsequently shows areas of pigmentation and depigmentation because of retinal pigmentary degeneration. The electroretinogram shows no response to light stimuli. The ocular disorder may be associated with mental retardation and epilepsy as well as cataract and keratoconus. This is the only congenital ocular condition with severe visual loss in which the external eyes appear normal. In ocular or oculocutaneous albinism and total loss of color vision (achromatopsia), vision is somewhat better, although nystagmus is present. Congenital glaucoma with its tearing, irritated eyes and subsequent ocular enlargement, congenital cataract, and various failures of development, such as microphthalmia, all manifest abnormalities on external examination. The absence of pupillary

constriction to light in Leber disease distinguishes it from a rare disorder in which there is near blindness during the first year of life and eventual normal visual development; this disorder arises presumably from failure of normal myelination of the optic nerve.

One type of Leber disease progresses to complete blindness; the other type appears stationary. Histologically the condition seems to occur because the sensory retina does not develop. There are oval-shaped, abnormal nuclei in the outer nuclear layer and abnormal fine structures of the inner segment, and there is a lack of basal foldings in the retinal pigment epithelium.

Vitelliruptive degeneration. Vitelliruptive degeneration (vitelliform degeneration, Best disease) is an autosomal dominant disorder with onset at birth or shortly thereafter in which the central retinal region is occupied by a bright orange deposit that looks like the yolk of a "sunny-side up" fried egg (Fig. 16-14). The electro-oculogram is decreased, and there is a mild disturbance of dark adaptation. Tests indicate a generalized

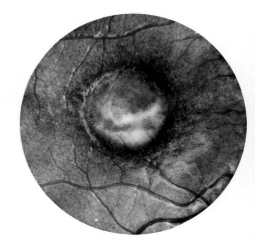

Fig. 16-14. Vitelliruptive degeneration in a 9-year old girl with normal vision.

involvement of the retinal pigment epithelium, although the lesion appears to be confined to the central retinal region. Vision is normal as long as the "sunny-side up" appearance continues. At a variable age from 7 to 15, the material is dispersed ("scrambled"), and scarring and pigmentary changes occur with loss of central vision. The fundus lesion may spare the central retina or may be entirely absent. However, although the eyes may appear normal, all affected individuals have an abnormal electro-oculo-gram.

Drusen. Retinal drusen, which are colloid or hyaline bodies, occur either secondary to a variety of changes in the choroid that affect the pigment epithelium or as a familial abnormality of the retinal pigment epithelium. (Drusen of the optic disk [p. 366] are a different and unrelated disorder.)

Secondary drusen occur commonly as a senile change and have been seen in association with systemic diseases such as angioid streaks, recurrent polyserositis, scleroderma, and Rendu-Osler disease. They occur almost universally with aging, particularly in the peripheral eye-grounds. Secondary drusen are often, but not invariably, seen in disciform degenerations of the central retina. Degenerative drusen usually form in eyes that are becoming phthisical.

Secondary drusen caused by conditions other than aging may occur adjacent to areas of choroidal abnormality, such as malignant melanoma (see Fig. 15-10). Senile drusen tend to involve the equatorial to peripheral retina, whereas familial drusen affect both the posterior pole and the periphery.

Familial drusen are divided into three stages on the basis of their ophthalmoscopic appearance. Initially, during the first to third decade, drusen appear as small, discrete spots slightly pinker than the surrounding fundus. At this early stage they are demonstrated more clearly by fluorescein angiography than by ophthalmoscopy. Initially they are nearly equal in size and appearance. Eventually the dots assume a bright yellow color, and larger ones tend to appear.

During the fourth decade, the dots increase in number, become more whitish, vary in size, and tend to cause elevation of the overlying sensory retina. The last is best appreciated with biomicroscopy and a contact lens (p. 175). During this second stage, there is a tendency to calcification, formation of minute pigment clumps that increase in size, and atrophy of pigment epithelial cells (Fig. 16-15).

In the third stage, beginning in the fifth or sixth decade, the drusen become confluent and plaque formation occurs, particularly in the central retina. Pigment proliferation is common, and there may be secondary degeneration of the overlying retina.

The defects in the retinal pigment epithelium caused by drusen commonly lead to subretinal neovascularization and subsequent disciform retinal degeneration. Serous elevation of the central retina with

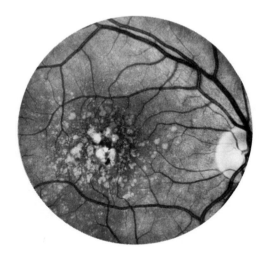

Fig. 16-15. Drusen of the central retina of the right eye. Several of the central drusen are calcified, and there is some pigment proliferation.

"leaking" subretinal areas may precede neovascularization.

Fundus flavimaculatus. Fundus flavimaculatus consists of multiple, round and linear, fishtaillike, yellow or yellow-white lesions, usually involving the posterior fundus (Fig. 16-16). The flecks vary in size, shape, outline, density, and apparent depth. The abnormality is transmitted as an autosomal recessive disorder and occasionally as an autosomal dominant one.

The disorder has its onset in the first or second decade and may follow several courses. There may be an initial loss of vision before central retinal changes are obvious, and it is sometimes difficult to determine the cause of the visual loss. Eventually deposits appear in the atrophic central retina, and the diagnosis is evident. Atrophy of the central retina usually ushers in the disease (Stargardt disease), but occasionally it appears after the flecks develop. In some patients who never develop an atrophic central retinal lesion, visual loss occurs because of incidental direct involvement of the fovea with a deposit, which causes secondary changes in the overlying receptors.

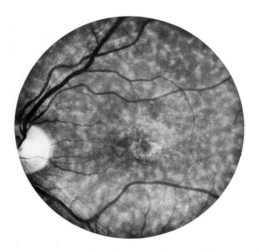

Fig. 16-16. Fundus flavimaculatus with central atrophic lesion (Stargardt disease).

The deposits usually first appear in the perimacular area and are isolated with fairly sharp borders and variable shapes, many of them linear and fishtaillike. Clusters of fresh lesions appear from time to time, and older lesions eventually disappear. The older lesions are less sharply demarcated, appear less dense, and show a greater tendency toward confluence.

Fluorescein angiography does not demonstrate the early lesions, since fresh lesions do not fluoresce. Hyperfluorescence is seen only at the sites of old lesions. The fuzzy, irregular hyperfluorescent blotches at such sites are entirely different from the discrete, sharply outlined hyperfluorescent areas seen with drusen.

Fundus albipunctatus. Fundus albipunctatus is a rare autosomal recessive disorder characterized by dotlike, yellowish white lesions of uniform size located deep in the retina and particularly concentrated at the midperiphery of the fundus. The dotlike deposits usually increase in number but occasionally may decrease or even disappear.

Progressive retinitis albipunctatus presents a similar ophthalmoscopic picture at its onset. However, the electroretinogram is extinguished, and there is a markedly elevated rod threshold with dark adaptation. Eventually bone spicule pigmentation, vascular attenuation, and optic atrophy develop as in related pigmentary dystrophies of the retina.

Lamina basalis choroideae. This is the Bruch membrane (p. 15), previously called the lamina vitrea. It is composed of the basement membrane of the retinal pigment epithelium and the basement membrane of the endothelium of the choriocapillaris. It has inner and outer collagen layers, which sandwich a layer of elastic tissue. It separates the retina and choroid and acts as a permeable membrane between the choriocapillaris and the retina. Drusen (p. 343) of the retinal pigment epithelium rest upon the membrane and have been incorrectly designated as arising from it. Ruptures of the elastic layer occur prominently in angioid streaks and are seen microscopically in disciform degeneration of the central retina (p. 346) and in myopia (p. 435).

Angioid streaks. Angioid streaks consist of a bizarre network of reddish to brown striations that, on ophthalmoscopic examination, appear to lie between the sensory retina and the choroid. The condition is bilateral, but ocular involvement is not symmetrical. Both sexes are affected equally.

In a typical case, the fundus presents a more or less complete peripapillary ring, with offshoots extending toward the equator in a radial distribution (Fig. 16-17). In the early stages, the streaks usually appear red but later may assume a gray, brown, or black color. The striations are flat, serrated, and may be several times wider than a retinal vein. They gradually taper off toward the periphery of the fundus, where they appear as thin lines. They do not branch dichotomously,

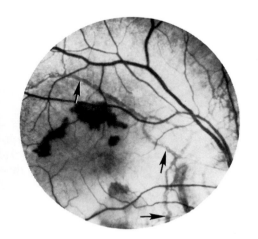

Fig. 16-17. Marked angioid streaks *(arrows)*. There has been subretinal neovascularization with bleeding and early development of disciform degeneration.

as do retinal vessels, and they give the appearance of cracks in dry mud.

Angioid streaks occur primarily in pseudoxanthoma elasticum (of Grönblad and Strandberg, p. 562) and fibrodysplasia hyperelastica (of Ehlers-Danlos, p. 562). In these diseases there is a degeneration of the elastic tissue portion of the Bruch membrane, which ruptures and secondarily calcifies. Secondary causes include sickle cell anemia (5%) (p. 552), osteitis deformans (of Paget), and rarely, acromegaly, hypercalcemia, and lead poisoning. Those conditions with generalized elastic tissue disease may show concurrent vascular hypertension because of involvement of elastic tissue in the walls of arteries.

Ocular changes are asymptomatic until subretinal vascularization occurs. This is often heralded by a retinal hemorrhage followed by disciform central retinal degeneration (p. 346). There is no effective treatment.

Subretinal neovascularization. New blood vessels arising from the choroid and extending between the Bruch membrane and the retinal pigment epithelium (Fig. 16-18) cause visual loss in disciform degeneration of the central retina, degenerative myopia, presumed ocular histoplasmosis, and angioid streaks.

Initially, a break in the Bruch membrane is followed by separation of the retinal pigment epithelium from the Bruch membrane in this area. This is followed by growth of a capillary plexus from the choroid that extends rapidly, with the appearance of large vessels from the periphery. Generally, the capillary network does not increase in size once large blood vessels appear.

The capillary network causes hemorrhage and exudation into the sensory retina along with loss of vision. Eventually it becomes organized with fibrous tissue and proliferated retinal pigment epithelium, and the capillary bed is obliterated.

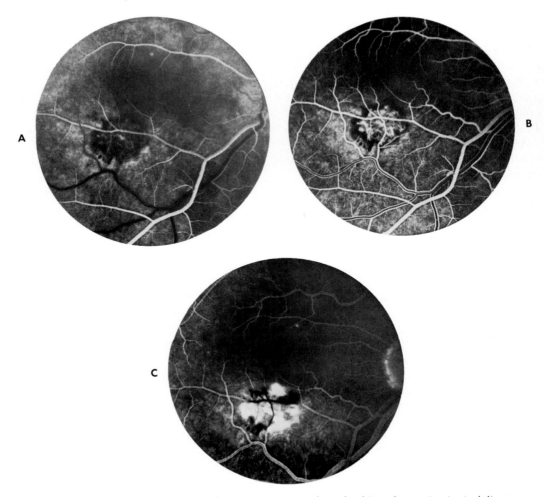

Fig. 16-18. A subretinal neovascular net in presumed ocular histoplasmosis. **A,** A delicate tracery of fine blood vessels beneath the sensory retina. **B,** In the midvenous retinal phase the blood vessels are filled. **C,** In the delayed fluorescein view the neovascular net leaks fluorescein.

Photocoagulation of the initial break in the Bruch membrane and retinal pigment epithelium detachment may prevent the neovascularization. The break must be in an area other than the fovea centralis, or the photocoagulation itself will destroy central vision. Once neovascularization has started, photocoagulation must destroy the entire vascular network inasmuch as partial destruction stimulates additional blood vessels.

Disciform degeneration of the central retina. This is a common cause of poor vision in the elderly (Kuhnt-Junius disease). Both sexes are affected equally, most often in the seventh and eighth decades. The lesion is usually preceded by drusen (p. 343) involving the central retina. Perhaps one fourth of these individuals develop a detachment of the retinal pigment epithelium and go on to develop a disciform degeneration. Of these, about one third develop a similar lesion in the fellow eye.

Typically, an elderly patient in good general health develops a serous separation of the retinal pigment epithelium. Foveal central vision is severely impaired, but extrafoveal vision is spared. Shortly thereafter, a subretinal hemorrhage develops, and the blood often breaks through into the sensory retina. There may be striking, yellowish white deposits at the posterior pole often arranged in an annular pattern surrounding the central retina. After approximately 1 year the lesion is converted to a fibrous mass, and vision is reduced to a level of 1/60 (3/200). Treatment is unsatisfactory. Photocoagulation of extrafoveal pigment epithelium detachment or extrafoveal neovascularization may prevent progression of the lesion.

Central retinal (macular) degenerations

We have seen (p. 30) that the central retina is located temporal to the optic disk and surrounds the fovea centralis. The fovea centralis contains the cones mainly responsible for visual acuity and color vision. The area is involved in the same vascular, inflammatory, and degenerative diseases that affect the retina and underlying choroidal vasculature elsewhere. Several factors so modify disease in the central retina that its abnormalities are often considered apart from diseases of the remainder of the retina. A minute lesion that would not affect visual function if located peripherally may cause a severe loss of visual acuity. Additionally, the spreading of the inner layers of the retina to expose the cones in the fovea centralis favors swelling of the outer plexiform layer of the retina (called the Henle layer in this region). This swelling is seen particularly in neuroretinitis with the formation of a circular area of deposits surrounding the fovea centralis. The optical system of the eye focuses light energy in this region, so that degeneration of the area may follow unwise exposure to the light of the sun as occurs in eclipse retinopathy. Moreover, the central retinal area, for reasons as yet unexplained, appears to be preferentially involved in a variety of degenerative conditions.

Abnormalities confined to the fovea centralis and causing decreased visual acuity have been classified broadly as central retinal degenerations. For the most part, the lesions are easily seen with the ophthalmoscope. Degeneration of the central retina can be divided into primary and secondary types. The primary type results from a genetically transmitted defect. It is familial, bilateral, and progressive. The main types include vitelliruptive degeneration and fundus flavimaculatus (p. 344). Drusen may be transmitted as an autosomal dominant defect and initiate the detachment of the retinal pigment epithelium, leading to disciform degeneration of the posterior pole (p. 346).

Primary central retinal degenerations also include abnormalities with central nervous system involvement. Central nervous system involvement arises because of abnormalities affecting the ganglion cells of both the retina and the brain. Degenerations include amaurotic familial idiocy (Tay-Sachs disease, p. 483) and Batten ceroid neuronal lipofucinosis. Involvement of the central nervous system frequently leads to early death, and many cases are not diagnosed, because the fundi have not been examined.

The secondary type follows vascular, inflammatory, or degenerative disease, is commonly unilateral, and frequently does not progess after the cause has been removed. The secondary type is at times amenable to therapy, although in many diseases, particularly vascular degenerations, therapy is not successful.

The secondary group of central retinal degenerations occurs because of severe ocular trauma, inflammation involving the central retinal area, distant inflammation causing edema of nerve fibers in direct contact with the vitreous body, and vascular disease affecting the area.

The foveal changes associated with a decreased blood supply from the choriocapillaris are diagnosed as senile retinal degeneration. Visual acuity diminishes gradually, and involvement of one eye precedes involvement of the other by months or years. Ophthalmoscopic examination may indicate minimal change even though there is severe visual loss. There may be fine pigmentary deposits at the posterior pole with discrete, minute, yellowish exudative areas. There may be drusen of the retinal pigment epithelium (p. 343).

Medical therapy is of no value. The visual loss occurs because of unknown factors that may include diminution of blood supply to the fovea centralis, premature deterioration of cones, loss of elastic tissue in the Bruch membrane, and similar mechanisms. Function cannot be restored to the delicate cones once it is lost. Some patients obtain useful vision with telescopic lenses, special magnifying lenses, and similar optical aids. Although the proportion of patients who obtain satisfaction is disappointingly small, each patient should have a trial opportunity with these lenses before it is concluded that they are of no use. Physicians must reassure these patients that the condition will not progress to complete blindness. Although central vision is lost, the disease never involves the peripheral retina sufficiently to eliminate so much of the peripheral vision that the patient becomes helpless.

PRERETINAL FIBROSIS

Fibrosis over the surface of the internal limiting membrane of the retina ranges from translucent wrinkling to extensive periretinal cellular proliferation.

The condition has been called premacular fibrosis, preretinal vitreous membrane, surface wrinkling retinopathy, and (after retinal detachment surgery) macular pucker. It may occur after accidental trauma, eye surgery, retinal vascular disease, and inflammation and with any of the conditions that cause retinitis proliferans. In most instances there is a break in the internal limiting membrane with proliferation of glial cells arising from the optic nerve, from Müller cells, or from retinal astrocytes. The condition is triggered by separation of a posterior vitreous with subsequent disruption of the internal limiting membrane. A cellular membrane of variable thickness then proliferates on the inner surface of the retina. Unlike vitreous membranes (p. 360), which are acellular unless inflammatory in origin, preretinal fibrosis has a well-defined cellular structure.

FLUID-SEPARATING RETINAL LAYERS

The smooth continuity of the retina lining the globe may be disturbed by a number of abnormalities (see outline). Giant cysts in the outer plexiform layer of the sensory retina give rise to retinoschisis. Traction, holes, or exudation beneath the sensory retina may separate it from the pigment epithelium in retinal

---

Layers separated by fluid in various retinal abnormalities

In sensory retina (retinoschisis)
Between sensory retina and pigment
    epithelium (retinal detachment)
    Vitreous traction
    Hole(s) in sensory retina
    Serous choroidopathy
Between pigment epithelium and choroid
Elevation of both sensory retina and
    pigment epithelium
    Tumor (equivalent) of choroid

separation or detachment. Fluid between the Bruch membrane and the choriocapillaris may cause a detachment of the retinal pigment epithelium. Both the sensory retina and pigment epithelium may be elevated by tumors and fluid in the choroid—a secondary detachment.

Retinoschisis

Retinoschisis develops because of splitting of the sensory layers of the retina, usually in the outer plexiform layer. Two forms occur: (1) X chromosome–linked, in which splitting occurs in the nerve fiber layer and which affects the central and peripheral retina, and (2) peripheral, which does not involve the central retina. Central vision is affected late, if at all, and a defect in the peripheral visual field is the main sign.

Prognosis in retinoschisis is good. It seems likely that in many instances it remains undiagnosed indefinitely. In advanced cases, however, visual acuity may be lost. The development of a break in the retina may lead to retinal detachment.

Retinoschisis, in its early stages, appears to be an exaggeration of cystoid degeneration of the retina. If the sclera of the area is indented, the affected retina appears to have lost some of its transparency (white with pressure). In later stages the inner layer forms a fixed, smooth, convex, sharply limited, transparent elevation.

If the condition is stationary, no treatment is indicated, and annual ophthalmoscopic and perimetric examinations are advised. Progression may be limited when necessary by photocoagulation, surface diathermy, or cryotherapy at the advancing edge of the elevation in normal retinal tissue or in the area of the elevated retina.

X chromosome–linked juvenile retinoschisis. This is an X chromosome recessive disorder in which initially there appears to be a cystlike structure involving the fovea centralis. In the early stages it has a spokelike appearance with the hub corresponding to the foveola. Later the radial folds disappear and are replaced by a nonspecific atrophic appearance. In about one half of the patients there is a peripheral retinoschisis, often in the inferior temporal region. There are silver-gray glistening spots scattered throughout the retina in all cases. The vitreous contains veils, most often in the periphery.

Vision may be normal initially and may gradually deteriorate to about 6/60 (20/200) at puberty. Strabismus and nystagmus may occur, but most commonly the condition is detected when the child fails to pass vision tests on entering school. A subnormal electroretinographic b-wave occurs with a normal electrooculogram. There are no signs in carrier females.

Peripheral retinoschisis. This usually begins as a cystic degeneration of the extreme retinal periphery, most commonly the inferior temporal quadrant. It extends nasally to encompass the entire periphery, and the cysts consolidate to form a huge elevation.

Retinal separation (detachment)

The invagination of the primary optic vesicle gives rise to two primitive retinal layers: the outer pigment epithelium and an inner sensory layer. A potential space is present between these layers except at the optic nerve and at the ora serrata. Traction upon or formation of a hole in the inner sensory layer permits the accumulation of fluid between the two primitive layers of the retina, which separate, causing loss of retinal function (Fig. 16-19). The subretinal fluid that accumulates between the two primitive retinal layers contains more protein than does the vitreous and is derived in large part from blood plasma.

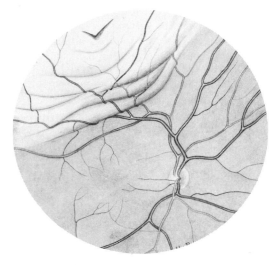

Fig. 16-19. Retinal detachment with a horseshoe-shaped hole in the superotemporal quadrant. (From Newell, F. W.: In Walters, W., editor: Lewis-Walters practice of surgery, vol. 4, New York, 1974, Harper & Row, Publishers, Inc.)

Serous retinal separation occurs secondary to the formation of breaks or holes in the sensory layer of the retina or because of separation of this layer at the ora serrata, a retinal dialysis, or disinsertion. Retinal breaks occur because of degenerative changes in either the retina or the adjacent vitreous body or because of ocular trauma. Retinal disinsertion, in which the sensory retina is stripped from the ora serrata, occurs mainly in young individuals as either a congenital or a traumatic defect.

Retinal separations occur more commonly in men than in women, in eyes with degenerative myopia, and in the elderly. The separation tends to be bilateral in about one third of the patients with retinal degenerative changes. The time interval between separation in the first and then in the second eye may be as long as 10 years. The role of ocular trauma is obvious when there is a direct ocular contusion or a penetrating injury with a retinal break in an otherwise healthy retina. Often, however, the history of trauma is obscure, and enough degenerative changes are present in each eye to account for the retinal separation. In such eyes the role of trauma in precipitating the detachment is difficult to assess, particularly if the trauma has not involved the eye directly. Retinal separation may occur after an uncomplicated cataract extraction, but it is seen more often if vitreous humor has been lost during surgery. Congenital cataract extraction is prone to be complicated by retinal separation that may occur many years after surgery.

Retinal breaks may follow penetrating ocular injuries, but in other instances the cause of the break is not clear. They may result from the vitreous adhering in a localized area of the retina and the remaining vitreous body retracting. Some arise from degenerative changes following minute retinal or choroidal vascular obstructions, or they may follow retinal inflammations. In youthful eyes the rupture of a congenital retinal cyst is an etiologic factor, whereas in senile eyes there may be rupture of peripheral degenerative cysts.

The two main premonitory symptoms of retinal separation are (1) photopsia, or flashes of light without retinal stimulation by light caused by vitreous traction on the retina, and (2) a sudden shower of black dots in the peripheral visual field arising from a minute vitreous hemorrhage at the point of a retinal break. In many patients, premonitory symptoms are either absent or ignored, and the first symptom is a progressive defect in the visual field corresponding to the area of detachment.

The diagnosis of retinal separation is based on the ophthalmoscopic appearance of the retina. Indirect ophthalmoscopy may be combined with scleral depression, and the examiner may study the retina from the optic disk to the ora serrata. Maximal pupillary dilation is required—10% phenylephrine and 1% tropicamide (Mydriacyl) are frequently used. The peripheral retina is also studied with a biomicroscope and a contact lens containing prisms that allow visualization of the periphery.

On ophthalmoscopic examination the detached retina appears dark red to gray, and the normal choroidal pattern cannot be seen. The retina may be thrown into folds that change in location or shape with changes in position of the eye or the head. Fixed folds, the result of alterations in the vitreous body, do not change with position. The retinal vessels are dark red in the area of detachment and have an undulating course over its surface. The arteries and veins appear to have blood of the same color.

Retinal breaks are recognized by the bright red reflex of the choroid shining through the grayish, opaque veil of surrounding detached retina. Additional holes may be found in areas of attached retina. Horseshoe-shaped tears with their base anterior are most common in the superior temporal quadrant near the equator. Small round holes may be found anywhere but are frequently seen in the extreme peripheral retina. Retinal dialysis usually occurs in the inferior quadrants, and it is most often single, semilunar, and at the extreme retinal periphery. Retinal detachments with hole formation are readily diagnosed. However, in serous detachments, holes are not found in 5% to 15% of the patients, depending on the skill of the observer.

Visual field examination delineates the extent of retinal separation and indicates whether or not the separation regresses with bed rest.

The most important differential point is the solid detachment caused by tumor, particularly malignant melanoma of the choroid (p. 311). Failure of the detachment to regress with bed rest, the darker color, the failure to transilluminate, and the usual absence of hole formation serve to characterize tumor formation.

The treatment of serous retinal detachment is essentially surgical and is directed toward closure of breaks in the retina and absorption of subretinal fluid. Once the diagnosis has been established, treatment must be started immediately.

Retinal breaks are closed by producing an area of chorioretinitis in the region of the defect so that adhesions forming between the edges of the break and the underlying choroid will obliterate the opening. The inflammation is produced by the application of intense cold ($-80°$ C) to the sclera in the region of the hole. Subretinal fluid is often removed by perforating the choroid, but it will absorb spontaneously if the pigment epithelium is brought into contact with the retinal hole.

A variety of procedures are employed to decrease the size of the sclera so that a smaller or shrunken retina will fit the smaller scleral shell. In shortening procedures, one or more quadrants of the sclera are shortened. This may be combined with buckling of a segment of sclera (plombage) with a material such as silicone sponge to cause further indentation of the choroid. Alternatively, an encircling rod (cerclage) may be placed around the circumference of the eye at the equator.

Failure to obtain anatomic reattachment of the retina usually is caused by failure to obliterate the causative retinal break or because the retina has shrunk. Because of the frequency with which the fellow eye is involved, every attempt must be made to secure correction, even if several reoperations are required.

Secondary retinal detachment. Both the pigment epithelium and the sensory retina may be elevated by malignant choroidal melanomas, which cause a solid detachment. Additionally, the tumor may be associated with a serous fluid between the pigment epithelium and the retina either in the region surrounding the tumor or distant from the tumor. Severe uveitis may cause secondary retinal detachments either through vitreous traction or because of an exudative reaction from the choroid. In eclampsia or sudden severe vascular hypertension from other causes, a transudate may elevate the retina. Vitreous traction bands from whatever cause may elevate the retina without causing any tear (nonrhegmatogenous).

Detachment of the retinal pigment epithelium. Clinically this lesion is most significant as a stage in the development of disciform degeneration of the central retina (p. 346). It is postulated that the initial stage is a lesion in the choroid with increased permeability of the choriocapillaris permitting serous fluid to collect beneath the retinal pigment epithelium. This lesion is usually round, sharply circumscribed, and surrounded by a circumscribed light reflex. Fluorescein angiography indicates accumulation of fluid in the area. The serous fluid then enters into the subretinal space, causing a localized detachment. There may be hemorrhage with extension of blood into the sensory retina. Ultimately there is degeneration of the pigment epithelium and sensory retina.

INJURIES

Contusions and retinal breaks. Contusion may cause a variety of injuries (p. 191), including retinal breaks that lead to retinal separation. A traumatic retinal break occurs in an otherwise healthy retina—it is usually single, often horseshoe shaped, and located in the superior temporal quadrant. Eyes that have been subject to severe contusions should be studied carefully 3 and 6 months after the injury to be certain a retinal break has not developed. It is necessary to study the fundus with wide pupillary dilation and to direct particular attention to the periphery.

Commotio retinae. Commotio retinae is a contrecoup phenomenon in which the posterior pole develops edema and hemorrhages because of a blunt contusion of the anterior segment. Vision is markedly reduced and often does not improve. Ophthalmoscopically there is an edema that obscures the underlying retina. It may disappear spontaneously or may be followed by atrophy of the retina and choroid.

Central retinal hole. Central retinal hole is a term applied to round, red defects of the fovea centralis that measure about ¼ disk diameter in size and are associated with marked reduction in vision. Ophthalmoscopically, they appear to be holes in the retina, yet retinal separation follows only exceptionally. Examination with a biomicroscope indicates that the majority of them are cysts with a translucent anterior wall. There is no treatment.

Lacerations of the retina. Lacerations of the retina are usually associated with loss of vitreous and considerable disorganization of the globe. Retinal separation is uncommon following such injury inasmuch as the trauma stimulates proliferation of glial tissue, which closes the defect.

Purtscher injury. Purtscher injury is a rare abnormality in which the sudden increase in intravascular pressure associated with crushing injury of the chest causes hemorrhages and edema of the retina.

Fat emboli. Fat emboli of the retinal blood vessels may be seen in fractures of long bones. They cause localized areas of grayish retinal edema often with diminished visual acuity, which tends to improve.

Radiant energy. The cornea and the lens transmit long visible light rays (red) and infrared with nearly 100% efficiency (p. 98). These rays are usually absorbed by the retinal pigment epithelium, and the energy is dissipated by the choriocapillaris. They may cause injury to the retina if (1) the exposure is of long duration and continuous, (2) the energy is at particular wavelengths, (3) the pupil does not constrict to limit the amount of energy entering the eye, (4) the eye is nearly emmetropic so that the rays come to focus on the fovea centralis, (5) the retina is sensitized by vitamin A depletion, or (6) the retina is sensitized by drugs.

The classic type of such damage follows observation of a solar eclipse, in which the pupil is dilated because of low light intensity and infrared rays are focused on the fovea centralis.

Light damage (photic retinopathy) to the retina may occur in those who gaze at the sun as part of sun worship or in a psychosis. Marked pupillary constriction may prevent injury. A lesion that appears endemic in American servicemen at some military installations seems to be caused by either sun gazing or a central serous choroidopathy (p. 308). Infants with hemolytic anemia, in whom light oxidizes the bilirubin in the skin, must have their eyes protected during phototherapy.

The mechanism of injury is not known. The damage may be produced by levels of energy that seem to be easily dissipated by the choriocapillaris. Metabolic or electrolytic changes in the retina are a possible cause, and retinol (p. 93) has a lytic effect on some cell membranes.

Retinal poisons and toxins. Chloroquine and the phenothiazines (p. 141) in large doses cause a pigmentary degeneration of the central retina. Topical administration of epinephrine eye drops in aphakic eyes also causes a maculopathy with loss of vision. In susceptible persons a small amount of quinine may cause severe vasoconstriction of retinal arteries with the central field reduced to 5° to 10° in diameter.

TUMORS
Retinoblastomas

Retinoblastomas are malignant tumors that arise most commonly from the inner nuclear layer of the retina, less commonly from the ganglion cell and nerve fiber layer, and exceptionally from the outer nuclear layer. The incidence is between 1:14,000 (Holland) and 1:23,000 (Michigan). The tumor may be present at birth but usually occurs at about 1½ years and is rarely seen in adults. Retinoblastomas are characterized by origination from multiple foci within the eye and, in about one third of the patients, involve both eyes. Children with hereditary retinoblastoma may develop secondary primary neoplasms (1:50), particularly osteogenic sarcoma of long bones.

Rarely, chromosome analysis in infants with multiple defects in addition to retinoblastoma shows a deletion of the long arm of chromosome 13. This is the only instance known in humans in which a specific chromosomal abnormality prezygotically and consistently predisposes to a specific tumor.

Retinoblastoma of both eyes is transmitted as an autosomal dominant characteristic. Unilateral retinoblastomas are rarely hereditary (20%); they most commonly are sporadic and will not be transmitted. Multiple discrete tumors in one eye suggest a hereditary basis.

If a parent or one or more siblings of the retinoblastoma patient is affected, there is a 40% chance that each of the patient's children will receive the mutant gene, and bilateral retinoblastoma is likely. The unaffected subject in this hereditary situation has a chance (1:8) of being a carrier of the mutant gene but has no chance of having the tumor. There is about a 1:20 chance of having a child with retinoblastoma. In a family with one affected child and no other members with retinoblastoma, there is a 1.1% chance of subsequent children being affected. It is imperative in such a situation that both parents be examined for evidence of the tumor that has regressed spontaneously.

Usually the tumor is first diagnosed when it has protruded far forward into the vitreous body, filling the entire globe, and is visible in the eye as a grayish yellow reflex behind the lens. Often by this time the pupil is fixed and the eye is blind; the term "cat's eye" has been applied to the clinical appearance.

Less frequently, an esotropia or exotropia occurs because of poor vision. Tumor necrosis may cause a red, painful eye that may or may not have glaucoma.

The most important diagnostic step to be taken when retinoblastoma is suspected in one eye is careful ophthalmoscopic examination of the opposite eye with the pupil widely dilated and, if necessary, the child anesthetized. All portions of the retina must be inspected, and particular attention should be directed to the periphery. Careful study of the fellow eye, when there is no involvement, must be carried out at 6- to 8-week intervals until late childhood.

The tumor appears as a pale pink or white mass (Fig. 16-20) with newly formed blood vessels on its surface. There may be multiple independent tumors or implantation growth on the iris, cornea, or vitreous. The vitreous may contain multiple globules of dull white tumor seeds. When tumor necrosis occurs, nuclear DNA is released and becomes complexed to calcium to form radiopaque masses. These appear as pearly white sharply defined areas on the surface of the tumor or as chalky white areas with poorly demarcated edges when deeper. The DNA-calcium depo-

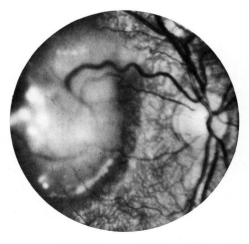

Fig. 16-20. Retinoblastoma of the right eye in a lightly pigmented 1-year-old infant. The tumor projects into the vitreous and casts a shadow on the adjacent retina. There is calcification visible at the apex of the tumor.

sition is pathognomonic of retinoblastoma and can be detected by x-rays in about 75% of the cases. Ultrasonography provides echoes compatible with calcium.

The ratio of aqueous humor lactic dehydrogenase to serum lactic dehydrogenase is greater than 1:50 in most, but not all, cases of retinoblastoma. Increased ratios rarely appear in eyes that do not contain retinoblastomas. Alternatively, a normal ratio may be found in eyes that do contain retinoblastomas. The danger of extraocular seeding of the tumor must be considered when aqueous humor is removed from an eye containing a tumor. The phosphoglucose isomerase level may also be increased in the aqueous humor. In some patients the serum carcinoembryonic antigen level is increased.

Treatment. Unilateral retinoblastomas are often far advanced when diagnosed, and enucleation including as long a section of the optic nerve as possible is the treatment of choice. Immediately after removal of the eye frozen sections of the optic nerve should be studied to be certain that no tumor extends beyond the point of excision. If there is no evidence of orbital tumor, an implant is used. If tumor is found in the optic nerve remaining in the orbit, the orbit should be treated with radiation similar to that used when the tumor is diagnosed in the fellow eye.

Bilateral retinoblastomas are best treated by enucleation of the most-involved eye and radiation therapy to the opposite eye combined with chemotherapy. (When both eyes are involved with far-advanced tumors, it is probably kindest to the patient and to all concerned to proceed with bilateral enucleation, because radiation is almost certain to destroy an eye with an advanced tumor.) By using isotopes, one may apply radiation locally.

Photocoagulation is used to treat retinoblastomas involving less than one third of the retina. The therapy does not sterilize tumor nests that are invisible ophthalmoscopically and is often used after radiation when there is activity in the main tumor mass. Since the tumor itself is too pale to absorb much light energy, treatment must be directed to the surrounding choroid.

Prognosis. The prognosis is related to the number and size of the tumors and to whether they are located anterior or posterior to the equator. They are classed as follows: (I) solitary or multiple tumors, none over 4 disk diameters in size at or behind the equator; (II) solitary or multiple tumors, 4 to 10 disk diameters in size behind the equator; (III) tumors anterior to the equator; (IV) solitary or multiple tumors larger than 10 disk diameters in size; (V) massive tumors involving over half of the retina and vitreous seeding. Most tumors fall into group V.

Unilateral tumors in groups I to IV have a good prognosis; the mortality of those in group V is about 17%. Bilateral tumors in groups I to III have a good prognosis; bi-lateral tumors in group V have a 13% mortality. Approximately 80% of the deaths are caused by metastatic disease. Malignant neoplasms, either radiation induced or outside the radiation field, account for the remainder of the deaths.

Other tumors

Vascular malformations of the retinal blood vessels, Coats disease (p. 328), phakomatoses (p. 327), and assorted tumors may occur. Hyperplasia of the retinal pigment epithelium may cause a localized black area in the fundus or may occur congenitally as grouped pigmentation (p. 326). Neoplastic transformation of the retinal pigment epithelium is rare.

BIBLIOGRAPHY

Appen, R. E., Wray, S. H., and Cogan, D. G.: Central retinal artery occlusion, Am. J. Ophthalmol. **79:** 374, 1975.

Azar, P., Jr., Gohd, R. S., Waltman, D., and Gitter, K. A.: Acute posterior multifocal placoid pigment epitheliopathy associated with an adenovirus type 5 infection, Am. J. Ophthalmol. **80:**1003, 1975.

Bellhorn, M. B., Friedman, A. H., Wise, G. N., and Henkind, P.: Ultrastructure and clinicopathologic correlation of idiopathic preretinal macular fibrosis, Am. J. Ophthalmol. **79:**366, 1975.

Campbell, C. J., and Wise, G. N.: Photocoagulation therapy of branch-vein obstructions, Am. J. Ophthalmol. **75:**28, 1973.

Char, D. H., and Herberman, R. B.: Cutaneous delayed hypersensitivity responses of patients with retinoblastoma to standard recall antigens and crude membrane extracts of retinoblastoma tissue culture cells, Am. J. Ophthalmol. **78:**40, 1974.

Clarkson, J. G., Green, W. R., and Massof, D.: A histopathologic review of 168 cases of preretinal membrane, Am. J. Ophthalmol. **84:**1, 1977.

Cleasby, G. W.: Idiopathic focal subretinal neovascularization, Am. J. Ophthalmol. **81:**590, 1976.

Conway, B. P., and Welch, R. B.: X-chromosome-linked juvenile retinoschisis with hemorrhagic retinal cyst, Am. J. Ophthalmol. **83:**853, 1977.

Cotlier, E.: Cafe-au-lait spots of fundus in neurofibromatosis, Arch. Ophthalmol. **95:**1990, 1977.

Cross, H. E., and Bard, L.: Electro-oculography in Best's macular dystrophy, Am. J. Ophthalmol. **77:**46, 1974.

Deutman, A. F.: The hereditary dystrophies of the

posterior pole of the eye, Assen, Netherlands, 1971, Van Gorcum and Co.

Deutman, A. F., and Lion, F.: Choriocapillaris non-perfusion in acute multifocal placoid pigment epitheliopathy, Am. J. Ophthalmol. **84:**652, 1977.

Devesa, S. S.: The incidence of retinoblastoma, Am. J. Ophthalmol. **80:**263, 1975.

Fine, S. L., Patz, A., Orth, D. H., and others: Subretinal neovascularization developing after prophylactic argon laser photocoagulation of atrophic macular scars, Am. J. Ophthalmol. **82:**352, 1976.

Flynn, J. T., O'Grady, G. E., Herrera, J., and others: Retrolental fibroplasia, Arch. Ophthalmol. **95:**217, 1977.

Gass, J. D. M.: Stereoscopic atlas of macular diseases; diagnosis and treatment, ed. 2, St. Louis, 1977, The C. V. Mosby Co.

Gitter, K. A., Cohen, G., and Baber, B. W.: Photocoagulation in venous occlusive disease, Am. J. Ophthalmol. **79:**578, 1975.

Glaser, J. S., Savino, P. J., Sumers, K. D., and others: The photostress recovery test in the clinical assessment of visual function, Am. J. Ophthalmol. **83:**255, 1977.

Gragoudas, E. S., Chandra, S. R., Friedman, E., and others: Disciform degeneration of macula, Arch. Ophthalmol. **94:**755, 1976.

Hadden, O. B., and Gass, J. D. M.: Fundus flavimaculatus and Stargardt's disease, Am. J. Ophthalmol. **82:**527, 1976.

Hollenhorst, R. W., Jr., Hollenhorst, R. W., Sr., and MacCarty, C. S.: Visual prognosis of optic nerve sheath meningiomas producing shunt vessels on the optic disk, Mayo Clin. Proc. **53:**84, 1978.

Holt, W. S., Regan, C. D. J., and Trempe, C.: Acute posterior multifocal placoid pigment epitheliopathy, Am. J. Ophthalmol. **81:**403, 1976.

Horton, W. A., Wong, V., and Eldridge, R.: Von Hippel–Lindau disease; clinical and pathological manifestations in nine families with 50 affected members, Arch. Intern. Med. **136:**769, 1976.

Jacobson, D. R., and Dellaporta, A.: Natural history of cystoid macular edema after cataract extraction, Am. J. Ophthalmol. **77:**445, 1974.

Jampol, L. M., Isenberg, S. J., and Goldberg, M. F.: Occlusive retinal arteriolitis with neovascularization, Am. J. Ophthalmol. **81:**583, 1976.

Jampol, L. M., Wong, A. S., and Albert, D. M.: Atrial myxoma and central retinal artery occlusion, Am. J. Ophthalmol. **75:**242, 1973.

Kalina, R. E., and Forrest, G. L.: Proliferative retrolental fibroplasia in infant retinal vessels, Am. J. Ophthalmol. **76:**811, 1973.

Krill, A. E., and Archer, D. B.: Krill's hereditary retinal and choroidal diseases, vol. 2, New York, 1977, Harper & Row, Publishers, Inc.

L'Esperance, F. A., Jr.: Ocular photocoagulation; a stereoscopic atlas, St. Louis, 1975, The C. V. Mosby Co.

Maloney, W. F., Robertson, D. M., and Duboff, S. M.: Hereditary vitelliform macular degeneration, Arch. Ophthalmol. **95:**979, 1977.

McPherson, A., editor: New and controversial aspects of vitreoretinal surgery, St. Louis, 1977, The C. V. Mosby Co.

Merin, S., and Auerbach, E.: Retinitis pigmentosa, Surv. Ophthalmol. **20:**303, 1976.

Mizuno, K., Takei, Y., Sears, M. L., and others: Leber's congenital amaurosis, Am. J. Ophthalmol. **83:**32, 1977.

Norton, E. W. D.: The past 25 years of retinal detachment surgery, Am. J. Ophthalmol. **80:**450, 1975.

Patz, A., Fine, S., and Orth, D.: Sights and sounds in ophthalmology. Vol. 1: Diseases of the macula, St. Louis, 1976, The C. V. Mosby Co.

Reese, A. B.: Tumors of the eye, ed. 3, New York, 1976, Harper & Row, Publishers, Inc.

Roth, A. M.: Retinal vascular development in premature infants, Am. J. Ophthal. **84:**636, 1977.

Ryan, S. J., Jr.: Cystoid maculopathy in phakic retinal detachment procedures, Am. J. Ophthalmol. **76:**519, 1973.

Swartz, M., Herbst, R. W., and Goldberg, M. F.: Aqueous humor lactic acid dehydrogenase in retinoblastoma, Am. J. Ophthalmol. **78:**612, 1974.

Teeters, V. W., and Bird, A. C.: The development of neovascularization of senile disciform macular degeneration, Am. J. Ophthalmol. **76:**1, 1973.

Tolentino, F. I., Schepens, C. L., and Freeman, H. M.: Vitreoretinal disorders; diagnosis and management, Philadelphia, 1976, W. B. Saunders Co.

West, C. E., Fitzgerald, C. R., and Newell, J. H.: Cystoid macular edema following aphakic keratoplasty, Am. J. Ophthalmol. **75:**77, 1974.

Wise, G. N.: Clinical features of idiopathic preretinal macular fibrosis, Am. J. Ophthalmol. **79:**349, 1975.

Wise, G. N.: Congenital preretinal macular fibrosis, Am. J. Ophthalmol. **79:**363, 1975.

Wise, G. N.: Relationship of idiopathic preretinal macular fibrosis to posterior vitreous detachment, Am. J. Ophthalmol. **79:**358, 1975.

Woldoff, H. S., Gerber, M., Desser, K. B., and Benchimol, A.: Retinal vascular lesions in two patients with prolapsed mitral valve leaflets, Am. J. Ophthalmol. **79:**382, 1975.

Wyhinny, G. J., Apple D. J., Guastella, F. R., and Vygantas, C. M.: Adult cytomegalic inclusion retinitis, Am. J. Ophthalmol. **76:**773, 1973.

Zweng, H. C., and Little, H. L.: Argon laser photocoagulation, St. Louis, 1977, The C. V. Mosby Co.

Chapter 17

THE VITREOUS BODY

The vitreous body (pp. 36 and 90) occupies the vitreous cavity and is a transparent intraocular tissue that has the physical properties of a gel. It has a volume of about 4.5 ml. It accounts for two thirds of the volume of the eye and three fourths of the weight. Normally it fills the entire vitreous cavity, and vitreous fibrils insert into and blend with the fibrillary material of the internal limiting lamina of the retina (Fig. 17-1). There are firm attachments to the ora serrata and to the margin of the optic disk. The vitreous cortex, the outer surface, may be divided into an anterior and posterior hyaloid. The anterior hyaloid is hollowed to receive the posterior convexity of the lens, and a few fibers may extend between the anterior vitreous hyaloid and the posterior capsule of the lens. The posterior hyaloid lines the entire retina. This cortical layer contains a few large flat cells (hyalocytes) that function as connective tissue macrophages and a collagen network that extends fanlike into the central vitreous. The central vitreous contains a much finer fibrillar meshwork than the cortex. Additionally, it contains hyaluronic acid in which a large amount of water is suspended. Centrally an ill-defined area extends from the disk to the lens and contains many fewer fibrils, which in embryologic life transmitted the hyaloid vascular system (canal of Cloquet).

The vitreous body is a true physiologic and biologic gel. Disease, aging, and injury disturb the delicate factors that balance water in suspension, and the vitreous liquefies. With the loss of the gel structure fine fibers, membranes, and cellular aggregates become visible, although they are nearly transparent. With disease, blood vessels may grow from the surface of the retina or optic disk into the vitreous, and blood may fill the vitreous cavity. One of the most exciting developments in ophthalmology in the past decade has been vitrectomy, the mechanical removal of severe opacities and membranes by means of cutting, aspiration, and replacement of the cloudy vitreous with Ringer solution. The absence of vitreous seems not to damage the adjacent retina, but cataract may form.

SYMPTOMS AND SIGNS OF DISEASES

Abnormalities of the vitreous body manifest themselves by three main symptoms: (1) decreased vision from membranes or opacities ("floaters") in the vitreous; (2) visualization of material floating in the vitreous ("floaters"); and (3) flashes of light noted when the eyes move, often with the eyes closed (photopsia). The floaters occur because of visualization of cells or cellular remnants in the vitreous and may be observed in normal eyes. Photopsia arises from traction of the vitreous upon the retina and

357

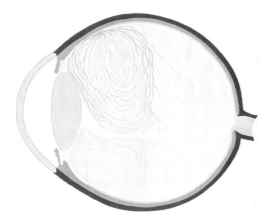

Fig. 17-1. The vitreous body. The surface of the vitreous anterior to the ora serrata is the anterior hyaloid; that adjacent to the retina is the posterior hyaloid. The anterior vitreous fibrils are oriented perpendicular to the ora serrata, and those posterior are parallel to the retina.

may be a sign of actual or impending retinal hole formation (p. 348). Additionally, shrinkage of the vitreous causes a variety of entoptic phenomena that are observed with the eyes closed or in the dark. As the eyes move, the shrunken vitreous gently bumps the retina, initiating a nervous impulse and perception of light.

The vitreous body is studied with the indirect ophthalmoscope and a convex lens so that opacities are visible against the red background of the fundus. It may be studied with a biomicroscope and either a −40 diopter lens or a −50 diopter contact lens equipped with inclined mirrors to study the ocular periphery. Gross vitreous opacities can be seen with a direct ophthalmoscope and a convex lens.

DEGENERATIONS

Liquefaction (synchysis). This degenerative condition occurs in aging, in myopia, and after injuries and inflammation of the eye. The vitreous body becomes partially or completely fluid, creating the appearance of delicate membranes or strands floating freely in the fluid. The condition arises from dehydration of the vitreous fibrillar structure, which then floats in the released water. These particles float across the visual line, impair vision, and may be extremely vexing. They are easily visible with the ophthalmoscope or slit lamp. The symptoms may be minimized by wearing of an appropriate lens for any ametropia present, but no treatment will restore the integrity of the vitreous.

Vitreous detachment. The vitreous body is firmly attached in the area surrounding the optic nerve (p. 36). With liquefaction the posterior hyaloid may be stripped from the retina and create a fluid-filled, optically empty space between the retina and the posterior surface of the vitreous body. The original site of attachment between the posterior hyaloid and the margin of the optic disk is often marked with a ring-shaped opacity. Vitreous detachment occurs most commonly in middle-aged individuals who suddenly notice a relatively large, fixed floater near the point of fixation. As the individual attempts to fix upon the floater, it darts out of the field of vision. There may be associated subjective lightning flashes (of Moore), so that with the eyes closed or in a dark room a sudden movement of the eye causes a flash of light, which results from the vitreous body striking the retina. On examination, one may see the floater in front of an optically empty space adjacent to the posterior retina. The fellow eye usually becomes involved within a few months. There is no effective treatment, although the floater tends to become less conspicuous with time.

Vitreous adhesion syndromes. Vitreous adhesion is a destructive phenomenon in which contraction of the vitreous causes traction upon the retinal areas to which it is abnormally attached. Shrinkage in the peripheral region may cause a horseshoe-shaped tear, with the flap held open by the persistent attachment of vitreous. Traction in the region of the ora serrata may be a factor in the production of peripheral retinal holes or retinal dialysis.

Hereditary degenerations. The three main forms of inherited vitreal-retinal degeneration are: (1) X chromosome–linked juvenile retinoschisis, inherited as an X chromosome–linked recessive trait; (2) hyaloideotapetoretinal degeneration of Goldmann-Favre; and (3) dominantly inherited hyaloideoretinopathy of Wagner. Additionally, vitreous degeneration is seen in hereditary degenerative myopia (p. 435), the facial-clefting syndromes, and some retinal and peripheral degenerative diseases.

X chromosome–linked juvenile retinoschisis is apparent at birth. The sensory retina in the region of the fovea centralis splits with the nerve fiber and internal limiting lamina on the inner side and with the photoreceptors and their nuclei adjacent to the pigment epithelium. Although the cause is different, the central retinal region that has a stellate lesion with radiating spokes looks similar to cystoid central retinal edema. Retinoschisis is sometimes present in the lower temporal quadrant along with veils in the vitreous. Vision gradually diminishes to the level of about 6/60 (20/200). This is probably the most common type of juvenile central retinal degeneration.

Hyaloideotapetoretinal dystrophy of Goldmann-Favre is an autosomal recessive progressive disorder in which there are vitreous veils with central and peripheral retinoschisis, tapetoretinal degeneration (p. 340), and complicated cataracts. This disorder leads ultimately to blindness.

Dominantly inherited hyaloideoretinopathy of Wagner in itself does not cause blindness. It is associated with liquefaction and destruction of the vitreous with grayish white preretinal membranes, myopia, cataracts, retinal separation, and retinal pigmentation and depigmentation. A similar condition is also found in association with cleft palate, flat facies, and epiphyseal hypoplasia.

VITREOUS OPACITIES

Many foreign substances may be suspended in the vitreous body: (1) exogenous material, such as parasites or foreign bodies, or (2) endogenous substances, such as leukocytes or erythrocytes from the blood or pigment, tumor cells, cholesterol, or calcium salts. All give rise to the symptoms of floaters and may cause a severe reduction in vision.

Muscae volitantes. These physiologic opacities are universally present. They consist of residues of the primitive hyaloidal system of vessels. They may be seen while one is viewing a brightly illuminated field, such as a cloudless sky or a pastel-shade wall. They drift in and out of the visual field and dart from the field of vision when one attempts to fixate on them directly. Some patients require reassurance about the universality of their occurrence. Correction of ametropia makes them more difficult to observe.

Hemorrhage. The moment of a retinal break may be signalled by a minute hemorrhage into the vitreous body as vitreous traction causes a tear in the sensory retina that ruptures a retinal blood vessel. The sudden shower of floaters is a signal for immediate examination to locate any retinal break and close it before a retinal separation occurs.

Bleeding into the vitreous arises from rupture of fragile new-formed blood vessels originating from the optic disk or retinal capillaries, from trauma, from inflammations, from tumors, and from rupture of a subhyaloid retinal hemorrhage secondary to a subarachnoid hemorrhage. The blood may be localized, evenly dispersed throughout the vitreous body, or distributed in sheets. In youth absorption may be rapid, but recurrent hemorrhages are followed by fibrous membranes in the vitreous body. The symptoms depend on the location of the vitreous hemorrhage. Peripheral hemorrhage causes floaters, whereas blood in the visual line causes a marked reduction in vision. Vitreous hemorrhage causes permanent visual loss because of persistent opacification, inflammation, glaucoma, siderosis, or fibrous tissue proliferation and contraction along with retinal detachment.

Vitrectomy through the pars plana (p. 30) provides a mechanical method for removal of diseased or opacified vitreous and membanes. The procedure may be complicated by additional bleeding at the time of the operation or immediately thereafter. There may be cataract formation, retinal injury or detachment, production of glaucoma, and development or worsening of rubeosis iridis.

Vitreous membranes. Vitreous membranes appear clinically as thick, rubbery, well-defined structures lining the posterior surface of a detached vitreous. They usually have a yellow-ochre appearance but are rarely brown from migrating retinal pigment epithelial cells. The membranes are composed of degenerating red blood cells and a delicate matrix of collagen. Some membranes contain phagocytic cells. Blood in the vitreous stimulates a phagocytic invasion and proliferation of fibrous vitreous membranes. The retina behind such membranes is often well preserved, although its details may be obscured by the membrane.

Asteroid hyalosis. This is a senile, mainly uniocular phenomenon that predominantly affects males, in which hundreds to thousands of stellate or discoid ("snowball") opacities are suspended throughout or in a portion of a solid vitreous. They appear creamy white when viewed with the ophthalmoscope and sparkle like Christmas ornaments in the illumination of a biomicroscope. The opacities consist of various calcium-containing lipids and appear to arise from degeneration of vitreous fibrils. They are suspended in vitreous of normal viscosity. There are no symptoms, treatment, or associated disease.

Cholesterolosis bulbi. This abnormality was known during much of the twentieth century as synchysis scintillans. However, the vitreous need not be liquefied, and the crystals may occur in the iris and retina. Cholesterol crystals occur in blind eyes along with retinal separation, may be secondary to severe ocular disease or injury, and are mainly observed in enucleated eyes. If the lens is removed, the crystals may be observed both in the anterior chamber and in the vitreous cavity.

Persistent hyperplastic primary vitreous. The primary vitreous (p. 77) is a fibrillar meshwork that bridges the area between the lens vesicle and inner wall of the optic cup and carries the hyaloid vessel system. At the 11-mm stage (see Fig. 1-45) it is invaded by mesoderm and intermingles with the elaborate vasa hyaloidea propria. The hyaloid system begins to atrophy at the 60-mm stage, and by the eighth month of gestation the process is completed, leaving only minute remnants seen as muscae volitantes.

Failure of the hyaloid artery to regress, combined with hyperplasia of the posterior portion of the vascular meshwork of the embryonic lens (tunica vasculosa lentis), produces persistent hyperplastic primary vitreous. This monocular condition occurs in full-term infants. The eye fails to develop, is smaller than the fellow eye, and the initially clear lens becomes opaque. Immediately behind the lens is a pinkish-whitish fibrous tissue mass that may vary in size from a small plaque to one entirely covering the posterior surface of the shrunken lens. The ciliary processes are elongated and seem to extend to the mass. The equator of the lens is smaller than normal. The anterior chamber is shallow. The tissue at the back of the lens is vascular, and the vessels radiate from the center. The posterior capsule may rupture, causing swelling of the lens and a secondary glaucoma. Spontaneous hemorrhages occur deep in the vitreous chamber and in the posterior chamber. Buphthalmos may develop.

The elongation of the ciliary body, the microphthalmos, the rupture of the posterior lens capsule, and spontaneous hemorrhage occurring in one eye of a full-term, normal-weight infant distinguish the condition from retinoblastoma, retrolental fibroplasia, retinal dysplasia, and congenital cataract.

Early removal of the lens is necessary to preserve the eye. Useful vision is rarely obtained; but without the surgery, the eye is destined to enucleation because of hemorrhage and lens rupture. Preferably, the lens is removed with the retrolenticular membrane by means of a suction-aspiration-cutting instrument introduced through the pars plana. Patients should be operated on as early as possible (4 to 6 weeks of age).

PROLAPSE OF THE VITREOUS

After opening or removal of the posterior lens capsule, the anterior hyaloid may herniate into the anterior chamber. The severity of the herniation varies from a delicate break in the anterior hyaloid to nearly complete filling of the anterior chamber with vitreous. If an intact anterior hyaloid adheres to the corneal endothelium, a bullous keratopathy (p. 254) develops because of failure of the corneal endothelium to maintain corneal hydration. Treatment must be directed to surgical separation of the hyaloid from the cornea. In addition, a prolapse of vitreous through the pupil may block the passage of aqueous humor from the posterior chamber to the anterior chamber (iris bombé) and cause a secondary glaucoma. This is treated mainly by pupillary dilation but may require removal of the vitreous.

Loss of vitreous at the time of intraocular surgery is a serious complication, because the interposition of vitreous between wound edges may lead to faulty healing. Additionally, the firm adhesions of the base of the vitreous to the ora serrata and peripheral retina combined with its forward displacement may cause external traction upon the retina and result in retinal separation. Ophthalmic surgeons aim to prevent such a vitreous loss by maintaining a soft eye and avoiding pressure on it. Vitreous loss is treated by means of an anterior vitrectomy to assure that no vitreous is between the wound edges and no traction is upon the vitreous base.

VITRECTOMY

Removal of the vitreous and replacement with Ringer solution (which is soon

Table 17-1. Indications for vitrectomy

  I. Persistent vitreous opacity with legal blindness
   A. Hemorrhage
   B. Vitreous amyloidosis
   C. Preretinal membranes
   D. Vitreous membranes and strands
 II. Complications of cataract extraction
   A. Vitreous touch with bullous keratopathy
   B. Pupillary block glaucoma
   C. Loss of vitreous
   D. Incarceration of vitreous in wound with traction
III. Endophthalmitis with vitreous abscess
IV. Trauma
   A. Anterior chamber reconstruction
   B. Intraocular nonmagnetic foreign bodies
 V. Complicated retinal detachments
   A. Vitreous adhesion syndromes
     1. Massive vitreous retraction
     2. Localized traction
     3. Transvitreal membranes
   B. Giant retinal tears
VI. Persistent hyperplastic primary vitreous

replaced by the body fluids) is indicated in patients with vitreous opacities causing legal blindness or in patients with complications of intraocular surgery, inflammation, trauma, or complicated retinal separations (Table 17-1). Additionally, vitrectomy is often performed as preretinal membranes are stripped from the posterior hyaloid. Many legally blind patients who benefit from the procedure are not aware of the improvement possible. However, the primary disorder causing the abnormal vitreous in such patients may have seriously damaged other ocular structures so that substitution of a clear vitreous would not improve vision.

The procedure is of no value if the retina is not functional, but cataract or severe opacification of the vitreous may make evaluation of retinal function difficult. An ideal patient is able to visualize his own retinal tree with a penlight moving against the lower eyelid (entoptic visualization). Bright-flash electroretinography should be normal. The visual-evoked potential to bright flash should be normal. The pupillary response and light projection should be normal. The anterior chamber angle and iris should be free of new blood vessels; glaucoma should not be present.

Unfortunately, ideal surgical candidates are difficult to find. Light projection is often poor, but light perception must be present. Prognosis is poor if electroretinography evokes no response. Generally, rubeosis of the iris or anterior chamber angle is a contraindication. Dense membranes attached to the retina or generalized retinal detachment is associated with a poor prognosis. Eyes becoming soft and disorganized (phthisical) respond poorly. Generally, about half of the patients respond with improvement of vision. Inasmuch as the lens may have to be removed in the course of the procedure, the procedure may not be indicated if vision is good in the fellow eye.

Successful vitrectomy requires simultaneous suction from the eye and infusion of an equal amount of Ringer solution into the eye. The flow rate is in the range of 6 ml/minute. The infusion-aspiration is combined with one of several types of

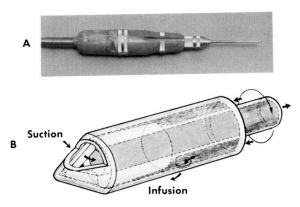

Fig. 17-2. A, The suction infusion vitreous cutter. **B,** Schematic drawing of the cutting tip. Vitreous is aspirated into the cutting port of an outer stationary tube and cut by the sharp edges of the inner rotating tube. It is then aspirated through the inner tube out of the eye. Simultaneously, the intraocular volume removed is replaced by an infusion of Ringer solution, which enters the eye through a small opening at the side of the outer tube. (Courtesy Robert Machemer.)

rotating or chopping cutters (Fig. 17-2). (Ultrasound fragmenters, although useful in lens extraction, are usually not helpful in vitrectomy.) The intraocular pressure must be maintained; a pressure of between 25 and 35 mm Hg is considered optimal. Generally, one of two approaches is used. The aphakic eye may be entered through a corneoscleral incision and through the pupil. If the lens is present, the operation is usually carried out through a scleral incision in the pars plana about 5 mm posterior to the corneoscleral limbus in the temporal quadrant slightly above or below the horizontal meridian with its long ciliary artery. A cataractous lens is removed with the same or a slightly modified instrument.

The procedure is carried out under microscopic control, with the use of a contact lens to neutralize the corneal refraction and to view the vitreous and retina. Many types of cutters have been designed to cut membranes without traction upon the retina.

The operations may be divided into those in which the anterior vitreous is removed and those in which both the anterior and posterior vitreous are removed. Preretinal membranes may be removed at the same time (Fig. 17-3). The most common complication following the operation is aggravation of a rubeosis iridis or a persistent glaucoma. The cell membranes of erythrocytes (ghost cells) may obstruct the passage of aqueous humor through the trabecular meshwork, giving rise to glaucoma. There is usually an initial vitreous hemorrhage. The cells cannot enter the anterior chamber when the lens is present; but after lens extraction and vitrectomy with rupture of the anterior hyaloid face, these cells are free to circulate throughout the eye. The condition may occur in as many as one third of the eyes having vitrectomy–lens extraction. Every effort must be made to irrigate adequately the vitreous cavity at

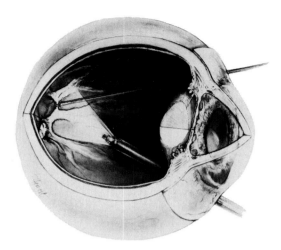

Fig. 17-3. Vitrectomy with a self-contained illuminating system together with the suction infusion vitreous cutter. The surgeon views the interior eye through a microscope and contact lens. A hook strips the preretinal membrane from the posterior hyaloid. (Courtesy Ronald G. Michels.)

the time of surgery in order to remove all of the cells.

BIBLIOGRAPHY

Gitter, K. A., editor: Current concepts of the vitreous, St. Louis, 1976, The C. V. Mosby Co.

Irvine, A. R., and O'Malley, C., editors: Advances in vitreous surgery, Springfield, Ill., 1976, Charles C Thomas, Publisher.

Knobloch, W. H.: Inherited hyaloideoretinopathy and skeletal dysplasia, Trans. Am. Ophthalmol. Soc. **73:**417, 1975.

Machemer, R.: Vitrectomy; a pars plana approach, New York, 1975, Grune & Stratton, Inc.

Michels, R. G., and Schacklett, D. E.: Vitrectomy technique for removal of retained lens material, Arch. Ophthalmol. **95:**1767, 1977.

Peyman, G. A., Huamonte, F. U., and Goldberg, M. F.: One hundred consecutive pars plana vitrectomies using the vitrophage, Am. J. Ophthalmol. **81:**263, 1976.

Tolentino, F. I., Schepens, C. L., and Freeman, H. M.: Vitreoretinal disorders; diagnosis and management, Philadelphia, 1976, W. B. Saunders Co.

Treister, G., and Machemer, R.: Results of vitrectomy, Am. J. Ophthalmol. **84:**394, 1977.

Chapter 18

THE OPTIC NERVE

The optic nerve is morphologically and embryologically a nerve fiber tract of the central nervous system. Posterior to the lamina cribrosa its axons are sheathed in a thin layer of doubled plasmalemma derived from oligodendrocytes that form the myelin covering. The nerve is composed mainly of the axons of the ganglion cells of the retina that synapse in either the lateral geniculate body (vision) or the pretectal region (pupil). In the retina the fibers are bare axons that constitute the nerve fiber layer of the retina, but behind the lamina cribrosa they are myelinated. In addition to fibers directly related to visual and pupillary activity, there are autonomic fibers and efferent fibers coursing to the retina that may have a feedback regulatory function.

The optic nerve may be divided into the following parts: (1) intraocular, (2) orbital, (3) intracanalicular, and (4) intracranial. The nonmyelinated intraocular portion contained within the scleral canal may be divided into three parts: (1) inner retinal, (2) middle choroidal, and (3) outer scleral. The retinal portion is seen ophthalmoscopically (p. 176) as the optic disk. A central depression, the physiologic cup with its edges concentric to those of the disk, is lined with glial tissue, which may be sparse, so that the ophthalmoscopist can see the perforations of the lamina cribrosa or abundant (Berg-meister) papilla (p. 78). The nerve fiber bundles are separated into columns by small fibrous astrocytes. The lamina cribrosa begins at the level of the choroidal layer, where it is composed mainly of astrocytes, collagenous connective tissue, and small blood vessels. Considerable attention is directed to the blood supply of the intraocular portion of the optic nerve because of its involvement in glaucoma and papilledema.

Within the orbit the optic nerve is surrounded by a continuation of the cranial meninges: an external dura mater, an intermediate arachnoid, and an internal pia mater, which is a thin, vascularized connective tissue sheet. The collagenous pia sheath enters the nerve and divides and subdivides myelin nerve fiber bundles into columns. The pia septa are always separated from isolated neural elements by a continuous layer of fibrous astrocytes.

Within the orbit to the level of the lamina cribrosa the pia mater provides the optic nerve blood supply. At the scleral level short posterior ciliary arteries provide the blood supply, whereas the retinal surface is supplied by the branches from the central retinal artery.

The intraocular portion of the optic nerve that is visible with the ophthalmoscope is the optic papilla, or optic disk (papilla is a misnomer inasmuch as the disk is at the same level as the retinal nerve fiber layer). The ophthalmoscopic appearance of the disk is described on p. 176. A vertical line through the center of the foveola divides the retina into nasal and temporal portions; all nerve fibers nasal to this line decussate in the optic chiasm (see Fig. 1-42). Temporal fibers do not decussate.

SYMPTOMS AND SIGNS OF OPTIC NERVE DISEASE

The main symptom of optic nerve disease is loss of vision. If fibers composing the papillomacular bundle, which arise from the fovea centralis, are involved, there is decreased visual acuity, often with disturbances of color vision. (The central retina provides some 90% of the fibers of the optic nerve [see Fig. 1-26].) Involvement of fibers anterior to their decussation in the chiasm causes defects in the vision of one eye only unless there is separate involvement of the fellow optic nerve. Interference with nerve conduction in the chiasm or in the optic tract causes visual defects in both eyes.

Conduction defects in the optic nerve cause an afferent pupillary defect (p. 286) of the involved eye.

Pain is a prominent symptom only in retrobulbar neuritis, in which there is pain deep in the orbit when the eye is moved or when pressure is applied to the globe. The pain is combined with loss of vision and a normal-appearing disk. In papilledema there is often no disturbance of vision, and the diagnosis is based on ophthalmoscopic observation. Diagnosis in optic atrophy is based on correlation of an abnormal visual field with an abnormal optic disk.

Ophthalmoscopy plays a major role in the diagnosis of optic nerve abnormalities inasmuch as the optic disk may be viewed directly. The central artery and vein are located at the center or slightly to the nasal side of the disk. A small whitish depression is located at the center of the disk (optic cup, physiologic cup), and through this one may sometimes view the lamina cribrosa. Surrounding the cup is a pink area of tissue composed of nerve fiber bundles, columns of glial cells, and capillaries, giving rise to a pink appearance. The margins of the optic disk are usually regular. However, in some normal eyes the pigment epithelium and choroid do not extend to the disk, and a crescent of sclera is visible. The transparent nerve fiber layer of the sensory retina passes over the sclera to the optic disk. In other eyes the retinal pigment epithelium terminates short of the disk so that the choroid is visible.

Attention is directed particularly to the size and shape of the physiologic cup, the surface of the disk and its color, pulsation of the central retinal vein, and the regularity of the disk. Measurement of the visual acuity and determination of the visual fields are essential to accurate diagnosis. The variety of diseases affecting the optic nerve is extremely large (p. 372), and accurate diagnosis requires a complete history, neurologic examination, evidence of systemic disease, and awareness of the large variety of diseases that may cause similar findings.

The cup-disk ratio (see Fig. 20-3) is the ratio of the horizontal width of the physiologic optic cup to the horizontal diameter of the entire disk. Its main significance is in the diagnosis and management of glaucoma. A marked difference in the ratio between the two eyes is suggestive of glaucoma.

The optic nerve head has a dual blood supply from the retinal circulation and the posterior ciliary arteries. The surface of the optic disk is nurtured mainly by retinal arteries, whereas the deeper portion derives its blood supply from the posterior ciliary arteries. Neovascularization of the surface of the optic disk occurs in diabetes mellitus, branch and central vein occlusion, obstruction or insufficiency of the internal carotid artery, pulseless disease (Takayashu disease), and similar conditions. These vessels seem to be derived from the posterior ciliary arteries rather than from the retinal blood vessels.

DEVELOPMENTAL ANOMALIES

Hyaloid artery. The hyaloid artery provides nutrition of the lens during the first 10 weeks of fetal development. After the retinal fissure closes, the hyaloid artery enters the eye at the optic cup and then atrophies. Occasionally a short stub of this vessel projects into the vitreous body from the center of the optic disk. It is usually of no clinical significance, although rarely it causes a recurrent vitreous hemorrhage. At the 100-mm stage of fetal development, the hyaloid artery forms a fusiform enlargement, the bulb, from which arise retinal vessels. The bulb is surrounded by a small mass of neurologic cells, the Bergmeister papilla, which may proliferate and slightly elevate the central portion of the disk. Failure of the hyaloid artery to regress gives rise to persistent primary vitreous (p. 360). As one gazes at a bright blue sky, the minute residual fragments of the hyaloid system (muscae volitantes, p. 359) may be seen as faint threads.

Drusen. Two types of drusen affect the intraocular portion of the optic nerve. Giant drusen are astrocytic hamartomas that usually occur with tuberous sclerosis (p. 327). Ordinary drusen are basophilic, laminated, calcareous acellular accretions. They often cause field defects but rarely affect central vision. Rarely, hemorrhage on the disk, vitreous, or adjacent retina occurs.

Drusen have been described in association with angioid streaks (p. 345) (Fig. 18-1), pigmentary degenerations of the retina (p. 340), optic atrophy, and renal dysfunction. They autofluoresce in blue

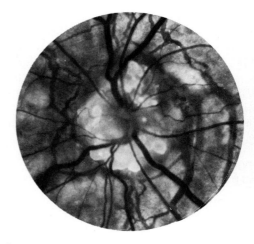

Fig. 18-1. Drusen (hyaline bodies) of the optic disk, which have been described as resembling tapioca pudding. In addition, angioid streaks are present; they are deeper than retinal vessels and do not extend to the disk.

light and fluoresce readily so that angiography is helpful in identifying their occurrence within the optic nerve. Drusen of the retinal pigment epithelium (p. 345) are not related to optic nerve drusen in any way.

Conus. In conus, or congenital crescent, the choroid and retinal pigment epithelium do not extend to the disk. A large white semilunar area of sclera is thus seen adjacent to the disk, most commonly below in the region of the primitive retinal fissure. Defective vision, hyperopic astigmatism, and visual field defects are often present. The retinal blood vessels may be displaced to the periphery of the disk or to its lower portion.

A myopic crescent, which has a similar appearance, is located at the temporal side of the disk, is not present at birth, and is associated with degenerative myopia.

Colobomas of the optic disk. Incomplete closure of the retinal fissure of the developing optic nerve gives rise to an optic

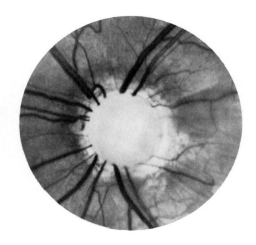

Fig. 18-2. Coloboma of the optic disk in a 19-year-old man with 6/12 (20/40) vision. This condition is transmitted as an autosomal dominant defect. Patients are particularly prone to develop a central serous choroidopathy that suggests a communication between the subretinal space and the subarachnoid space.

nerve defect that varies from a deep physiologic cup to a pit in the optic disk to a deeply excavated optic nerve (Fig. 18-2) to a defect involving the optic nerve and a coloboma of the choroid and iris (p. 290). There may be associated ocular defects and failure of the eye to develop normally. The condition is mainly unilateral, but bilateral colobomas of the optic disk occur as an autosomal dominant hereditary defect.

Pits in the optic disk are probably incomplete colobomas of the optic nerve. They are usually single and are located in the inferior temporal margin of the optic disk. The pit is darker than the surrounding tissue and is usually round or oval. The pit may be shallow or as deep as 8 mm. It is from one-eighth to one-third the size of the disk. A small central scotoma is often present. In some 30% of the patients a typical serous chorioretinopathy (p. 308) develops.

Hypoplasia of the optic disk. Failure of the axons of ganglion cells to develop or

to reach the disk gives rise to a small atrophic disk that is often, but not invariably, associated with decreased size of the optic foramen. It may be unilateral or bilateral, and vision is usually severely reduced. It occurs in otherwise normal eyes, in microphthalmos, and in hydrocephalus.

Myelinated nerve fibers. Myelination of the optic nerve begins at the optic chiasm and reaches to the lamina cribrosa at birth. Sometimes the process does not stop there but continues over the retinal surface (Fig. 18-3). Ophthalmoscopy reveals an area of white, opaque, glistening appearance with soft, feathered edges usually continuous with the optic disk.

The area of myelination involves only a small sector of the retina and does not extend beyond the second arteriolar bifurcation. The absence of pigment proliferation, the feathery edges, and the normal visual field differentiate myelinated nerve fibers from chorioretinitis. Rarely, a patch of myelinated nerve fiber is seen on the surface of the retina, and the area surrounding the optic nerve is normal. There are no symptoms or treatment.

OPTIC NEURITIS

The optic nerve may be involved in inflammatory, degenerative, or demyelinating disease any place in its course, from the ganglion cells in the retina to the synapse of these fibers in the lateral geniculate body. The causes of optic neuritis (Table 18-1) are approximately the same irrespective of the portion of the nerve involved. The main symptom is loss of visual acuity along with a central scotoma. In retrobulbar neuritis the inflammation affects the optic nerve behind the optic disk. The ophthalmoscopic appearance of the disk is normal, although optic atrophy (p. 371) may follow. If the inflammation involves the intraocular portion of the nerve, the abnormality

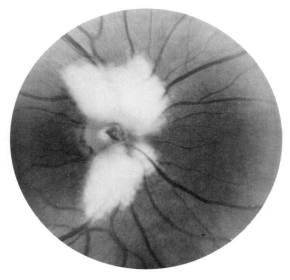

Fig. 18-3. Myelinated nerve fibers on the inner surface of the sensory retina.

Table 18-1. Some causes of optic neuritis

Infections: ocular (acute keratitis, purulent uveitis, chronic uveitis), orbital cellulitis, meningitis, encephalitis, syphilis, tuberculosis, coccidiomycosis, bacterial endocarditis
Vessels: giant cell arteritis, periarteritis nodosa, pulseless disease, arteriosclerosis
Demyelination: multiple sclerosis, acute disseminated encephalomyelitis, neuromyelitis optica (Devic disease), diffuse periaxial encephalitis (Schilder disease), diffuse cerebral sclerosis (Krabbe disease, Pelizaeus-Merzbacher syndrome, metachromatic leukodystrophy)
Toxicity: methanol, disulfiram (Antabuse), iodochlorhydroxyquin (Entero-Vioform), ethambutol, chloramphenicol, organic insecticides
Nutrition: starvation, avitaminosis (pellagra, beriberi, pernicious anemia)
Heredity: Leber's disease?
Metabolism: diabetes mellitus, thyroid disease
Miscellaneous: blood loss, lactation

is called papillitis, and inflammatory changes of the disk are evident ophthalmoscopically. When the disk and the retina are both involved, the condition is termed neuroretinitis.

Optic neuritis may be an acute or a chronic process characterized by loss of central vision and development of a central scotoma demonstrated by visual field examination (see Fig. 5-6). The loss of vision varies from a slight depression to complete loss of light perception. The loss of vision may occur abruptly over a period of a few hours, and recovery may be equally rapid. In other patients the visual decrease develops slowly. The disease is usually unilateral, but the second eye may be subsequently involved.

A similar loss of vision with a central scotoma without obvious cause may occur in edema of the central retina. In optic neuritis, however, an afferent pupillary defect (p. 286) is present. Additionally, color vision is much more severely affected in optic neuritis than in retinal edema. Directing the light from a penlight into the eye for 10 seconds does not further impair vision in optic neuritis, whereas vision is reduced two or more Snellen lines in central retinal edema.

Retrobulbar inflammation of the optic nerve in the posterior portion of the orbit where it is in close relationship with the superior rectus and medial rectus muscles gives rise to pain on movement of the eye. There may be tenderness on palpation. This pain combined with loss of central vision, a central scotoma, and the absence of any ophthalmoscopic changes often suggests the diagnosis of retrobulbar neuritis. If the causative agent is removed or if the condition occurs in the course of a demyelinating disease, the inflammation may run its course in 2 to 6 weeks, and a complete recovery ensues. However, a residue of optic atrophy affecting the papillomacular bundle may remain and be combined with decreased visual acuity.

An optic neuritis involving the intraocular portion of the optic nerve causes hyperemia and edema of the disk, known as papillitis. Central vision is reduced, and a central scotoma is present. The disk appears smaller than normal because of diminished contrast with the surrounding retina. The disk margins are obscured, and there is dilation of retinal veins. The physiologic cup is obliterated. Flame-shaped hemorrhages may occur on the surface of the disk and the adjacent retina. In severe inflammations retinal deposits occur, and these may be grouped about the fovea centralis in an oval (circinate) pattern. The edema of the disk seldom exceeds 2 diopters. With persistence of the swelling there may be glial tissue proliferation from the disk along the retinal vessels, and any subsequent atrophy is classed as "secondary" (p. 372). Ophthalmoscopically, early papilledema and early papillitis appear the same, but there is early loss of vision in papillitis. Additionally, papillitis is unilateral, the disk is never elevated more than 2 diopters, and there may be inflammatory cells in the adjacent vitreous.

The cause of optic neuritis is often impossible to determine. About 15% of patients who develop multiple sclerosis have optic neuritis as the initial event, and additional symptoms develop within 4 years. About one third of patients with established multiple sclerosis develop optic neuritis sometime in the course of their disease. Even though there is no history of visual impairment in multiple sclerosis, the visual-evoked potential (p. 104) may be impaired.

In severe inflammations of the retina or the choroid, there is often an extension of the inflammatory process to the optic nerve. The primary disease dominates the clinical picture, and the optic neuritis is of histologic interest.

Vitamin B deficiency may give rise to a bilateral optic neuritis, particularly in individuals in whom alcohol is the main source of calories. Vision improves if vitamin B is provided, even though the alcohol consumption is unrestricted. Patients with pellagra, beriberi, or pernicious anemia may have a similar bilateral optic neuritis.

Diabetic neuropathy, exophthalmic thyroid disease, severe hemorrhage, lactation, infectious diseases, and toxic substances may be associated with optic neuritis. Sinus disease and foci of infection are considered unlikely causes, although in previous years the spontaneous improvement often seen in optic neuritis was attributed to treatment of these infections.

Treatment must be directed to the cause. In those numerous instances in which a cause cannot be demonstrated, the main reliance is on systemic or retrobulbar administration of corticosteroids and vitamin B.

Pseudoptic neuritis. Either pseudoptic neuritis or pseudopapillitis is the name given to congenital abnormalities of the optic disk in which the disk margins are blurred by the heaping up of nerve fibers, accentuated by an excess of glial tissue. The disk has a dirty, grayish appearance with ill-defined margins, frequently most marked on the nasal side. It occurs commonly in hyperopic eyes. There is no interference with vision, and the blood vessels are normal. The condition is not progressive and requires no treatment.

PAPILLEDEMA

The optic nerve is surrounded by the meningeal sheath of the brain. Increased intracranial pressure may thus be transmitted to the subarachnoid space surrounding the optic nerve. The combination of increased pressure in the central retinal vein and the venous drainage of the disk and possibly blockage of axonal transport (p. 95) at the lamina cribrosa causes a passive edema of the optic nerve and disk that does not interfere with vision in its early development.

Papilledema (Fig. 18-4) begins at the superior and inferior disk margins, then involves the nasal side, and finally involves the temporal portion of the disk. The physiologic cup is obliterated, the central vessels on the surface of the optic disk are displaced forward, the retinal veins are markedly dilated, and there is nearly always a loss of spontaneous or induced venous pulsation. The swollen disk displaces the sensory retina and causes enlargement of the physiologic blind spot on perimetric measurement. Hemorrhages may occur on the surface of the disk and in the nerve fiber layer of the retina. These may break through into the vitreous body. A retinal edema develops, often combined with exudates in the central retinal region. In the early stages, visual acuity is not affected, in contrast to inflammations of the optic nerve. If papilledema persists, there is ultimate interference with visual acuity and the development of a secondary type of optic atrophy. Fluorescein angiography may be

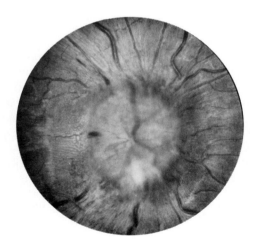

Fig. 18-4. Chronic papilledema in a 33-year-old woman with benign cerebral hypertension. Vision was 6/6 (20/20) in each eye, and the condition disappeared spontaneously.

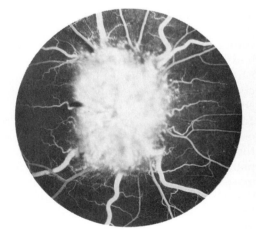

Fig. 18-5. Fluorescein angiography of papilledema. Dye shows the dilated veins and outlines the hemorrhages. There is fluorescein leakage, which never occurs from normal optic disk vessels.

used to distinguish between pseudoptic neuritis and actual pathologic involvement of the optic disk (Fig. 18-5).

The severity of papilledema is often proportionate to the increase in the intracranial pressure. However, papilledema is not an invariable accompaniment of increased intracranial pressure. When papilledema fails to develop when the intracranial pressure is increased, the subarachnoid space surrounding the optic nerve is probably not in free communication with the intracranial subarachnoid space. In similar fashion, if there is a block in the brain stem in a patient with increased intracranial pressure, there may be papilledema with low pressure demonstrated on lumbar puncture.

Brain tumors located below the tentorium are considered to be more likely to produce papilledema than those located above. Papilledema may occur in blood dyscrasias and in hypertensive cardiovascular disease. In hypertensive cardiovascular disease the occurrence of cotton-wool spots in the retina and the arteriolar constriction serve to distinguish hypertensive papilledema from that caused by intracranial neoplasms. Papilledema is seen in pseudotumor cerebri, congenital hydrocephalus, craniosynostosis (p. 246), and following head injury. Pulmonary insufficiency, particularly that associated with cystic fibrosis of the pancreas, may cause the condition.

Papilledema is usually bilateral. Marked unilateral swelling of the optic disk is most likely caused by an inflammation that involves the nerve between the globe and the exit of the central retinal vein. Vision is reduced, and a central scotoma is present. When unilateral optic atrophy occurs before a condition causing papilledema to develop, the atrophic nerve does not swell.

Treatment must be directed to the cause. Persistent papilledema is asso-

ciated with eventual loss of vision and secondary optic atrophy. Decompression procedures are indicated to preserve vision.

OPTIC ATROPHY

Optic atrophy is the end result of diseases or injuries of the optic nerve (Table 18-2) causing loss of axis cylinders and myelin sheaths. The pia septa widen to compensate for the loss, and gliosis with proliferation of astrocytes occurs. There is always an associated change in the visual field or the visual acuity, or both. If the lesion causing the optic atrophy is in the retina, an ascending optic atrophy occurs, terminating in the lateral geniculate body. Descending optic atrophy follows diseases involving optic nerve fibers anterior to their synapse in the lateral geniculate body.

The chief symptom of optic atrophy is loss of central or peripheral vision. The failure to demonstrate a defect by means of confrontation fields does not exclude a field defect that may require extremely small stimuli to detect.

The atrophy is called primary if there is no evidence of preceding edema or inflammation. It is called secondary if there is glial proliferation on the surface of the disk causing blurred, irregular disk margins. The same conditions may be responsible for either a primary or a secondary optic atrophy; the sole difference is an inflammatory or edematous disturbance of the disk that occurs before the onset of the optic atrophy.

In primary optic atrophy the number of nerve fiber bundles in the optic nerve is reduced, and there is a rearrangement of the remaining disk astrocytes into dense parallel layers across the nerve head. The disk margins are distinct; and although there appears to be a loss of capillaries, they are demonstrated on fluorescein angiography. The atrophy may be complete or partial. The ophthalmoscopic appear-

Table 18-2. Etiologic classification of optic atrophy

I.   Glaucoma
II.   Retinal ganglion cell or nerve fiber disease
A. Pigmentary degeneration of the retina
B. Chorioretinal degenerations, inflammations, atrophy
III. Inflammation
A. Demyelinating disease
B. Meningitis, encephalitis, abscess
C. Tabes dorsalis
D. Optic neuritis (Table 18-1)
E. Metastatic septicemia
IV.   Ischemia
A. Arterial occlusive disease: retina, disk, nerve, or tract
1. Arteriosclerosis
2. Giant cell vasculitis
3. Lupus erythematosus
B. Blood loss
C. "Soft" glaucoma
V.   After papilledema
VI.   Toxicity
A. Chemical: arsenic, lead, methanol, ethanol, quinine, tobacco, chloroquine, ethambutol, chloramphenicol
B. Vitamin B deficiency: beriberi, pellagra, pernicious anemia
VII. Nerve tumors: juvenile pilocytic astrocytoma ("glioma")
VIII. Compression
A. Tumors: neoplasm, aneurysm
B. Bony overgrowth: Paget disease, craniosynostosis
C. Adhesions: opticochiasmic arachnoiditis
IX.   Heredity
A. Leber disease
B. Congenital disease
C. Behr disease
D. Glucose-6-phosphate dehydrogenase deficiency—Worcester variant

ance does not parallel the severity of the visual field loss.

Glaucoma (p. 392) is the chief cause of primary optic atrophy. After central artery occlusion or after quinine poisoning, the optic nerve may appear to be waxy white, and the retinal vessels may appear as small white chords. In the late stages of retinal pigmentary degeneration the disk appears to have a yellowish waxy color with attenuated arteries crossing it. In lesions limited to the central retina the atrophy involves only the papillomacular bundle at the temporal margin of the optic disk.

Secondary optic atrophy. Secondary optic atrophy is preceded by swelling of the optic disk, arising either from papil-ledema or papillitis. Ophthalmoscopically, the disk margins appear blurred, the lamina cribrosa is obscured, and there is gliosis over the surface of the disk extending to the retina. The blood vessels may be obscured and their course distorted by scar tissue.

OPTIC NERVE TUMORS

Retinoblastomas and malignant melanomas of the choroid may extend to involve the optic nerve, but primary optic nerve tumors are uncommon.

Melanocytoma. A melanocytoma of the optic disk (Fig. 18-6) is a maximally pigmented nevus that usually occurs on the inferior temporal portion of the optic disk but may cover the entire disk. It occurs

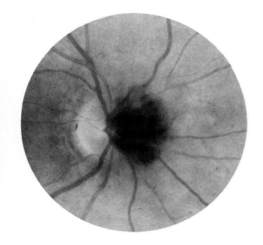

Fig. 18-6. Melanocytoma of the optic disk of the right eye.

mainly in deeply pigmented individuals and is benign with a low malignant potential.

Juvenile pilocytic astrocytoma (glioma). This tumor occurs most commonly in the first decade of life. The orbital portion of the optic nerve is solely involved in about one half of the instances, whereas the tumor is both orbital and intracranial in the remainder. Loss of vision occurs wherever the tumor is located. Additionally, orbital involvement causes proptosis. About 10% of patients with gliomas of the optic nerve have neurofibromatosis.

Meningioma. Meningiomas of the optic nerve either arise in the meninges surrounding the nerve or extend from the cranial cavity. They produce proptosis, optic atrophy, and visual loss. Neurofibromatosis is present in about 16% of the patients, who are predominantly women (5:1). Meningiomas surrounding the optic nerve and sphenoid ridge meningiomas extending into the orbit may produce supernumerary dilated shunt vessels on the surface of the optic disk (p. 337).

BIBLIOGRAPHY

Cant, J. S.: The optic nerve, St. Louis, 1972, The C. V. Mosby Co.

Dailey, M. J., Smith, J. L., and Dickens, W.: Giant drusen (astrocytic hamartoma) of the optic nerve seen with computerized axial tomography, Am. J. Ophthalmol. 81:100, 1976.

Glaser, J. S., editor: Symposium of the University of Miami and the Bascom Palmer Eye Institute. Vol. 9: Neuro-ophthalmology, New York, 1978, Harper & Row, Publishers, Inc.

Hayreh, M. S., and Hayreh, S. S.: Optic disc edema in raised intracranial pressure, Arch. Ophthalmol. 95:1237, 1977.

Quigley, H. A., and Anderson, D. R.: The histologic basis of optic disk pallor in experimental optic atrophy, Am. J. Ophthalmol. 83:709, 1977.

Riznia, R. A., and Price, J.: Recovery of vision in association with a melanocytoma of the optic disk, Am. J. Ophthalmol. 78:236, 1974.

Sacks, J. G., O'Grady, R. B., Choromokos, E., and Leestma, J.: Pathogenesis of optic nerve drusen, Arch. Ophthalmol. 95:425, 1977.

Savell, J., and Cook, J. R.: Optic nerve colobomas of autosomal-dominant heredity, Arch. Ophthalmol. 94:395, 1976.

Chapter 19

THE LENS

The lens is a transparent, avascular, biconvex structure held in position behind the pupil by the zonular fibers (p. 37). It has a single layer of epithelium beneath its anterior surface and is entirely surrounded by the capsule, the basement membrane of the epithelium. (The epithelial nuclei of the posterior capsule are located on the nuclear bow and anterior subcapsular layer after their migration to obliterate the embryonic lens vesicle.) A central nucleus formed by the oldest fibers is surrounded by a cortex that consists of more recently formed lens fibers. New lens fibers continuously form at the equator and lose their nuclei as they migrate inward and become increasingly dense. Because the lens has no blood vessels, its metabolism is mainly anaerobic. It is not inert, however, and remains relatively dehydrated, has actively multiplying cells at the equator, synthesizes lens proteins and membranes from amino acids derived from posterior chamber aqueous humor, and maintains a concentration gradient with high potassium, glutathione, ascorbic acid, and inositol levels.

The lens and the cornea are the main refracting surfaces of the eye (p. 104). The inherent elasticity of the lens causes it to become more spherical when zonular fibers relax after the ciliary muscle contracts to provide increased refractive power (accommodation, p. 105). Because of compression of mature fibers in the central nucleus, the lens gradually loses its inherent elasticity, and usually by the age of 45 years the change in shape in response to ciliary muscle contraction is too slight to provide adequate additional refractive power for near work (presbyopia, p. 437).

The lens is transparent because it contains few nuclei and because its components have approximately the same index of refraction. Any loss of transparency is called cataract, or a lens opacity, a term less ominous to a patient. Cataracts result from protein denaturation, increased molecular weights of proteins, water clefts and vesicles between lens fibers, and proliferation and migration of lens fibers and capsular epithelium.

SYMPTOMS AND SIGNS OF DISEASES OF THE LENS

The symptoms of diseases of the lens relate entirely to vision. In presbyopia, accommodation decreases and near vision fails. With cataract formation a decrease of vision for far and near may occur. In nuclear sclerosis the index of refraction of the lens increases, thus increasing the refractive power of the anterior segment. This increase may cause myopia, in which the patient unexpectedly is able to read without glasses, although the myopia reduces uncorrected distance visual acuity. Central lens opacities may split the visual axis and cause an optical defect in which two or more blurred images are formed, a monocular diplopia. Opacities caused by increased water content may migrate or disappear, improving vision. The coincidence of better vision in a patient receiving a proprietary medication to treat cataract has led to a number of cataract remedies, all ineffective.

Ophthalmoscopic examination with a convex lens (+10) and the pupil widely dilated shows cataracts as dark opacities against the red background of the fundus reflex. Appreciation of details and location of the opacity usually require examination with a biomicroscope. Examination using a penlight and a condensing lens (+20) indicates only gross abnormalities.

If the lens is dislocated, the iris loses support and becomes tremulous, the condition of iridodonesis; the anterior chamber is deeper. The catatropic image reflected from the anterior lens surface is lost. If a lens is dislocated into the vitreous body, it may be seen with the ophthalmoscope in the region to which it has gravitated as a dark sphere that magnifies the retina beneath it or as a black globule if cataractous.

DEVELOPMENTAL ANOMALIES
Coloboma

In coloboma there are one or more minute notches at the equator of the lens. The disorder occurs as a congenital absence of a segment of zonule, progressively in the course of hereditary disorders such as Marfan or Refsum disease, or after blunt trauma. The absence of a sector of zonular fibers relaxes the corresponding lens equator, which becomes a chord rather than an arc of a circle. A retinal detachment may occur. Restora-

tion of the defective zonule is not possible.

Spherophakia (microphakia)

In spherophakia the lens is small and has increased anterior and posterior curvature. The zonular fibers are easily visible with pupillary dilation, and since the iris lacks support, it is tremulous (iridodonesis). Subluxation of the lens is common, apparently because the stretched zonule weakens and breaks. Angle-closure glaucoma occurs when the small lens causes a pupillary block. The increased refractive power of the lens causes myopia.

Spherophakia may be part of an autosomal recessive syndrome (Weill-Marchesani), which is characterized by short stature, short stubby fingers, joint stiffness, and mental retardation. The syndrome is a hyperplastic form of congenital mesodermal dystrophy, in contrast to the Marfan syndrome, which is a hypoplastic defect. Treatment by sector iridectomy is directed mainly toward the prevention of a pupillary-block glaucoma.

Lenticonus

Lenticonus is a sporadic disorder, rarely inherited as an autosomal recessive characteristic, in which a cone forms at the anterior pole of the lens. Ophthalmoscopically a dark disk ("oil globule") reflex is visible in the pupillary area. Males are predominantly involved. Anterior lenticonus with familial hemorrhagic nephritis (Alport syndrome) occurs with spherophakia and cataract.

An abnormal increase in curvature of the anterior or, more commonly, of the posterior surface of the lens (lentiglobus) is usually unilateral and causes an oil-globule ophthalmoscopic appearance.

Ectopia lentis

When the lens loses the support provided by the zonular fibers, it dislocates

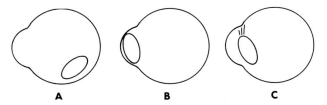

Fig. 19-1. A, Dislocation of the lens into the vitreous cavity. **B,** Dislocation of the lens into the anterior chamber, an abnormality that leads to pupillary-block glaucoma. **C,** Subluxation of the lens with the remaining zonular fibers acting as a hinge.

either into the vitreous cavity or into the anterior chamber (Fig. 19-1). If some, but not all, of the zonular fibers remain attached, they act as a hinge so that the lens is subluxated from its usual position. Examination indicates the anterior chamber to be deeper than normal and the iris to be tremulous. The symptoms are mainly optical, since absence of a major refracting element causes the eye to become markedly hyperopic and to lose the accommodation provided by the lens. Migration of a dislocated lens into the anterior chamber causes an acute secondary glaucoma. A glaucoma may occur with a lens in the vitreous cavity, although the mechanism is unclear. A subluxated lens eventually may become dislocated, but not inevitably.

The same conditions are responsible for either subluxation or dislocation: ocular contusion, particularly in an individual with latent syphilis; deliberate dislocation, an ancient (and unwise) surgical procedure (couching); and a variety of hereditary diseases. These include aniridia, Marfan syndrome (p. 561), homocystinuria (p. 494), spherophakia (Weill-Marchesani), cutis hyperelastica (Ehlers-Danlos), proportional dwarfism, oxycephaly, Crouzon disease, Spengel deformity, and Sturge-Weber syndrome. Rarely, an autosomal recessive defect causes ectopia lentis without other somatic changes.

Spectacles or contact lenses are used to correct the optical defect. Lens extraction is difficult, complications are common, and the visual results are often poor.

Marfan syndrome. The Marfan syndrome (p. 561) (arachnodactyly, dystrophia mesodermalis hypoplastica) is a widespread abnormality of connective tissue transmitted as an autosomal dominant defect. Ectopia lentis occurs in many cases. The lens is often subluxated upward and temporally so that its equator can be seen in the pupil. Severe myopia is common. Hypoplasia of the iris, miosis, and anterior chamber anomalies (see Fig. 29-1) may be present. The systemic manifestations include aortic dilation, dissecting aneurysms of the aorta, muscular underdevelopment, femoral and diaphragmatic hernias, and multiple skeletal defects, particularly arachnodactyly (spider fingers).

Homocystinuria. Homocystinuria (p. 494) is a widespread autosomal recessive abnormality characterized by dislocation of the lens, sometimes by mental retardation, and by the excretion of an excessive amount of homocystine in the urine. The latter defect is qualitatively detected by a cyanide nitroprusside test of the urine; cystinuria and homocystinuria are differentiated by paper electrophoresis. Excessive amounts of homocystine in the urine result from a deficiency in the enzyme cystathionine synthetase, which converts homocystine and serine to cystathionine.

Ectopia lentis is progressive, and the dislocated lens commonly causes a pupillary-block glaucoma. Myocardial infarction, stroke, and other manifestations of arterial or venous thrombosis are common. Other signs include fair hair and skin, skeletal abnormalities, and malar flush. Many clinical features suggest Marfan syndrome, but demonstration of the inborn error of metabolism distinguishes the two conditions. Therapy with a low-methionine diet, folate, and pyridoxine to reduce blood and urine homocystine levels seems to have no clinical effect other than occasional behavioral improvement.

LENS-INDUCED OCULAR DISEASE

In addition to the glaucoma resulting from deformities or displacement of the lens (p. 375), secondary glaucoma may result from hypermaturity of the lens (phacolytic glaucoma) or from rapid swelling of the lens (phacogenic glaucoma). Rupture of the lens capsule may be followed by uveitis; or there may be systemic hypersensitivity to lens protein after an extracapsular lens extraction, so that liberation of lens protein in the fellow eye with cataract removed causes a severe intraocular inflammation (endophthalmitis phacoanaphylactica).

Phacolytic glaucoma. In some eyes with hypermature cataract, large mononuclear phagocytes filled with lens material obstruct the trabecular meshwork, causing a secondary open-angle glaucoma intractable to medical treatment. The possibility of this glaucoma leads surgeons to remove cataracts before they become hypermature even though other ocular diseases may preclude restoration of good vision.

Phacogenic glaucoma. A rapid swelling of the lens follows hydration of lens fibers in senile intumescent cataract and also follows either surgical or accidental rupture of the lens capsule. A secondary an-gle-closure glaucoma may ensue, particularly if the anterior chamber is already shallow. The glaucoma must first be controlled medically, and then the lens must be removed.

Lens-induced uveitis. Accidental traumatic rupture of the lens capsule liberates lenticular protein within the eye. Although lens proteins are relatively poor antigens, uveitis, sometimes complicated by glaucoma, may develop. Mutton-fat keratic precipitates, posterior synechiae, and, rarely, a cyclitic membrane form. Treatment consists of lens extraction and corticosteroid administration. Sometimes after extracapsular cataract extraction the eyes appear to be sensitized to lens protein. Extracapsular lens extraction with retention of lens material in the second eye then may cause an endophthalmitis (endophthalmitis phacoanaphylactica).

Retention of the lens nucleus or of fragments of the nucleus in the vitreous cavity after extracapsular lens extraction causes a severe uveitis. The material must be removed from the eye by means of vitrectomy.

CATARACT

A cataract is any opacity in the crystalline lens. Acquired cataract is a common disorder. In the Framingham, Massachusetts study, 15% of persons aged 52 to 85 years had cataracts that reduced their visual acuity to 6/9 (20/30) or less. Some 300,000 to 400,000 cataract extractions are done annually in the United States, and it is estimated that 5 to 10 million individuals become visually disabled each year because of cataract. Patients who refuse surgery for operable cataracts constitute the second largest group of blind individuals in the United States.

No classification of cataract is entirely satisfactory. Most cataracts can be loosely described as congenital, senile, traumatic, or secondary to a systemic or ocular disorder (Table 19-1). The most signifi-

Table 19-1. Etiologic classification of cataract

I. Eye otherwise healthy and no systemic disease
    A. Nearly all senile cataracts
    B. Most cataracts in adults
    C. Many hereditary and congenital cataracts
II. Cataract combined with other ocular disorders but no systemic abnormalities
    A. Congenital and hereditary abnormalities (cyclopia, colobomas, microphthalmia, aniridia, persistent primary vitreous [retained hyaloid vasculature], heterochromia iridis)
    B. Acquired defects and delayed hereditary abnormalities
        1. Miscellaneous ocular diseases (glaucoma, uveitis, retinal separation, pigmentary degeneration of retina, myopia, ocular neoplasms)
        2. Oculopathy of prematurity (cataracts develop at age 3 years)
        3. Toxicity (corticosteroids systemically or topically, ergot, naphthalene, dinitrophenol, triparanol [MER-29], topical anticholinesterase, chlorpromazine)
        4. Ocular trauma
            a. Contusion (Vossius ring [pigment on anterior capsule], posterior subcapsular cataract)
            b. Laceration
            c. Retained intraocular foreign body (iron: siderosis; copper: chalcosis)
            d. Electromagnetic radiation
                (1) Infrared (iris absorption with heat coagulation of underlying lens, also true exfoliation of lens capsule)
                (2) Microwaves (focused high energy, a heating effect)
                (3) Ionizing radiation (cataractogenic dose varies with energy and type, younger lens more vulnerable)
            e. Anterior segment necrosis after retinal detachment surgery
III. Cataract and systemic disorders (associated ocular defects common)
    A. Generalized
        1. Embryopathies (induced in utero)
            a. Maternal infection (rubella first trimester of pregnancy [associated deafness and heart disease], other viruses [cytomegalovirus, mumps, vaccinia, variola, poliomyelitis possible], toxoplasmosis, syphilis)
            b. Maternal drug ingestion, radiation
            c. Chromosomal abnormality (Down syndrome)
        2. Marfan syndrome (arachnodactyly, ectopia lentis, mesodermal hypoplasia)
        3. Mandibulo-oculofacial dyscephaly ("bird face")
        4. Retinal pigment epithelium degenerations (Laurence-Moon-Biedl: retinitis pigmentosa, obesity, polydactyly, hypogenitalism, deafness, ataxia, oligophrenia)
        5. Systemic infections causing uveitis with complicated cataract
    B. Cutaneous
        1. Atopic dermatitis (15 to 25 years of age)
        2. Rothmund syndrome (onset 3 to 6 months)
        3. Incontinentia pigmenti (Werner) (often with uveitis)
        4. Congenital ichthyosis or ectodermal dysplasia
        5. Siemen syndrome
    C. Metabolic
        1. Diabetes mellitus (growth-onset diabetes)
        2. Galactosemia (usually shortly after birth: transferase or kinase deficiency)
        3. Lowe syndrome (oculocerebrorenal syndrome)
        4. Hypocalcemia (with tetany)
        5. Fabry disease
        6. Refsum disease
    D. Neurologic
        1. Hepatolenticular degeneration (sunflower cataract)
        2. Spinocerebellar ataxia, oligophrenia (Marinesco-Sjögren)
        E. Muscular
            1. Myotonic dystrophy (20 to 30 years of age)

Table 19-1. Etiologic classification of cataract—cont'd

   F. Osseous
      1. Mandibulofacial dysostosis
      2. Osteitis fibrosa and skin pigmentation
      3. Stippled epiphysis
      4. Oxycephaly
   G. Chromosomal abnormalities
      1. Down syndrome
      2. 13-15 trisomy
      3. Cockayne syndrome

Table 19-2. Methods of classifying cataract

   I. According to age at onset
     A. Congenital
     B. Infantile
     C. Juvenile
     D. Adult
     E. Senile
  II. According to location of opacity in lens
     A. Nuclear
     B. Cortical
     C. Capsular: posterior or anterior (rare)
     D. Subcapsular: posterior or anterior (rare)
 III. According to degree of opacity present
     A. Immature: transparent lens fibers are present
     B. Intumescent: swelling of lens with fluid clefts
     C. Mature: entire lens has become opaque
     D. Hypermature: liquefaction of the opaque lens fiber occurs (morgagnian cataract)
     E. After-cataracts: capsular remains after lens has been removed
 IV. According to rate of development
     A. Stationary
     B. Progressive
  V. On basis of biomicroscopic appearance
     A. Lamellar
     B. Coralliform
     C. Punctate and many others
 VI. On basis of etiology (Table 19-1)

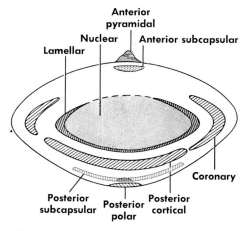

Fig. 19-2. Locations of various cataracts.

cant clinical points include: (1) severity of visual impairment; (2) whether visual improvement will follow surgery if required; and (3) whether a systemic disease is present and, if present, whether it is related to the development of the cataract. Many methods of classifying cataract are used (Table 19-2).

Acquired cataract

Acquired cataracts include those that occur sporadically as a result of toxins, systemic disease, injury, damage from intraocular inflammation, and aging. Many abnormalities cause characteristic morphologic changes that may be distinguished by biomicroscopic examination (Fig. 19-2).

Symptoms. The chief symptom of acquired cataract is a gradual decrease of vision that is not associated with pain or inflammation of the eye. Double vision in one eye (monocular diplopia) may be caused by the lens opacity splitting light bundles, but this disappears with further decrease in vision.

Vision is often better with dilation of the pupil and in dim illumination. Posterior subcapsular cataracts involve the visual line, and often vision is markedly reduced in bright light. Patients may complain of spots in the visual field that, unlike those arising from vitreous floaters, remain fixed and do not dart about with movements of the eye. In nuclear cataracts there is often an increase in the refractive power of the lens, so that patients are able to read without glasses.

Examination. Examination of the lens with the ophthalmoscope may indicate a gross opacity filling the pupillary aperture or an opacity silhouetted against the red background of the fundus. A nuclear opacity is located centrally and usually appears larger than a posterior subcapsular opacity. A peripheral cortical opacity gives rise to the appearance of irregular spokes with a clear center. Dilation of the pupil is necessary to examine the lens adequately.

Ocular examination is particularly directed toward finding evidence of injury or inflammation to account for the lens opacity. Roentgenographic examination to demonstrate a metallic foreign body is indicated if there is a history of ocular injury followed by lens opacity. General physical examination and laboratory studies seldom suggest the cause. The main differential diagnosis involves aging, toxins, diabetes mellitus, or other systemic disorders such as hypocalcemia, myotonic dystrophy, or skin disease. Nonspecific senile types of cataract occur more commonly in patients with diabetes mellitus than in others.

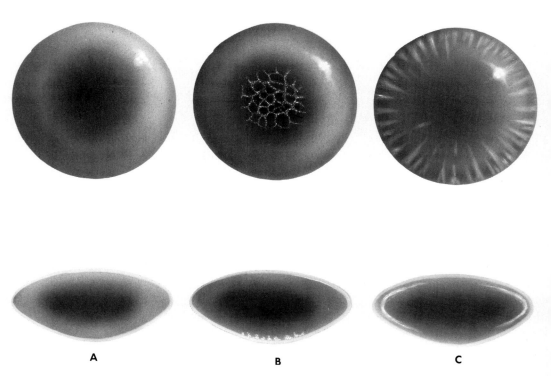

Fig. 19-3. Appearance of various types of senile cataracts. **A,** Nuclear sclerosis. **B,** Nuclear sclerosis and posterior subcapsular cataract. **C,** Nuclear sclerosis and anterior and posterior cortical cataracts.

Special types. A large variety of acquired types of cataract have been described: senile, toxic, traumatic, diabetic, and hypocalcemic. Some have a characteristic appearance in their early stages, but with progression it is not possible to distinguish the various types.

In the Framingham, Massachusetts study, individuals with senile cataract were more likely to have increased serum phospholipid and high nonfasting blood glucose levels, as well as high blood pressure. As expected, aging-related factors were also present.

With aging, the proteins of lens fibers increase in molecular weight, and the lens gradually becomes less transparent. Opacities associated with aging may be divided into those involving the nucleus, the cortex, and the posterior capsule (Fig. 19-3). Often changes occur concurrently in these regions.

Nuclear, or hard, cataract is an accentuation of the normal condensation process in the lens nucleus. It becomes evident at about the age of 50 years and progresses slowly until the entire nucleus is opaque. Often the earliest change is an increase in the index of refraction of the lens so that there is a decrease in hyperopia or an increase in myopia. The gradual progress of this lens opacity may be associated with improved near vision. This may lead the patient to believe erroneously that vision is permanently improved—"second sight." However, as the opacity progresses, vision for both near and far gradually deteriorates. Inasmuch as the opacity is located in the visual line, the vision may vary with the pupillary diameter.

A cortical, or soft, cataract involves the lens cortex. Lens fibers are either opaque or hydrated, giving rise to clefts that run radially to create a spokelike pattern. These opacities tend to involve the equatorial region initially. They may become very marked without interference with vision. Gradually, however, the opacities involve the central area, causing decreased visual acuity.

A posterior subcapsular opacity is the most common type of senile change. It develops gradually and causes the posterior capsule to appear as beaten gold. Inasmuch as the visual axis is obscured early, the opacity causes a disproportionate loss of vision for its density and size.

Toxic cataract. Permanent and transient lens opacities may be produced in experimental animals, particularly weanlings, by various sugars, electrolyte disturbances, and endocrine and dietary deficiencies. For the most part, the correlation with human cataract is remote, although galactose cataract (p. 390) occurs in infants (as well as the susceptible experimental animal) who, because of absence of the enzymes for their galactose metabolism, accumulate high levels of galactose alcohol (dulcitol) in their lenses.

The corticosteroids systemically administered in high doses for long periods, especially in arthritis patients, cause posterior subcapsular opacities in susceptible individuals. Prolonged topical administration has the same effect with considerable individual variation. The opacity begins at the posterior pole as a highly refractile, multicolored dot that interferes with vision. Peripheral cortical opacities then develop, but vision is seldom so decreased as to require cataract extraction. Patients who have ulcerative colitis or asthma and receive quantities of the drugs comparable to the quantities received by arthritis victims seldom develop lens opacities.

Miotic drugs (p. 119), particularly anticholinesterases, used topically to treat glaucoma (p. 400) or accommodative esotropia (p. 420), produce anterior subcapsular opacities. These seldom progress, and they can be distinguished from aging changes only by prospective studies.

High doses of chlorpromazine produce a star-shaped figure composed of granular deposits in the anterior capsular region of the lens. There are similar deposits in the cornea and an associated photosensitivity.

Traumatic cataract. Contusion of the eye may cause a posterior subcapsular cataract many months after the original injury, even though the lens capsule has not been grossly injured.

Rupture of the lens capsule invariably causes a cataract. If the opening is microscopic in size, there may be a minute linear opacity corresponding to the opening. More commonly, however, an initial posterior subcapsular opacity extends forward to involve the entire lens, and grayish lens material extrudes into the anterior chamber. An inflammation of varying severity results, and in individuals less than 25 years of age the entire lens may be autolyzed. In patients older than 25 years the nucleus remains and causes a continuing inflammation.

The effects of a foreign body within the lens depend on its size and rate of oxidation. Glass and plastics are well tolerated. Iron and copper cause characteristic opacities.

Diabetic cataract. Diabetic cataract is an uncommon type of lens opacity that occurs in poorly controlled growth-onset diabetes mellitus in the second decade of life. The opacity closely resembles "sugar" cataracts in experimental animals. The opacities are bilateral and cortical, predominantly involve the anterior and posterior subcapsular region, and consist of minute dots of varying size, usually called "snowflakes." A diabetic cataract may go to complete opacity (maturity) in less than 72 hours.

Adults with diabetes mellitus have a slightly earlier onset of senile cataract than do nondiabetic patients. Surgery is usually uncomplicated, but retinopathy may impair vision.

Sugar cataracts have been extensively studied in experimental animals (p. 90). This type of cataract follows an increase in sugars (or pentoses given experimentally) in the lens. The excess sugar within the lens is reduced by aldose reductase (p. 90) to its alcohol (glucitol is glucose alcohol, also called L-sorbitol; dulcitol or galcitol is galactose alcohol). The lens capsule is relatively impermeable to sugar alcohols. Because of the excess sugar alcohol (polyol) the lens imbibes water, causing an osmotic imbalance. Eventually increased sodium and decreased potassium levels and decreased glutathione levels lead to cataract formation. Topical administration of aldose reductase inhibitors prevents the cataract in rats.

In some strains of mice a hereditary deficiency of sodium-potassium adenosinetriphosphatase (Na-K ATPase) with failure of the cation pump causes cataract formation.

Medical treatment. No treatment will restore the denatured protein of the cataractous lens to its original transparent state. However, lens vacuoles may at times disappear spontaneously and give rise to a transient improvement in vision. Because of this spontaneous improvement, many remedies have been used; but there is no evidence that they are of value.

During the period of decreasing vision, frequent and accurate refraction will maintain vision at the best possible level. When minute opacities involve the axial area, dilation of the pupil by means of a weak solution of phenylephrine (Neo-Synephrine 2.5%) or 2% homatropine may provide visual improvement. Pupillary dilation must not be used in patients with a shallow anterior chamber in whom there is danger of precipitating angle-closure glaucoma (p. 404).

Surgical treatment. Cataract extraction is indicated in the following instances: (1) when the opacity has advanced to the stage where a visual defect interferes with an individual's vocation or avocation, and (2) if the lens threatens to cause a secondary glaucoma or uveitis.

Vision is evaluated in terms of both eyes with the best possible correcting lenses worn. As long as there is adequate vision in one eye, surgery is seldom indicated in the poorer eye. Cataract extraction is often not recommended if either eye has corrected vision of better than 6/24 (20/80). There are many exceptions, however, and the vision required by an active middle-aged individual may be quite different from that required by a sedentary elderly person.

Many surgeons advocate surgery for advanced monocular cataract in active individuals irrespective of the vision in the opposite eye. Binocular vision may be restored postoperatively by means of a contact lens (p. 442) on the operated eye or, less commonly, by an intraocular lens.

The cataract may cause glaucoma because of increased size or release of a toxic fluid in hypermaturity that causes macrophages to block the trabecular meshwork. Any opening in the lens capsule releases material into the anterior chamber that causes a uveitis and sometimes a secondary glaucoma.

Cataract surgery is usually contraindicated in any disease of the anterior or posterior ocular segment that has destroyed vision and makes lens extraction unlikely to provide improvement in vision. If light projection, color vision, and two-point discrimination are faulty, cataract extraction probably will not materially improve vision.

An acquired cataract may be removed in one of two ways: (1) by removal of the entire lens, including its capsule (intracapsular extraction); or (2) by removal of the anterior capsule, nucleus, and cortex, with retention of the posterior capsule (extracapsular extraction). The intracapsular procedure has been the method of choice for more than 40 years. In the past decade the development of instruments to simultaneously infuse and aspirate fluid from the eye at the same rate combined with mechanical dissolution of the lens material has stimulated renewed interest in extracapsular extraction.

Adequate anesthesia and ocular muscle immobility (akinesia) are the most important factors in successful surgery. Akinesia of the orbicularis oculi muscle is produced by means of a block of the facial nerve just anterior to the tragus or by infiltration of the muscle fibers with a local anesthetic. An anesthetic is also injected into the muscle cone and causes anesthesia of the eye (retrobulbar injection) and akinesia of the extraocular muscles. Following the retrobulbar injection, massage of the globe for 5 minutes reduces the intraocular pressure and decreases the danger of vitreous loss. General anesthesia is often used, particularly if an intraocular lens is implanted.

For the customary *intracapsular lens extraction,* an incision is made at the superior corneoscleral limbus. A portion of the iris may be removed, sparing the sphincter (peripheral iridectomy), or the peripheral and central portions of the iris may be excised (sector iridectomy). A sector iridectomy causes a cosmetic defect. Although the peripheral iridectomy provides a cosmetically pleasing eye with a round pupil, it may be associated with more postoperative complications.

The zonular fibers supporting the lens may be dissolved with the proteolytic enzyme alpha-chymotrypsin in individuals less than 60 years of age. In patients older than 60 years the zonule may be stripped by use of counterpressure. Preferences for surgical management vary widely among surgeons. The lens capsule and underlying lens substance are frozen to a low-temperature probe, and the entire lens is lifted from the eye. Lens forceps may be used, but this instrument is used less commonly than previously. The incision is closed carefully with fine sutures; as many as 10 or 12 are currently used. With careful wound closure, the patient is permitted out of bed within a few hours after surgery. Systemic complications are rare.

In the *extracapsular extraction* a large portion of the anterior lens capsule is excised, and the lens nucleus is removed from the eye. The incision at the corneoscleral limbus is smaller than that used for intracapsular extraction. The remaining cortex is then removed by irrigation, which is sometimes facilitated by suction. A secondary membrane (after-cataract) consisting of posterior capsule and sometimes proliferated anterior capsule and retained lens cortex occurs commonly (33%), so that many surgeons routinely open the posterior capsule at the time of the initial procedure. The advantageous separation between the anterior chamber and the vitreous cavity by the posterior capsule is lost by this opening.

In general, a soft (cortical) cataract is best removed by one of the variants of mechanical disruption of the lens and aspiration. The procedure requires a small (3-mm) incision, and the patient may leave the hospital promptly. The procedure is particularly useful in cataracts, whatever type, that occur before the age of 50 years and have no nuclear sclerosis. After 50 years of age the degree of sclerosis of the nucleus determines whether or not the procedure is used. The procedure is difficult and tedious in patients with hard amber nuclei. It is contraindicated in glaucoma, in corneal endothelial disease, in subluxated lenses where the vitreous humor is firm, and after severe uveitis. Irritation from nuclear remnants that accidentally fall into the vitreous may necessitate a vitrectomy. In-

sertion of an intraocular lens requires a larger incision than that used in phacoemulsification and related procedures. Damage to the corneal endothelium by vibration of a sclerotic nucleus may cause a severe bullous keratopathy (p. 270).

Removal of the lens causes a marked reduction of the refractive power of the eye (aphakia, p. 438) and impairment of the efficiency of the eye as an optical instrument. The most evident change is a severe hyperopia that cannot be neutralized by accommodation, because the lens is absent. Additionally, spherical and chromatic aberration and magnification of retinal images are increased. Irregular closure and faulty position of the incision may cause astigmatism. The larger pupillary aperture caused by a sector iridectomy causes increased size of diffusion circles on the retina and diminution of the depth of focus. Additionally, the correcting lenses worn in aphakia are maximally effective only when the patient looks through the optical center of the lens. With spectacle correction there is an annular area of blindness from 30° to 60° in the field of peripheral vision, and objects dart in and out of this field of vision. Because of the magnification, patients have a moderately difficult time of adjustment to the glasses, particularly in walking. Conversely, because of the magnification, they are frequently able to read unusually small print. Since accommodation is absent, it is necessary to wear bifocal or trifocal lenses; and because of the decreased depth of focus, the range of clear vision for near is limited. Usually the refraction following a cataract extraction does not stabilize for several months, and a final type of lens is not prescribed until then.

Contact lenses in aphakia. Many of the optical disturbances caused by aphakia may be minimized, although, not eliminated, with contact lenses. Because of the interruption of the nerve supply by the corneal incision, contact lenses appear to be somewhat better tolerated by cataract patients than by other patients. Conversely, many patients are unable to wear contact lenses successfully because of age, hemiplegia, parkinsonism, rheumatoid arthritis, or mental deterioration.

Prolonged-wear soft contact lenses may be used in patients who are unable to insert and remove hard contact lenses. It is not possible to use the lenses in patients who have glaucoma, dry eyes, vitreous touching the cornea, or more than 3 diopters of astigmatism. Patients are fitted after all sutures are removed and the refraction has become stable.

About one quarter of the eyes develop superficial vascularization that extends 1 or 2 mm into the cornea, usually superiorly. In patients with preexisting corneal vascularization, a soft contact lens aggravates the condition or causes vessels not previously carrying blood (ghost vessels) to carry blood. Poor fitting may cause epithelial edema, which may be corrected by more accurate fitting.

Inasmuch as soft contact lenses do not correct astigmatism, this must be corrected by means of spectacles. Additionally, since the aphakic eye cannot accommodate, this must also be provided by correction.

Intraocular lens implantation. Insertion of a clear acrylic lens in the pupillary space at the time of lens extraction is popular. The lenses are currently (1978) limited to experimental use by qualified investigators in fully informed patients. When first introduced (1949), the lenses were not fixed in the pupillary space and were easily dislocated. Subsequent lenses (1960) touched the corneal endothelium and caused a bullous keratopathy, which necessitated their removal. Present lenses seem to avoid these problems, but long-term results are unknown. Possible problems include loss of trans-

parency of the plastic or dissolution of the supporting loops or nylon suture used with some lenses for support. Operations for retinal separation are more difficult because of poorer visualization of the peripheral fundus through an intraocular lens.

Inasmuch as the long-term characteristics of the plastics are unknown, patients should be more than 70 years of age and unlikely to use a contact lens successfully. An intraocular lens is used in some individuals who have an advanced cataract in one eye and good vision in the fellow eye in order to provide binocular vision.

The lenses are contraindicated in patients who have only one eye with potentially useful vision, in patients who have axial myopia of more than 7 diopters, and in patients who have had a poor operative result in the fellow eye. Corneal endothelial dystrophy is a contraindication, as is proliferative diabetic retinopathy, glaucoma, or retina detachment in the fellow eye. Patients require careful postoperative management and must be available for convenient follow-up.

Two main types of lenses are used: (1) anterior chamber lenses and (2) pupillary lenses (Fig. 19-4). The second type may be held in place by the peripheral lens capsule and proliferating connective tissue from the posterior iris after extracapsular lens extraction. Alternatively, it may be sutured to the iris or held in position by means of loops in front and back of the iris.

A wide variety of shapes and sizes are available. The refractive power of the lens is determined by measurement of the refractive power of the cornea with a keratometer and by measurement of the length of the eye by ultrasonography. Less desirable is an estimate based on the power of the correcting lens used before cataracts developed.

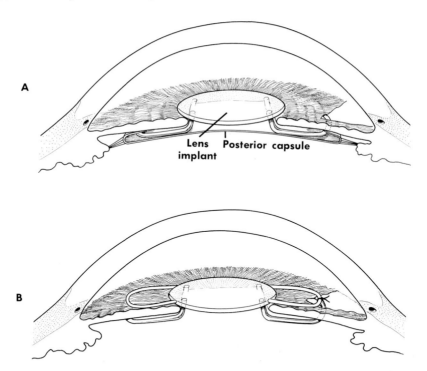

Fig. 19-4. Intraocular lens. **A,** The anterior chamber lens may be held in position by two loops in the capsular bag after extracapsular cataract extraction. **B,** Four loops bridge the iris for support following intracapsular cataract extraction. The upper loops are tied together through the iridectomy opening.

The major complication of intraocular lenses relates to mishaps in which the corneal endothelium remains in contact with the lens, causing bullous keratopathy. Furthermore, insertion of the lens requires an additional operative step that may increase operative complications. Cystoid central retinal edema may be more common after a lens is inserted than when no lens is inserted.

The use of such lenses in children is debatable, because over the next 60 or 70 years the implant lens may become opaque. However, I believe that, although the lenses are not indicated in children with bilateral congenital cataracts, they are indicated in some youths with severe lacerations of one eye that require reconstruction of the anterior segment and lens removal.

Complications. Cataract extraction may be associated with many complications that interfere with a successful result. At the time of surgery the lens capsule may rupture before the lens is removed, and the operation is converted to an inadvertent extracapsular extraction. Unlike the planned extracapsular extraction, the anterior capsule is removed inadequately or not at all. The cortex freed with capsule rupture may cause uveitis and may lead to the complications of intraocular inflammation.

Pyogenic bacteria introduced into the eye at the time of surgery cause a panophthalmitis; fungi cause an endophthalmitis.

Loss of vitreous humor at the time of surgery previously caused both immediate and delayed complications, ranging from faulty wound closure to updrawn pupil to late retinal detachment. Apposition of the vitreous face to the corneal endothelium may give rise to localized areas of corneal edema combined with cystoid central retinal edema (p. 336), which interferes with vision. Many of the complications caused by loss of vitreous or apposition with the cornea have been eliminated by vitrectomy.

Faulty apposition of the wound edges may prevent the reforming of the anterior chanber and thus produce peripheral anterior synechiae and an angle-closure type of secondary glaucoma. Loss of the anterior chamber 7 to 14 days after lens extraction may be caused by a fistula or an internal cyclodialysis. The trabecular meshwork may be damaged and consequently produce glaucoma. Faulty wound healing may cause inclusion of epithelium in the anterior chamber, leading to epithelium covering the surface of the iris and the posterior surface of the cornea. This complication may be noted many weeks after the cataract operation when there is an onset of tearing of the eye. Treatment is often unsatisfactory.

Cystoid central retinal edema (p. 307) is an abnormality in which the capillaries nurturing the central retina become permeable to large molecules and cause edema of the fovea centralis and surrounding retina. The edema may occur after apparently uncomplicated lens extraction without apparent cause. It occurs somewhat more frequently after lens implantation than after intracapsular lens extraction and is least common in extracapsular extraction. There is no effective treatment, but the edema often resorbs spontaneously 6 to 12 months after its onset.

Congenital cataract

At least 90% of the general population have minute nonprogressive lens opacities that do not impair vision. Many hereditary cataracts are recognized by their characteristic morphology, and their main clinical importance lies in not confusing them with those caused by trauma or disease. These opacities consist of multiple, fine, irregularly shaped opacities in the central or peripheral areas of the lens. The diagnosis is based on their morphologic characteristics as seen with a biomicroscope.

Attention is directed to cataracts severe enough to impair vision. The questions that arise include: (1) Does the opacity involve one or both eyes? (2) Does the visual decrease prevent normal schooling? (3) Are there associated ocular defects? (4) Are there associated systemic defects? (5) Are the lens opacities progressive? (6) What is the cause?

General physical examination shortly after birth should indicate a red fundus reflex, which indicates whether the lens opacity occurred before or after birth. If a red fundus reflex is not seen with the ophthalmoscope, careful examination should be done with the pupils dilated with a mixture of 2-5% phenylephrine and 0.5% cyclopentolate. Ocular examination of infants may be facilitated by allowing a hungry baby to nurse or by immobilization by wrapping in a sheet. The fundus may be studied through an infant-size goniolens (Koeppe) that also permits visualization of the lens and anterior chamber angle.

Monocular cataract seldom requires treatment. On occasion lens extraction may be required because of lens-induced glaucoma or intraocular inflammation, but sensory amblyopia usually limits corrected vision to 6/60 (20/200) or less.

Visual acuity is difficult to assess in infants, but if opticokinetic nystagmus can be elicited, visual acuity likely will be more than 6/18 (20/60) and surgery will not be required. If retinal blood vessels can be seen with an ophthalmoscope with the pupils dilated, surgery will likely not be required.

Nystagmus, retinal or choroidal abnormalities, microphthalmia, and strabismus reduce the likelihood of good postoperative vision. However, dense cataracts are often removed despite associated ocular defects inasmuch as the 6/60 (20/200) corrected vision is far better than preoperative vision. Conversely, corrected vision of 6/6 (20/20) with aphakia is not more effective than 6/18 (20/60) vision with the lens and accommodation intact.

Systemic defects should be identified and the progression of the lens opacity observed. The medical and ocular history of other members of the family should be obtained. A family study is most rapidly initiated by examining the eyes of those accompanying a young patient. Hearing should be tested. The occurrence of supernumerary fingers and toes, gross abnormality in the development of the bones of the face or skull, or disproportion of the bones of the extremities should be noted. Flaccidity of the muscles should be investigated. Evidence of mental retardation and delayed physical development should be sought, particularly with reference to delayed psychomotor development such as failure to sit, stand, or talk at anticipated age levels.

Laboratory studies may include patient and maternal studies for antibodies against rubella, cytomegalovirus, toxoplasmosis, and syphilis. Pharyngeal secretions in the affected infant may contain the rubella virus (and infect susceptible individuals in waiting rooms and hospitals). Some 0.5% to 2.0% of newborn infants demonstrate the typical inclusions of cytomegalovirus disease, but only some 0.03% are affected. Galactosemia is excluded by appropriate enzyme testing (p. 390). A reducing substance may be present in the urine. Commercial test tapes are specific for glucose and do not indicate other reducing substances in the urine. Homocystinuria may cause cataract, although it more commonly causes ectopia lentis. It is excluded by means of the cyanide nitroprusside test. A positive test requires chromatography. Reducing substance and albumin may occur in the urine in the oculocerebrorenal (Lowe) syndrome, a moderately common cause of congenital cataract. Aminoaciduria occurs in a variety of congenital disorders associatied with cataract. Chromosome analysis (p. 476) is indicated if there are widespread systemic defects in addition to cataracts.

Special types. Special types of congenital cataract include lamellar (zonular) and those associated with maternal rubella, occulocerebrorenal (Lowe) syndrome, mental retardation (Sjögren), Down syndrome (mongolism), and galactosemia.

Lamellar (zonular) cataract. The lens grows throughout life by forming successive layers (p. 37). Lens fibers may become opaque because of a transient disturbance; with further growth of the lens, these fibers migrate centrally as deep concentric lamellar, or zonular, cataracts. Lamellar cataract is a common type of cataract and may develop up to 1 year af-

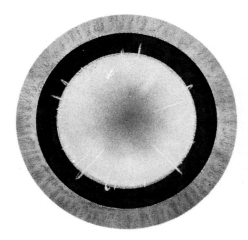

Fig. 19-5. Lamellar cataract with riders.

ter birth (Fig. 19-5). It is usually bilateral and is often transmitted as a dominant trait without any other abnormality. It consists of a series of concentric thin sheets (lamellae) of opacities surrounded by clear lens. There may be ⊃-shaped riders that extend along the edge from the anterior surface of the opacity to its posterior surface. Depending on the density of the opacity, vision may be good or markedly reduced. Vision may become worse at puberty, necessitating surgery. A unilateral lamellar cataract may follow contusion of the eye. Hypocalcemia in infancy causes a bilateral lamellar defect.

Maternal rubella. During pregnancy maternal rubella (p. 464) may cause widespread fetal ocular and systemic defects. The severity of the complications varies with different strains of the virus and is more severe the earlier in pregnancy the rubella occurs. The lens may be entirely opaque, or there may be a central pearly white opacity. Nystagmus, strabismus, corneal opacities, microphthalmia, retinal pigmentation, and glaucoma also occur. The pupil dilates poorly, and surgical results are often unsatisfactory. The lens may harbor the virus for up to 2 years after birth, and surgery with retention of infected lens substance may cause endophthalmitis.

Oculocerebrorenal (Lowe) syndrome. Lowe syndrome is a familial disease associated with a renal tubular lesion, a vitamin-resistant renal rickets, retarded physical and mental development, hypotonia, and cataracts or glaucoma. The cataract is present at birth, and several different types have been described: complete, nuclear, and posterior polar. Glaucoma may occur independently or may be associated with cataract. There are aminoaciduria, albuminuria, and intermittent glycosuria. Bony and constitutional changes occur, and there may be many constitutional signs. Only affected males have been described (p. 496).

Congenital cataract with mental retardation (Sjögren). Congenital cataract with mental retardation is an autosomal recessive abnormality in which the cataract develops during the first year of life and deficient mental development takes place after the fourth year. The cataracts are usually lamellar and often progress to involve the entire lens. Skeletal deformities, epilepsy, and deafness have been reported. Congenital cataract, spinocerebellar ataxia, and mental retardation (Marinesco and Sjögren) are transmitted as an autosomal recessive disorder, and consanguinity of the parents is frequent. There may be widespread bony and central nervous system changes.

Down syndrome. Down syndrome (mongolism, p. 477) is a frequent type of mental retardation associated with widespread systemic and ocular defects. There is both physical and mental retardation. The stature is small, the face is round and mongoloid in appearance, the skull is small, there is obesity, hypogenitalism is common, and there is generalized laxity of ligaments and hypotonia. The intelligence quotient is between 20 and 50.

The eyes are widely separated, and the palpebral fissures are narrow and run obliquely down and inward. Epicanthus (p. 202) is common. The free edge of the upper eyelid is markedly arched. The iris is light blue, sometimes with speckled white or light-colored dots in the ciliary portion (Brushfield spots). Brushfield spots may occur in normal infants but are said to be present at birth in all mongoloid infants. They tend to disappear with increasing pigmentation of the iris.

Various types of cataract may occur: lamellar, posterior polar, sutural, and peripheral. For the most part, the opacities are not marked. Nystagmus may occur, and high myopia is common.

Two types of chromosomal abnormality occur (p. 476). The most common is trisomy of chromosome pair 21, resulting in a total of 47 chromosomes. The involvement of children of older mothers is related to the tendency for nondisjunction of older ova. The other type of chromosomal anomaly is translocation, in which nonhomologous chromosomal segments are exchanged. This abnormality appears to be genetic and occurs in children of younger mothers.

Galactosemia. Galactosemia (p. 497) is a hereditary abnormality in which there is impairment of the enzymatic conversion of galactose to glucose. Lactose (milk sugar) is enzymatically hydrolyzed in the intestinal tract to glucose and galactose. Galactose is converted in the liver to glucose by two series of reactions. It is first phosphorylated by the enzyme galactokinase to yield galactose-1-phosphate.

ATP + D-galactose →
$\qquad$ ADP + D-galactose 1-phosphate

Galactose-1-phosphate is converted to uridyl diphosphogalactose by one of two reactions. In adults, but not infants, the reaction is catalyzed by galactose-1-phosphate uridylyltransferase.

D-Galactose 1-phosphate + UTP ⇌
$\qquad$ UDP–D-galactose + PP$_i$

In infants it is catalyzed by hexose-1-phosphate uridylyltransferase.

UDP–D-glucose + D-galactose 1-phosphate ⇌
$\qquad$ UDP–D-galactose + D-glucose 1-phosphate

Two clinical types are recognized. Deficiency of galactokinase is uncommon. It is characterized by increased plasma galactose levels, galactosuria, and less severe cataracts than in the transferase deficiency.

In the more common type of galactosemia, there is a deficiency of hexose-1-phosphate uridylyltransferase. Infants deficient in the enzyme are unable to metabolize the galactose in their diet, which is derived from milk lactose (composed of galactose and glucose). The children are normal at birth but soon develop feeding problems, with vomiting, diarrhea, and failure to thrive. Rarely, cataracts may be present at birth; but more commonly, bilateral cataracts form in previously clear lenses. In the early stages an oily drop appears in the center of the lens. A zonular cataract may develop. Treatment involves exclusion of milk and other sources of galactose from the diet. Cataract, mental retardation, and liver impairment may be avoided by early recognition of the disorder. Mothers of children with galactosemia should exclude sources of milk from their diets in subsequent pregnancies. Visual results are usually good after surgery when it is required.

Surgical treatment. When the lens opacity completely prevents view of the fundus, surgery is carried out much earlier in life than it would be otherwise. The lens may be removed any time after the sixth month. The selection of the procedure is governed to some degree by whether the eye is of normal size and whether the pupil can be widely dilated.

If the pupil dilates widely and the eye is of normal size, an opening may be made in the anterior capsule with a needle-knife. The lens is broken up with the knife, ultrasound, or an infusion-suction cutter (p. 362) and aspirated. The incision is small, and usually no iridectomy is necessary. If the pupil does not dilate well or if the eye appears small, a sector iridectomy is done, often with one of the rotating cutters (Douvas rotoextractor), and customary lens aspiration is performed. Often a long-term type of soft contact lens is used postoperatively.

Complications. The complications after surgery for congenital cataract include the following.

Glaucoma may be caused by pupillary block resulting from postoperative iridocyclitis or peripheral anterior synechiae caused by delayed formation of the anterior chamber.

Retinal separation, previously a common cause of blindness following congenital cataract surgery, is now rare. It usually occurred 20 or more years after the operation.

Loss of vitreous humor at the time of surgery frequently leads to retinal detachment and to an occluded pupil. Vitreous humor in the anterior chamber interferes with the absorption of lens cortex and often results in persistent cortex in the anterior, with an unsatisfactory visual result. To avoid many of the problems of vitreous loss, the anterior vitreous may be removed by vitrectomy after the posterior capsule is opened.

Results. The visual results of surgery for congenital cataract are often poor because of ocular defects associated with lens opacities. In one series of 233 eyes, 35.5% had vision of 6/12 (20/40) or better, whereas 25% had vision of 6/60 (20/200) or less, and 6% were blind. In another series, only 11% obtained a vision of 6/24 (20/80) or better, whereas 42% had vision of less than 6/60. Some 37% of patients with congenital cataracts were found to have serious associated ocular defects.

BIBLIOGRAPHY

Binkhorst, C. D.: Evaluation of intraocular lens fixation in pseudophakia, Am. J. Ophthalmol. **80:**184, 1975.

Cleasby, G. W., Fung, W. E., and Webster, R. G., Jr.: The lens fragmentation and aspiration procedure (phacoemulsification), Am. J. Ophthalmol. **77:** 384, 1974.

Farnsworth, P. N., Burke, P., Dotto, M. E., and Cinotti, A. A.: Ultrastructure abnormalities in Marfan's syndrome lens, Arch. Ophthalmol. **95:**1601, 1977.

Fasanella, R. M., editor: Eye surgery; innovations and trends, pitfalls, complications, Springfield, Ill., 1977, Charles C Thomas, Publisher.

Garcia-Castineira, S., Dillon, J., and Spector, A.: Detection of bityrosine in cataractous human lens protein, Science **199:**897, 1978.

Gasset, A. R., Lobo, L., and Houde, W.: Permanent wear of soft contact lenses in aphakic eyes, Am. J. Ophthalmol. **83:**115, 1977.

Havener, W. H., and Gloeckner, S. L.: Atlas of cataract surgery, St. Louis, 1972, The C. V. Mosby Co.

Jaffe, N. S.: Cataract surgery and its complications, St. Louis, 1976, The C. V. Mosby Co.

Jaffe, N. S.: Suggested guidelines for intraocular lens implant surgery, Arch. Ophthalmol. **94:**214, 1976.

Jaffe, N. S., and Duffner, L. R.: Iris-plane (Copland) pseudophakos, Arch. Ophthalmol. **94:**420, 1976.

Jensen, A. D., Cross, H. E., and Paton, D.: Ocular complications in the Weill-Marchesani syndrome, Am. J. Ophthalmol. **77:**261, 1974.

Kelman, C. D.: Phacoemulsification and aspiration; the Kelman technique of cataract removal, Birmingham, 1975, Aesculapius Publishing Co.

Manschot, W. A.: Histopathology of eyes containing Binkhorst lenses, Am. J. Ophthalmol. **77:**865, 1974.

O'Day, D. M.: Fungal endophthalmitis caused by *Paecilomyces lilacinus* after intraocular lens implantation, editorial, Am. J. Ophthalmol. **83:**130, 1977.

Ramsey, M. S., Fine, B. S., Shields, J. A., and Yanoff, M.: The Marfan syndrome; a histologic study of ocular findings, Am. J. Ophthalmol. **76:**102, 1973.

Sommer, A.: Cataracts as an epidemiologic problem, Am. J. Ophthalmol. **83:**334, 1977.

Troutman, R. C.: Microsurgery of the anterior segment of the eye, St. Louis, 1977, The C. V. Mosby Co.

Wilensky, J. T., editor: Intraocular lenses; transactions of the University of Illinois Symposium on Intraocular Lenses, New York, 1977, Appleton-Century-Crofts.

Chapter 20

THE GLAUCOMAS

The glaucomas (Table 20-1) are a family of ocular diseases in which increased intraocular pressure may cause optic atrophy with excavation of the optic disk and characteristic loss of visual field. The degree of increased pressure that causes organic change is not the same in every eye, and some individuals may tolerate for long periods a pressure that would rapidly blind another. There are two major factors involved in the visual loss of glaucoma: (1) the intraocular pressure, which depends on the rate of production of aqueous humor and the ease of exit of the aqueous humor through the trabecular area, which provides the homeostatic control of the level of the intraocular pressure, and (2) the resistance of the intraocular portion of the optic nerve to the development of optic atrophy. This relates to its configuration, the adequacy of its blood supply, axoplasmic transport (p. 95), and unknown factors.

Glaucoma is customarily divided into open-angle and closed-angle types. If the cause is evident, glaucoma is designated as secondary, but if the cause is unknown, as primary. In open-angle glaucoma the aqueous humor has free access to the trabecular meshwork, the drainage apparatus in the anterior chamber angle. In angle-closure glaucoma the root of the iris is in apposition to the trabecular meshwork, and aqueous humor cannot leave the eye. This occurs in eyes that have an anatomically shallow anterior chamber, and angle closure involves one of several mechanisms: (1) direct mechanical block by the root of the iris, (2) increased size or edema of the ciliary body pressing the root of the iris forward against the trabecular meshwork, or (3) pupillary block in which the aqueous humor does not pass through the pupil but accumulates in the posterior chamber causing the iris to balloon forward to block the chamber angle.

Primary open-angle glaucoma is a disease of unknown cause previously called simple glaucoma, chronic glaucoma, glaucoma simplex, compensated glaucoma, and wide-angle glaucoma. It is characterized by three abnormalities: (1) increased intraocular pressure, (2) atrophy of the optic disk with characteristic excavation ("cupping"), and (3) typical visual field defects with an open anterior chamber angle.

Primary angle-closure glaucoma is a disorder in which an anatomic abnormality displaces the iris root anteriorly so that the anterior chamber is shallow and the entrance to the chamber angle is narrow. In the past it has been called acute glaucoma, congestive glaucoma, uncompensated glaucoma, or narrow-angle glaucoma. It is present only when the angle is closed and aqueous humor cannot escape from the eye.

Secondary glaucoma may be of the

Table 20-1. Classification of the glaucomas

I. Primary
   A. Open-angle
   B. Angle-closure
      1. Pupillary block
      2. Ciliary body block
      3. Mechanical block
II. Congenital
   A. Developmental
   B. Secondary to persistent hyperplastic vitreous, neurofibromatosis, aniridia, and so on
   C. Autosomal recessive disorder
III. Secondary
   A. Open-angle mechanism
      1. Uveal tract–related
         a. Inflammation, heterochromia iridis
         b. Pigment dispersion
         c. Glaucoma cyclitic crises
         d. Essential iris atrophy
         e. Malignant melanoma
         f. Anterior chamber epithelization
      2. Trauma
         a. Angle recession, hemorrhage
         b. Contusion injury, vitrectomy
      3. Lens-related
         a. Dislocation
         b. Phacolytic and phacogenic
         c. Oculocerebrorenal (Lowe) syndrome
         d. Pseudoexfoliation of lens capsule(?)
      4. Miscellaneous
         a. Corticosteroid-induced
         b. Increased episcleral venous pressure
         c. Thyrotropic exophthalmos
         d. Retinopathy of prematurity
         e. Alpha-chymotrypsin glaucoma
         f. Hemosiderin, ghost cells
   B. Angle-closure mechanism
      1. Ciliary body block and mechanical block
         a. Intumescent lens
         b. Neovascularization of the iris
         c. Penetrating injuries with flat anterior chamber
         d. Postoperative flat anterior chamber
         e. Anterior displacement of iris-lens diaphragm (malignant glaucoma)
         f. Ciliary body tumors
      2. Pupillary block
         a. Inflammatory adhesions of iris to lens or vitreous face (in aphakia)
         b. Vitreous block (in aphakia)
         c. Intraocular lens block
         d. Anterior dislocations of lens

open- or closed-angle type. Secondary open-angle glaucoma occurs after systemic or topical corticosteroid administration, with increased episcleral venous pressure in conditions such as carotid-cavernous sinus fistula, after trauma, and with inflammation. Secondary angle-closure glaucoma occurs with anterior displacement of the iris-lens diaphragm from increased size of the lens (intumescence), with adhesions between the iris and lens that cause a pupillary block, or with tumor or swelling of the ciliary body.

Tearing, photophobia, and blepharospasm characterize infantile glaucoma. In this disorder the increased intraocular pressure arises from a congenital, occasionally hereditary disorder in which the anterior chamber retains its fetal configuration with the root of the iris attached to the trabecular meshwork or the trabecular meshwork covered by a membrane. The treatment is surgical.

SYMPTOMS AND SIGNS

The symptoms of angle-closure glaucoma are mainly related to a sudden intermittent increase in intraocular pressure. There may be repeated attacks of ocular pain and blurred vision occurring after a prolonged time in darkness, such as at the movies, after emotional upset, or after similar factors that cause pupillary dilation. The rapid increase in intraocular pressure causes a subepithelial edema of the cornea with blurred vision and rainbows surrounding street lights (iridescent vision). The initial attacks are often spontaneously relieved by pupillary constriction during sleep or in bright illumination. After repeated attacks or without previous symptoms, an acute angle closure may occur with reduced vision and a red, painful eye. Severe prostrating pain, often unilateral, may be confused with migraine, impending rupture of a carotid artery aneurysm, and similar causes of hemicrania. There may be nausea, vomiting, and symptoms suggestive of an acute surgical abdominal condition.

Angle-closure glaucoma is diagnosed on the basis of (1) increased intraocular pressure and (2) closed anterior chamber angle. When the chamber angle is not closed, the pressure is normal, unless there have been a number of preceding attacks that have damaged the trabecular meshwork.

Open-angle glaucoma is often symptomless. Usually the intraocular pressure slowly increases over several years or more, and although it may reach a high level, corneal edema and ocular pain do not occur. In the early stages of disease the range of peripheral vision (the peripheral isopters) is not affected, and the changes can be demonstrated only by careful measurement of visual function in the area surrounding the point of fixation. Measurement of the visual fields by confrontation is of little diagnostic value until late in the disease when the visual field becomes extremely constricted. Accommodation may be decreased, with premature presbyopia or frequent changes of lenses. Optic atrophy, excavation, and nasal displacement of the blood vessels are common, and the size of the physiologic cup is increased.

METHODS OF EXAMINATION

Intraocular pressure is measured indirectly (ocular tension) by determining the ease with which the eye is indented or the cornea flattened (p. 395). Angleclosure glaucoma is distinguished from open-angle glaucoma by means of a contact lens containing a prism or a mirror and examination of the angle with a microscope. The changes in the optic disk are evaluated by means of an ophthalmoscope or by means of a biomicroscope and a concave lens to neutralize the refraction of the cornea. Visual field changes are measured by perimetry with particular attention directed to the area about 15° from the point of fixation.

Inasmuch as the ocular tension in an individual with glaucoma may be normal at the time of examination, a number of tests have been developed to induce an increase in the intraocular pressure to distinguish the glaucoma patients from the normal population. Pupillary dilation is mainly used in the diagnosis of angleclosure glaucoma (p. 399), whereas the topical epinephrine test is sometimes used in open-angle glaucoma (p. 404). The water drinking test, although widely used, does not adequately distinguish the glaucoma patient from the normal one.

Tonometry. The intraocular pressure is measured by means of a tonometer. There are two basic types: (1) contact, in which the instrument is placed on the anesthetized eye, and (2) noncontact, in which an air pulse is used. The Schiøtz tonometer (Figs. 20-1 and 6-5) is an indentation tonometer that measures the amount of corneal deformation produced by a given force. The Goldmann applanation tonometer (see Fig. 6-5) measures the force necessary to flatten a given area of the cornea. Other tonometers use an electronic sensor in the tip. With contact tonometers the cornea must first be anesthetized by the instillation of a local anesthetic such as tetracaine. The indentation tonometer measures the ease with which the globe is indented by the plunger of the instrument. A soft eye is easily indented and a low pressure is found, whereas a hard eye is indented with greater difficulty and a higher pressure is found. The amount of indentation has been calibrated in enucleated eyes in millimeters of mercury pressure. (The weight of the tonometer also displaces blood from the uvea, and the volume varies in different eyes.)

The applanation tonometer is influenced by fewer extraneous factors than indentation tonometry, but it requires greater experience and more costly equipment.

The noncontact tonometer flattens the cornea with an air pulse, which increases the reflected light from the cornea. The time required to produce complete corneal flattening is measured electronically, and a computer in the instrument provides a digital readout of the pressure.

Normal individuals have a mean intraocular pressure of about 15 mm Hg ± 3 mm. Untreated glaucomatous eyes with field loss have a mean intraocular pressure of 24 mm Hg ± 5 mm. Intraocular pressure tends to increase with aging and to be higher in women than in men.

Tonography. Tonography measures the rate at which the intraocular pressure decreases when the eye is compressed by means of an indentation tonometer resting upon it. The weight of the tonometer resting upon the eye expresses aqueous humor through the outflow channels, causing an increase in the amount of indentation by the plunger of the instrument. Inasmuch as the tonometer has been calibrated by determination of the volume of the indentation, the difference between the volume at the beginning and at the end of the test is equal to the amount of aqueous humor expressed from the eye minus the amount of aqueous humor produced by the ciliary body while the tonometer rested upon it. Clinically, tonography is carried out by allowing an electronic tonometer to rest upon the eye for 4 minutes while recording the pressure response on a galvanometer. The results are expressed as the coefficient of the facility of outflow (C), the microliters of aqueous humor expressed from the eye per minute per milimeter of mercury of intraocular pressure. The decay curve of the coefficient of outflow facility is essentially the slope of this curve. Values of more than 0.20 are considered normal. Values of less than 0.11 occur almost exclusively in glaucoma. In

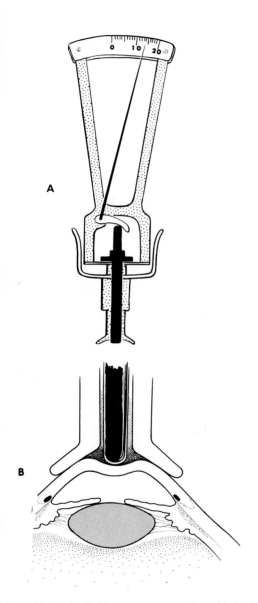

Fig. 20-1. A, Schiøtz tonometer in which the plunger, in black, measures the ease of indentation of the cornea. **B,** Indentation of the anesthetized cornea by the plunger of the tonometer in order to measure ocular tension.

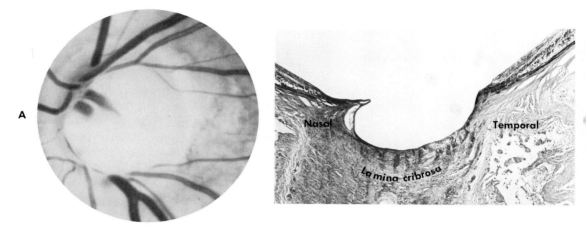

Fig. 20-2. **A,** Glaucomatous optic atrophy with excavation of the optic cup in the left eye. The normal rim of nervous tissue on the temporal side of the optic disk is displaced toward the lamina cribrosa. The blood vessels are displaced nasally. **B,** Histologic section of advanced optic atrophy and glaucomatous excavation ("bean pot" excavation). The lamina cribrosa is characteristically bowed away from the eye.

the range of 0.12 to 0.19 additional studies are necessary to exclude glaucoma. The following ratio (glaucoma index) is of value in suggesting glaucoma:

$$\frac{\text{Intraocular pressure}}{\text{Coefficient of the facility of outflow}}$$

A value greater than 100 occurs in 95% of open-angle glaucoma patients.

In angle-closure glaucoma, tonometry shows normal values between attacks, but there may be little outflow when the angle is closed.

Ophthalmoscopy. In glaucoma the examination of the ocular fundus is directed particularly to the appearance of the optic disk (Fig. 20-2). The nerve fibers at the optic disk receive their main blood supply from small branches of the partial arterial circle of Haller-Zinn derived from the posterior ciliary arteries. These small optic disk branches are subjected to the intraocular pressure, and it has been hypothesized that they are compromised by chronic increase of the intraocular pressure, causing nerve fiber degeneration. The superior and inferior temporal

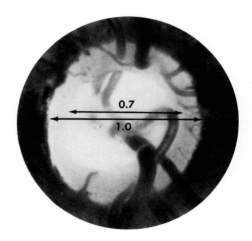

Fig. 20-3. The cup/disk ratio is the ratio between the horizontal diameter of the optic cup and the horizontal diameter of the optic disk. In this illustration, the cup/disk ratio is 0.7/1.0.

nerve fibers of the optic disk are most vulnerable to increased intraocular pressure, and the initial disk changes in glaucoma occur there.

The optic disk is usefully studied with stereoscopic visualization and magnification obtained with a Hruby or corneal contact lens combined with a biomicroscope. Stereoscopic photographs using a fixed parallax may document changes. The optic disk is evaluated with respect to the ratio between the horizontal diameter of the physiologic cup and the horizontal diameter of the entire disk (Fig. 20-3) and to the uniformity of the rim of optic nerve surrounding the physiologic cup. The physiologic cup usually appears as a white, gray, or reddish white color distinctly lighter than the surrounding optic nerve. In glaucoma the ratio of cup to disk (p. 396) usually exceeds 0.5, and a difference of more than 0.2 between the two eyes should suggest the possibility of glaucoma. The rim of the optic nerve should be uniform in size and color. Hemorrhage on the optic nerve rim is an uncommon but important sign of acute decompensation of the disk vasculature in glaucoma.

In a typical glaucomatous cup the retinal vessels are displaced to the nasal half of the disk, and they disappear at an undercut edge of the excavated optic disk. The disk appears whiter than normal, the physiologic cup extends to the margin of the disk, and a rim of the optic nerve is partially or completely absent. The cup slopes away from the temporal margin of the disk onto a concave floor where gray stippling of the cribriform plate is seen. The nasal slope is much steeper than the temporal slope.

Retinal vein occlusion may be induced by increased intraocular pressure, and ophthalmoscopy must document spontaneous or induced pulsation of the central retinal vein and the absence of pathologic arteriovenous crossings (p. 547).

Perimetry. The appearance of the optic disk must be correlated with the function in the peripheral and central fields of vision. Perimetry (p. 161) is particularly valuable in diagnosing early open-angle glaucoma and in documenting progression of the disease and effectiveness of therapy. The field defect is often proportionate to the amount of nerve atrophy present. The skilled examiner may anticipate perimetric changes by the ophthalmoscopic appearance of the optic disk. However, nuclear sclerosis of the lens may give the optic disk a false appearance of redness; thus, perimetry should not be neglected because of normal-appearing disks. The visual field defect in glaucoma is often transient and present only when the intraocular pressure is increased. As optic nerve damage progresses, the defect becomes permanent.

The nasal visual field is most susceptible to change in glaucoma. It corresponds to axons entering the temporal side of the optic nerve from the temporal periphery. These fibers arc above and below the large mass of fibers from the fovea centralis and do not cross the horizontal midline. With increased intraocular pressure, a group of axons arising from an arc-shaped area of the retina lose their function, causing a typical arcuate island of blindness called an arcuate scotoma. The fibers in the temporal periphery are also involved and cause a depression in the peripheral nasal field. The field defects in glaucoma are demonstrated on a tangent screen using small white test objects. The Goldmann hemispherical perimeter more sensitively controls test conditions. The central retinal fibers are relatively more resisitant to the increased pressure, and good visual acuity may be retained despite advanced glaucoma.

Gonioscopy. The opaque sclera and corneoscleral limbus prevent direct inspection of the angle of the anterior chamber. It is possible to see this area by means of a contact lens and mirror (Figs. 20-4 and 20-5) or a contact lens combined with a prism. This method of inspection is of particular diagnostic importance inasmuch as findings in the angle are the

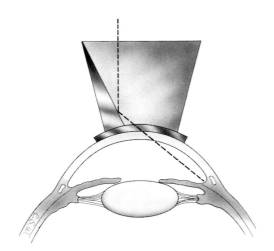

Fig. 20-4. Gonioscopy of the anterior chamber angle. The mirror may be rotated to inspect the entire circumference of the angle.

basis for distinction between angle-closure glaucoma and open-angle glaucoma. Angle-closure glaucoma cannot be diagnosed definitely unless the angle is observed to be closed when the intraocular pressure is increased. However, earlier self-limited attacks of angle-closure may have produced adhesions between the iris and the angle (peripheral anterior synechiae, goniosynechiae), which suggest the diagnosis. Gonioscopy has also been used in the development of an effective surgical procedure for congenital glaucoma and in the diagnostic and therapeutic evaluation of many types of secondary glaucoma.

GENETICS OF GLAUCOMA

Primary open-angle glaucoma has a multifactorial, or polygenic, inheritance. Autosomal dominant, autosomal recessive, and X chromosome–linked inheritance is described. The children and

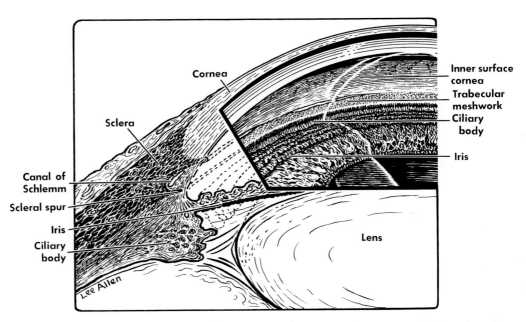

Fig. 20-5. Correlation of chamber angle anatomy with gonioscopic appearance. The trabecular meshwork, which opens into the canal of Schlemm, is bounded anteriorly by the Schwalbe line and posteriorly by the scleral spur. (Courtesy Lee Allen.)

siblings of glaucomatous patients tend to have a higher intraocular pressure, lower facility of outflow, a cup/disk ratio of more than 0.3, and increased intraocular pressure when topical corticosteroids are administered. Diabetes mellitus, myopia, and large optic cups are also risk factors that increase the likelihood of developing optic nerve disease with increased pressure.

Most patients with open-angle glaucoma develop increased intraocular pressure and a decreased outflow facility following the topical administration of 0.1% dexamethasone four times daily for 6 weeks. Continued increase in the intraocular pressure leads to optic nerve atrophy with excavation and a typical visual field defect, and the dexamethasone must be discontinued. It is postulated that the response to topical corticosteroids is genetically determined, so that those who respond with a marked increase in pressure have a genotype with a similar allele pair for high pressure (P^H or gg). Those who do not respond have a similar allele pair for low pressure (P^L or nn), whereas those with an intermediate response are heterozygous for high and low pressure. Those who are homozygous for a high pressure response tend to have positive glucose tolerance tests and low serum protein-bound iodine and tend to be nontasters of phenylthiourea.

Angle-closure glaucoma has a multifactorial inheritance related in the main to the size of the anterior ocular segment.

Congenital, or infantile, glaucoma is transmitted as an autosomal recessive characteristic. Boys are affected twice as often as girls. Cardiac, auditory, and cerebral defects may also be present.

PRIMARY OPEN-ANGLE GLAUCOMA

In primary open-angle glaucoma (simple glaucoma, glaucoma simplex, compensated glaucoma, chronic glaucoma, or chronic simple glucoma) there is a path-

ologic increase in the intraocular pressure in the absence of an obstruction between the trabecular meshwork and the anterior chamber (see Fig. 2-3). The increased intraocular pressure leads to a characteristic atrophy and excavation of the optic disk and typical defects of the visual field. In the United States open-angle glaucoma is one of the chief causes of blindness in adults. It occurs because of an abnormality of the trabecular meshwork that impairs the flow of aqueous humor between the anterior chamber and the canal of Schlemm. There are varying degrees of severity, and unquestionably, many individuals have mild forms of the disease without knowing it.

Symptoms and signs. Open-angle glaucoma tends to manifest itself after the age of 35 years. It has no particular sex predisposition. Open-angle glaucoma may occur in myopic as well as hyperopic eyes, but it is more frequent in myopic individuals. External examination of the eye does not indicate an abnormality such as that which may be recognized in angle-closure glaucoma.

Open-angle glaucoma is characterized by an almost complete absence of symptoms and a chronic, insidious course. Halos around lights and blurring of vision do not occur unless there has been a sudden increase in intraocular pressure, and many patients never have visual difficulties. Form vision remains good until late in the course of the disease; thus, measurement of visual acuity is of no value as a screening test. As the decrease progresses, a premature presbyopia or a more rapid than normal decrease in accommodative power occurs. Additionally, there may be a fairly rapid increase in hyperopia.

Diagnosis. The diagnosis of open-angle glaucoma depends on demonstration of an increased intraocular pressure combined with characteristic changes in the visual field and optic nerve. The increased intraocular pressure precedes the optic nerve and visual field changes by many years, and it is important that the abnormality be diagnosed before such changes occur. Gonioscopy indicates that the aqueous humor has access to the trabecular meshwork at times when the intraocular pressure is increased.

A difference in size of the physiologic cup of the optic disk of each eye may be the first sign. The cup in the eye with the higher pressure is wider and deeper than the other. After initial enlargement the central cup gradually extends to the lower temporal rim of the optic disk or, less commonly, to the superior temporal rim. The blood vessels overlying this region show a sharp abnormal bend at the rim. The normal pink color of the cupped peripheral portion of the disk is lost, and the disk becomes atrophic.

Provocative testing. The intraocular pressure varies slightly with respiration, heartbeat, and activity. During the day there may be variations in pressure of 4 or 5 mm Hg in healthy persons and more than 10 mm Hg in glaucoma patients. Inasmuch as the ocular tension in an individual with glaucoma may be normal when he is examined, a number of tests have been developed to induce an increase in the intraocular pressure in order to distinguish the glaucoma patient from the normal population. The topical epinephrine test appears to be the most useful of these tests.

These tests are by no means foolproof, and even known glaucoma patients with optic atrophy may react negatively. Such tests are indicated in patients with (1) an intraocular pressure of 21 mm Hg or more, (2) a coefficient of outflow of less than 0.18, (3) a ratio of intraocular pressure/coefficient of outflow facility greater than 100, (4) optic nerve changes suggestive of glaucoma, and (5) field changes suggestive of glaucoma. Provocative tests permit an increased suspicion of glaucoma than is possible if one waits for unequivocal signs of optic atrophy.

Epinephrine test. This test appears useful in distinguishing patients with suspicious ocular changes who will develop optic nerve disease from patients with similar signs who will not. The pressure is first measured, and 1% or 2% epinephrine is instilled once in one eye; then the pressure is measured again 4 hours later. A decrease of over 5 mm Hg in the treated eye, corrected for changes in the untreated eye, suggests the possibility of developing optic nerve changes.

Water-drinking test. The water-drinking test is probably the most common provocative test used in the diagnosis of open-angle glaucoma. The patient is instructed not to use ocular medications for 48 hours before the test. The intraocular pressure is measured, preferably in the morning while the patient is fasting. The patient then drinks 14 ml of water per kg body weight (1 liter in a 70 kg adult) within 4 minutes, and the ocular tension is measured at 15-minute intervals until the pressure stops rising. An increase in the intraocular pressure of more than 8 mm Hg indicates glaucoma. If tonography is done 45 minutes after the ingestion of water, some 94% of glaucoma patients will have a ratio of intraocular pressure/coefficient of facility outflow of more than 100.

Medical treatment. In contrast to the treatment of angle-closure glaucoma, which can be surgically cured, the treatment of open-angle glaucoma is mainly medical. Open-angle glaucoma is treated medically unless the pressure cannot be controlled, as indicated by persistently increased intraocular pressure and by progression of the optic nerve atrophy with associated visual field defects. Treatment is directed toward increasing outflow of aqueous humor from the anterior chamber, decreasing secretion of aqueous humor, or both.

Medical treatment of open-angle glaucoma presents the same difficulties as treatment of all chronic diseases that have no symptoms. Miotic drugs may aggravate the visual loss caused by incipient cataract or, in younger individuals, induce ciliary muscle spasm with painful excessive accommodation. Patients have difficulty in remembering to take their medications, a problem often aggravated when different medications are prescribed for multiple daily use.

In well-controlled glaucoma, examination is usually indicated three times a year. The tension must be measured and the optic disks studied. At least once a year perimetry and gonioscopy must be repeated. In poorly controlled glaucoma, in which the intraocular pressure is persistently increased and there is progressive optic nerve involvement, more frequent examination is necessary.

Primary open-angle glaucoma is treated with cholinergic-stimulating drugs, particularly pilocarpine (p. 118); anticholinesterase drugs, particularly echothiophate iodide (p. 119); adrenergic receptor–stimulating compounds, particularly epinephrine (p. 123); and carbonic anhydrase inhibitors, particularly acetazolamide (p. 127). The traditional medication used is pilocarpine drops in concentrations of 1% to 4%. Therapy should begin with the smallest possible concentration that will maintain normal pressure and prevent optic nerve defects. The concentration is increased gradually as the disease becomes refractory to the effects of the pilocarpine. Pilocarpine is used because it facilitates the aqueous outflow in open-angle glaucoma. Because of its miotic effect on the pupil, it is also used in the management of angle-closure glaucoma. Pupillary constriction often decreases vision in patients with minor cataracts; in individuals less than 40 years of age it often causes ciliary muscle spasm with aching pain in the eyes and artificial or increased myopia from excessive accommodation, and because of this it is poorly tolerated. Epinephrine drops may often be usefully substituted.

Topical instillation of epinephrine in a ¼% to 2% solution decreases secretion of aqueous humor and improves aqueous outflow. This is moderately irritating to the eye and may cause black adrenochrome pigmentation of the conjunctiva and maculopathy in aphakic eyes. Epinephrine solutions are used either alone or in combination with cholinergic-stimulating drugs, often pilocarpine.

Eserine (¼%) and organophosphates, mainly echothiophate iodide ($^1/_{16}$%, ⅛%, ¼%), may be used, although the latter may lead to anterior subcapsular lens opacities. Echothiophate iodide depletes systemic pseudocholinesterases, may cause abdominal distress, and should not be used in many systemic diseases (p. 119).

Carbonic anhydrase inhibitors reduce the secretion of aqueous humor by the ciliary processes. Acetazolamide is the drug commonly used (p. 128). The drug is effective 2 hours after administration; its maximum action lasts for 6 hours. It must be administered every 6 hours to be continuously effective. Paresthesia, with numbness and tingling of extremities, anorexia, and other side effects often require reduction of the dose or substitution of other carbonic anhydrase–inhibitor compounds.

Many drugs are currently being studied for treatment of open-angle glaucoma. New delivery systems make it possible to instill medication once weekly. Currently a variety of beta-adrenergic agonists and antagonists (p. 124) are being studied, as are synthetic tetrahydrocannabinol analogues. Biotransformation involving activation of inactive compounds instilled into the eye underlies study of other drugs, particularly dipivalyl epinephrine. Explanation of the therapeutic action of drugs on intraocular pressure is complicated by the pressure-reducing effects of compounds considered as having opposite pharmacologic actions. Thus, both blockers and agonists of the adrenergic system lower intraocular pressure.

In contrast to the low ocular concentration in the eye after systemic administration, high concentrations follow topical administration. Some believe these large concentrations inhibit or destroy ocular receptors so that the glaucoma becomes constantly more difficult to control. Thus, control with the lowest possible drug concentration is desirable.

Surgical treatment. If the intraocular pressure can be maintained at a normal level by means of drugs, and if there is no progress in the severity of the glaucoma as judged by the ophthalmoscopic appearance of the optic disk and by the absence of progressive visual field defects, open-angle glaucoma is treated medically. If the intraocular pressure cannot be controlled medically and there is progress in the visual field defects and in the severity of optic atrophy, surgery is indicated. Surgery is also indicated in patients who do not use their medication because of simple noncompliance, defective intelligence, or unreliability.

The main surgical procedure in open-angle glaucoma is a filtering operation, of which there are many variations. All are based on forming a fistula between the anterior chamber and the subconjunctival space through which aqueous humor will flow. The opening may be made by means of a trephine that is 1 or 2 mm in diameter. Alternatively, an incision may be made into the anterior chamber, and the anterior or posterior lip may be removed so that the wound edges are not adjacent and will not be closed by cicatrix. Cauterization by heat of the scleral wound edges also prevents the wound from closing. The scleral openings into the anterior chamber are combined with a complete or peripheral iridectomy or with inclusion of a portion of the iris in the scleral wound.

Trabeculectomy has recently become popular and in many centers is the operation of choice. An operating microscope is used, and a superficial flap of sclera is fashioned to expose the scleral side of the trabecular meshwork. A portion of the meshwork is then excised and the scleral flap replaced. A filtering bleb often develops after surgery. The chief advantage of the operation is the immediate formation of the anterior chamber after the procedure; this prevents the development of peripheral anterior synechiae. Excessively low pressure (hypotension), cystic conjunctival blebs, cataract, and corneal endothelial disorders occur less commonly after trabeculectomy than after other filtering operations. The level of pressure after the procedure is somewhat higher, however.

EARLY GLAUCOMA OR INCREASED INTRAOCULAR PRESSURE WITHOUT GLAUCOMA?

In this situation the intraocular pressure is "elevated" in an individual with a normal open angle, optic nerve, and visual field. Some individuals will develop optic atrophy and cupping, although most will not. Some physicians call the situation early primary open-angle glaucoma and emphasize the importance of prompt treatment. Other physicians insist that the alarm caused by designating the condition glaucoma is unwarranted in that only 5% to 10% of the patients who have intraocular pressure between 22 and 30 mm Hg ever develop frank glaucoma within 5 to 10 years. Inasmuch as the tolerance of the optic nerve to increased pressure varies widely and the drugs used in treatment have deleterious effects, it remains debatable as to whether these eyes are glaucomatous and should be treated. The epinephrine test (p. 400) suggests two populations, but widespread testing is required for confirmation. Even though the disks of a patient are normal, most ophthalmologists in the United States regard patients with pressures of 30 mm Hg or more as being vulnerable to optic atrophy. Some regard 25 mm Hg as the dividing point. Most patients with pressures consistently between 21 and 29 mm Hg do not develop a glaucomatous field loss within 5 to 10 years. However, patients with a family history of glaucoma who have optic disks with large physiologic cups, diabetes mellitus, or myopia probably should be treated if their pressure is 25 mm Hg or more. Because of this tendency of pressure to increase with age and the generally higher pressures in women, the choice of treatment must be made on an individual basis. Drugs such as acetazolamide and cholinesterase compounds are not indicated, but topical epinephrine is most useful and may be supplemented with pilocarpine if necessary.

SECONDARY OPEN-ANGLE GLAUCOMA

The secondary open-angle glaucomas include many abnormalities in which the intraocular pressure is increased to a level incompatible with continued normal function of the eye. These may be unilateral, or both eyes may be involved, but usually to a different extent. The majority are related to ocular trauma and inflammation, but a number of special types occur.

Special types. Lens abnormalities may produce either a secondary open-angle or a secondary angle-closure glaucoma. Occasionally an intact lens dislocated in the vitreous body will be associated with an open-angle glaucoma, the mechanism of which is not evident. Hypermaturity and rupture of the lens capsule cause a glaucoma through the release of lens polypeptides or protein, giving rise to a uveitis with secondary glaucoma (p. 377).

A carotid-cavernous sinus fistula (p. 531) increases the episcleral venous pressure with increased intraocular pressure. Thyrotropic exophthalmos may increase intraocular pressure by a mechanism that does not involve the episcleral veins but limits ocular motility. Changes in position of the eyes will give false tonometry readings. Corticosteroid glaucoma follows topical and sometimes systemic administration of corticosteroid preparations. It may be self-limited and may also give rise to severe optic nerve atrophy and cupping with persistently increased intraocular pressure.

Iridocyclitis may cause a secondary glaucoma through obstruction of the trabecular meshwork by inflammatory cells and debris (p. 302).

Heterochromic iridocyclitis is a nongranulomatous chronic anterior uveitis associated with a secondary glaucoma and frequently a posterior subcapsular cataract. Both the glaucoma and the cataract with which the uveitis is associated may be aggravated by corticosteroids used locally in the treatment of the uveitis. Iridocyclitis may cause a depigmentation of the iris, and some believe that a heterochromic iridocyclitis is not a distinct clinical entity (p. 293).

Glaucomatocyclitic crisis is an acute inflammation of the uveal tract in which the signs of an acute increase in intraocular pressure predominate. There is corneal edema with blurring of vision and marked decrease in the coefficient of outflow facility. The disease is distinguished from angle-closure glaucoma in that the angle is open. The inflammation may be confined to the trabecular meshwork with minimal inflammatory signs.

The pigment dispersion syndrome is an abnormality in which uveal pigment is deposited on the endothelium in a vertical line (Krukenberg spindle), markedly colors the trabecular meshwork, and is associated with transillumination defects of the iris.

Contusion of the eye results in a marked immediate increase in intraocular pressure that persists for 30 to 45 minutes.

If hemorrhage follows contusion, a secondary glaucoma may ensue. It arises from blockage of the trabecular meshwork by breakdown products of erythrocytes and macrophages containing hemoglobin products. Contusion may result in tears in the ciliary body and recession of the chamber angle. The majority of such eyes do not develop glaucoma. Some develop what clinically appears to be monocular open-angle glaucoma from 1 month to 10 years after the injury.

Exfoliation of the lens capsule occurs in two conditions. True exfoliation occurs in glassblowers' cataract, in which the iris absorbs infrared energy and transmits it to the lens capsule, causing a splitting of the zonular lamellae. Pseudoexfoliation is an unusual abnormality in which the lens capsule, mainly in a zone between the pupillary area and the equator, is involved with a deposition of a flaky translucent material that is also found surrounding conjunctival blood vessels. Patients with this condition have a slightly higher incidence of glaucoma than the normal population, but the significance is not known. About one half of those who respond to instillation of cyclopentolate (Cyclogyl) with increased intraocular pressure develop open-angle glaucoma.

PRIMARY ANGLE-CLOSURE GLAUCOMA

Angle-closure glaucoma is an abnormality in which the intraocular pressure increases because the outflow of aqueous humor from the anterior chamber is mechanically impaired by contact of the iris with the trabecular drainage meshwork and the peripheral cornea. The condition has been designated in the past as narrow-angle, acute congestive, and uncompensated glaucoma. No term is ideal inasmuch as the intraocular pressure is normal when the angle is open and glaucoma occurs only when a major portion of the angle is closed. If the iris remains in contact with the trabecular meshwork, adhesions result (peripheral anterior synechiae or goniosynechiae), and there is an impairment of aqueous outflow. Both eyes are involved, although one eye may develop symptoms several years before the fellow eye. There is a familial tendency to shallow anterior chambers.

The disease arises because of an inherited anatomic defect that causes a shallow anterior chamber. The peripheral iris often inserts on the extreme anterior edge of the ciliary body, causing the anterior chamber angle to be shallow and placing the iris close to the trabecular meshwork. The cornea is often small in diameter, and the eye is hyperopic. The lens is closer to the cornea than usual, and with the normal increase in size of the lens with aging, it becomes ever closer. The iris appears to bow forward so that it seems to closely parallel the posterior convexity of the cornea (Fig. 20-6). This may be observed by shining a penlight into the anterior chamber from the temporal side of the eye. A shadow, which is not present in the normal eye, is cast by the nasal portion of the relatively convex iris.

Increased intraocular pressure occurs when there is anterior displacement of the peripheral iris. This anterior displacement causes it to isolate the trabecular meshwork from the anterior chamber, preventing the exit of aqueous humor. Three conditions operating singly or together may cause this displacement.

1. The flow of aqueous humor through the pupil is impaired, causing aqueous to accumulate in the posterior chamber. This pupillary block (iris bombé) causes increased pressure in the posterior chamber so that the peripheral iris balloons forward. Mechanical crowding of the angle by the iris isolates the trabecular drainage apparatus from the anterior chamber.

2. Dilation of the pupil causes the iris to

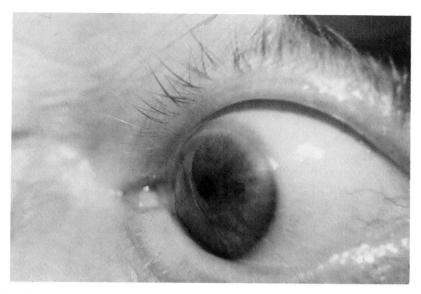

Fig. 20-6. Shallow anterior chamber angle observed from the temporal side. The diagnosis of angle-closure glaucoma requires observation of a closed-angle when the tension is elevated.

become thicker and crowd into the drainage apparatus, preventing aqueous outflow.

3. Edema or increased volume of the ciliary body pushes the peripheral iris forward so that it closes the trabecular meshwork—a ciliary block angle-closure.

Patients who have an anterior chamber with a depth of 2.5 mm or less are likely candidates for the development of angle-closure glaucoma. The shallow anterior chamber may be recognized by the decreased distance between the posterior surface of the cornea and the anterior surface of the iris. Patients with such predisposition may go for many years without symptoms, and it may be impossible to provoke an increase in intraocular pressure or a decrease in aqueous outflow by means of pupillary dilation. With the gradual increase in size of the lens, however, the margin of safety decreases, and such patients may have attacks of increased intraocular pressure when they are elderly. Many patients with a shallow anterior chamber never develop symptoms of an acute increase in intraocular pressure. Such eyes, however, must be observed with caution to avoid an acute angle-closure episode. Patients should be warned, particularly concerning symptoms of blurry and hazy vision that may be combined with iridescent vision and pain.

Provocative testing. In angle-closure glaucoma, provocative testing is done by combining dilation of the pupil with gonioscopy. Angle-closure glaucoma is present only when the combination of increased intraocular pressure and closure of the angle occurs. Inasmuch as dilation of the pupil may induce an acute increase in intraocular pressure, the test is performed cautiously on only one eye at a time, and the pupil is constricted before the patient is released. The pupillary dilation is usually brought about by instillation of an easily neutralized mydriatic such as 5% eucatropine or 1% tropicamide (Mydriacyl) sometimes combined with 2.5% phenylephrine. Placing the patient in a dark room for 60 minutes is a physiologic method of inducing pupillary dilation. Primary open-angle glaucoma as well as angle-closure glaucoma may respond to pupillary dilation by cycloplegics with an increase in intraocular pressure, but such tests are more often positive in angle-closure glaucoma. An increase in intraocular pressure of 8 mm Hg or more is generally considered pathognomonic. Tonography indicates a decrease of 25% to 30% in the coefficient of the facility of outflow. The angle must be observed with the gonioscope to be closed at the time the intraocular pressure is increased in order to be certain that the abnormality is angle-closure glaucoma.

Prodromal or intermittent angle-closure glaucoma. This occurs in individuals in whom there is a spontaneous relief of increased intraocular pressure when the pupil constricts. Such individuals have a shallow anterior chamber. There are intermittent episodes of blurring of vision that may or may not be associated with ocular pain. On occasion the ocular pain is severe and has been confused with impending rupture of an intracranial aneurysm or with migraine. The attacks are usually spontaneously terminated by the miosis caused by bright illumination or by the miosis of sleep.

If the patient is seen during a period of attack, the intraocular pressure may be markedly increased, but congestive signs are minimal. These patients may develop peripheral anterior synechiae with a decreased coefficient of facility of outflow. Between attacks there are no symptoms, but dilation of the pupil often increases the intraocular pressure 8 mm Hg or more or reduces the coefficient of facility of outflow 25% to 30%. Gonioscopy indicates that the angle is closed when the pressure is increased.

Acute angle-closure glaucoma. This glaucoma is often preceded by many attacks of prodromal or intermittent angle-clo-

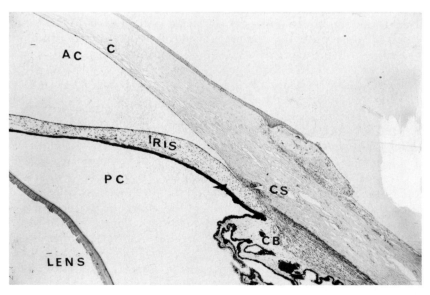

Fig. 20-7. Angle-closure glaucoma with anterior synechiae excluding the anterior chamber, *AC,* from the trabecular area and the canal of Schlemm, *CS.* The posterior chamber, *PC,* is larger than normal. *C,* Cornea. *CB,* Ciliary body. (Hematoxylin and eosin stain; ×38.)

sure glaucoma. Initially there is blurred, iridescent vision, but spontaneous relief does not occur, the intraocular pressure continues to increase, and the symptoms become more severe. A ciliary type of injection (Table 20-2) is present, and there may be profuse lacrimation. Subepithelial corneal edema is marked, and epithelial bullae form, giving the cornea a steamy appearance. The blood-aqueous barrier breaks down, and there is increased protein in the aqueous humor. The blood vessels of the iris stroma are dilated, and the pupil is in middilation and does not react to light. Severe systemic symptoms include nausea, vomiting, malaise, and signs suggestive of an acute abdomen. The symptoms may be aggravated by systemic absorption of drugs used in the treatment of the acute angle-closure attack.

If the attack persists, peripheral anterior synechiae form between the root of the iris and the cornea (Fig. 20-7). After several days, these synechiae nearly destroy the drainage meshwork. Adhesions (posterior synechiae) form between the iris and the lens, and if the attack is not relieved, necrosis of the sphincter pupil-

lae muscle results in a permanently semidilated pupil. Fluid vesicles form in the anterior subcapsular region of the lens. If the condition is untreated, vision progressively deteriorates and a blind, painful eye develops. Optic atrophy with pallor of the nerve occurs relatively early and excavation occurs late in the glaucoma.

Chronic primary angle-closure glaucoma. This is a common type of glaucoma in which the patient never has a severe acute congestive attack but has intermittent periods of increased pressure. Symptoms may be absent, or there may be periodic episodes of mild congestion and iridescent vision. The iris gradually occludes the trabecular meshwork that begins above, but peripheral synechiae are not seen. Eventually, pressure is at a level of 40 to 60 mm Hg. Gonioscopy is essential to establish the basis for the disease and to distinguish it from open-angle glaucoma. Peripheral iridectomy is curative. Gonioscopy at the time of iridectomy should show that the angle is open and not closed with peripheral anterior synechiae.

Diagnosis. The diagnosis of angle-

Table 20-2. Differential diagnosis of angle-closure glaucoma

	Angle-closure glaucoma	Acute iritis	Acute conjunctivitis
Pain	Severe, prostrating	Moderate to severe	Burning, itching
Injection	Ciliary type that is more intense near the corneoscleral limbus and fades toward fornices; not constricted with 1:1,000 epinephrine; vessels do not move with conjunctiva, are violet in color; individual vessels not distinguishable		Conjunctival type that is most intense in fornices and fades toward limbus; eye whitened with 1:1,000 epinephrine; vessels superficial, move with conjunctiva, are bright red; individual vessels evident
Pupil	Semidilated, does not react to light	Miotic, reaction delayed or absent	Normal
Cornea	Steamy, iris details not visible	Usually clear with deposits on posterior surface sometimes visible	Clear and normal
Secretion	Watery	Watery	Stringy pus
Onset	Sudden	Gradual	Gradual
Vision	Markedly reduced	Slightly reduced	Normal
Intraocular pressure	Increased	Normal or soft	Normal

closure glaucoma requires abnormally increased intraocular pressure and a closed angle demonstrated by gonioscopy. Acute iritis and acute conjunctivitis are disorders to be distinguished (Table 20-2).

Treatment. Angle-closure glaucoma with an acute increase in intraocular pressure presents a difficult problem in management. The type of treatment is often governed by the duration of the attack before normalization of the intraocular pressure and whether there has been permanent damage to the trabecular meshwork. The intraocular pressure is reduced by oral administration of carbonic anhydrase inhibitors or if necessary by intravenous infusion of mannitol (p. 128). Once the intraocular pressure is less than 50 mm Hg, the pupil becomes responsive to miotics, and the attack is usually corrected within several hours. The organophosphates must not be used, because they cause edema of the ciliary body with a ciliary block mechanism.

The angle-closure mechanism may be eliminated by a peripheral iridectomy in which the accumulation of aqueous humor in the posterior chamber is eliminated. This opening prevents the pressure in the posterior chamber from exceeding that of the anterior chamber and prevents physiologic iris bombé entirely. After control of the attack, the iridectomy is done when signs of ocular congestion have disappeared. It is not customary to operate on both eyes at the same time, but the fellow eye may well be operated on during the same hospital admission.

In patients with shallow angles who have never had an attack of angle-closure glaucoma, an iridectomy would probably ensure freedom from an attack. However, inasmuch as the individual may not live long enough to develop an attack and if pupillary dilation does not induce increased intraocular pressure, the surgeon and the patient are usually reluctant to undertake intraocular surgery for a disease that is at best potential.

In a patient who is having intermittent symptoms with spontaneous relief, an iridectomy is indicated. A peripheral iridectomy is the operation of choice. This is carried out in the superior temporal quadrant through a small scratch incision. A small opening is made in the iris, and the corneoscleral wound is closed with sutures so as to be watertight. The eye tolerates the procedure well, provided the anterior chamber does not remain flat postoperatively, a complication avoided by careful wound closure.

The iridectomy may be done with a laser rather than through a surgical incision. After topical anesthesia, a localized area of the iris is caused to bulge forward by means of mild laser burns. When this area is no longer in contact with the anterior lens capsule, its central portion is perforated by a much stronger laser beam. Multiple applications may be necessary, and iris perforation may be impossible when markedly pigmented.

Malignant glaucoma (ciliary block glaucoma) may occur after surgery for angle-closure glaucoma or after a filtering procedure for open-angle glaucoma in an individual with a shallow anterior chamber. The anterior chamber becomes shallow or obliterated, and the intraocular pressure is increased. This may occur immediately after the operative procedure or as late as 1 year later. Miotics aggravate the condition. Initial treatment consists of pupillary dilation with phenylephrine and atropine combined with acetazolamide and intravenous infusion of mannitol. After 5 days, if the anterior chamber does not deepen, vitreous humor is aspirated from the anterior vitreous cavity and air is injected into the anterior chamber. If vitreous aspiration does not cure the malignant glaucoma, the lens is extracted. If the anterior chamber remains flat after surgery, a partial anterior vitrectomy with an infusion-aspiration cutter may be curative (p. 362).

SECONDARY ANGLE-CLOSURE GLAUCOMA

Secondary angle-closure glaucomas arise in a variety of situations in which aqueous humor is prevented from free access to the trabecular meshwork. Ciliary block and mechanical block occur, particularly in complicated surgical procedures, penetrating injuries of the eye, and intumescence of the lens. Mechanical obstruction of the angle occurs with an anterior chamber of normal depth in epithelial downgrowth and rubeosis of the iris. The pupillary-block mechanism is evident in posterior synechiae, in vitreous block in aphakia, and in anterior dislocation of the lens.

Failure of the anterior chamber to reform after cataract or glaucoma procedures and other anterior segment surgery or after a penetrating injury of the eye is a serious complication inasmuch as the root of the iris comes into contact with the trabecular meshwork. If the condition persists, peripheral anterior synechiae form, and a secondary glaucoma occurs that is particularly recalcitrant to treatment. The condition is far easier to prevent by careful closure of ocular wounds than it is to treat once it is established.

After injury or anterior segment surgery, particularly lens extraction complicated by faulty wound healing, there may be downgrowth of conjunctival or corneal epithelium into the eye. This causes a single sheet of epithelium to cover the trabecular meshwork, iris, and ciliary processes and causes a severe glaucoma, often intractable to treatment.

Neovascular glaucoma (rubeosis iridis) complicates diabetic retinopathy and retinal venous occlusion. It arises from newly formed blood vessels on the surface of the iris and in the trabecular meshwork and closes off the drainage angle (p. 86). Swelling of the lens (intumescence) closes off the angle with forward displacement of the root of the iris. Ciliary body tumors cause glaucoma by a similar mechanism.

Secondary angle-closure glaucoma caused by pupillary block arises because of vitreous or an intraocular lens blocking the pupillary aperture after lens extraction in which there is not an adequate peripheral iridectomy. Inflammatory adhesions of the iris to the lens or to the vitreous face in aphakia may also give rise to a pupillary block. Anterior dislocation of the lens blocks the pupil and causes a similar secondary glaucoma.

CONGENITAL GLAUCOMA

Congenital glaucoma occurs with developmental anomalies that are manifest at birth. The congenital glaucomas may be divided into primary, or infantile, glaucoma with anomalies in the angle of the anterior chamber, aniridia (p. 290), and glaucoma associated with systemic disorders such as neurofibromatosis or Sturge-Weber-Dimitri syndrome (p. 327). The defects interfere with drainage of the aqueous humor, causing an increase in intraocular pressure, which in turn causes stretching of the elastic coats of the eye with marked enlargement of the globe (total staphyloma [Fig. 20-8, buphthalmos]) and optic atrophy with excavation. The human globe is subject to this stretching only until about the age of 3 years. Glaucoma occurring after this age does not cause enlargement of the globe and follows a course similar to adult glaucoma. Some authors use the term *juvenile glaucoma* for the open-angle glaucoma occurring after the age of 3 years.

Infantile glaucoma is transmitted as an autosomal recessive characteristic. Boys are affected more often than girls, and the disease is bilateral in 75% of the cases. Cardiac, auditory, and cerebral defects may also be present. Signs of infantile

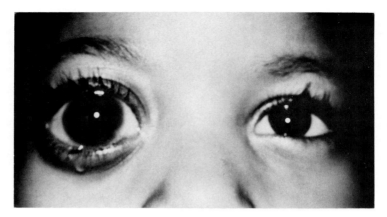

Fig. 20-8. Marked enlargement of the right eye of a 3-year-old girl with infantile glaucoma.

glaucoma may be present and even far advanced at birth, or become apparent before the child has reached the age of 3 months. The earliest symptoms are tearing of the eyes, blepharospasm, and sensitivity of the eyes to light. Examination indicates a subepithelial corneal edema with a ground-glass appearance that obscures the pattern of the iris. The corneal diameter increases from 10.5 to 12 mm or more, and tears appear in the Descemet membrane as glassy lines on the back surface of the cornea. The anterior chamber is deeper than normal. The intraocular pressure is best measured with a pneumatographic or air tonometer without general anesthesia to avoid the increased intraocular pressure associated with ketamine or the decreased intraocular pressure of halothane anesthesia. In infants with subepithelial corneal edema or a cornea that measures more than 10.5 mm in diameter, increased intraocular pressure must be excluded.

Infantile glaucoma may arise from a congenital defect in which there is retention of the fetal state of the anterior chamber angle. The trabecular meshwork inserts into the anterior portion of the ciliary body. The peripheral iris is hypoplastic and inserts abnormally forward, often into the trabecular meshwork itself. Gonioscopy shows the abnormality.

The preferred surgical treatment of infantile glaucoma is the goniotomy procedure, in which an incision is made into the region of the trabecular meshwork under direct visual control by using a gonioscope. Trabeculotomy may be effective if goniotomy fails.

Patients must be carefully observed postoperatively to be certain the glaucoma is controlled. Intraocular pressure must be measured and the corneal diameters carefully measured with attention directed to tears in the Descemet membrane.

BIBLIOGRAPHY

Anderson, D. R., and Braverman, S.: Reevaluation of the optic disk and vasculature, Am. J. Ophthalmol. **82:**165, 1976.

Anderson, D. R., Drance, S. M., Galin, M. A., and others: Symposium on glaucoma; transactions of the New Orleans Academy of Ophthalmology, St. Louis, 1975, The C. V. Mosby Co.

Becker, B., Shin, D. H., Cooper, D. G., and Kass, M. A.: The pigment dispersion syndrome, Am. J. Ophthalmol. **83:**161, 1977.

Becker, S. C.: Clinical gonioscopy; a text and stereoscopic atlas, St. Louis, 1972, The C. V. Mosby Co.

Campbell, D. G., Simmons, R. J., and Grant, W. M.: Ghost cells as a cause of glaucoma, Am. J. Ophthalmol. **81:**441, 1976.

Chandler, P. A., and Grant, W. M.: "Ocular hypertension" vs open-angle glaucoma, Arch. Ophthalmol. **95**:585, 1977.

Chumbley, L. C., and Brubaker, R. F.: Low-tension glaucoma, Am. J. Ophthalmol. **81**:761, 1976.

Fishbein, S. L., and Schwartz, B.: Optic disc in glaucoma, Arch. Ophthalmol. **95**:1975, 1977.

Gorin, G., editor: Ophthalmology series. Vol. 1: Clinical glaucoma, New York, 1977, Marcel Dekker, Inc.

Hart, W. M., Jr., and Becker, B.: Visual field changes in ocular hypertension, Arch. Ophthalmol. **95**:1176, 1977.

Hoskins, H. D., Jr., and Gelber, E. C.: Optic disk topography and visual field defects in patients with increased intraocular pressure, Am. J. Ophthalmol. **80**:284, 1975.

Kass, M. A., Becker, B., and Kolker, A. E.: Glaucomatocyclitic crisis and primary open-angle glaucoma, Am. J. Ophthalmol. **75**:668, 1973.

Kerman, B. M., Christensen, R. E., and Foos, R. Y.: Angle-closure glaucoma; a clinicopathologic correlation, Am. J. Ophthalmol. **76**:887, 1973.

Kimura, R.: Color atlas of gonioscopy, Baltimore, 1974, The Williams & Wilkins Co.

Kirsch, R. E., and Anderson, D. R.: Clinical recognition of glaucomatous cupping, Am. J. Ophthalmol. **75**:442, 1973.

Kolker, A. E., and Hetherington, J.: Becker-Shaffer's diagnosis and therapy of the glaucomas, St. Louis, 1976, The C. V. Mosby Co.

Krupin, T., Mitchell, K. B., and Becker, B.: Cyclocryotherapy in neovascular glaucoma, Am. J. Ophthalmol. **86**:24, 1978.

Layden, W. E., and Shaffer, R. N.: Exfoliation syndrome, Am. J. Ophthalmol. **78**:835, 1974.

Lichter, P. R., and Henderson, J. W.: Optic nerve infarction, Am. J. Ophthalmol. **85**:302, 1978.

Luntz, M. H., and Livingston, D. G.: Trabeculotomy ab externo and trabeculectomy in congenital and adult-onset glaucoma, Am. J. Ophthalmol. **83**:174, 1977.

Merritt, J. C.: Malignant glaucoma induced by miotics postoperatively in open-angle glaucoma, Arch. Ophthalmol. **95**:1988, 1977.

Phelps, C. D., and Watzke, R. C.: Hemolytic glaucoma, Am. J. Ophthalmol. **80**:690, 1975.

Radius, R. L., and Maumenee, A. E.: Optic atrophy and glaucomatous cupping, Am. J. Ophthalmol. **85**:145, 1978.

Shin, D. H., Kolker, A. E., Kass, M. A., and others: Long-term epinephrine therapy of ocular hypertension, Arch. Ophthalmol. **94**:2059, 1976.

Troutman, R. C.: Microsurgery of the anterior segment of the eye. Vol. 1: Introduction and basic techniques, St. Louis, 1974, The C. V. Mosby Co.

Watson, P. G., and Barnett, F.: Effectiveness of trabeculectomy in glaucoma, Am. J. Ophthalmol. **79**:831, 1975.

Chapter 21

OCULAR MOTILITY

A normal pair of eyes is so aligned that an object in space is imaged simultaneously on each retina and perceived singly. The eyes remain parallel in all directions of gaze except when they converge on a nearby object. This ocular alignment involves two interrelated mechanisms: (1) a sensory retinocerebral apparatus engaged in elaborating a sensation in response to excitation of a unit area of retinal surface, and (2) a motor system subsidiary to the sensory system to provide clear, distinct vision and binocular fixation. These form a single indivisible entity, although clinically the sensory and motor systems may be considered separately. An abnormality in either mechanism may lead either to faulty alignment of the eyes or to a visual abnormality.

A complicated terminology is used to describe the motor-sensory relationships.

TERMINOLOGY

Visual line. The visual line (axis) is an imaginary line that connects an object in space (fixation point) with the fovea centralis. In normal eyes, the visual lines intersect at the fixation point and there is binocular fixation. If the visual lines are not directed to the same fixation point, then fixation is by one eye only. The line of direction is a line that connects an object in space with the retina. It cor-

responds to the visual line when it connects an object with the fovea centralis.

Retinal correspondence. Whenever a retinal area is stimulated by light, the stimulus is perceived as being of a certain intensity and form and is localized in a subjective visual direction. The directional value is an intrinsic property of the stimulated retinocerebral elements that elaborate the visual impulse. The foveas of each eye have the same subjective directional value so that a visual object imaged on each appears as a single object. All retinocerebral elements that have the same subjective directional value are called *corresponding retinal points*. Images from corresponding retinal points are perceived as a single image. Images from noncorresponding points (disparate points) are seen as double (diplopia). For the retinocerebral system to unify images from corresponding retinal points the images must be sufficiently similar in size, brightness, and clarity to permit sensory unification. Images that provide dissimilar contours, unequal luminance, or different colors to corresponding retinal points are not perceived singly but give rise to conflict and confusion (retinal rivalry).

The retinal correspondence of the two eyes is not absolute, and within a narrow band, stimulation of slight disparate horizontal retinocerebral elements causes transmission of a single image. When disparate horizontal retinocerebral elements are stimulated simultaneously, the fusion of such disparate images results in perception of the visual object in three dimensions (stereopsis) Stereopsis occurs only through the use of the two eyes and is restricted to maximum distances of about 125 to 200 meters. Monocular clues provide additional information concerning depth perception. These include motion parallax (when one looks at a scene with one eye and moves one's head or eye, further objects move more than closer objects), linear perspective (parallel railroad tracks seem to approach each other in the distance), overlays of contours (interposition of closer object in front of more distant object), highlights, shadows, size of known objects, and color of more distant objects (bluish haze of more distant mountains).

Sensory fusion. This is the retinocerebral unification of images from corresponding retinal points of each eye into a single visual percept.

Motor correspondence. The nerve impulse to perform an eye movement is always integrated and coordinated and sent equally to corresponding muscles of each eye (Hering's law of motor correspondence). Isolated impulses to the muscles of one eye or to a single ocular muscle do not occur. Thus, whenever the eyes rotate, corresponding muscles receive equal innervational impulses to contract or relax.

Motor fusion. The divergence and convergence (p. 109) movements align the eyes in such a way as to ensure and maintain binocular fixation and binocular vision, or fusion.

Vergences. These are simultaneous rotations of both eyes in opposite directions. Thus, they consist of convergence or divergence (p. 102) stimulated mainly by accommodation. In accommodation, objects remain focused on the retina as

they are moved nearer to the eyes because of the increase in refractive power of the lens in response to contraction of the ciliary muscle (p. 12). In convergence, the eyes turn inward because of contraction of each medial rectus muscle and relaxation of the lateral recti muscles. Accommodation is associated with a balance between convergence and divergence so that the line of direction of each eye remains directed to the same fixation object.

Fusional vergence. This term is applied to the delicate movements of convergence or divergence that occur when an object is imaged on slightly disparate horizontal parts of the retina. These movements are elicited by double vision to bring about stereopsis.

Fusion-free position. This is the position of an eye when it is covered or when vision is otherwise obscured so as to eliminate binocular vision.

Duction movements. These are movements of one eye: adduction (movement nasalward), abduction (movement templeward), sursumduction (elevation), deorsumduction (depression), excycloduction (rotation of upper pole of cornea templeward), and incycloduction (rotation of upper pole of cornea nasalward). Movements in an oblique direction, such as up and in or down and out, are combinations of horizontal and vertical movements (p. 106).

Strabismus. Strabismus (heterotropia, squint, walleyes, or cross-eyes) is that condition in which the visual axes of each eye are not directed simultaneously to the same fixation point. It may be divided into (1) paralytic (noncomitant), in which one or more muscles are weakened, their normal action is impaired by mechanical or restrictive factors, or their nervous connections are impaired, and (2) comitant, in which there is no primary muscle impairment. Secondary overaction or underaction of individual muscles in comitant strabismus may simulate a noncomitant strabismus.

A heterotropia is a manifest deviation of one eye from its normal position that occurs despite both eyes being open and uncovered. Esotropia refers to medial deviation of the eye. Exotropia refers to lateral deviation of the eye. Hypertropia refers to upward deviation. The higher rather than the lower eye is designated, so that in an example in which the right eye is higher and the left eye lower, the abnormality is described as a right hypertropia. Cyclotropia refers to torsional deviation in which the upper end of the vertical corneal meridian leans temporally (excyclotropia) or nasally (incyclotropia).

Strabismus is termed intermittent or periodic when there are periods when the eyes are parallel, and it is termed constant when the eyes are never parallel. Strabismus is monocular when the same eye always deviates and the fellow eye always fixates. It is alternating when either eye fixates while the fellow eye deviates. An accommodative strabismus is one in which the degree of crossing varies with the amount of accommodation. A sensory strabismus is one in which some abnormality in image formation causes the deviation.

Comitance. This refers to equal deviation in all directions of gaze. A noncomitant deviation is one in which the deviation varies in different directions of gaze. Nonparalytic strabismus is initially comitant but may become noncomitant because of secondary contracture, overactions, and inhibition of muscles. A paralytic strabismus is always noncomitant initially but eventually may become comitant, thus making it difficult to determine the paretic muscle(s).

Heterophoria. This is a tendency for the eyes to deviate that is prevented by fusion mechanisms. When fusion is interrupted, the eyes are not parallel. Esophoria refers to medial deviation, exophoria to lateral deviation, and hyperphoria to upward deviation.

Orthophoria. This is that ideal condition in which the eyes are parallel without fusion in distance fixation and have the proper convergence in near vision.

DIAGNOSTIC MEASURES

The different tests available to study strabismus may be confusing. Worse, they may lead to the erroneous conclusion that diagnosis and treatment should be delayed until the patient is old enough to cooperate in subjective testing, thus allowing poor vision from disuse (strabismic amblyopia) or other sensory abnormalities to develop. Examination and treatment are indicated in any infant whose eyes are not aligned at all times during waking hours after the age of 6 months. Diagnostic measures emphasize two major areas: (1) the ocular deviation and (2) the visual (sensory) status.

Cover-uncover test. The presence or absence of a deviation is determined by the

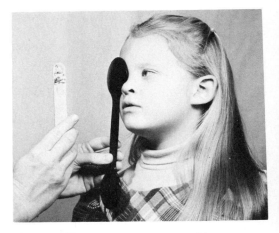

Fig. 21-1. The cover-uncover test with an accommodative target. The individual fixes on details on the target, and the eye is covered for a few seconds and then uncovered. The test should be done for near and distance fixation and with and without correcting lenses.

cover-uncover test (Fig. 21-1). First, the examiner looks at the patient and estimates which eye is being used for fixation. The patient's attention is then directed to a fixation target such as a small picture or letters (a light should not be used). The test should always be done for both distance and near fixation. The eye that appears to be fixing is covered for a few seconds using the palm of one's hand or an occluder of some sort. As the eye is covered, attention is directed to the uncovered eye (Fig. 21-2). If there is no movement, binocular fixation was present before covering. If the uncovered eye moves to achieve fixation, a manifest deviation was present before covering. Attention is then directed to the covered eye as it is uncovered. If there is a movement to achieve fixation (fusional movement) and no movement of the previously uncovered eye, then heterophoria is present. If there is no movement of either eye and the eye that was covered is deviated, then an alternating heterotropia is present. If the eye that was covered assumes

fixation and the fellow eye deviates, then a nonalternating monocular heterotropia is present, and the eye that was covered is preferred for fixation.

This test is of more than theoretic importance. If a heterophoria is present, then the patient has binocular vision. If strabismus is present, the individual either is seeing double or is suppressing the image from one eye.

Prism and cover test (alternate cover test). If the cover-uncover test indicates that either a heterophoria or a heterotropia is present, the prism and cover test is used to measure how much deviation is present. As the patient maintains fixation, one eye is covered and then uncovered as the fellow eye is immediately covered. Attention is directed to the movement made by the covered eye as it is uncovered. If the eye has been turned inward while under the cover and moves outward to fix when it is uncovered, either an esophoria or an esotropia is present. If the eye has been turned outward under the cover, it will move inward when the cover is removed,

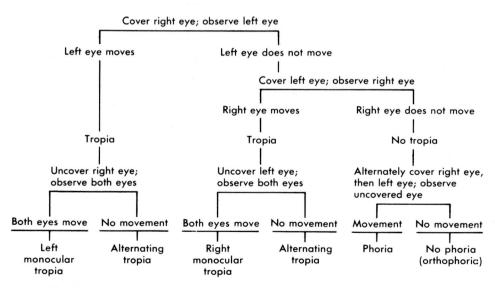

Fig. 21-2. Diagnosis of phorias and tropias by using the cover-uncover test.

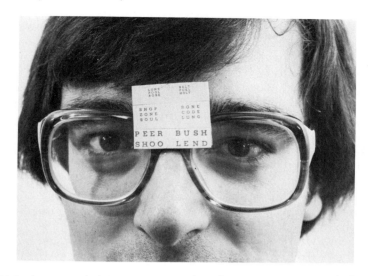

Fig. 21-3. Accommodative target mounted on the examiner's spectacle frames.

and an exophoria or an exotropia is present.

As the eye is uncovered, it moves to place the fixation object on the fovea (movement of redress). The eye moves in the direction opposite the deviation; thus, if the basic deviation is nasalward, the movement of redress is templeward. Prisms of increasing strength are then placed in front of one eye until the movement of redress is neutralized. The movement is neutralized because the prisms move the image of the fixation object onto the retina. To ensure maximal accommodation, small pictures or letters (Fig. 21-3) are used for near fixation and the 6/9 (20/30) line is used for distance fixation. The test is carried out with the patient wearing correcting lenses and without correction at near and far. The cover-uncover test must be done first to distinguish between a phoria and a tropia.

Corneal reflection test. The degree of deviation may be estimated by observing the reflection of light from the cornea of the deviating eye. The cornea has a diameter of approximately 11.5 mm, and each millimeter of displacement of the reflec-

tion is equal to about 7° of deviation of the visual axes. Thus, if the reflection from the deviating eye is at the corneoscleral limbus, the deviation is about 38.5° (11.5/2 × 7).

The test is more accurately performed by having the patient fixate on a small light with the examiner on the side of the deviating eye. Prisms are then placed in front of the fixating eye until the light reflection is centered in the deviated eye.

NONCOMITANT STRABISMUS

Noncomitant strabismus is a misalignment of the visual axes that arises from paresis (weakness), paralysis, or restriction of one or more ocular muscles. It is characterized by limitation of ocular rotation in the field of action of the involved muscle. There is less or no deviation in the field of action of uninvolved muscles. The deviation is greater when the involved eye is used for fixation than when the normal eye is used for fixation. When the normal eye fixes, the involved eye is in the position of primary deviation. When the involved eye fixes, the normal eye is in the position of secondary deviation. The secondary deviation (involved eye fixing) is greater than the primary deviation because the involved eye requires an excess innervational impulse to maintain fixation with impaired musculature, and this excess impulse is distributed to the normally acting muscles of the fellow eye (Hering's law of motor correspondence) and causes an overaction.

In general, a noncomitant strabismus in an adult with previously single binocular vision causes double vision (diplopia), which is most marked when the individual turns his eyes into the field of action of the affected muscle. In those without binocular vision, diplopia does not occur and thus is not found in many congenital paralyses that interfere with the development of binocular vision in infancy.

To minimize diplopia the face may be turned, the chin elevated or depressed, and the head tilted to the right or left shoulder (ocular torticollis). In paralysis of the medial and lateral recti muscles, the face is turned toward the field of action of the paralyzed muscle, but the head is not tilted. Thus with paralysis of either the right medial rectus or the left lateral rectus muscle, the face will be turned to the left. When the face is turned to the left, the eyes move so that the right medial rectus and the left lateral rectus muscles are not contracting. With the face turned in this direction, diplopia is absent or minimal.

Because of the multiple actions of the four cyclovertical muscles (p. 106), the head position is more complicated. The chin is elevated in palsy of the elevator muscles and depressed in palsy of the depressor muscles. Except in superior oblique muscle palsy, the head is tilted toward the shoulder on the side of the affected muscle and the face slightly turned in this direction. With superior oblique muscle involvement, the head is tilted toward the shoulder on the side of

the normal eye, the face is turned slightly in this direction, and the chin is depressed. When the head is tilted toward the shoulder on the side of the involved eye, this eye turns upward.

Structural anomalies of ocular muscles, conjunctiva, or the Tenon capsule cause many signs of noncomitant strabismus. In thyroid myopathy (p. 509), muscles on the inferior surface of the eye may become fibrosed and lose their elasticity so that the eye cannot rotate upward. In blowout fractures of the orbit (p. 248), the tissues in the inferior portion of the orbit may be trapped in the maxillary sinus, and the eye cannot rotate upward (p. 106). Diagnosis requires demonstration of a physical restriction to ocular rotation.

In the forced duction test, the conjunctiva is anesthetized with a topical anesthetic reinforced by 5% cocaine solution on a cotton pledget applied to the conjunctiva near the corneoscleral limbus. This conjunctiva is then grasped with toothless forceps, and the eye is passively rotated to determine its freedom of movement. Children may require general anesthesia.

The retraction syndrome (of Stilling-Türk-Duane) appears to arise because an innervational disturbance causes the lateral rectus muscle to contract instead of relaxing when the medial rectus muscle contracts. Electrical activity in the lateral rectus muscle may be decreased or absent in abduction. This leads to limited or absent abduction, restriction of adduction, retraction of the globe, and narrowing of the palpebral fissure when adduction is attempted. There may be elevation or depression of the globe in adduction. Women are more commonly affected than men (60%), and the left eye is more commonly affected than the right eye (73%); the condition is bilateral in some (18%). Ocular abnormalities include cataracts, iris and pupil anomalies, persistent hyaloid artery, cataract, and choroid colobomas. Labyrinthine deafness, facial defects, cleft palate, and malformations of the external ear, hands, and feet occur.

Too short a tendon of the superior oblique muscle or contracture of the muscle after injury makes the ipsilateral inferior oblique muscle appear paralyzed, because the eye cannot be elevated when adducted.

The diagnosis of the specific muscle involvement in a paralytic strabismus may be difficult. The history may indicate the cause to be head injury, tumor, aneurysm, or thyroid oculopathy. The onset of multiple sclerosis (p. 538) may be associated with muscle palsy. Myasthenia gravis (p. 568) may be limited to ocular muscles.

COMITANT STRABISMUS (NONPARALYTIC)

In comitant strabismus there is no muscle weakness; therefore, the angle of deviation is initially the same in all fields of gaze.

Comitant esotropia

The two main types of comitant esotropia are accommodative and nonaccommodative (Table 21-1). Additionally, there are combinations of these forms.

Accommodative esotropia. Accommodation (p. 105) is the process by which the eye increases in refractive power. Accommodative esotropia is an excessive inward deviation associated with accommodation. When the child accommodates to maintain a clear image of an object, the eyes converge an abnormal amount, and the result is esotropia.

There are two types of accommodative esotropia: (1) refractive and (2) nonrefractive. Both types have their onset after the age of 1 year, usually between 2 and 3 years. The onset is abrupt in a child who has previously had straight eyes. The deviation is brought about by an attempt to visualize objects clearly, and the

amount of crossing varies with activity and fatigue. There is often a family history of ocular deviation. The esotropia is often intermittent initially and then develops into a constant type.

Examination indicates inward deviation of the eye, and this may be demonstrated with the cover-uncover test. A point of light for fixation may not stimulate accommodation adequately to demonstrate an intermittent accommodative deviation, but use of a small picture for fixation that requires accommodation makes the deviation evident. The angle of deviation, however, may be different for near and far fixation and upward or downward gaze (incomitance). Early in the development of the deviation there may be double vision, but this may quickly disappear, because the image originating in the deviating eye is suppressed.

Refractive accommodative esotropia. This is caused by uncorrected hyperopia combined with inadequate motor fusion for divergence. The uncorrected hyperopia requires excessive accommodation to maintain a clear retinal image, and this evokes excessive convergence. The inadequate motor fusion causes the inward deviation to become manifest (esotropia). If the motor fusion is adequate, the inward deviation remains latent (esophoria). Generally, a full correction of the hyperopia with glasses is all that is required. Miotics (p. 118) may be substituted in uncooperative patients or to permit vacation activities without glasses. Ocular muscle surgery is not indicated.

Nonrefractive accommodative esotropia. This is caused by a faulty synkinesis between accommodation and convergence (accommodative-convergence/accommodation ratio [AC/A], p. 423). The effort to accommodate causes an excessive convergence. There is a small refractive error that may be hyper-

Table 21-1. Comitant esotropia

I. Accommodative
    A. Onset after 1 year (average, 2½ years)
    B. Familial
    C. Normal or high accommodative-convergence/accommodation ratio (AC/A)
    D. Sensory mechanisms often normal
    E. Ocular deviation
        1. Same or greater for near than far
        2. Initially intermittent but tending to become constant
        3. Decreased by convex lenses (which decrease accommodation)
    F. Treatment: decrease accommodative stimulus
        1. Full hyperopic correction
        2. Bifocal lenses
        3. Miotics
II. Nonaccommodative—excessive muscle tone (tonic convergence)
    A. Congenital
        1. Onset at birth
        2. Familial
        3. Abnormal sensory mechanisms common
            a. Strabismic amblyopia
            b. Abnormal retinal correspondence
            c. Defective fusion mechanism
        4. Ocular deviation
            a. Nearly equal for near and far
            b. Does not vary with accommodation
        5. Treatment
            a. Exclude neurologic and ocular disease
            b. Prevent abnormal sensory mechanism
                (1) Mainly patching of eye with better vision
                (2) Pleoptics
            c. Surgery
    B. Sensory interference
        1. Onset after disease or injury
        2. Possibly hereditary eye disease
        3. Defective vision in one or both eyes
            a. Marked anisometropia   d. Retinal disease
            b. Corneal opacity   e. Optic nerve or tract disease
            c. Cataract
        4. Ocular deviation
            a. Equal for near and far
            b. Monocular fixation using eye with better vision
        5. Treatment
            a. Lenses if anisometropic (contact lenses, if necessary, as in monocular aphakia)
            b. Cosmetic surgery to straighten eyes
            c. Correction of condition causing defective vision, if possible
III. Combined accommodative and nonaccomodative
    A. Onset following neglected accommodative esotropia
    B. Abnormal sensory mechanisms common
    C. Ocular deviation
        1. Monocular fixation
        2. Tends to increase initially; exotropia common with aging
    D. Treatment
        1. Avoid neglect of accommodative esotropia
        2. Surgery

opic or myopic. However, with the refractive error fully converted, there is a significant inward deviation of the eyes at near.

Treatment is by means of full correction of any refractive error combined with bifocal correction for near vision. This may be combined with topical instillation of anticholinesterase drugs in each eye. The anticholinesterase drugs decrease the angle of deviation by facilitating ciliary muscle action and thus facilitating peripheral accommodation. Since the drug facilitates accommodation, fewer nerve impulses are required. This decreases motor impulses to the medial recti muscles, there is less convergence during accommodation, and esotropia no longer occurs.

Often 0.06% echothiophate (Phospholine Iodide, p. 119) combined with 10% phenylephrine (p. 123) is used. Phenylephrine (an adrenergic agonist) prevents the development of cysts on the pupillary border that may become so large as to interfere with vision. Echothiophate binds pseudocholinesterase and may simulate an acute abdomen in children; there may be prolonged apnea after administration of succinylcholine as a muscle relaxant in general anesthesia.

Orthoptic training (p. 428) is of value in teaching the child to maintain parallelism without lenses. It involves elimination of suppression and development of motor fusion in divergence. This is not always an easy task, because a child may suppress the image of the deviating eye.

Nonrefractive accommodative esotropia does not require surgery.

Accommodative esotropia may be combined with a nonaccommodative esotropia, and then surgery must be directed to the nonaccommodative portion of the esotropia.

Nonaccommodative esotropia. Nonaccommodative esotropia (Fig. 21-4) may involve one of several mechanisms. Many patients have no obvious abnormality of ocular image formation or perception, and an anatomic factor cannot be demonstrated. The deviation appears shortly after birth. There is frequently a familial history of strabismus. The deviation is often more than 50 diopters and is the same for both near and distance. There may be a short period in which there is alternate fixation, but the deviation tends to become monocular. The angle of deviation tends to remain relatively constant and is not modified by corrective lenses or by anticholinesterase agents. Amblyopia (p. 426) and abnormal retinal correspondence (p. 428) commonly develop. The children rarely develop stereopsis or fusion even after early surgery to align the visual axes.

Often there is cross-fixation, with the infant using the left eye to look to the right and the right eye to look to the left. This fixation pattern encourages equal use of the eyes and discourages the development of amblyopia and abnormal retinal correspondence. Cross-fixation may lead to the erroneous belief that a lateral rectus muscle palsy is present, since the child cross-fixates rather than abducts his eyes. The cross-fixation is distinguished

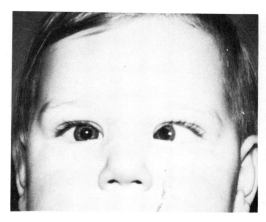

Fig. 21-4. Esotropia with the right eye fixing and the left eye deviating.

from bilateral lateral rectus muscle paralysis with limited abduction, in which the head turns spontaneously or when one eye is covered. Under general anesthesia in lateral rectus muscle paralysis there is no spontaneous abduction during the induction or recovery stages, and the eyes are not in a divergent position in surgical planes of anesthesia.

Congenital nystagmus associated with esotropia may be accompanied by a position of the eyes in which the amplitude of the oscillation is reduced when the eyes are turned to the right or the left. Thus, the fixing eye may be strongly adducted in the position of least nystagmus. The condition is called the nystagmus blockage, or compensation, syndrome, because the fixing eye is put into a position with minimal nystagmus. This type of esotropia usually has its onset in early infancy and is preceded by nystagmus. There may be pseudoparalysis of the lateral recti muscles and, as the fixing eye moves from adduction to abduction, there is a nystagmus. Usually both eyes are in the convergent position.

In the treatment of nonaccommodative esotropia it is important (1) to evaluate the neurologic status of the child to exclude cerebral palsy, and (2) to exclude cataract, unequal refractive errors, and retinal and choroidal disease. Treatment must be started by 6 months of age. Spontaneous improvement does not occur. In cases in which amblyopia has developed, the abnormality is treated by occlusion of the habitually fixing eye to force use of the nonfixing eye. This is essential to develop central vision in each eye (p. 158). Patching converts monocular strabismus to an alternating type. This conversion, a sign of visual improvement, may upset parents who believe that the crossing involved only one eye. Surgery is recommended during the first year of life.

Sensory interference. Children born with an abnormality that interferes with clear ocular images often develop esotropia. A severe monocular deviation is present for both near and far vision from the beginning, and the child uses the better eye. It is important to diagnose the cause of the sensory disturbance, and if the individual cannot develop central vision because of a cataract or a retinal disorder, he should not be treated for amblyopia (p. 426). A life-endangering retinoblastoma (p. 353) may cause sensory interference and esotropia.

When retinal disease is present, cosmetic alignment of the eyes is the only treatment of value. This may be delayed until just before the child enters school inasmuch as there is no likelihood of providing binocular vision. The eyes tend to deviate outward in later life, and surgery to make the eyes parallel in childhood may accelerate the development of exotropia (consecutive exotropia).

Combined esotropia. Combined accommodative and nonaccommodative esotropia most commonly follows a neglected accommodative esotropia. A monocular deviation tends to develop, with an excessive tonic convergence and strabismic amblyopia. The esotropia thus consists of two components: an accommodative deviation, which may be treated with spectacles and anticholinesterase drugs, and a nonaccommodative component. Often surgery is indicated to correct the nonaccommodative portion of the esotropia. Treatment must also be directed toward correction of the amblyopia.

Comitant exotropia

Outward deviations (exodeviations) (Table 21-2) of the eyes differ not only in direction from esodeviations but also in progression, prognosis, and nature of the underlying sensorial adaptation. The usual type begins as an exophoria, becomes an intermittent exotropia, and sometimes (75%) progresses to a manifest exotropia. Secondary exodeviations occur

Table 21-2. Comitant exotropia

I. Exophoria→intermittent exotropia→constant exotropia
  A. Onset at birth to 5 years
  B. Familial
  C. Sensorial mechanisms proportional to bionocularity established before constant exotropia (often normal)
  D. Deviation
    1. Greater for far than near
    2. Phoria measures as much as tropia
    3. Aggravated by fatigue
  E. Treatment
    1. Tropias: surgery
    2. Phorias: observe for progression
II. Acquired exotropia
  A. Variable age of onset
  B. Deteriorated esotropia; surgical overcorrection of esotropia (consecutive exotropia)
  C. Sensory impairment common
  D. Ocular deviation
    1. Equal for near and far
    2. Convergence poor
    3. Usually monocular fixation
  E. Treatment: surgery
III. Uncorrected myopic exotropia
  A. Onset after 5 years
  B. Familial
  C. Uncorrected myopia present
  D. Sensory mechanisms normal
  E. Ocular deviation
    1. Greater for far than near
    2. Initially intermittent but tends to become constant
  F. Treatment: stimulation of accommodation by correcting myopia with lenses

---

as the result of reduced visual acuity in one eye and follow esotropia either spontaneously or after surgery (consecutive exotropia). Individuals with uncorrected myopia do not accommodate for clear vision at near, and the inadequate impulse to converge may cause an exotropia relieved by correcting the refractive error. In craniosynostosis (p. 246) the deformity of the skull places the eyes far apart, and there is often inadequate convergence with an exotropia.

Exophoria → intermittent exotropia → constant exotropia. This is the most common type of exodeviation. It begins at birth to 5 years, rarely (5%) thereafter. Initially it is a large-angle exophoria elicited by the cover-uncover test. The phoria is greater at distance than at near fixation. This period of binocularity is important in allowing normal visual development, and thus amblyopia and abnormal retinal correspondence are not as common in this disorder as in nonaccommodative types of esotropia. With growth, an intermittent exotropia occurs, first at distance and then at near, brought about by fatigue and visual inattention. Suppression with inhibition of fusion leads to a constant exotropia.

Treatment is usually surgical when there are long periods of manifest deviation. Correction of myopia increases accommodation of near and provides sharp retinal images that encourage fusion. Surgical correction is indicated in infants who develop an early exotropia of more than 20 diopters with little tendency to periods of parallelism. In adults with a large-angle exotropia, surgery is indicated as soon as the diagnosis is established. In exotropia-exophoria, surgery should be deferred until it is established that the condition is progressing or until binocular vision is uncomfortable.

Acquired comitant exotropia. Acquired exotropia occurs because of defective vision developing in one eye or because of a deteriorated exophoria.

Deteriorated exophoria-exotropia. Patients with this condition initially have an alternating exophoria-exotropia that is either untreated or neglected. The divergence is delayed until the age of 10 to 12 years. Before that age, an intermittent alternating exophoria-exotropia is present. The deviation subtly becomes constant, initially for distance and then for near. The exotropia (Fig. 21-5) may become marked for both near and far, and attention may not be directed to the deviation until it is marked for near. Visual acuity is good, but often fusion is poor, and ab-

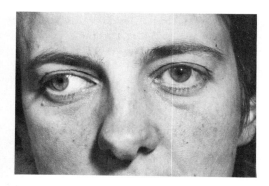

Fig. 21-5. Exotropia in an adult that began as a large-angle exophoria, passed through a stage of intermittent exotropia, and then became a constant exotropia with suppression of the image in the deviating right eye.

normal retinal correspondence may be present. The deviation may be monocular. Convergence is impaired.

Sensory impairment exotropia. Decreased vision in one eye often leads to exotropia. If the sensory loss occurs in infancy an esotropia occurs, but with passing years the eye diverges. This happens in strabismic amblyopia. As the eyes pass from esotropia to exotropia, there is a phase in which they are parallel, and this leads to the naive belief that the esotropia has disappeared spontaneously. The eyes continue to diverge, finally developing a constant exotropia that may recur after surgery. In an older person an esotropia does not develop, but early, after visual impairment, the eye diverges.

Uncorrected myopic exotropia. This is a relatively uncommon disorder that arises because of uncorrected myopia, which decreases the need for accommodation for near work. The decrease in accommodative effort minimizes normal convergence, so the eyes tend to turn outward. Inasmuch as most infants are hyperopic at birth, the condition occurs after visual acuity has developed, and sensory anomalies are uncommon. It may occur in myopic adolescents who prefer

poor vision to wearing glasses. There may be a family history of myopia. Symptoms are minimal. The blurred vision arising from myopia prevents appreciation of the diplopia. Examination reveals an intermittent outward deviation of the eyes, which becomes constant if the condition is neglected. The wearing of concave lenses to correct the myopia is all that is required. Young individuals often prefer contact lenses.

ACCOMMODATIVE-CONVERGENCE/ ACCOMMODATION RATIO

In fixation on distant objects the visual axes are directed straight ahead. Fixation on an object closer to the eyes than 20 feet requires simultaneous adduction of each eye to maintain single vision. The result is convergence of direction of the visual axes. The meter angle is the unit of measurement of convergence. One meter angle is the amount of convergence required for the eyes to fixate an object located in the median plane 1 meter distant (Fig. 21-6). Thus, if the fixation distance is 1 meter, the individual must converge 1 meter angle to maintain fixation with both eyes. Numerically, this is the reciprocal of the fixation distance in meters. For example, if the fixation distance is ½ meter there are 2 meter angles of convergence, or if the fixation distance is ¼ meter there are 4 meter angles of convergence.

Accommodative convergence is measured in prism diopters and is related to the distance between the eyes (interpupillary distance) and the fixation distance. It is the product of the number of meter angles of convergence and the distance between the eyes in centimeters. Thus, if an individual fixates an object ⅓ meter distant, he exerts 3 meter angles of convergence, and if the interocular distance is 5.5 cm he will exert 16.5 diopters of accommodative convergence. The amount of accommodation the normal eye must exert at ⅓ meter is the reciprocal of the distance in meters and thus is 3 diopters.

In the example provided above, the individual's accommodative-convergence/accommodation ratio (AC/A) would be 16.5/3, or reduced, 5.5/1. With an excess or deficiency of accommodative convergence for a particular amount of accommodation, the ratio is abnormal. A high AC/A is related to excessive convergence for near. A patient with esotropia and a high AC/A will have greater deviation for near than for far. A patient with exotropia and a high AC/A will have less deviation for near than for far. The converse is true if the AC/A ratio is reduced. Any deviation of the eyes that is greater for near than for far is considered to involve primarily the convergence mechanism. Conversely, all deviations that are greater for far than for near involve primarily the divergence mechanism.

The AC/A ratio may be measured by one of several methods. First, the interpupillary distance must be measured.

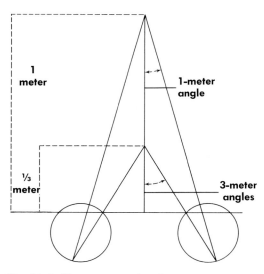

Fig. 21-6. The meter angle of convergence. At 1 meter the eyes must converge 1 meter angle. If the eyes are 5.2 cm apart, they must exert 5.2 diopters of accommodative convergence.

Then the phoria or tropia is measured at both near and far with the patient having full optical correction. The following equation is then used:

$$\frac{AC}{A} = \text{Interpupillary distance (in cm)} + \frac{\text{Deviation for near} - \text{Deviation for far}}{\text{Accommodation at near}}$$

Inward deviations are positive numbers, and outward deviations are negative numbers. Thus, if the interpupillary distance was 5 cm and the deviation for near was 10 prism diopters of esophoria and for far 4 prism diopters of esophoria, the equation would read:

$$\frac{AC}{A} = 5.0 + \frac{10 - 4}{3}$$

$$(\text{Accommodation at near}) = 5.0 + \frac{6}{3} = 7.0$$

Alternatively, a gradient method may be used in which the amount of deviation for near is measured first with full correction and then with a concave lens over the correction. The following formula is then used:

$$\frac{AC}{A} = \frac{\text{Deviation with concave lens} - \text{Deviation without concave lens}}{\text{Power concave lens}}$$

The AC/A ratio is not affected by eye muscle surgery or orthoptic training. Cycloplegics increase the ratio, and miotics, such as anticholinesterases, lower the ratio. Bifocals decrease the need for accommodation when viewing near objects, and thus excess accommodative convergence does not occur. Spectacle-corrected refractive errors change the patient's near point of accommodation and thus affect the AC/A ratio.

A AND V SYNDROMES

A and V syndromes are ocular deviations in which the angle of deviation is more marked on looking either upward or downward. In the A type of deviation the visual axes are closer to each other in upward gaze. In the V type of deviation the visual axes are closer together in downward gaze. Thus an A-esotropia is greater looking upward than downward and a V-esotropia is greater looking downward than upward. In A-exotropia, the exotropia is greater looking downward than upward, and a V-exotropia is greater looking upward than downward.

The cause of the abnormality is debated. In V types of esotropia and exotropia there is often, but not always, overaction of both inferior oblique muscles (N VI). In A types of deviation there may be overaction of the superior oblique muscles. The overaction of the inferior oblique muscle is noted by having the patient look to the right or to the left and observing the upward deviation of the adducting (turned in) eye. Overaction of the superior oblique muscle is noted by the downward deviation of the adducting eye. However, A and V patterns occur without anomalies of the oblique muscles. Physiologically, the visual lines tend to converge in downward gaze so that V patterns, in some cases, may be caused by overaction of the horizontal muscles.

A frequency as high as 50% has been established. V-pattern esotropia is the most common, followed by A-esotropia, V-exotropia, and A-exotropia. Surgery is directed to the muscles believed to be implicated. In V-pattern anomalies with overaction of the inferior oblique muscles, these muscles may be weakened. This may be combined or followed by recession or resection of the lateral recti and medial recti muscles. To enhance the effect of these procedures, the new insertion of the horizontal muscles are often displaced upward or downward. In both exotropia and esotropia the medial recti muscles are always displaced toward the apex of the A or V, thus upward in A pat-

terns and downward in V patterns. The lateral recti muscles are displaced away from the apex, irrespective of whether a horizontal recession or resection is done.

PSEUDOSTRABISMUS

Pseudostrabismus is a condition in which the eyes appear to be crossed although they are in reality perfectly aligned. The appearance arises because of an extra fold of skin at the inner canthus of each eye (epicanthus) (see Fig. 8-2), because of a broad, flat nose, because the eyes are unusually close together, or because of an oval palpebral fissure, as in Orientals. Each of these conditions conceals some of the white sclera at the medial side of the eye and simulates the appearance of the eyes turning inward. The cover-uncover test indicates that the eyes are parallel, and the sole treatment is reassurance of the parents. As the child's face grows, the appearance of strabismus disappears.

The center of the pupil may not correspond to the visual axis, so that when the eye fixates on a penlight the reflection from the cornea is not centered. When the reflection is nasal, a positive kappa angle

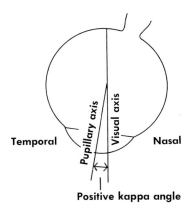

Positive kappa angle

Fig. 21-7. The kappa angle created when the visual line is not in the anatomic center of the pupil. When the visual line is nasal, a positive (common) kappa angle is present. When the visual line is temporal (rare), a negative kappa angle is present.

(Fig. 21-7) is present and, if large enough, produces the appearance of an exodeviation. If the reflection is temporal, a negative kappa angle is present and may simulate the appearance of an esodeviation.

SUPPRESSION

Suppression is that condition in which the image arising on the retina of one eye does not enter consciousness. Marksmen, microscopists, and others who use one eye may, without conscious effort, intermittently ignore the image from the nonfixing eye. In contrast, in strabismus the stimulation of noncorresponding points on the retinas creates a retinal rivalry in which there is cortical suppression of the image arising from the deviating eye to avoid diplopia. There are suppression scotomas in the deviating eye that correspond to the foveal area and to the abnormal fixation point. Visual acuity may be good in each eye when used separately, but the image of the eye that is not being used is suppressed.

AMBLYOPIA

Vision may be divided into (1) form vision, originating in the cones of the fovea centralis, and (2) peripheral vision.

Normal development of binocular vision requires binocular, synchronous use of the fovea centralis during a critical period that occurs during the early years of life. In the monkey, unilateral deprivation of vision for as short a period as 2 weeks during the first 12 weeks of life causes the cells in the binocularly innervated lateral geniculate body to be up to 30% smaller than those in the adjacent nondeprived layers. In cats deprived of vision in one eye, binocularly driven cells are absent, so that the cortex receives some 90% of its input from the nondeprived eye. The input from the deprived eye appears to arise from synaptic inhibition, and in cats intravenous administration of a gamma-amino butyric acid receptor blocker makes visual cortical neurons accessible to stimulation by the deprived eye.

Clinically, amblyopia is a condition in which there is a unilateral or bilateral decrease in form vision not fully attributable to organic ocular abnormalities. It is caused by form vision deprivation, abnormal binocular interaction, or both, and may be reversible in appropriate cases by therapeutic measures (Table 21-3). In addition to reducing visual acuity, amblyopia reduces contrast sensitivity, light

Table 21-3. Classification of amblyopia

Cause	Mechansim	
	Deprivation of form vision	Abnormal binocular interaction
Functional		
Strabismus	Yes	Yes
Anisometropia	Yes	Yes
Visual deprivation		
Binocular occlusion	Yes	No
Bilateral high hypermetropia	Yes	No
Organic ocular disease		
Congenital nystagmus	Yes	No
Monocular occlusion (cataract, leukoma, iatrogenic)	Yes	Yes
Malorientation of retinal receptors	Yes	No

Modified from von Noorden, G. K.: Mechanisms of amblyopia, Adv. Ophthalmol. **34:**93, 1977, S. Karger, Basel.

flicker, and stereoscopic depth perception and produces a condition in which the visual responses are comparable to those in the dark-adapted eye, where rod mechanisms predominate. As might be anticipated from the defect in visual fixation, following (pursuit) movements are impaired. Because of crowding of details when more than one letter is viewed, the visual acuity of the amblyopic eye is better when letters are viewed singly rather than in a series. Examination of the amblyopic eye indicates no decrease in vision in decreased illumination, whereas an eye with an organic disease may show a marked decrease.

Diagnosis of strabismic amblyopia in infants and extremely young children is difficult. Measurement of the degree that the habitually fixing eye is preferred for fixation as compared with the habitually deviating eye suggests the diagnosis. The habitually fixating eye is covered and then uncovered. If it immediately resumes fixation, amblyopia is probably present. If, however, the normally deviat-

ing eye is able to hold fixation through the next blink of the eyelids, amblyopia is not likely.

The reversibility of amblyopia depends on the maturity of the visual system at the onset and the duration of the abnormal visual experience. Treatment is by occlusion of the better eye (Fig. 21-8) to force use of the poorer eye. Because of the sensitivity of the visual system in infants to deprivation during the first year of life, patching should follow a pattern of 3 days sound eye and 1 day amblyopic eye. Between 1 and 3 years of age the sound eye may be patched 4 days and the amblyopic eye 1 day. Patients must be examined at least once every 2 weeks, since fixation preference and amblyopia shift rapidly. After 3 years the patching period may be extended provided visual acuity is monitored frequently. Patching is usually carried out for at least 3 months before it is concluded that there will be no improvement in vision. If vision decreases after patching is terminated, patching should be reinstituted until the visual improvement continues. Often this requires intermittent occlusion into the teen years.

Prolonged atropinization of one eye or patching of one eye for disease or injury should also be avoided in infants and children under 5 years of age. If atropinization is required, the sound eye should also be atropinized so as not to produce a sensory imbalance. Occlusion amblyopia is reversible, but if occlusion is prolonged during visual immaturity, a permanent iatrogenic amblyopia may be induced.

When amblyopia is combined with eccentric fixation, the initial step is to induce normal foveal fixation. The better eye may be patched and the amblyopic eye covered with a red filter until fixation becomes central. Patching of the good eye continues until maximal improvement of visual acuity is attained.

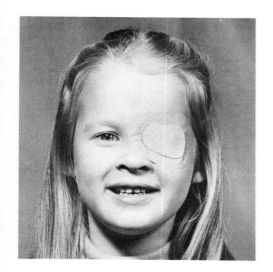

Fig. 21-8. Occlusion of the better eye to force use of the poorer eye in strabismic amblyopia.

ECCENTRIC FIXATION

Eccentric fixation is a monocular condition (usually) in which the fovea centralis is not used for fixation. A special ophthalmoscope (Visuscope), which projects a fixation target on the fundus, may indicate that an area adjacent to the fovea centralis is used for fixation rather than the fovea centralis. In such instances the condition of eccentric fixation is said to be present. The retinal area selected for fixation varies widely, and the more distant it is from the fovea centralis the poorer the vision. Severe eccentric fixation is evident if an eye remains deviated when the fellow eye is covered. The prognosis for visual improvement is much poorer when amblyopia is associated with eccentric fixation.

ANOMALOUS RETINAL CORRESPONDENCE

Anomalous retinal correspondence is a binocular condition in which corresponding points on the two retinas do not have the same relative direction in space. It may be regarded as an attempt to restore binocular cooperation to eyes that have misalignment of the visual axes. Thus the foveas of the two eyes have different directional values, or the fovea of one eye is aligned with an extrafoveal region of the fellow eye. Abnormal retinal correspondence involves directional values of the two eyes and may sometimes be associated with normal visual acuity.

The angle formed by the visual lines of each eye is the angle of strabismus. The objective angle of strabismus is that angle measured by the prism cover test (or a similar test). The subjective angle is that angle in which the patient indicates his perception of the direction of the visual lines in each eye. If the subjective angle and the objective angle of strabismus are different, then anomalous retinal correspondence is present. If the patient's subjective angle is zero, then the anomalous retinal correspondence is harmonious. If the subjective angle is not zero and does not equal the objective angle, the anomalous retinal correspondence is nonharmonious or disharmonious. When the subjective angle and objective angle are the same, then normal retinal correspondence is present.

MICROTROPIA

The term *microtropia* is applied to unusually small deviations that cause sensory abnormalities such as amblyopia, abnormal retinal correspondence, suppression of central vision, and defective stereopsis. The cover test shows no ocular movement of redress and, except for the sensory abnormalities, strabismus is not present. However, when the cover test is repeated with a 4^Δ prism with its base either in or out, there is no recovery movement of either eye. A severe anisometropia may be present, and examination with the Visuscope indicates nonfoveal fixation. In children up to 5 years of age with anisometropia, amblyopia is treated by occluding the fixing eye. Microtropia is present in nearly all nonaccommodative comitant esotropic patients after corrective surgery and accounts for the absence of binocularity.

ORTHOPTICS

Orthoptists participate in the diagnosis and medical correction of sensory and motor anomalies of the eyes. In the United States they are college-trained individuals who have a specialization in orthoptics certified by the American Orthoptic Council. Almost universally, orthoptists are sponsored by physicians or universities. Their diagnostic studies consist of the steps that have been mentioned: (1) detection of a deviation, (2) measurement of the deviation by objective and subjective test, and (3) study of the sensory and motor cooperation between the two eyes. Therapy is carried out to correct amblyopia and AC/A abnormalities, and to improve fusional abilities.

TREATMENT OF STRABISMUS

The treatment of comitant strabismus is directed toward (1) development of normal visual acuity (p. 155), (2) correction of the deviation of the eyes, and (3) superimposing the retinal images to provide fusion and stereopsis.

Correction of deviation. The deviation is corrected by several methods. The accommodative portion of any strabismus requires lenses and not surgery. Surgery usually does not permit patients with comitant strabismus to discard spectacles required to correct astigmatism or accommodative defects or required to support the prisms needed to neutralize small residual deviations.

Patients with an abnormal accommodative-convergence/accommodation ratio may need only bifocal lenses or anticholinesterase drugs. In many patients with phorias, prisms incorporated into the lenses will be helpful; others may benefit from orthoptic exercises. The stimulation of latent fusion may bring about parallelism in some patients.

Surgery is indicated if maximal improvement cannot be accomplished medically and a significant deviation remains. Most instances of strabismus with a small angle do not require surgery but do require continued care to maintain normal central vision.

Choice of surgical procedure. Selection of the proper surgical procedure in cases of strabismus involves considerable judgment. In general, it is undesirable to weaken a normally acting muscle; it is more desirable to strengthen an underacting muscle. When vision is equal in the two eyes, it is desirable to perform symmetric surgery, normally carrying out the same surgical procedure in each eye rather than limiting the surgical correction to one eye. Usually, the better the fusion, the less surgery is required to achieve a cosmetic and functional result. When vision is markedly decreased in one eye, however, it is impossible to achieve a functional result, because surgery will not restore vision to the eye.

In comitant esotropia in which vision is approximately equal in the two eyes and in which correspondence is normal, bilateral resections of the lateral recti muscles or bilateral recessions of the medial recti muscles may be performed.

In patients with comitant esotropia in which vision in one eye is poor, the best results are probably achieved by resecting the lateral rectus muscle and recessing the medial rectus muscle in the amblyopic eye. If this is not adequate to achieve parallelism, a similar procedure may be carried out in the opposite eye.

In alternating exotropia, each lateral rectus muscle is recessed if the divergence is mainly for distance and the eyes are parallel for near, provided vision and fusion are good. If the exotropia is monocular, the deviation the same for near and far, and fusion poor, the initial procedure is recession of the lateral rectus muscle and resection of the medial rectus muscle in one eye.

The surgeon's aim is to perform the minimal procedure that will correct the strabismus. However, some patients require several procedures. This commonly occurs because correction of a horizontal or vertical deviation revealed anomalies that could not be diagnosed earlier. Usually at least 6 months should elapse between procedures to permit the correction to stabilize.

BIBLIOGRAPHY

Burian, H. M., and von Noorden, G. K.: Binocular vision and ocular motility; theory and management of strabismus, St. Louis, 1974, The C. V. Mosby Co.

Cogan, D. G.: Neurology of ocular muscles, ed. 2, Springfield, Ill., 1956, Charles C Thomas, Publisher. (A classic.)

Foster, R. S., Metz, H. S., and Jampolsky, A.: Strabismus and pseudostrabismus with retrolental fibroplasia, Am. J. Ophthalmol. **79:**985, 1975.

Foster, R. S., Paul, T. O., and Jampolsky, A.: Management of infantile esotropia, Am. J. Ophthalmol. **82:**291, 1976.

Helveston, E. M.: Atlas of strabismus surgery, St. Louis, 1977, The C. V. Mosby Co.

Metz, H. S., and Schwartz, L.: Treatment of A and V patterns by monocular surgery, Arch. Ophthalmol. **95:**251, 1977.

Miller, N. R.: Solitary oculomotor nerve palsy in childhood, Am. J. Ophthalmol. **83:**106, 1977.

Parks, M. M.: Ocular motility and strabismus, New York, 1975, Harper & Row, Publishers, Inc.

Pratt-Johnson, J. A., Barlow, J. M., and Tillson, G.: Early surgery in intermittent exotropia, Am. J. Opthalmol. **84:**689, 1977.

Symposium: Recent advances in strabismus management, Trans. Am. Acad. Ophthalmol. Otolaryngol. **79:**703, 1975.

Von Noorden, G. K.: Nystagmus compensation (blockage) syndrome, Am. J. Ophthalmol. **82:**283, 1976.

Von Noorden, G. K.: Update on amblyopia, editorial, Am. J. Ophthalmol. **82:**147, 1976.

Von Noorden, G. K.: Mechanisms of amblyopia, Adv. Ophthalmol. **34:**93, 1977.

Von Noorden, G. K., and Maumenee, A. E.: Atlas of strabismus, St. Louis, 1973, The C. V. Mosby Co.

Von Noorden, G. K., Morris, J., and Edelman, P.: Efficacy of bifocals in the treatment of accommodative esotropia, Am. J. Ophthalmol. **85:**830, 1978.

Chapter 22

OPTICAL DEFECTS OF THE EYE

Parallel rays of light that enter the eye are refracted by the anterior and posterior surfaces of the cornea, pass through the anterior chamber, are refracted by the various zones of the lens, and come to a focus. The position of this focus is determined by the combined refractive power of the cornea, the lens, and the surrounding media. The length of the eye determines whether the focus is in front of the retina as in myopia, upon the retina as in emmetropia, or whether the retina intercepts converging rays before they reach a focus as in hyperopia.

The diopter, the unit of measurement in optics, is equal to the reciprocal of the focal length of a lens in meters. The cornea has a focal distance of 0.0233 meter, and its refractive power is 1/0.0233 or 43 diopters. The refractive power of the lens at rest is about 17 diopters, with extremes of 12 and 22 diopters. The total refractive power of the eye is about 58 diopters, with extremes of 53 and 64 diopters. The axial length of the normal globe varies from 22 to 27 mm, with a mean of 24 mm. Accommodation in youthful individuals (p. 105) increases the refractive power of the lens to a maximum of about 33 diopters.

Refractive errors occur because the refractive power of the anterior segment is disproportionate to the length of the eye. Usually these two elements are correlated so that long eyes have less and short eyes have more refractive power to minimize any refractive error (Fig. 22-1). Thus, it is an oversimplification to regard the myopic eye as one that is too long or a hyperopic eye as one that is too short. Instead, the refractive power of the anterior segment and the length of the globe are not correlated. For the most part, refractive errors of less than 5 diopters are considered to be biologic variations, and the various components of the refractive system of the anterior segment and length of the globe follow a binomial distribution. Refractive errors of more than 5 diopters are generally considered to be pathologic and to result from developmental abnormalities, the origin of which is largely unknown.

SYMPTOMS AND SIGNS OF REFRACTIVE ERROR

The cardinal sign of a refractive error is decreased visual acuity, which is entirely corrected by means of lenses. If vision cannot be corrected to normal by means of lenses, the eye must be considered abnormal and an organic cause found to explain the decrease in vision. In myopia, vision is often decreased for distance and normal for near. In hyperopia, vision may be normal or decreased for both near and far. Inasmuch as accommodation may compensate for hyperopia, often no rela-

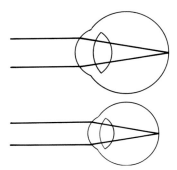

Fig. 22-1. The emmetropic eye. The refractive power of the anterior segment is so correlated with the length of the eye that parallel rays of light are focused on the retina. The eye on the left has much more refractive power than the eye on the right, although both are emmetropic. If such a difference were present in the right and left eyes, there would be a difference of image size, called aniseikonia (p. 439).

tionship exists between vision without lenses and the severity of the hyperopia.

Many different symptoms are attributed to refractive errors. Inasmuch as vision and the eyes prominently figure in psychologic attitudes, symptoms may be difficult to interpret. Thus, ocular discomfort is a vague symptom referring to almost any unexplained sensation occurring in or about the eyes. Asthenopia is the term usually used to denote pain or aching around the eyes, burning and itchiness of the eyelids, ocular fatigue, and headaches.

Headache, irrespective of its cause, is commonly and erroneously attributed to refractive errors. If a refractive error contributes to headache, then the discomfort should be related to sustained use of the eyes and relieved when the eyes are not used. It is unlikely that a headache present on awakening in the morning can be ascribed to excessive use of the eyes the evening before. Additionally, symptoms that occur even after prolonged use of the eyes are not necessarily ocular in origin.

This is particularly true of those individuals living in unpleasant situations from which there is no escape, who develop tension headaches that they attribute to the use of the eyes. Migraine (p. 154) is never caused by a refractive error.

EMMETROPIA

Emmetropia is that optical condition in which rays of light parallel to the visual axis on entering the eye are brought to a focus on the fovea centralis when no accommodation is exerted (Fig. 22-1). There is an exact correlation between the refractive power of the anterior segment and the axial length of the eye. Clinically, emmetropia rarely occurs, because the components of refraction are usually not entirely correlated.

AMETROPIA

Ametropia is that condition in which the refractive power of the cornea and lens and the length of the globe are not correlated (Fig. 22-2). Hyperopia, myopia, or astigmatism may be present, or astigmatism may be combined with hyperopia or myopia.

Hyperopia. Hyperopia is that refractive condition of the eye in which, with accommodation suspended, parallel rays of light are intercepted by the retina before coming to focus (Fig. 22-3).

The condition arises because the refractive power of the anterior segment is inadequate for the length of the globe, or the globe is too short for the amount of refractive power present. Accommodation (p. 105) increases the refractive power of the anterior segment and may compensate for hyperopia and provide normal vision. At birth normal eyes are hyperopic, but the small eye is compensated by increased refractive power of the cornea and lens. Gradual decrease in hyperopia occurs with growth of the eye.

Pathologic degrees of hyperopia may occur with an abnormally small eye,

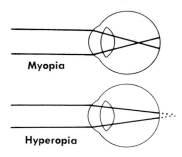

Fig. 22-2. Major types of refractive error (ametropia).

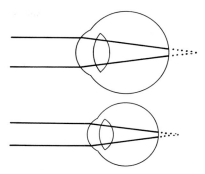

Fig. 22-3. Hyperopia. Both eyes are hyperopic even though the refractive power of the eye on the left is more than that on the right. Accommodation may increase the refractive power of the anterior segment in hyperopia so that a distinct image is formed on the retina.

which may range in size down to an extreme microphthalmia. A tumor in the ocular muscle cone indenting the eye, subretinal fluid at the posterior pole, or an intraocular tumor that elevates the retina may induce hyperopia by displacing the fovea centralis toward the cornea. Often such a primary disease simultaneously decreases vision. Reduction of the radius of curvature of the cornea or lens, or displacement of the lens backward into the vitreous body reduces the refracting power of the anterior segment and may cause an excessive degree of hyperopia. In aphakia, in which the lens is absent, hyperopia is marked, and there is also loss of the accommodation provided by the lens.

Hyperopia may be symptomless or cause ocular fatigue related to use of the eyes. If the refractive error is neutralized by accommodation, vision is normal. There is no direct relationship between the symptoms and the degree of accommodation required to neutralize a hyperopia that is present. Since a portion of accommodation must be used to neutralize the refractive error for distance and additional accommodation is required for near work, the symptoms may be more marked for near work than for distance.

There are no specific signs of hyperopia. The cornea may appear smaller than normal, and the globe itself may appear small. This should not be confused with the appearance caused by a narrow interpalpebral fissure. Hyperopia that exceeds 5 diopters may be associated with blurring of the disk margin, called pseudoneuritis or pseudopapillitis. The disk is not elevated, but the margins appear indistinct and the physiologic cup is absent. This condition is distinguished from early papilledema by the normal caliber of veins, their pulsation, and the absence of retinal edema, or hemorrhages. Inflammation of the optic nerve at the level of the disk is usually unilateral (papillitis, p. 367) and causes decreased vision with a central scotoma.

Hyperopia is classified as follows:

1. Total hyperopia is the amount of hyperopia present with all accommodation suspended, a condition produced by paralysis of the ciliary muscle by means of a cycloplegic drug (p. 440).

2. Manifest hyperopia is the maximum hyperopia that can be corrected with

a convex lens with accommodation active and vision normal.

3. The difference between total and manifest hyperopia is the latent hyperopia.

Since accommodation for near is related to convergence of the eyes, the increased accommodation required to neutralize hyperopia may stimulate an excessive degree of convergence. This excessive convergence is manifested as a tendency for the eyes to deviate inward (esophoria or esotropia, p. 418).

The treatment of hyperopia requires analysis of the interrelation of the symptoms, the visual acuity, and the muscle balance. If visual acuity is good, muscle balance is normal, and there are no symptoms, correction of the hyperopia is not necessary, irrespective of its severity. Conversely, convex lenses are prescribed when visual acuity is decreased, when a convergence excess is present, or when hyperopia creates symptoms.

Myopia. Myopia is that optical condition in which rays of light entering the eye parallel to the visual axis come to a focus in front of the retina (Fig. 22-4). The condition occurs (1) because the refractive power of the anterior segment is too great for the length of the eye or (2) be-

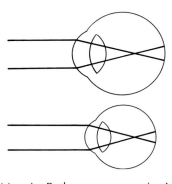

Fig. 22-4. Myopia. Both eyes are myopic. Accommodation increases the refractive power of the anterior segment and aggravates the myopia rather than neutralizes it.

cause the eye is too long for the refractive power present. Inasmuch as the refractive power of the anterior segment is already too great for the length of the globe, accommodation, which shifts the focal point even farther anterior, blurs vision even more.

Myopia may be divided into two types: (1) physiologic myopia and (2) pathologic, or degenerative, myopia. Physiologic myopia, the most common type, occurs because of failure in correlation of the refractive power of the anterior segment with the length of the globe.

Pathologic myopia refers to any myopia in which there are degenerative changes in the choroid and retina. There is an excessive growth of the eye in all dimensions, with a myopia that exceeds 6 diopters (axial myopia). Commonly, pathologic myopia, previously called progressive or malignant myopia, tends to increase rapidly during adolescence. Unlike physiologic myopia, which stabilizes when growth is attained, pathologic myopia continues to increase in adulthood, causing eventual impairment of vision because of choroidal and retinal changes.

An increase in the refractive power of the crystalline lens (lenticular myopia) increases the refractive power of the anterior segment. The increased refractive power originates in the nucleus of the lens and is known as nuclear sclerosis. Such a change occurs at an early stage in the development of senile cataract (p. 379). Initially, vision may be improved with concave lenses, but with increasing opacification of the lens, vision decreases. Individuals who have lost their accommodation (presbyopia, p. 437) and who are able to read without lenses were either myopic previously or have developed nuclear sclerosis.

The chief symptom of myopia is a decrease of distance vision. Each myopic eye has a point, a finite distance in front of the eye, that is in conjugate focus with the retina. An object placed here is imaged distinctly on the retina. If there are 4 diopters of myopia, this point is ¼ meter (25 cm) in front of the eye. An individual with a moderate degree of myopia is thus able to see nearby objects without correction. In more marked degrees of myopia the near point in conjugate focus with the retina is so close to the eye that excessive convergence is required to direct both eyes on the object, and sustained near work is uncomfortable.

The decreased amount of accommodation required for near work in uncorrected myopia may be associated with a decreased amount of convergence, giving rise to a convergence insufficiency along with a tendency for the eyes to deviate templeward (p. 423).

Ophthalmoscopic examination in pathologic myopia may indicate a fluid vitreous body, an abnormal optic disk, and atrophy of the retinal pigment epithelium and choriocapillaris (Fig. 22-5). A myopic crescent of the optic disk appears as a

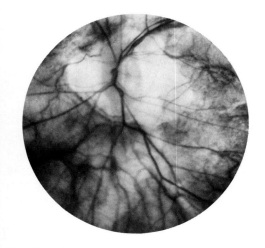

Fig. 22-5. The ocular fundus in pathologic myopia. There is atrophy of the choriocapillaris and depigmentation of the retinal pigment epithelium. The sclera is bared in the region surrounding the optic disk, and the choroidal blood vessels (mainly veins) are easily seen.

white area of sclera adjacent to the temporal side of the optic disk. Sometimes the nasal margin of the disk is obscured by retinal tissue extending over it. The retinal pigment epithelium may have decreased pigment, so that the choroidal vessels are distinctly seen. Atrophy of the choriocapillaris and the depigmentation permit visualization of stark white sclera. Proliferation of retinal pigment may simulate chorioretinitis. Atrophy of the choriocapillaris that nurtures the fovea centralis causes a loss of central vision. Pigment proliferation in the region of the fovea centralis (Fuchs spot) occurs between the ages of 30 and 50 years and markedly reduces visual acuity. There may be subretinal neovascularization. Myopic degeneration of the peripheral retina may lead to retinal hole formation and subsequent retinal separation.

Myopia is neutralized by concave lenses. Lenses should be prescribed for patients dissatisfied with poor visual acuity. Wearing correcting lenses has no apparent effect on the progression of myopia. A decrease in myopia requires a decrease in the axial length or refractive power of the eye, and this does not occur spontaneously.

If a concave lens has more refractive power than necessary to neutralize the myopia, accommodation may provide distinct vision. Such individuals may show an apparent decrease in myopia when proper lenses are prescribed. The use of a contact or bifocal lens does not affect the progression of myopia. Incorrectly fitted contact lenses may temporarily modify the corneal curvature and thus temporarily decrease the severity of myopia. The refractive error reverts to its previous state after use of the contact lenses is discontinued.

Inasmuch as physiologic myopia is a variation in growth, nearly any remedy may be associated with the termination of the growth process, and credit is often given to the therapy. However, nearly all studies of myopia treatment have been anecdotal. Controlled studies, or double-masked methods, and adequate experimental designs have been ignored. When sound experimental studies have been conducted, treatment to decrease or eliminate myopia has been found to be ineffective.

Pathologic myopia is uncommon in the United States. Treatment is based mainly on general hygienic measures of adequate nutrition and exercise and the avoidance of excessive amounts of any single activity, including near work. Affected children need not withdraw from school, limit the amount of school work, or use textbooks with large type unless defective visual acuity makes this desirable. There is no evidence that faithful wearing of corrective lenses or the use of contact lenses has any effect on the course of myopia. It is not necessary to insist that adolescents wear lenses at all times to correct their myopia.

Astigmatism. Astigmatism is an optical condition in which the refracting power of a lens (or an eye) is not the same in all meridians. Thus, if the refracting power of the eye is 58 diopters in the vertical and 60 diopters in the horizontal meridian, two diopters of astigmatism would be present. Parallel rays of light would not focus at a point, but there would be one focal line corresponding to the 60-diopter meridian and another corresponding to the 58-diopter meridian. The distance separating these focal lines is the conoid of Sturm (Fig. 22-6).

Ocular astigmatism may be myopic, hyperopic, or mixed. In myopic astigmatism, both focal lines are in front of the retina. In hyperopic astigmatism, both focal lines are intercepted by the retina before reaching a focus. In mixed astigmatism, one focal line is focused in front of the retina and the other focal lines would have a focus behind the retina if it were

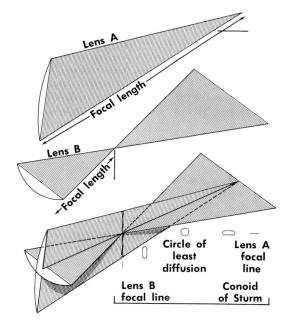

Fig. 22-6. Refraction by two cylindrical lenses, *A* and *B*, of unequal strength. Parallel rays of light are focused as a line rather than as a point. The combination of two cylindrical lenses of unequal power forms two major focal lines corresponding to their refractive power. The distance between the focal lines is the conoid of Sturm. A circle of least diffusion is located between the focal lines at an area where the diverging and converging tendency of the light rays is the same. It is located between the two focal lines and is closer to the stronger cylinder in proportion to the strength of the component cylinders.

not intercepted. In simple myopic astigmatism, one focal line is on the retina and the other is in front. In simple hyperopic astigmatism, one focal line is on the retina and the other would be behind it if it were not intercepted by the retina.

Astigmatism usually occurs because of a difference of curvature of the vertical and horizontal meridians of the cornea. This may arise as a biologic variant, from the weight of the upper eyelid resting upon the eyeball, from surgical incisions into the cornea, from trauma and scarring

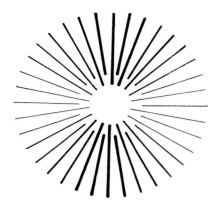

Fig. 22-7. The astigmatic dial as seen by a patient with astigmatism. The thick black lines are focused on the retina, whereas the thin lines lie in front of the retina.

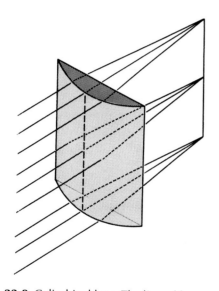

Fig. 22-8. Cylindrical lens. The line of focus parallels the axis of the lens.

of the cornea, or from tumors of the eyelid such as a chalazion (p. 209) pressing upon the globe. An extreme form of curvature astigmatism, frequently irregular, arises in keratoconus (p. 257), in which the cornea becomes cone shaped with the apex of the cone below the center of the cor-

nea. Minor degrees of astigmatism may occur from variations in the radius of curvature of the lens. This condition is seen in patients who wear hard contact lenses that neutralize corneal astigmatism, uncovering the astigmatism of the lens.

The symptoms of astigmatism vary considerably. A distinct retinal image cannot form (Fig. 22-7), but the circle of least diffusion is imaged. Some believe that small degrees of astigmatism are particularly prone to give rise to the symptoms of ocular discomfort because of this constantly changing accommodation. Small degrees of astigmatism cause no obvious external signs. Marked degrees of astigmatism may cause the optic disk to appear elliptic in shape rather than circular. In irregular astigmatism there may be scars and other abnormalities in the cornea.

Astigmatism is neutralized by cylindrical lenses (Fig. 22-8). The amount of astigmatism that should be corrected is debated. Some believe that even minor degrees of astigmatism necessitate correction. If, however, visual acuity is good and there are no symptoms, correction is not indicated. Hard contact lenses may be used to correct irregular astigmatism. If irregular astigmatism cannot be corrected with contact lenses and if vision is markedly reduced, consideration should be given to a corneal transplant to substitute a regular refractive surface for the diseased cornea.

Presbyopia. Accommodation (p. 105) increases the refractive power of the anterior segment through an increased curvature and thickness of the lens. The change in the shape of the lens occurs because of its inherent elasticity in response to contraction of the ciliary body, which causes relaxation of the zonule (p. 39). With each year of life the lens loses some of this elasticity, and there is less accommodation. Generally, there are about 14 diopters of accommodation at the age of 10 years and only 2 diopters of accommodation by the age of 50 years. The decrease occurs gradually, but with only 2 diopters of accommodation, objects viewed closer than ½ meter from the eye are blurred.

The optical condition of decreased accommodation is known as presbyopia. The loss of accommodation occurs in all individuals, irrespective of their refractive error. However, a myopic individual may compensate for presbyopia by removing the lens that corrects his distance vision. Presbyopia is aggravated in a hyperopic individual if the lens that corrects the hyperopia is removed.

The chief symptom of presbyopia is inability to see near work distinctly. This is aggravated in dim illumination and with small print. The individual is frequently annoyed at having to place reading matter farther away from his eyes than previously. The use of nearly all accommodation for clear near vision may cause ocular discomfort. There are no external signs of presbyopia except the general appearance that indicates that the individual is more than 40 years old.

Presbyopia is treated by means of convex lenses added to the distance correction. The power of the lens required for clear vision for near work varies with an individual's habits, age, occupation, length of arms, and accustomed distance of doing near work. Generally, the weakest possible convex lenses are prescribed to permit the individual to carry on vocational and avocational tasks. Bifocal or trifocal lenses are prescribed not as an aggravating additional burden to the middleaged, but so that it will not be necessary to wear a separate pair of lenses for near and for far. If an individual requires lenses for distance, bifocal or trifocal lenses should be worn as early as they are indicated. When an individual does not become accustomed to bifocal lenses relatively early in the development of presbyopia, he frequently suffers unnecessary symptoms in trying to accustom himself to bifocal lenses in later years. If distance lenses are not required, an individual may get along nicely with lenses that correct the presbyopia solely. However, because of the restricted focus of reading lenses, many individuals who do not need a distance correction wear bifocal lenses so that distant objects can be seen without removing the lenses.

Aphakia. When the crystalline lens is not in the visual axis, rays of light entering the eye are refracted solely by the cornea. Surgical removal of the lens is the common cause of aphakia, but dislocation of the lens out of the pupillary area may occur in systemic disease, such as Marfan syndrome (p. 561), or after trauma. Since the lens is one of the two refracting portions of the eye, its removal causes severe hyperopia and a loss of accommodation.

The chief symptom is decreased vision for both far and near. Inasmuch as accommodation is not possible, there are no symptoms of ocular discomfort.

The condition may be diagnosed by the loss of the reflected image from the surface of the lens and by excessive movement of the iris because of loss of support by the anterior lens capsule (iridodonesis).

Aphakia is corrected by means of convex lenses. Because there is no lens, accommodation is not possible and an additional convex lens is for near work. When corrected with ordinary spectacle lenses, the image of the aphakic eye is 25% to 33% larger than that of the normal eye. If the fellow eye is normal, binocular vision is usually not possible because of the difference in size of the retinal images (aniseikonia, p. 439). The difference in image size may be reduced to somewhat less than 10% by means of a contact lens. Convex lenses are required for near vision in aphakic eyes corrected for distance with contact lenses. Intraocular lenses (p. 385) reduce the difference in image size to less than 2%, but convex lenses are required for near.

ANISOMETROPIA

Anisometropia is that condition in which the refractive error of each eye is different. Minor differences are nearly universal, but when there is a difference of more than 2 diopters, the difference in image sizes of the two eyes may be the cause of symptoms. Often such patients are asymptomatic until bifocal lenses are prescribed. When the eyes are turned downward to use the bifocal segment, the difference in power of the two lenses induces a vertical prism, so that the image from each eye is on a different level. This may give rise to marked symptoms that may be neutralized by prescribing the appropriate prism in the reading segment or by using separate lenses for near and distance.

Marked anisometropia is a common cause of amblyopia (p. 426) because of the developing infant's failure to use the eye with the greater refractive error. Failure of central vision to develop leads in turn to strabismus (p. 413). Even when the visual acuity is normal, binocular vision may fail to develop; then the anisometropia produces no symptoms, because the retinal image arising from one eye is suppressed (p. 426).

Aniseikonia. Aniseikonia is that condition in which the size or shape of the retinal images of the two eyes is different. A difference of 0.5 diopter in the refractive error gives rise to a retinal image size difference of about 1%. Most individuals can tolerate a difference of up to 5% without symptoms. Symptoms arise from aniseikonia only if binocular vision is present. Thus, many individuals who have a markedly different refractive error in the two eyes do not have symptoms, because they suppress the image arising from one eye. Patients may prefer to use one eye when reading or watching moving objects. They may complain of objects appearing tilted. All symptoms are entirely eliminated by covering one eye, as is true of all disorders of binocular vision.

Some 40 years ago and for 10 years thereafter, aniseikonia was intensively studied and corrected with specially ground lenses with different curvatures on their front and back surfaces to equalize the size of the retinal images. Today equalization may be accomplished by using contact lenses of different strengths neutralized by appropriate spectacle lenses to alter the size of images.

MEASUREMENT OF THE REFRACTIVE ERROR

The presence or absence of a refractive error may be estimated by a number of methods. Some refractive errors have characteristic symptoms, whereas symptoms of others may be misleading. Measurement of near and distance vision may indicate the probable refractive error present. There may be typical ophthalmoscopic signs evident, but the measurement of the severity of ametropia by means of the ophthalmoscope is unreliable.

Visual acuity. An impression of the degree of ametropia can be learned by measurement of the visual acuity. If vision is 6/6 (20/20) for distance, the patient is not myopic. If vision is 6/6 (20/20) for distance and poorer than this for near, the patient is either presbyopic or has hyperopia not compensated for by accommodation. If vision is less than 6/6 (20/20) for distance but normal for near, the patient may be myopic. Patients with hyperopic astigmatism with the cylinder axis at 90° often see the horizontal bars of letters such as E, F, and Z more clearly than they do the vertical bars of letters such as N, H, and K. The condition is reversed when the astigmatism is about 180°.

Measurement of distance visual acuity by using a pinhole lens in patients who do not wear correcting lenses will indicate whether decreased vision is the result of an organic disease or refractive error. If vision is not improved with a pinhole lens, the decreased vision is likely the result of an organic disease.

Ophthalmoscopy. The estimation of ametropia by means of the ophthalmoscope may be inaccurate unless the examiner is presbyopic and unable to accommodate. However, in hyperopia the disk may appear smaller than normal, and a pseudopapillitis may occasionally be present. In myopia the disk may appear larger than normal. In pathologic myopia a scleral myopic crescent may be present, there may be attenuation of the retinal pigment epithelium with a prominent choroidal pattern, and there may be areas of pigment proliferation. In astigmatism the optic disk may appear oval rather than round.

Retinoscopy. Retinoscopy is an objective method of measurement of the refractive error. It is extremely accurate when carried out by a skilled examiner. The basic principle is to substitute lenses in front of the patient's eye so that emerging rays of light from his retina are brought to a focus at the examiner's eye. The light is directed into the patient's eye by means of a light source that has an aperture for observation.

Retinoscopy (skiascopy) constitutes the single most valuable method of examination for the measurement of ametropia. It is the only method that is of value in children and in individuals with poor discrimination or who respond slowly.

Recently a variety of refracting machines have become available that electronically provide the results of retinoscopic measurement. Even with their assistance, however, the examiner must measure the visual acuity with lenses and provide reading correction for presbyopic patients.

Subjective methods. The many subjective methods for estimating refractive errors depend largely on the patient's responses to changes in lenses. In one common method, called fogging, a convex lens, much in excess of that required for distinct vision, is placed in front of the eyes until accommodation relaxes to improve vision. The power of the convex lens is then reduced until vision is at about the level of 6/12 (20/40). The patient's attention may then be directed to an astigmatic dial and a concave cylinder placed with its axis at right angles to the axis he finds most dark. Subjective testing requires discrimination of moderately small changes in vision by an individual who has moderately rapid reaction times and is most accurate in presbyopia.

Keratometry. The keratometer is an instrument for measuring the anterior curvature of the cornea. In principle, the size of a corneal image created by an object of known size located a fixed distance from the cornea is measured. It is now used to measure the cornea curvature ("K" reading) in order to aid in the selection of a properly fitted contact lens.

Cycloplegia. As has been seen, accommodation may cause the refractive power of the eye to vary by as much as 15 diopters between the condition of the eye at rest and when actively accommodated in youth. Paralysis of accommodation by means of drugs (cycloplegia) permits measurement of the refractive error uncomplicated by changes in accomodation. Cycloplegia is indicated in children, in patients with strabismus, when spasm of accommodation is suspected, and in patients with cloudy media in whom retinoscopy through the undilated pupil is not possible.

Inasmuch as adequate ophthalmoscopic examination is not possible through the undilated pupil, many physicians insist that a complete eye examination include pupillary dilation. In many adults, pupillary dilation (mydriasis) is all that is required. In younger individuals, cyclo-plegia and pupillary dilation are required. The chief precautions are not to dilate the pupil of a patient predisposed to angle-closure glaucoma (Chapter 20) and to constrict the pupils of all adult patients at the conclusion of the examination.

OPTICAL DEVICES

Spectacle lenses may provide convex or concave spherical correction combined with cylindrical lenses and bifocal and trifocal additions in a variety of sizes and shapes. Additionally, prisms may be incorporated into the lenses to compensate for muscle imbalance. Lenses may be case hardened or plastic to resist breaking and have various metallic salts incorporated to alter light transmission.

Spectacle lenses generally have the following functions: (1) improving vision by correction of refractive errors; (2) relieving symptoms by changing the amount of accommodation required; (3) making the eyes parallel by correcting an error of refraction, or by changing the amount of accommodation required, or by incorporating neutralizing prisms; (4) protecting the eye from mechanical trauma or radiant energy; or (5) compensating of subnormal vision by providing magnification.

Refractive errors are neither induced nor prevented by wearing spectacle lenses. Refractive errors are not aggravated or corrected by wearing improper lenses or by not wearing lenses at all. (However, accommodative types of esotropia and exotropia may be corrected by the appropriate lens [p. 418].) Previously, some individuals preferred blurred vision to wearing spectacles, but now contact lenses are usually worn. Some patients complain of ocular discomfort but refuse to wear correcting lenses; there is little help for them.

Lenses to relieve the symptoms arising from excessive accommodative effort are prescribed to treat abnormalities of the accommodative-convergence mechanism; they may not improve visual acuity. Children with either divergence or convergence anomalies arising from disorders in accommodative convergence should wear lenses to prevent intermittent crossing of one eye, which is often associated with suppression of the image in that eye and results in interference with binocular function.

Impact-resistant lenses. All optical lenses sold in the United States, unless specifically excluded by the prescriber, must be tested to resist the impact of a ⅝-inch diameter steel ball dropped from a height of 50 inches. Such impact-resistant glass lenses are either chemically treated or case hardened by heating followed by cooling. Although plastic lenses do not shatter, they scratch more easily than glass lenses. However, some individuals prefer them because of their lighter weight. Ordinary impact-resistant lenses do not meet the safety requirements of industry, which requires a minimum thickness of 5 mm combined with industrial-type frames.

Spectacle frames manufactured in the United States are constructed with fire-retardant material, but some frames manufactured abroad are flammable. A frame constructed with a posterior lip so that the lens cannot be displaced toward the wearer's eye provides additional protection.

Colored lenses. Most colored lenses are manufactured by dissolving metallic oxides in glass or plastic so that certain wavelengths of light are absorbed by the lens and others are reflected or transmitted. Infrared radiation is difficult to protect against, and in the United States the steel- and glass-making industries use manufacturing methods that prevent infrared exposure of the worker. Ultraviolet radiation is mainly absorbed by the cornea and may cause a painful superficial keratitis (p. 197). Skiers, sailors, and others exposed to high levels of ultraviolet radiation should wear colored lenses to protect the cornea. Lenses designed for industrial protection should be used solely within that industry inasmuch as they may markedly reduce visual acuity in other situations.

Colored lenses should not be worn at night, because they reduce the amount of light entering the eye. Individuals with defective color perception may further

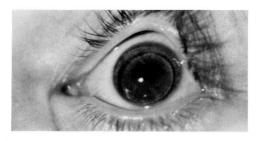

Fig. 22-9. Corneal contact lens. The lens floats on the precorneal tear film and is outlined by shadows.

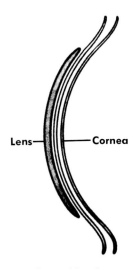

Lens——   ——Cornea

Fig. 22-10. An aspherical hard contact lens with a back surface that exactly parallels the surface of the cornea. (From Gasset, A. R.: Contact lenses and corneal diseases; a programmed course, New York, 1976, Appleton-Century-Crofts.)

reduce their color vision by wearing amber or pink lenses. Deeply tinted lenses provide much comfort to patients with albinism, photophobia, aversion to light, cone disorders, and conditions in which the pupil is dilated or the iris absent. However, bright sunlight cannot harm normal eyes and, although dark glasses may make vision more comfortable, they are not necessary.

Contact lenses. Contact lenses are worn beneath the eyelids and in front of the cornea (Fig. 22-9). They may be hard or soft. Hard lenses may be corneal or corneoscleral. The corneal lens may be rigid or semiflexible. Soft lenses have diameters (12.5 to 15 mm) greater than the corneal diameter, and they adapt to the curvature of the eye, a feature that makes them unsuitable for correction of severe astigmatism. In addition to correction of refractive errors, soft contact lenses are also used to treat corneal inflammations and degenerations (bandage lens).

Hard corneal lenses have a diameter of 8 to 9 mm and are ground with a concave inner surface (base curve) and a convex outer surface (Fig. 22-10). The curvature of the inner surface usually corresponds to the curvature of the cornea as measured by keratometry (p. 440), whereas the curvature of the outer surface varies with the refractive power required to correct the visual acuity. In general, hard lenses are more uncomfortable than soft lenses and require adaptation by progressive increase in wearing time. Some individuals are unable to tolerate them. Additionally, hard lenses are more likely to cause corneal injury and produce temporary changes in corneal curvature. But they provide better vision than the soft variety. Corneoscleral lenses require a mold of the anterior segment, and they are now reserved for treatment of severe disease, such as ocular erythema multiforme.

Soft contact lenses cover both the cornea and anterior sclera and are much more easily tolerated than hard lenses. Oxygen-permeable soft lenses may be worn continuously under close medical supervision with removal for cleaning every 30 to 90 days. Soft lenses are much more useful for occasional wear (such as sports activity) and are lost less frequently than hard lenses. Their major defect arises from poor correction of visual acuity in some individuals, particularly those with severe astigmatism Occasionally the astigmatism may be neutralized by wearing one soft contact lens over another. A problem of the soft lenses is their hydrophilic composition; they combine with lens-cleaning solutions, medications, and chlorinated water in swimming pools and then gradually release these compounds into the eye. Fluorescein and bengal rose stain soft lenses. Because of their hydrophilic property, soft contact lenses can be used to release medications gradually into the eye in the treatment of glaucoma.

Contact lenses are indicated to improve vision in keratoconus and in conditions, such as corneal scarring, that cause irregular astigmatism. They may be advantageous after cataract extraction. Contact lenses are valuable in the management of some cases of conjunctival scarring to prevent exposure keratitis, corneal drying, and injury.

Contact lenses occasionally cause injury to the eye. Directions for sterilizing soft contact lenses must be followed exactly. Contact lenses, except those made of silicone and the extremely thin soft contact lenses, which are permeable to oxygen, separate the corneal epithelium from the atmospheric oxygen necessary for its metabolism (p. 82). After such contact lenses have been worn for a period, minute abrasions of the epithelium and subepithelial edema develop. The subepithelial edema is known as a Sattler veil and is identical with the edema ob-

served after sudden increase in intraocular pressure. Infection may be introduced into the cornea by means of a contact lens, and ocular disease may be neglected by patients who believe their symptoms are caused by wearing contact lenses. Some soft lens wearers develop excess mucus, ocular itching, and giant papillae in the tarsal conjunctiva of the upper eyelids that resemble vernal conjunctivitis.

Soft spots of calcium deposit may develop in soft contact lenses ("lensopathy"), particularly in aphakic patients and in patients with diseased corneas. These may be removed as a corneal body by using a fine needle or by soaking in a chelating agent, or they may necessitate substitution of a different brand of soft lens or a hard lens. Frequent boiling may cause some soft lenses to be coated with mucus, which can be minimized by using an enzymatic cleaner.

Intraocular lenses. A lens may be placed in the plane of the pupil at the time of cataract extraction (p. 385) to substitute for the optical power of the lens removed. Many different lens shapes and surgical techniques are used. Surgeons vigorously debate the indications, the superiority of the intraocular lens or permanent-wear soft contact lenses, and whether the additional step at the time of lens extraction is indicated.

Reading aids for the partially sighted. Many magnifying devices that increase the size of the retinal image are available to compensate for subnormal vision. The two basic devices are (1) a Galilean telescope to produce an enlarged virtual image of a distant object in the same plane as the object itself, and (2) an optical device to decrease the distance of an object from the reader, usually by means of a magnifier lens. This may be in the form of a spectacle lens, stand magnifier, projection magnifier, or television reader.

Diagnosis of the ocular condition that causes subnormal vision and an understanding of the occupational needs of the individual must be correlated with the selection of the mode of correction. Some patients may benefit from use of a mydriatic, others from use of a miotic. Some individuals with central retinal degeneration require high illumination, whereas others with various forms of cone degeneration see better in reduced illumination. Many patients who could be benefitted become discouraged at the long process of fitting and selection, and many practitioners lack the patience and the special equipment and optical devices required for testing.

A hand magnifier may be extremely useful. Some patients benefit from the use of a jeweler's loupe. Successful use of reading aids is correlated with the cause of loss of vision and the motivation and personality of the patient. Patients with visual reduction caused by vitreous hemorrhage and retinitis proliferans do poorly as compared with those who have isolated central retinal lesions. Optimistic, self-reliant patients accept optical aids much better than those who are hostile, pessimistic, and sedentary.

BIBLIOGRAPHY

Allansmith, M. R., Korb, D. R., Greiner, J. V., and others: Giant papillary conjunctivitis in contact lens wearers, Am. J. Ophthalmol. **83**:697, 1977.

Binder, P. S., and Worthen, D. M.: Clinical evaluation of continuous-wear hydrophilic lenses, Am. J. Ophthalmol. **83**:549, 1977.

Gasset, A. R., and Kaufman, H. E., editors: Soft contact lens, St. Louis, 1972, The C. V. Mosby Co.

Karlin, D. B., and Curtin, B. J.: Peripheral chorioretinal lesions and axial length of the myopic eye, Am. J. Ophthalmol. **81**:625, 1976.

Klein, R. M., and Curtin, B. J.: Lacquer crack lesions in pathologic myopia, Am. J. Ophthalmol. **79**:386, 1975.

Sloan, L. L.: Reading aids for the partially sighted; a systematic classification and procedure for prescribing, Baltimore, 1977, The Williams & Wilkins Co.

Sloan, L. L., Habel, A., and Feiock, K.: High illumination as an auxiliary reading aid in diseases of the macula, Am. J. Ophthalmol. **76**:745, 1973.

Sloan, L. L., Habel, A., and Ravadge, F.: Basic test kit for selection of reading aids for the partially sighted, Am. J. Ophthalmol. **78**:1014, 1974.

Weinberg, R. J.: Deep corneal vascularization caused by aphakic contact lens wear, Am. J. Ophthalmol. **83**:121, 1977.

PART FOUR

Systemic diseases and the eye

Chapter 23

INFECTIOUS OCULAR DISEASES AND GRANULOMAS

The globe and ocular adnexa may be inflamed by invasion of almost any microbial organism. Only the conjunctiva and the eyelids have lymph drainage. Thus, the globe and orbital contents may be relatively unprotected when exposed to an infectious agent. Additionally, the eyes of a compromised host may be susceptible to infections that rarely occur in the normal individual. Many microbial agents considered to be noninfectious will cause ocular inflammation if introduced in sufficient quantity into the cornea or the interior eye. Alternatively, rather than producing an infectious process, they may cause an immune reaction.

In general, if an infecting organism causes skin lesions elsewhere, it may often involve the skin of the eyelids with a marked swelling. Additionally, the conjunctiva may be inflamed. The glands of the eyelids may be infected, causing chalazia, hordeola, or blepharitis. Introduction of pathogenic organisms into the conjunctival sac often causes conjunctivitis. If introduced in adequate quantities, organisms that infect other mucous membranes in the body will cause conjunctivitis. Loss of the corneal epithelium, which acts as a barrier to most infections, may result in bacterial, viral, or fungal ulcers. Preauricular adenopathy occurs particularly in suppurative infections of the eyelids and in adenovirus keratoconjunctivitis.

The introduction of infectious agents directly into the eye either by accidental trauma or surgery may give rise to an immediate inflammation as the result of the multiplication of bacteria. A more delayed reaction may be caused by the introduction of fungi. An immune reaction may develop. Involvement of the brain and the cranial nerves may give rise to ocular muscle palsies and optic neuritis.

The topic of infectious ocular disease has previously been considered in discussions of inflammations of the eyelids, conjunctiva, cornea, and uveal and retinal tracts. Because modern therapy has made infectious diseases a rarity, they are often not recognized when they do occur. Conversely, cancer chemotherapy and immune suppression after transplant have made the eye susceptible to inflammations that were previously rarely seen.

BACTERIAL INFECTIONS

Bergey's Manual of Determinative Bacteriology is a standard reference for bacterial classification and taxonomy. The eighth (1974) edition has radically departed from earlier editions in that it no

Table 23-1. Classification of bacteria that may cause ocular disease

---

Kingdom Procaryotae
  Division I. The cyanobacteria
  Division II. The bacteria
    Part 5. The spirochetes
      Family I. Spirochaetaceae
        Genus III. *Treponema,* sp. *pallidum* (chancre, iridocyclitis, chorioretinitis, gumma, tabes dorsalis, optic atrophy)
        Genus V. *Leptospira,* sp. *interrogans*
    Part 7. Gram-negative aerobic rods and cocci
      Family I. Pseudomonadaceae
        Genus I. *Pseudomonas,* sp. *aeruginosa* (necrotic keratitis)
      Uncertain genera
        Genus *Brucella,* sp. *melitensis* (goats); *abortus* (cows); *suis* (sows); *ovis* (sheep); *canis* (dogs) (uveitis? keratitis nummularis [coin-shaped]? optic neuritis?)
        Genus *Bordetella,* sp. *pertussis* (ocular hemorrhages)
        Genus *Francisella,* sp. *tularensis* (necrotic conjunctival ulcer [Parinaud syndrome])
    Part 8. Gram-negative facultatively anaerobic rods
      Family I. Enterobacteriaceae
        Genus I. *Escherichia* (keratitis, panophthalmitis)
        Genus IV. *Salmonella* (keratitis, panophthalmitis)
        Genus VI. *Klebsiella* (keratitis, panophthalmitis)
        Genus X. *Proteus* (keratitis, panophthalmitis)
        Genus XI. *Yersinia,* sp. *pestis* (hemorrhagic chemosis)
      Uncertain genera
        Genus *Haemophilus,* sp. *influenzae* (conjunctivitis, orbital abscess in children); uncertain species: *aegyptius* (Koch-Weeks) (conjunctivitis)
    Part 10. Gram-negative cocci and coccobacilli
      Family I. Neisseriaceae
        Genus I. *Neisseria,* sp. *gonorrhoeae* (ophthalmia neonatorum); *meningitidis* (petechiae, ecchymosis, panopththalmitis); *sicca* (conjunctivitis)
        Genus III. *Moraxella,* sp. *lacunata; nonliquefaciens* (indolent ulcer, conjunctivitis)
        Genus IV. *Acinetobacter* (endophthalmitis, conjunctivitis) (Tribe Mimeae, sp. *polymorpha* obsolete)
    Part 14. Gram-positive cocci
      Family I. Micrococcaceae
        Genus I. *Micrococcus,* sp. *luteus* (conjunctivitis)
        Genus II. *Staphylococcus,* sp. *aureus* (sty, blepharitis, conjunctivitis, keratitis, panophthalmitis); *epidermidis* (conjunctivitis)
      Family II. Streptococcaceae
        Genus I. *Streptococcus* (21 sp.), sp. *pyogenes* (conjunctivitis); *pneumoniae* (acute hypopyon keratitis, dacryocystitis); *anginosus* (beta-hemolytic streptococcus) (pseudomembranous conjunctivitis, acute hypopyon keratitis, uveitis?)
    Part 15. Endospore-forming rods and cocci
      Family I. Bacillaceae
        Genus I. *Bacillus,* sp. *subtilis* (surgical contaminant); *anthracis* (necrotic ulcer of eyelids)
        Genus III. *Clostridium* (300 sp.), sp. *botulinum* (paralysis N III, IV, V); *tetani* (miosis, orbicularis oculi spasm)
    Part 17. Actinomycetes and related organisms
      Coryneform group (unresolved classification problems)
        Genus I. *Corynebacterium,* sp. *diphtheriae* (membranous comjunctivitis with necrosis, postdiphtheritic paralysis [N VI and accommodation N III]); *xerosis* (in foamy secretion from inner canthus in the elderly)
      Family I. Actinomycetaceae
        Genus I. *Actinomyces,* sp. *israelii* (Streptothrix) (dacryocanaliculitis)
      Family II. Mycobacteriaceae
        Genus I. *Mycobacterium,* sp. *tuberculosis* (uveitis, lupus vulgaris, phlyctenules, periphlebitis); *leprae* (anterior uveitis and keratitis [lepromatous: cutaneous], ocular muscle paralysis [tuberculoid: neural])

Table 23-1. Classification of bacteria that may cause ocular disease—cont'd

Family VI. Nocardiaceae
    Genus   I. *Nocardia,* sp. *asteroides* (Leptothrix) (chorioretinal abscess in immune suppresion, keratitis, conjunctivitis, cat-scratch fever)
Part 18. The rickettsias
    Order I. Rickettsiales
    Genus   I. *Rickettsia,* sp. *prowazekii* (typhus fever); *rickettsii* (Rocky Mountain spotted fever)
    Order II. Chlamydiales
    Genus   I. *Chlamydia,* sp. *trachomatis* (VR 571, VR 572, VR 573: trachoma; VR 346, VR 575: inclusion conjunctivitis; VR 121: lymphogranuloma venereum); *psittaci* (psittacosis)

longer presents a hierarchy of bacteria but subdivides the bacteria into 19 different parts. Some of the major groups of bacteria and the ocular disorders they cause are shown in Table 23-1.

The spirochetes

Treponema pallidum. This spirochete causes acquired syphilis, usually by direct body contact, and congenital syphilis, in which the organism is transferred through the placenta of a pregnant syphilitic mother. Ocular involvement is seen mainly in patients who have had previous inadequate therapy with possible serologic reversal but continued infection.

Acquired syphilis. Acquired syphilis is divided into primary, secondary, and tertiary stages. The incubation period is 2 to 4 weeks, rarely as long as 90 days. The initial lesion is a chancre, usually on the external genitalia, rarely on the conjunctiva or the eyelids. The *Treponema* may be demonstrated by dark-field microscopic examination.

The iris and the ciliary body are involved early in the secondary stage and late in the tertiary stage. A severe iridocyclitis is usually (75%) associated with a skin rash and occurs in the fourth to the sixth month after the chancre. Broad, flat posterior synechiae occur between the stromal layer of the iris and the lens and not between the pigmented epithelium and the lens, as is usual in uveal inflammation.

The tertiary stage of syphilis occurs 10 or more years after the chancre, or it may never occur. It is characterized by a small number of organisms, extensive parenchymal destruction, gumma formation, and connective tissue proliferation.

Tabes dorsalis is a degenerative disease of the central nervous system characterized by signs of involvement of the posterior columns and the cranial nerves. White men are most commonly affected. The disease progresses slowly for 10 to 20 years. Ataxia is common, as is posterior root pain, "lightning pain," with paroxysmal attacks at night involving the legs, abdomen, arms, and face. There is impairment of deep sensibility and position sense and loss of vibratory sense. Pupillary signs (p. 284) are important for recognizing continued central nervous system progression. Slight inequality in size of the pupils and a sluggish reaction may be the only signs. Argyll Robertson pupils (p. 286) are diagnostic of tabes dorsalis.

Congenital syphilis. Congenital syphilis is an infectious disease caused by *Treponema pallidum.* The infection is acquired in utero and is characterized by massive systemic involvement without the occurrence of a primary lesion. Symptoms are usually present 2 to 6 weeks after birth, but a fatal pemphigus-like lesion may be present at birth. As a rule, a severe, persistent rhinitis develops, followed in a week by a maculopapular eruption. The infant's general nutrition suffers, and he is thin, snuffling, and irritable. Fissures about the mouth are uncommon but diagnostic.

Late signs of congenital syphilis include the Hutchinson triad of (1) pegged second dentition, particularly with the upper central incisors notched and enamel absent from the notched edge, (2) nerve-type deafness occurring about the time of puberty, and (3) interstitial keratitis. Other signs are collapse of the bridge of the nose as a result of necrosis of the nasal septum from syphilitic rhinitis, splenomegaly, lymphadenopathy involving the epitrochlear nodes, saber tibia, and exostosis of the tibia and the cranial bones.

Syphilitic interstitial keratitis is an infiltrative inflammation of the corneal stroma with an associated anterior uveitis. The disease, which affects boys predominantly (61%), occurs between the ages of 5 and 20 years. It commences with anterior uveitis, often preceded by minor ocular trauma. There is endothelial edema and deep staining with fluorescein. After about 2 or 3 weeks there is acute pain, photophobia, and lacrimation. The cornea is hazy, with circumcorneal injection. All corneal layers are affected, with edema of the epithelium and endothelium and cellular infiltration of the stroma. This stage of the disease is usually short and is followed by a period of vascular inflammation with invasion of the cornea from the periphery. The invading vessels, which appear to be pushing the haze in front of them, ultimately meet at the center of the cornea to form a "salmon patch." As soon as the vessels meet, symptoms and inflammation subside. When healing is complete, faint gray lines of empty blood vessels persist in the cornea. There may be late degenerative changes, with band keratopathy or keratoconus and secondary glaucoma. A penetrating corneal transplant will in many instances restore useful vision in healed interstitial keratitis.

Gram-negative organisms

Pseudomonas aeruginosa. This is an aerobic gram-negative rod, commonly present in soil and water, that may be isolated from wounds, burns, and urinary tract infections. There are a number of different strains. Proteolytic enzymes released by the bacteria cause a devastating keratitis (p. 261) with liquefaction of the cornea. Less commonly, as a surgical contaminant they cause panophthalmitis. Gentamicin, tobromycin, carbenicillin, polymyxin B, and colistin are inhibitory drugs.

Haemophilus influenzae. This is a gram-negative aerobic and facultative anaerobic coccobacillus- to rod-shaped organism that requires growth factors from blood for culture. It causes pneumonia, meningitis, and acute orbital inflammation in infants, usually by extension from a nasal sinus. It may cause conjunctivitis. Some strains are resistant to parenteral penicillin and ampicillin, and systemic infections require simultaneous administration of chloramphenicol until sensitivity of the organism to ampicillin is established.

Haemophilus aegyptius (Koch-Weeks bacillus) causes acute or subacute conjunctivitis in hot countries.

Neisseria. This genus includes two disease-producing species, *N. gonorrhoeae* and *N. meningitidis,* and several nonpathogenic species *(N. sicca)* that cause conjunctivitis.

N. gonorrhoeae. This is a gram-negative anaerobic or facultative anaerobic nonmotile diplococcus with at least four different antigenic types that causes inflammation of the mucous membranes of the urethra, anal canal, conjunctiva, pharynx, and endocervix.

The most serious ocular infection is a purulent conjunctivitis, which is a major cause of blindness, particularly in the Middle East. After an incubation period of 3 to 5 days there is an acute onset with a serious discharge that soon becomes purulent. Extreme conjunctival chemosis and periorbital edema prevent drainage of pus. The central cornea may perforate, leading to panophthalmitis or corneal scarring.

Ophthalmia neonatorum is the term applied to any conjunctival inflammation occurring during the first 10 days of life. The most common causes in the United States are *Chlamydia trachomatis* (inclusion conjunctivitis), *Streptococcus pneumoniae, Neisseria gonorrhoeae,* and species of the *Haemophilus* genus. The infection is acquired in the birth canal, and the risk of contamination increases with prolonged rupture of the membranes. Instillation of 1% silver nitrate (Credé prophylaxis) in the eyes of the newborn prevents gonococcal ophthalmia neonatorum but not the chlamydial type.

Despite the efficiency of 1% silver nitrate instillation in the eyes of the newborn, the gonococcus is again causing ophthalmia neonatorum in the United States. The main causes appear to be the higher incidence of gonorrhea and failure to instill silver nitrate. In some institutions where maternal gonorrhea is common, prophylactic antibiotics are administered at the beginning of labor. Meticulous attention must be directed to proper Credé prophylaxis. The disease is so serious that in any conjunctival inflammation of the newborn infant, the gonococcus must be excluded as a cause. Hourly local instillation of tetracycline should be combined with systemic penicillin and irrigation with saline solution to remove pus.

Gonorrheal conjunctivitis in the adult must be recognized and treated promptly. Gram staining permits identification of the gram-negative intracellular diplococcus some 48 hours before the results of cultures are available.

Gonococcemia is the most common extragenital complication. It occurs soon after infection or later during menstrua-tion. There is fever, polyarthralgia affecting the knees, wrists, and ankles, and skin lesions varying from petechiae to necrosis. There may be a catarrhal conjunctivitis or a severe acute iridocyclitis. Reiter syndrome (urethritis, arthritis, and ocular inflammation) is a more likely cause of this triad than gonorrhea, particularly in patients with histocompatibility antigen HLA-B27. Gonococcemia is diagnosed by culture or specific immunofluorescent antibody stains in blood, cerebrospinal fluid, synovial fluid, or skin lesions.

N. meningitidis. This is a gram-negative aerobic and facultative anaerobic organism that appears as a single coccus or in pairs. They are antigenetically divided into ABCDXYZ groups. Their natural habitat is the human nasopharynx, and they cause meningitis and bacteremia in susceptible individuals.

Ocular involvement during meningococcemia consists of conjunctival petechiae and ecchymosis. Intraocular embolization may cause a panophthalmitis with eventual shrinkage of the globe (phthisis bulbi), A purulent conjunctivitis may develop. Meningitis may be associated with ocular muscle paralysis and optic nerve inflammation. The organism may cause a purulent conjunctivitis in the absence of systemic infection and must be distinguished from the gonococcus by its cultural characteristics.

Gram-positive organisms

Gram-positive cocci. This group includes two important families: the Micrococcaceae with the widespread genus *Staphylococcus,* and the Streptococcaceae with the genus *Streptococcus,* which has numerous species.

Staphylococci. The staphylococci are gram-positive, toxin-producing, nonmotile organisms, typically occurring in irregular clusters.

Various strains of *S. aureus* can be recognized by the lysis produced by staphylococcal bacteriophages. Their pathogenicity is proportionate to their coagulase activity, but occasionally non-coagulase-producing pathogenic strains are seen. Most strains (80%) found in hospitals produce a penicillinase that inactivates benzylpenicillin, phenoxy-methylpenicillin, and ampicillin. However, most nonhospital strains are non-penicillinase-producing.

The skin is the common site of staphylococcal infection, and the organism is commonly found in sties and chalazia. Chronic blepharitis is often the result of continued staphylococcal infection and sensitivity to the organism. Staphylococcus conjunctivitis is less common than that caused by the *Streptococcus* and *Haemophilus* groups. The exotoxins in staphylococcus conjunctivitis produce minute corneal ulcers at the corneoscleral limbus (p. 266).

Streptococci. The streptococci are gram-positive, nonmotile microorganisms that are spherical or oval and tend to grow in chains. Only hemolytic streptococci (beta) are considered pathogenic; the nonhemolytic streptococci are saprophytic. Beta (hemolytic) streptococci have been divided into a number of well-defined serologic groups, the most important in human disease being group A. The manifestations of streptococcic disease vary markedly in different age groups.

Streptococci may cause a pseudomembranous conjunctivitis with a tendency for corneal involvement. Corneal invasion may be associated with hypopyon. These inflammations are readily treated with topical antibiotics. Diagnosis is usually based on culture, because chain formation does not commonly occur in ocular infections, and the organism may be confused with staphylococci.

Rheumatic fever (p. 564) rarely causes ocular manifestations. Glomerulonephritis caused by streptococci manifests itself in the eye only in the changes of vascular hypertension. Scarlet fever has no ocular signs except the occasional occurrence of ecchymoses and petechiae in severely ill patients after the rash appears on the second day.

Erysipelas is a recurrent, acute, hemolytic streptococcic infection of the skin of the middle-aged and elderly, usually involving the face and head. As a rule, the lesion spreads from a central focus to involve adjacent areas, which become red, glistening, swollen, and sometimes versicolored. The skin of the eyelids may be involved.

Streptococcus pneumoniae (pneumococci) are gram-positive oval- or coccal-shaped organisms that generally have tapered ends (lance-shaped) and grow in pairs. The organism is a common cause of corneal ulcers, with the lacrimal sac serving as a reservoir for chronic dacryocystitis (p. 236). Hypopyon is common, and the ulcer spreads across the cornea in a serpiginous pattern. Pneumococcus causes a mild, acute conjunctivitis, usually in children, and is rarely associated with chronic disease.

Acid-fast organisms

Mycobacterium. The genus *Mycobacterium* causes a number of chronic infectious granulomas in man and animals. There are a number of nonpathogenic species. The most important human diseases caused by members of the genus are tuberculosis and leprosy.

Mycobacterium tuberculosis is a nonmotile, encapsulated, rodlike organism that stains with difficulty, but once stained it resists decolorization with strong mineral acids (acid-fast). Human and bovine varieties are pathogenic for humans, whereas murine and piscine varieties cause tuberculosis in rodents and fish but not in humans. The avian (bird) variety rarely causes human disease.

The clinical and pathologic changes of

tuberculosis depend on the tissue involved and the degree of hypersensitivity of the host to the organism. Generally, the initial or primary lesion is an acute process, healing or progressing in a short time, and characterized in the main by an inconspicuous parenchymal lesion and massive tissue necrosis (caseation) of the draining lymph nodes. The postprimary lesion or reinfection occurs in an individual who has developed a hypersensitivity to the bacteria either because of previous infection or immunization with BCG (bacille Calmette-Guérin) vaccine. This lesion is more chronic than the primary type and is associated with severe parenchymal involvement with a minor effect on the regional lymph nodes.

As might be anticipated, inflammations of every portion of the eye and the adnexa have been attributed to tuberculosis. Because of the specific therapy now available, the diagnosis is made less frequently.

The skin of the eyelids may be involved in lupus vulgaris or, more rarely, in other cutaneous manifestations of tuberculosis, each of which may spread to the conjunctiva and the cornea.

Phlyctenular disease (p. 266) involves the conjunctiva and the cornea. In many instances it appears to be a response to sensitivity to tuberculoprotein (tuberculin) or other antigens and is responsive to local instillation of corticosteroids.

In the past, chronic uveitis was often considered tuberculosis when it occurred in an individual hypersensitive to tuberculin. Involvement of the anterior segment causes an insidious low-grade inflammation characterized by the development of mutton-fat keratic precipitates, by minute nodules at the pupillary margin (Koeppe nodules), and by a tendency to develop posterior synechiae. Posterior segment involvement causes an exudation of inflammatory cells into the vitreous body with destruction of the overlying

retina. A posterior polar cataract (complicated) frequently develops.

Retinal veins were considered a frequent site of involvement, with periphlebitis, combined neovascularization, and recurrent vitreous hemorrhage. Photocoagulation of the involved area of periphlebitis is helpful. Vitrectomy may be used to remove unabsorbed blood.

Leprosy (Hansen disease) is caused by an acid-fast rod, *Mycobacterium leprae,* similar to the agent that causes tuberculosis. There are about eleven million cases throughout the world, and about one third have eye complications. The infection involves predominantly the skin, superficial nerves, and nose and throat. It occurs as two principal types: (1) the lepromatous (cutaneous), with depressed cellular immunity and frequent ocular involvement, and (2) the tuberculoid (neural), with systemic resistance and ocular complications caused by neuroparalytic keratopathy (p. 266).

The eyes are usually involved late in the course of the lepromatous type of disease. There may be an initial superficial infection with conjunctivitis, episcleritis, or keratitis. Visual loss arises because of an insidious chronic iritis and granuloma formation. Eventually, complicated cataract and shrinkage of the globe occur. Involvement of the skin of the brows causes alopecia of the eyebrows, whereas facial nerve paralysis causes ectropion of the lower eyelids with weakness in elevation of the eyebrows.

The Rickettsias

This group contains two large orders, the Rickettsiales and the Chlamydiales. They are gram-negative organisms that can multiple only within living cells. For the most part the Rickettsiales are transmitted by arthropod vectors. The Chlamydiales are parasites of humans that are transmitted by contact.

Rickettsiales. These organisms occur in

various arthropods that transmit the disease to humans and cause an acute febrile illness usually associated with a skin rash. Vaccines have been prepared against some of the microorganisms, and delousing with DDT is effective prophylaxis. The tetracyclines and chloramphenicol are highly effective therapeutically.

The ocular changes caused by infections with this group have been best described in epidemic louse-borne typhus fever (*Rickettsia prowazekii* transmitted by the human louse, *Pediculus humanus*) and Rocky Mountain spotted fever (*Rickettsia rickettsii* transmitted by animal ticks). At the time of onset of the disease, conjunctival hyperemia may occur, sometimes with subconjunctival hemorrhages. Marked venous engorgement with edema of the disk and retina may occur during the second and third weeks of the fever. Venous engorgement may be so severe as to lead to retinal hemorrhages, which may burst into the vitreous body. Cotton-wool spots and arterial occlusion may be observed.

The diagnosis of rickettsial disease depends on clincial signs in an area where the diseases are endemic. The Weil-Felix test in rising titer is helpful, except in Q fever, where cross-antigens do not occur.

Chlamydiales. This order has but one genus, *Chlamydia*, divided into two species, *C. trachomatis* and *C. psittaci*. They are characterized by the development of a small elementary body, which changes into a large initial body that divides by fission. Daughter cells reorganize and condense to form an elementary body, which survives extracellularly to infect other host cells. The elementary body is not infectious. The initial body (inclusion cell) stains with Giemsa stain, but fluorescent antibody staining is more effective for diagnosis.

Trachoma. Trachoma (p. 222) is a chronic follicular conjunctivitis characteristically involving the upper eyelid and causing conjunctival and corneal cicatrization with severe visual disability. The disease has been recognized since antiquity and is probably the chief cause of blindness in the world. In the United States it is prevalent mainly in Indians in the Southwest. Rural children are infected, and the combination of poverty, lack of water, dryness, and dust causes severe infection. Conjunctival scarring leads to distorted eyelids, which scar the cornea and cause blindness.

Communicable ophthalmia is a mixed infection in which a chronic conjunctival inflammation caused by trachoma is combined with a chronic bacterial purulent conjunctivitis. Flies transfer the infection from one child to another, and the disease becomes recurrent. Control requires immediately available antibiotic therapy and fly control.

Inclusion conjunctivitis. This follicular conjunctivitis is caused by the agent that causes a nongonococcal urethritis and cervicitis (p. 221).

In the newborn infant, inclusion conjunctivitis has an incubation period of 5 to 12 days in contrast to gonorrheal ophthalmia, which occurs within 5 days of birth. The onset is acute. A purulent conjunctivitis develops rapidly, with intense infiltration of the conjunctiva, particularly of the lower eyelid. The infection is not prevented by Credé prophylaxis. Treatment is with tetracycline locally and erythromycin systemically for 6 weeks. The mother should be treated for cervicitis and the father for urethritis if necessary.

In the adult the same agent causes an acute follicular conjunctivitis with preauricular adenopathy. The follicles, unlike those of trachoma, are more marked in the lower eyelid and do not contain necrotic material. There is never corneal involvement, and the disease heals spontaneously without residual changes. The genitourinary tract serves as a reservoir for the infection. Treatment is by means of topically applied tetracycline ointment or drops and systemic tetracycline. Systemic erythromycin should be substituted for tetracycline in children whose permanent teeth have not erupted and in pregnant women.

Lymphogranuloma venereum. Lymphogranuloma venereum is a contagious venereal disease manifested by an initial vesicle that bursts, leaving a grayish ulcer followed by regional lymphadenitis that is frequently suppurative. Mild to severe constitutional signs may be present during the stage of adenitis.

Primary infection of the eyelid, occurring venerally or through accidental contamination in a laboratory worker, gives rise to an ulcerative lesion of the eyelid or conjunctiva with preauricular adenopathy (Parinaud oculoglandular syndrome). Hematogenous spread of the disease may cause uveitis, keratouveitis, or sclerokeratitis.

MYCOTIC INFECTIONS

Fungi are single-celled dimorphic (growth in two different forms under different environments) organisms characterized by the formation of mycelial filaments (hyphae) and the production of spores.

Oculomycosis is caused by many organisms that are opportunistic pathogens. The most virulent fungal infections may occur in patients with no apparent deficiency in resistance. Less virulent organisms select individuals who have some defect in resistance. Trauma is a factor in more than one half of such cases.

Fungi involve the eye in four main ways: (1) superficially to produce conjunctivitis, keratitis, and lacrimal obstruction; (2) by extension from infection in neighboring skin, nasal sinuses, or the nasopharynx; (3) by direct introduction into the eye during surgery or accidental trauma, particularly with plant material;

or (4) by hematogenous or lymphatogenous routes in patients with pulmonary, cutaneous, or generalized mycosis.

In recent years, histoplasmosis (p. 304) has been implicated as a common cause of uveitis. Patients with prolonged indwelling intravenous catheters who received systemic antibiotics in the treatment of complications of surgery have developed *Candida* endophthalmitis. Additionally, patients receiving immune-suppression agents following organ transplant may develop intraocular infections from fungi as well as viruses and other microorganisms for which there is no effective systemic therapy.

Superficial infection. Fungi may be introduced into the cornea (p. 264) by a foreign body or an epithelial abrasion, frequently from a tree branch or other vegetable matter. Instillation of corticosteroids may enhance the virulence of fungi or reduce tissue resistance to infection. A fluffy white spot appears in the cornea and melts into a shallow ulcer and hypopyon. Initially the corneal inflammation is deceptively mild, but there is marked ciliary and conjunctival congestion. Neovascularization does not occur. The inflammation gradually spreads to involve the entire cornea, which slowly melts and perforates.

The main causative organisms (p. 265) are *Aspergillus*, *Candida*, and *Fusarium* species. Treatment is by means of local nystatin, amphotericin B, natamycin (pimaricin), or flucytosine (p. 135). Medical therapy is frequently not effective, and the cornea does not heal until covered with a conjunctival flap.

A fungus conjunctival inflammation usually is diagnosed only when corneal involvement occurs. In tropical areas, *Rhinosporidium* may produce conjunctival polyps.

Unilateral, persistent tearing with patent lacrimal passages characterizes infections of the canaliculus. The lower canaliculus is usually involved. The punctum is dilated, and its edges are raised and inflamed. There is tearing and itching with a slight conjunctivitis medially. Diagnosis is commonly not made until a lacrimal probe grates against concretions of hardened colonies of fungi in the involved canaliculus.

The skin of the eyelids may be involved by any of the fungi that cause a dermatomycosis. Extension of fungus infection into the orbit may cause a cellulitis or because of involvement of the optic nerve, a retrobulbar neuritis. Some inflammatory granulomas of the orbit may also be caused by fungi.

Intraocular infection. Fungal endophthalmitis after intraocular surgery arises from fungal contamination by the air in the operating room, by the surgical instruments and solutions, or by the conjunctival sac and eyelids of the patient. Mucormycosis extends directly from the nasal pharynx in debilitated individuals with ketosis.

A variety of fungal infections of the inner eye are seen in patients with immune suppression after organ transplant. Presumed ocular histoplasmosis with a characteristic triad of hemorrhagic central retinal lesion combined with peripapillary and peripheral nonhemorrhagic lesions is a common disorder, particularly in the midwestern portion of the United States.

Fungal endophthalmitis has an incubation period of several weeks to several months and follows an indolent course. The anterior vitreous and uvea are predominantly involved, with a cloudy aqueous humor and hypopyon. The anterior vitreous may initially show a localized grayish green area with whitish masses resembling small balls of cotton. The pupils gradually become occluded with inflammatory mass, and the vitreous humor is converted to a granuloma. The therapeutic effect of antifungal agents is variable and unpredictable. However,

vitrectomy with removal of all visibly involved inflamed vitreous humor may be effective in saving the eye.

Slow, indolent progression distinguishes mycotic endophthalmitis from bacterial infection.

Orbital-cerebral phycomycetes. A rapidly lethal infection is caused by fungi such as *Basidiobolus, Mortierella, Mucor,* and *Rhizopus*. The nose or nasopharynx is the usual route of entry. The infection occurs in debilitated individuals with acidosis or ketosis, who develop facial swelling, proptosis, eyelid edema, and total ophthalmoplegia and blindness. Persistent coma develops, and death occurs within 1 week. Mucormycosis occurs in adults with diabetes mellitus, whereas other species may be the cause in debilitated infants or children who have diarrhea or vomiting that contributes to an acidosis. In mucor infections, hyphae are prominent in the choroid.

Immune suppression. Many fungi may cause a choroiditis or retinitis in patients receiving corticosteroids, azathioprine, and similar agents to suppress graft rejection. *Aspergillus* and *Candida* are most commonly involved. More uncommon are *Nocardia, Histoplasma, Coccidioides,* and others. Men are more commonly affected than women. An unrelated renal donor, increasing age, and leukopenia all predispose. Ocular involvement is not severe, and attention may be directed to the eyes because of decreased vision. The mild chorioretinitis excites minimal cellular reaction, and there is little tendency for extension. The eyes are often studied after death, and the organism is then identified.

Hematogenous *Candida* endophthalmitis may follow antibiotic therapy, immunosuppressive therapy, cardiac and abdominal surgery, use of intravenous catheters, and drug abuse. The organisms may be in the bloodstream without causing parenchymal involvement, and apparently they do not require treatment. However, systemic *Candida* may be diagnosed by the ocular lesions of *Candida* chorioretinitis, which reflect an underlying systemic candidiasis. The most common ocular lesion consists of multiple, white, cottonlike, circumscribed exudates with a filamentous border located in the chorioretina and extending into the vitreous with overlying vitreous haze. Additionally, hemorrhages have occurred with hypopyon, iritis, papillitis, and ciliary body abscess. Patients may be asymptomatic or have loss of vision combined with symptoms of intraocular inflammation. Typically, the histologic lesion is a combination of suppurative and granulomatous inflammation beginning in the choroid and extending into the retinal pigment epithelium and overlying retina. Amphotericin B is used to treat patients with ocular or systemic *Candida* infections, but patients with candidemia are not treated.

Presumed ocular histoplasmosis. Histoplasmosis is a mild to lethal systemic disease caused by *Histoplasma capsulatum*. It manifests itself mainly as an acute primary respiratory tract infection or as a chronic pulmonary disease with cavitation that resembles tuberculosis. Uncommonly the disease is disseminated, with widespread systemic involvement. Infection is common in rural dwellers of the Mississippi Valley and the great river valleys of South America, Africa, and Asia, but it is rare in Europe. The fungus is common in soil contaminated with bird droppings.

Ophthalmic interest in histoplasmosis arises because of the frequency with which typical fundus lesions occur in individuals with skin hypersensitivity to histoplasmosis in the absence of other causes. However, the fundus lesions do not occur in patients with clinical systemic histoplasmosis, and the ocular disease is designated as "presumed ocular histoplasmosis." The ocular lesion is found almost exclusively in whites, with a peak incidence in individuals between 30 to 40 years of age.

The triad of presumed ocular histoplasmosis consists of a lesion of the central retina (Fig. 23-1) combined with a healed (usually) chorioretinitis adjacent to the optic disk and a peripheral atrophic area ("histo spots") (Fig. 23-2).

There are multiple fundus lesions that vary in size from a minute dot to an area as large as the optic disk. Initially, these appear as yellowish orange oval or circular areas having indistinct, soft borders. The inflammation may disappear or progress, and areas of different degrees of activity are seen in different parts of the eye. There are no inflammatory cells in the vitreous, and the ocular disease may develop over a period of months.

The central retinal lesion is heralded by a collection of fluid between the choriocapillaris of the choroid and the Bruch

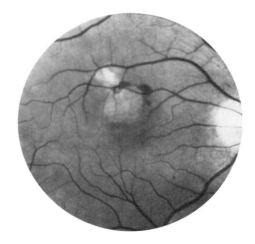

Fig. 23-1. Central retinal lesion of presumed ocular histoplasmosis in a 61-year-old woman in whom the lesion was inactive for many years. The dark material above is intraretinal blood; the inferior darkish material is greenish on ophthalmoscopy and constitutes some retinal neovascularization. The whitish material is edema.

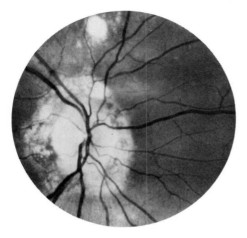

Fig. 23-2. Peripapillary chorioretinitis and the punched-out atrophic lesion of presumed histoplasmosis syndrome in a 33-year-old woman.

membrane that causes a metamorphosis with little or no decrease of visual acuity. Fluorescein angiography indicates subretinal neovascularization. A dark greenish gray circular or oval area reflects bleeding between the pigment epithelium and the Bruch membrane. Frank bleeding then occurs in the subretinal space and breaks into the sensory retina, often in a crescentic hemorrhage at the periphery of the lesion. Blood eventually spreads out into the sensory retina, causing loss of vision. The lesion eventually becomes inactive, with a hypertrophic pigmented scar. About half of the eyes have vision of less than 6/60 (20/200).

Both eyes are usually affected. There is early loss of vision from central retinal involvement followed by involvement of the second eye 1 month to 28 years (average 6⅔ years) later. Involvement of the peripheral retina may not be diagnosed. Most attention is directed to the central lesion, which interferes with vision. However, the lesions adjacent to the disk and peripheral lesions may show fluid accumulation but do not bleed.

Treatment is unsatisfactory. Complete destruction of the neovascular network (p. 345) by means of photocoagulation arrests the central lesion. Incomplete destruction stimulates more neovascularization. Photocoagulation cannot be directed to new blood vessels beneath the fovea centralis because it destroys the overlying retina. Amphotericin B used in systemic histoplasmosis is ineffective.

VIRAL INFECTIONS

Viruses are intracellular parasites that may infect and cause disease in all living organisms. Human viruses, which range in size from 17 nm (picornavirus) to 300 nm (poxvirus), demonstrate marked species and organ specificity. They contain macromolecular cores of either ribonucleic acid (RNA) or deoxyribonucleic acid (DNA) necessary for transcription of genetic information. They may contain only nucleic acid protected by a covering, the capsid, or they may have a lipid envelope and cytoplasm. Virus absorption of a cell surface is through specific carboxyl and sulfhydryl chemical groups. The virus enters the cell by pinocytosis and loses its protective covering. Thereafter, it depends on its host cell for all or a portion of its enzymatic requirements. The virus may remain latent in the cell without causing any sign, or it may be provoked into replication by a physiologic, biochemical, or environmental change or trauma (Table 23-2).

After the virus enters a susceptible cell, the cell nucleus is stimulated to produce interferon, which is released through the cell wall. The interferon enters other cells and stimulates them to release a transitional inhibitory protein that binds to cellular ribosomes and alters them in such a way that any virus RNA entering the cell is not translated, thus preventing the virus from replicating. Virus multiplication activates B and T lymphocytes; macrophages and polymorphonuclear leukocytes migrate to the area, producing

Table 23-2. Virus disease and the eye

Generic name and nucleic acid	Prototype virus	Systemic disease	Ocular disease
Herpesvirus (DNA)	*Herpesvirus hominis*		
	Type 1	Rarely, disseminated "cold sores"; encephalitis	Keratitis
	Type 2	Genital warts; encephalitis	Rarely keratitis
	Varicella-zoster	Chickenpox (children)	Vesicles of eyelids, conjunctiva
		Zoster (adults)	Ophthalmic zoster: keratitis, uveitis
	Epstein-Barr	Infectious mononucleosis	Conjunctivitis; uveitis; optic neuritis; dacryoadenitis
		Burkitt lymphoma (African children)	Orbital metastasis
	Cytomegalovirus	Brain damage	Necrotizing retinitis
Adenovirus (DNA) (31 human and 17 animal serotypes)	Types 1, 2, 3, and 5	Respiratory tract disease	None
	Type 4 (3, 14, and 21 rare)	Respiratory tract disease	None
	Types 3 and 7 (4 and 14 rare)	Pharyngoconjunctival fever	Conjunctivitis
	Types 8 and 19 (11 rare)		Epidemic keratoconjunctivitis
Poxvirus (DNA)	Variola	Smallpox	Keratitis
	Vaccinia	Vaccination	Keratitis
	Molluscum contagiosum	Multiple "warts"	Chronic conjunctivitis keratitis
Papovavirus		"Warts"	Keratitis ("wart" on eyelid)
Myxovirus (RNA)	Rubeola	Measles	Mild uveitis
Paramyxovirus (RNA)	Influenza	Influenza	Slight conjunctivitis
Arenovirus (RNA)	Togavirus: rubella	Mild evanescent rashes, fever	Acquired: none
		Pregnancy: fetus affected with deafness, heart defects	Congenital: microphthalmia, cataract, rubella retinopathy
Arbovirus (RNA)	Group A	Encephalitis; tick fever	Secondary to CNS syndromes
	Group B	Dengue; encephalitis	
	Group C		
	Ungrouped	Hemorrhagic fever	
Picornavirus (RNA)	Poliomyelitis	Flaccid limb or bulbar paralysis	Secondary to CNS involvement
	Hemorrhagic conjunctivitis	Radiculomyelitis	Hemorrhagic conjunctivitis

inflammation. The proteins of the virus capsid stimulate B lymphocytes to synthesize humoral (IgM, IgG, IgD) and secretory immunoglobulins (IgA). T lymphocytes produce cell-associated antibodies (IgE). Immunoglobulins are synthesized in lymph nodes, at body surfaces, and in inflammatory exudate. The ciliary body, uveal tract, and conjunctiva are sites of immunoglobulin synthesis. Even in the presence of neutralizing antibodies, however, a virus such as herpes simplex may spread from cell to cell. In herpesvirus disease, cell-mediated immunity is the most important means of defense. However, if this occurs in the corneal stroma, the tissue is disrupted and the immune complex appears to be responsible for the stromal keratitis (p. 363).

Virus diseases associated with petechial hemorrhages may show subconjunctival hemorrhage or ecchymosis of the eyelids. Iridocyclitis may occur with any viremia but may go undiagnosed because of the severity of the systemic disease. Viruses affecting the skin may involve the eyelid margin and cause a secondary chronic conjunctivitis or keratitis. Respiratory tract viruses may ascend the nasolacrimal duct to cause conjunctivitis or keratoconjunctivitis. Viruses that affect the mucous membranes, such as herpes simplex type 1, also affect the conjunctiva and corneal epithelium. Viruses affecting the central nervous system may interfere with the motor nerves to the eyes, resulting in strabismus. The optic nerve may be inflamed in neuritis or, less frequently, in papillitis.

The adenoviruses and herpesviruses infecting the conjunctiva and cornea may be cultured directly. Acute specimens are obtained by swabbing the conjunctiva or cornea with a moistened cotton-tipped applicator. Optimally, specimens are inoculated promptly into tissue culture. Virus particles may be recognized by electron microscopy, or the type of adenovirus may be determined by using a specific antiserum and fluorescent microscopy.

Herpesvirus. This is a group of DNA-type viruses grouped together mainly by their similarities when viewed with an electron microscope. The main members of the group are (1) *Herpesvirus hominis* type 1 (ocular, skin) and type 2 (genital), (2) varicella-zoster virus of children (chickenpox) and adults (zoster), (3) Epstein-Barr virus (infectious mononucleosis and Burkitt lymphoma), and (4) virus of cytomegalic inclusion disease. Monkey B disease is a subclinical herpes infection in monkeys but a fatal disease in the accidentally infected human being.

Herpesvirus hominis. *Herpesvirus hominis* includes two subtypes that are distinctly different. Type 1 produces lesions of the mouth, cornea, skin above the

waist, and central nervous system but not of the genitalia. Type 2 is transmitted as a venereal infection and involves the genitalia and the skin below the waist. However, in about one third of the patients in the age group 15 to 24 years, herpesvirus type 1 invades the genital region. Similarly, herpesvirus type 2 involvement of the mouth and cornea may be seen.

Herpes simplex virus type 2 is being implicated with increasing frequency as a cause of adult-onset keratoconjunctivitis. It is only slightly responsive to treatment with idoxuridine, and it causes a more severe inflammation of the eyes than type 1.

Primary infection usually occurs after the age of 6 months, when maternal antibodies have disappeared, and before the age of 5 years, by which time most individuals (90%) have been infected. As a rule, there is gingivostomatitis along with adenopathy, fever, and malaise. In most cases the primary infection either does not cause clinical signs or is so minor as not to be recalled. If eczema is present, a severe, widespread disease may occur (eczema herpeticum, Kaposi varicelliform eruption). Systemic infection in those without antibodies may cause meningoencephalitis. Visceral herpes simplex occurs in newborns infected by their mothers who have recurrent herpetic vulvovaginitis.

After the primary lesion, subsequent disease is entirely local and without systemic signs. Reactivation gives rise to vesicles on an erythematous base that occur at the same site in each individual. The most frequent manifestation is a fever blister (herpes labialis, herpes facialis, "cold sore"), which often involves a mucocutaneous junction. Reactivation causes an initial sensation of burning and irritation at the involved site followed by reddish papules that quickly vesiculate. The vesicles quickly become purulent (frequently with localized adenopathy), scale, and heal without a scar.

The eye may be the site of a primary infection in a child. More commonly it is the site of recurrent (reactivation) disease. Primary infection of the eye occurs in children and begins as a unilateral follicular conjunctivitis with a preauricular adenopathy and malaise. The disease may be confined to the conjunctiva, or the cornea may be involved with superficial punctate erosions or a single vesicle. Both types develop into a typical dendritic (branching) keratitis (p. 262).

Recurrent disease is triggered by fever, ultraviolet light, mechanical trauma, menstruation, emotional upsets, and allergy. There is an initial foreign body sensation in the eye, and the unfortunate experienced patient usually knows the disease has recurred. Vesicles are present early but are usually ruptured by the time the patient is seen, and a dendritic pattern can be demonstrated on the cornea with the instillation of 2% sterile fluorescein. Treatment (p. 263) is by mechanical removal of epithelium and administration of antiviral agents.

Chickenpox (varicella). Chickenpox is an acute contagious disease characterized by a vesicular xanthem involving predominantly the hands and trunk. It develops in crops over a period of 1 to 5 days, and is associated with malaise and fever. In adults a varicella pneumonia may develop. Vesicles may occur on the eyelids and rarely on the conjunctiva and the cornea. A mild iridocyclitis may occur.

Zoster. Zoster is an infectious process of the dorsal root or extramedullary cranial nerve ganglia and is characterized by a circumscribed vesicular eruption and neuralgic pain in the areas supplied by the sensory nerves extending to the affected ganglia. The causative virus is identical with that causing chickenpox. Zoster is probably caused by reactivation of latent virus and not by reinfection.

Varicella may constitute the response to infection in the nonimmune host, whereas zoster occurs in a host with a defect in resistance that permits activation of the latent virus. Zoster is most common after the age of 50 years, but also occurs in younger individuals. It may appear in the course of severe and debilitating systemic illness, and patients with lymphosarcoma and reticulum cell sarcoma are particularly susceptible.

Herpes zoster ophthalmicus is an inflammation of that portion of the gasserian ganglion receiving fibers from the ophthalmic division of the trigeminal nerve (N V). The disease is ushered in by a severe, unilateral, disabling neuralgia in the region of distribution of the nerve. Several days later there is a vesicular eruption with much swelling and tenderness. The vesicles rupture, leaving hemorrhagic areas that heal in several weeks and leave deep-pitted scars. Pain disappears in about 2 weeks, but in a small percentage of cases a postherpetic neuralgia persists that is resistant to treatment.

The eyelids may be swollen and tender, but involvement of the globe itself is seen in only about half of the patients. Ocular involvement is usually heralded by a vesicle on the tip of the nose, an area innervated, as is the cornea, by the nasociliary nerve (p. 68).

Zoster lesions of the cornea occur in two forms: (1) acute epithelial keratitis and (2) corneal mucous plaque keratitis. Acute epithelial keratitis is characterized by small, fine, multiple dendritic or stellate lesions in the peripheral portion of the cornea. They are always associated with conjunctivitis and resolve within 4 to 6 days. Corneal mucous plaque keratitis appears as a whitish gray, sharply defined plaque line on the surface of the cornea that can be lifted with ease. This line usually occurs 3 to 4 months after the onset of the cutaneous lesion.

Superficial and deep corneal opacities occur, combined with folds in the Descemet membrane and keratic precipitates caused by an anterior uveitis. The disease may persist for weeks and slowly regress, leaving a residue of round corneal infiltrates in the anterior corneal stroma. Secondary glaucoma occurs in about 20% of the patients, and paresis of extraocular muscles occurs in about 10%.

Treatment is often unsatisfactory. Elderly patients should not be exposed to children with chickenpox. Local corticosteroids and atropine appear helpful. In previously healthy individuals, systemic corticosteroids may relieve an attack and prevent postherpetic neuralgia. In debilitated patients, the corticosteroids may cause a fatal dissemination of the virus. The remote possibility that this might occur in an otherwise healthy patient leads many to believe corticosteroids are contraindicated. Many nonspecific remedies have been proposed.

Infectious mononucleosis. Infectious mononucleosis is a contagious disease with a benign, though frequently protracted, course; it is caused by the Epstein-Barr virus. Fever and pharyngitis occur initially, and there is associated lymphadenopathy and hepatitis with or without icterus. Atypical lymphocytosis is associated with some forms. There is a high serum concentration of heterophilic antibodies against sheep erythrocytes as well as development of antibodies against the Epstein-Barr virus.

Conjunctivitis with follicles, periorbital edema, uveitis, and optic neuritis, sometimes with papillitis, retinal edema, and hemorrhages, may occur. In some epidemics, lacrimal gland inflammation (dacryoadenitis) is prominent. It causes a red, painful swelling, with redness of the outer one third of the upper eyelid and a typically S-shaped curve of the upper eyelid margin. Involvement of the central nervous system may cause extraocular muscle paralysis, nystagmus, hemianopia, and disturbances of conjugate movement.

Treatment is symptomatic, and the disease is usually self-limited.

Cytomegalic inclusion disease. This is a widespread, frequently asymptomatic disease caused by a virus of the herpes group. Overt cytomegalic inclusion disease is relatively common in immune-compromised patients after organ transplant. Congenital infection causes mental retardation and sensorineural deafness in some 10% of newborns.

Infantile cytomegalovirus disease manifests itself by jaundice, hepato- and splenomegaly, purpura, and erythroblastic or hemolytic anemia. The neural lesions vary from a few cytomegalic cells to an extensive, multifocal, necrotizing, hemorrhagic and granulomatous encephalitis. These lesions may be followed by calcification. Some patients recover, but many have severe brain damage with mental deficiency and microcephaly. Epilepsy, cerebral palsy, hydrocephalus, and deafness may occur.

The ocular lesion varies from an isolated central retinal lesion, similar to that seen in toxoplasmosis, to a chorioretinitis with much disorganization of the globe (p. 339). Rarely, pigmentary retinal degeneration and perivascular retinal exudates are present. The diagnosis is based on the demonstration of larger than normal cells, with typical inclusions found in the urine, saliva, tears, or any tissue specimen. In the mother of an affected child, a complement-fixing antibody titer equal to or greater than 1:64 is diagnostic. The affected infant demonstrates a rising titer to either test after 4 months of age.

Occasionally an acute cytomegalic necrotizing retinitis produces irreversible damage and loss of vision. Men are affected more frequently than women. Transfusion, direct spread from other patients, and reactivation of a latent infection are postulated as causes. A cytomegalic viremia is fairly common in renal transplant patients judging by increasing titers of antibodies and excretion of the virus in the urine, but ocular infection is rare.

In renal transplant patients the infection is often superimposed upon a retina already damaged by vascular hypertension. There are large clumps of exudates, hemorrhages, and occlusion of retinal arteries and veins, which become sheathed. An optic atrophy may follow. The inflammation is self-limited, and effective therapy is not available.

Cytomegalic virus mononucleosis is an acute febrile illness with splenomegaly, hepatic involvement, and atypical lymphocytes. The heterophil test is negative, and Epstein-Barr antibodies do not develop.

Adenovirus. The group of adenoviruses is composed of at least 31 serologically distinct human types of large DNA viruses and 17 animal serotypes. The virus causes respiratory tract disease in infants and children and in military recruits.

Adenovirus types 8 and 19 cause epidemic keratoconjunctivitis in adults (pp. 222 and 263). In children, type 8 causes a systemic disease with fever, respiratory or gastrointestinal signs, and a conjunctivitis without corneal opacities. Adenovirus types 3, 4, and 7 usually cause an acute respiratory disease, pharyngoconjunctival fever, and simple follicular conjunctivitis. Adenovirus types 1, 2, 5, and others cause a febrile pharyngitis.

Pharyngoconjunctival fever. Pharyngoconjunctival fever is an acute sporadic or epidemic disease that affects all age groups, but predominantly children. It occurs at all seasons of the year but is more common in summer and is often associated with infection transmitted in swimming pools. The incubation period

is 5 to 7 days, and the disease persists 1 to 2 weeks. Clinical manifestations vary markedly in different individuals and epidemics. A usually mild nasopharyngitis is associated with a cervical or maxillary lymphadenopathy. A fever that may reach 39° C persists 3 to 14 days. Headache referable to the sinuses, catarrhal otitis, lassitude, malaise, and sometimes gastrointestinal disturbances occur.

The conjunctivitis is acute, sometimes monocular, and nonpurulent. Lymph follicle hyperplasia is most marked in the lower cul-de-sac. Congestion is most marked over the palpebral conjunctiva and spares the bulbar conjunctiva. Preauricular adenopathy may be present.

Adenovirus type 3 is most commonly implicated, but other types have been found to be a cause. The serum of affected patients contains group-specific complement-fixation bodies.

Epidemic keratoconjunctivitis. Adenovirus types 8 and 19 cause epidemic keratoconjunctivitis in the United States (p. 263). This is an acute infectious corneal disease spread by the ocular secretion or by eyedrops contaminated with secretions. In Japan, adenovirus type 8 causes an acute systemic disease in children with a conjunctivitis of varying severity without the production of permanent corneal opacities. The disease is usually associated with fever, malaise, gastrointestinal and upper respiratory symptoms, and a follicular conjunctivitis. Other children exposed to the disease develop the same disease, but exposed adults develop epidemic keratoconjunctivitis. An immunofluorescent test detects the adenoviral group antigen in conjunctival secretions. Treatment is symptomatic.

Molluscum contagiosum. Molluscum contagiosum is a tumor caused by a large poxvirus and is characterized by the development of multiple discrete nodules in the epidermal layer of the skin. The nodules are usually pearly white and painless, with an umbilicated center in which a small white cone can be seen. Humans are the only host of the virus; children are attacked most frequently, and the lesion is prevalent in some regions. The nodules may occur on the skin of the eyelids and on the eyelid margins. If on the eyelid margins, virus material may be released into the conjunctival sac and cause conjunctivitis or keratitis. Excision of the nodule is the treatment of choice. Histologically, large intracytoplasmic inclusion bodies occur within acanthotic epidermis.

Verrucae (warts). Verrucae are contagious viral tumors characterized by the development of one or more cutaneous masses with a cauliflowerlike appearance and a rough surface made up of many fine projections. When located on the eyelid margin, the lesions mechanically cause a chronic epithelial keratitis. The conjunctivitis is mild and, like the keratitis, nonspecific. Removal of the eyelid margin nodules is required to heal the keratitis.

Measles (rubeola). Measles is a contagious, infectious virus (RNA) disease characterized by prodromal symptoms of fever, cough, conjunctivitis, upper respiratory tract infection, and Koplik spots on the buccal mucosa, followed in 3 to 5 days by a maculopapular cutaneous rash. The conjunctivitis is nonpurulent and may be associated with Koplik spots, particularly on the semilunar fold. The cornea has multiple punctate epithelial erosions, which cause a severe photophobia. The photophobic patient is made more comfortable by either darkness or colored glasses. Local ocular treatment is not indicated in the absence of infection. Permanent corneal scarring does not occur unless there is secondary bacterial infection.

Not infrequently, measles or other acute contagious disease of childhood is the precipitating event in the appearance of strabismus. However, the primary cause of the squint is already present, and the disease seeems only to accelerate its appearance or to transform an intermittent type into a continuous type of strabismus.

Immunization has almost eliminated measles in the United States. During the incubation period, the administration of gamma globulin may prevent or modify the disease in the nonimmune individual. Subacute sclerosing panencephalitis (p. 540) is a slow virus infection caused by either the rubeola virus or a closely related virus.

Mumps. Mumps is an acute contagious virus (RNA) systemic disease characterized mainly by a painful enlargement of the salivary glands, most commonly the parotid gland, and, after puberty, by orchitis. Lymphocytic meningitis, pancreatitis, and involvement of other viscera occur rarely.

A transient corneal edema occurs commonly with a decrease in visual acuity. There are no associated ocular inflammatory signs. A uveitis or inflammation of the lacrimal glands may occur. The sole sign of meningeal involvement may be optic neuritis, or there may be widespread ocular signs from cranial nerve involvement.

Rubella (German measles). Rubella is a mild contagious disease characterized mainly by an evanescent, maculopapular skin eruption beginning on the face and neck, spreading to the trunk and extremities, and fading in 3 days. There may be mild pharyngitis and postauricular adenopathy, sometimes accompanied by slight fever, malaise, lassitude, and myalgia.

Conjunctivitis is common and consists of bilateral bulbar congestion that, unlike measles (rubeola) conjunctivitis, spares the tarsal area. Keratitis is exceptional.

Rubella causes severe congenital defects in infants of mothers who contract the disease early in pregnancy. The virus appears unique in interfering with the translation of DNA to RNA and subsequent polypeptide synthesis and organogenesis. Infection between the second and sixth week of pregnancy causes cardiac malformation and severe ocular malformations with microphthalmic cataract and pigment epithelium disorders. Infection any time during the first trimester of pregnancy up to the fifth month may be associated with deafness and mental retardation with extensive brain necrosis. A chronic virus infection may persist as long as 3 years after birth, causing further systemic deterioration as well as serving as a nidus of infection for pregnant mothers exposed in a physician's office.

Retinitis and congenital cataract are the most common ocular disorders. Microphthalmia follows infection early in pregnancy. Iris atrophy follows fetal uveitis and may make pupillary dilation almost impossible. Congenital glaucoma may occur.

The cataract is usually complete and bilateral. Aspiration of the cataract may be followed by a chronic endophthalmitis centered around lens remnants, with a severity proportional to the amount of lens cortex remaining in the eye. Inability to dilate the pupil complicates lens extraction, and a sector iridectomy, which is nearly always indicated, often results in significant visual improvement.

The retinitis appears as fine pigmentary deposits of greatest density in the central retinal region. The disks and blood vessels are normal. Fluorescein angiography shows a diffuse hyperfluorescence throughout the posterior eyegrounds reflecting a widespread abnormality in the retinal pigment epithelium. Vision remains normal.

Prevention of rubella infection in pregnant women will prevent rubella embryopathy. Boys as well as girls should be immunized with rubella vaccine to minimize transmission in childhood and the likelihood that pregnant women will be exposed. The vaccine can infect the fetus and may be used in sexually active women only when pregnancy can be excluded (as during menstruation or immediately after childbirth) and continued nonpregnancy can be assured for 3 months. After immunization, the hemagglutination-inhibition test indicates the presence or absence of immunity to rubella. The rubella vaccine currently available induces antibodies that are less stable than those acquired through natural infection, and it is doubtful if vaccination in childhood furnishes long-term immunity.

Poliomyelitis, rabies, and viral encephalitis. The viruses causing these diseases may affect the optic and motor nerves of the eye. Optic neuritis may occur, with direct invasion of the meningeal covering of the nerve, or papilledema may develop when there is increased intracranial pressure. Involvement of the motor nerves can give rise to a complete ophthalmoplegia that involves ocular movement and accommodation and produces pupillary dilation (N III). There may be bizarre types of motor involvement, with paralytic strabismus. All of these changes may occur as a presenting sign of intracranial involvement, but more often they occur late in the course of the infection.

Hemorrhagic conjunctivitis. This is a specific violent inflammatory conjunctivitis first seen in Africa in 1969 (at the time of the Apollo flight; thus it is called Apollo-eye). The infection has spread eastward and is now in Japan. It is apparently caused by a member of the picornavirus group (p. 223).

PROTOZOAN AND METAZOAN INFECTIONS

The animal kingdom may be divided into two subkingdoms, the protozoan and the metazoan. The protozoa are classically divided into amebas, flagellates, ciliates, and sporozoans. Diseases caused by protozoa include amebic dysentery, leishmaniasis, malaria, toxoplasmosis, and trypanosomiasis. The metazoa consist of all multicelled animals whose various types of cells are not generally capable of independent existence. The metazoa range in complexity from simply arranged sponges to the highly specialized structure of humans. Human infection by metazoa is chiefly by parasitic worms and some members of the phylum Arthropoda that are transmitters of disease. The larvae of flies are parasitic and may multiply in living tissue, causing myiasis. The adult fly is not a parasite.

The eye and adnexa may be affected by direct invasion by either the adult or larval form, by toxins elaborated by worms or released with death, or by impairment of the health of the host. Diagnosis is based on the recovery of the parasite and its larvae or eggs, on skin tests, and on other immunologic studies. A systemic eosinophilia occurs with massive invasion.

Protozoan infections

Toxoplasmosis. Toxoplasmosis is an infectious disease caused by an obligate intracellular protozoan, *Toxoplasma gondii*. The organism is capable of infecting a wide range of mammals, birds, and reptiles. The cat is its definite host. Transmission occurs readily after ingestion of toxoplasmosis cysts in meat or oocysts from cat feces.

Two main types of disease occur: (1) congenital and (2) acquired. The congenital disease is characterized by bilateral retinochoroiditis, hydrocephalus, convulsions, and other evidence of encephalomyelitis, such as cerebral calcifications demonstrated by roentgenographic examination. It occurs in infants whose mothers have no obvious illness during pregnancy but who are found to have antibodies to *T. gondii* when the disease is discovered in the infant. Severe disease in the infant occurs when the maternal infection is acquired during the first two trimesters. The main involvement is usually in the eyes and central nervous system, and there are wide variations in severity. Some infants mainly demonstrate visceral and muscular involvement. There is an inflammatory reaction and necrosis in the brain, with either single or multiple lesions. Disseminated organisms may be found, or pseudocysts may be formed that consist of parasites packed within a cell from which the nucleus has been extruded. With healing, calcification develops. There are associated signs of microcephaly or hydrocephaly, seizure disorders, and mental retardation.

The ocular lesion involves mainly the posterior pole of the eye and a characteristic retinitis with secondary involvement of the choroid (Fig. 23-3). The fovea is frequently destroyed, resulting in loss of central vision. The lesion is sharply

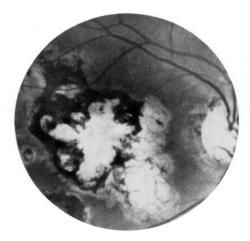

Fig. 23-3. Recurrent toxoplasmosis in a 39-year-old woman. Vision in this eye is counting fingers at 2 feet. There are a series of contiguous lesions, some with marked pigment proliferation and others so severe that the pigment epithelium has been destroyed and the sclera may be seen.

demarcated, with pigmented borders and atrophy of both the retina and the choroid, so that the white sclera is seen. There may be multiple lesions. Usually the vitreous body is clear, and there is no active inflammation. Because of the loss of central vision, there may be an associated esotropia, exotropia, or an ocular type of nystagmus. The mother and the infant have high IgM titers. Children of subsequent pregnancies are not affected.

The acquired form varies in severity from a mild febrile disturbance with lymphadenopathy to a severe, often fatal, disease with a maculopapular rash, pneumonitis, hepatitis, myocarditis, and encephalitis with fever and extreme prostration.

Several types of involvement have been described: (1) lymphoadenopathic, (2) exanthematous, (3) pneumonic, (4) meningoencephalic, and (5) ocular.

The ocular lesions of acquired toxoplasmosis vary considerably. The majority of inflammations reflect an activation of a congenital infection rather than acquired disease. The ocular inflammation occurs because of rupture of a pseudocyst and dissemination of the organisms in the course of or after healing of the congenital infection. The most typical fundus lesions are multiple, discrete, sharply defined areas of retinal and choroidal necrosis surrounded by proliferated pigment. More common is a nonspecific local or generalized intraocular inflammation involving either anterior or posterior ocular tissues. Posterior lesions cause many vitreous exudates and veils, whereas anterior lesions cause mutton-fat keratic precipitates, aqueous flare, posterior synechiae, and complicated cataract.

Diagnosis of the cause of the ocular inflammation may be based on the characteristic appearance of the fundus lesions. A high (1:4096) antibody titer for the Sabin-Feldman dye test, indirect fluoresent antibody test, or indirect hemagglutination test suggest a recent or present infection. A titer of 1:256 suggests a recent infection, and several specimens should be studied weekly. Lower titers suggest previous infection. The ocular inflammation that follows the rupture of cysts within the eye does not disturb systemic antibodies.

Individuals who lack any complement component in their system do not develop antibodies to toxoplasmosis and are at special risk. Acquired toxoplasmosis is seen increasingly often in debilitated and immune-suppressed individuals. Usually it affects the brain, myocardium, or lungs.

The treatment of choice for systemic toxoplasmosis is pyrimethamine (Daraprim) and sulfadiazine. Pyrimethamine is effective in therapy because it inhibits folic acid of the protozoa. To prevent bone marrow depression, folinic acid, which *Toxoplasma* cannot convert to folic acid, should be administered. The ocular disease in the absence of an acute systemic disease is usually treated with corticosteroids. Retrobulbar corticosteroids may cause a severe inflammation unless concomitant pyrimethamine therapy is provided.

Metazoan infections

The main metazoan infections of humans are caused by worms and flukes. The major conditions with ocular changes are caused by roundworms (nematodes) and tapeworms (cestodes). Generally, two types of infection occur: (1) the intestinal form, in which the mature worm is attached to the bowel wall, and (2) the visceral, or somite, form, in which the larva of the parasite is present in various tissues and organs.

Nematodes (roundworms). There are an estimated 500,000 species of nematodes that may become parasitic in virtually all arthropods, mollusks, plants, and vertebrates. Typically, they are elongated, cylindric worms that taper more or less at their head and tail and have a complete digestive tract and usually are different sexes. They vary from minute filiform objects to 1.5 mm in length. Most human infections are acquired by ingestion of the eggs, but hookworm and *Strongyloides* larvae actively invade the skin.

Ocular involvement occurs with the invasion of the eye by the larva of nematodes parasitic in lower animals, most commonly the roundworms of the dog and cat.

Visceral larva migrans. This term is applied to the invasion of nematode larvae into tissues other than the skin. The nematode of the dog and, less frequently, of the cat *(Toxocara canis* or *Toxocara cati)* are common causes of ocular disease. Visceral larva migrans also describes larval migration of *Ascaris lumbricoides* and other nematodes.

Children, particularly, become infected by eating dirt containing embryonated eggs. The eggs hatch in the duodenum, and the larvae then penetrate the intestinal wall, enter the venous circulation, and pass to the lungs, where they migrate across the pulmonary capillary beds, travel up the respiratory tree, and are swallowed to reach their final destination in the jejunum. Acute visceral larva migrans occurs mainly between 1 and 12 or 14 years of age, but an eye lesion may not occur until 6 to 9 years of age. The adult worm of nonhuman type cannot develop in the bowel, but the larva gives rise to hepatic, pulmonary, cerebral, and ocular signs. Infected children have fever, anorexia, chronic cough, vague pains, persistent eosinophilia, and hepatomegaly. The severity of the infection is proportionate to the number of eggs eaten. There may be no systemic signs, but a larva may lodge in the eye.

Larvae that lodge in the eye cause an intraocular granuloma that involves the central retina in a white, round lesion about the size of the optic disk (Fig. 23-4).

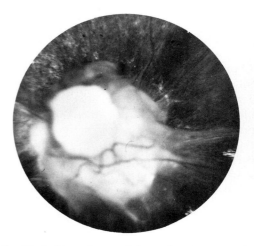

Fig. 23-4. Granuloma of the retina in toxocaris. The white mass extends into the vitreous cavity and obscures the optic disk.

Lines of stress in the retina radiate from the lesion. Occasionally the larvae can be seen. The lesion may be flat, or it may protrude into the eye. Rarely, an endophthalmitis develops, or multiple granulomas occur. Often by the time the eye lesion develops, the early history of visceral larva migrans is forgotten and the blood count is normal.

Antibody titers are markedly increased during the acute phase and are lower during the stage of ocular involvement. The tests are available from the Center for Disease Control in Atlanta, Georgia through local state departments of health. The tests are not specific, and skin-testing antigens are not standardized.

Treatment is supportive and symptomatic. Corticosteroids may minimize allergic reactions, and antibiotics may be useful in decreasing secondary bacterial infection. Animal pets should be dewormed.

Ascaris lumbricoides. *Ascaris lumbricoides* is the giant intestinal roundworm that affects children predominantly. There is no intermediate host, and infection occurs because of ingestion of eggs. The eggs hatch in the bowel, and the migrating larvae may be the cause of pneumonia, encephalitis, or meningitis. During this phase the larvae may cause intraocular inflammation that varies in severity from iridocyclitis to endophthalmitis. Ascaris larvae in the lungs break through the pulmonary capillaries to enter the air alveoli and then the upper respiratory tract, where they are swallowed and complete their development as mature worms in the intestinal tract.

In the bowel the worm may be asymptomatic or cause intestinal disorders varying in severity from mild colic to obstruction and perforation. Sensitization to the worms or their products may cause allergic manifestations, mainly asthma or urticaria.

The ocular inflammation of the larval migration is nonspecific but may be suspected because of the violent ocular tissue reaction often combined with an eosinophilia, depending on the number of worms in the circulation. Eyes that have been enucleated present the pathologic appearance of either Coats disease or endophthalmitis. The larvae are found in histologic sections.

Necator americanus. Necator americanus (common hookworm) is a nematode common in the southeastern United States. There is no intermediate host. In moist soil, eggs develop into larvae that readily penetrate the skin. The cutaneous invasion produces a severely pruritic cutaneous eruption, "ground itch." The larvae ultimately reach the lungs, enter the upper respiratory tract, and are swallowed to develop into mature worms in the intestinal tract. An anemia develops, along with malaise, fever, anorexia, and delayed development. The disease is diagnosed by discovery of ova in the stools. Treatment is with tetrachloroethylene.

The ocular signs are those described in visceral larva migrans. In the past, *Toxocara canis* infections were considered to be caused by the hookworm. The anemia may be associated with retinal hemorrhage.

Trichinosis. Trichinosis is an infestation of striated muscles by the larva of the nematode *Trichinella spiralis*, which infects a wide group of animals of which swine are the chief human reservoir.

The encysted larvae are ingested in undercooked pork and develop in the intestine into sexually mature adults. Eggs develop and hatch in the female nematode, which releases about 1,500 larvae over a 6-week period. The larvae enter the general circulation about 7 days after an individual has eaten infected meat, and they are widely distributed to all tissues. In severe infestations, there is muscle weakness and pain, remittent fever, and edema that is frequently localized to the orbit, prticularly the upper eyelid. Ocular muscle involvement causes pain on movement. There may be subconjunctival hemorrhage.

Diagnosis is based on muscle tenderness and associated eosinophilia. When these signs are associated with orbital edema, the diagnosis is most suggestive. The larvae may be found in biopsy specimens 10 days after infection. The intradermal skin test becomes positive about the third week after infection.

There is no specific therapy. Corticosteroids and ACTH suppress the acute manifestations of the disease.

Filariasis. The filariae are slender, threadlike nematodes that have a tendency to inhabit a particular part of the human body. The female worms produce embryos, microfilariae, which live in the blood or skin. Bloodsucking arthropods, their intermediate hosts, remove them to spread the infection.

ONCHOCERCA VOLVULUS. Ocular onchocerciasis, also called "river blindness," is a chronic filarial infection that occurs endemically in Mexico, Guatemala, Venezuela, and central Africa. It has been estimated to affect more than 20 million people and in some communities blinds as many as 20% of the adult population. The infection is transmitted from person to person by bites of infected black flies of the genus *Simulium*. Infected larvae are injected into the skin or subcutaneous tissue and give rise to nodules (cercoma) of pathognomonic appearance.

The microfilariae of *Onchocerca* swarm in the bulbar conjunctiva and may be seen as squirming, yellowish threads in the aqueous humor. A superficial punctate corneal inflammation occurs initially, followed by deep opacities without vascularization until they are so numerous as to cause epithelial degeneration. Inflammation of the iris is common, and generalized atrophy of the pigmented epithelium gives a spongy appearance to the iris. The lens is not invaded, but complicated cataract may follow uveal inflammation. There is a circumscribed degeneration of the posterior fundus similar to that seen in posterior choroidal atrophy. There is irregular deposition of pigment, perivascular sheathing, and an associated optic atrophy. The nature of the posterior segment lesion is variable. It occurs rarely in areas where there is adequate dietary vitamin A. A gross inflammatory lesion caused by death of the microfilaria is also seen.

Ocular treatment is largely symptomatic. Surgical excision of nodules is most important. Diethylcarbamazine (Hetrazan) is effective against the microfilaria but not the adult worm. Death of many microfilariae may lead to endophthalmitis. Suramin (Bayer 205) kills the adult worm, but it is very toxic. Control of the disease is being attempted by the use of insecticides to eliminate the vector.

LOA LOA. *Loa loa* (African eye worm) is a threadlike nematode 3 to 5 cm in length that lives in the subcutaneous tissue of humans, travels from place to place beneath the skin, and causes a creeping itch sensation. The disease is seen in the west and central parts of Africa. The worm is responsive to warmth, and in persons sitting before a fire, the worms move to the warm face and eyes.

The adult worm looks like a piece of surgical catgut beneath the conjunctiva or swimming in the anterior chamber. There is local irritation, congestion, and lacrimation, which disappears quickly when the worm moves to deeper tissues. The worm may be removed by capturing it with a ligature to prevent its escape. A topical anesthetic relieves symptoms.

Calabar swellings are painless, edematous, subcutaneous nodules that arise as an allergic reaction to metabolic products of the worm or from injured or dead worms. They tend to occur on removal to a cold climate. Systemic antihistamines give relief.

The microfilariae that do not cause ocular disease and some adult worms are destroyed by diethylcarbamazine, which may have to be administered repeatedly.

BANCROFT FILARIASIS. This disease is produced by *Wuchereria bancrofti,* a typical filarial worm that resides in lymph vessels and produces the lymph blockage known as elephantiasis. Physical signs result from inflammatory reactions caused by allergy to the worm and from obstruction of lymph vessels. Rarely, the eyelids or intraocular structures may be involved. Diethylcarbamazine is the drug of choice.

Cestodes (tapeworms). Tapeworm infections (cestodiasis) are of two types: (1) the intestinal form, in which the mature worm is attached to the bowel wall, and (2) the visceral, or somatic, form, in which the larval form of the parasite is present in various tissues and organs.

The intestinal type may cause no symptoms or only symptoms of gastrointestinal disturbances. The visceral type follows ingestion of tapeworm eggs, which, after hatching in the intestine, penetrate its wall, resulting in the spread of infection by the bloodstream.

The two main types of visceral involvement with tapeworms are (1) echinococcus, or hydatid, cysts and (2) cysticercosis.

Echinococcus cysts. Echinococcus cysts are produced by the larvae of *Echinococcus granulosis* a minute tapeworm of dogs and cats. Ingestion of the eggs by swine, cattle, or humans leads to echinococcus cysts of the liver, lungs, kidney, brain, eye, and other organs. The cyst development is slow and presents the symptoms of a slowly developing tumor. The contained fluid is highly irritating, and the cysts should not be evacuated. Orbital cysts, which are more common than intraocular cysts, cause a proptosis with related signs. The intraocular cyst appears as a white pea-sized mass within the vitreous body, or there may be a progressive, solid retinal detachment. Surgical excision is the only effective therapy, and care must be taken not to rupture the cyst and release toxic fluid.

Cysticercosis. Cysticercosis is infection with the cyst stage of the bladder worm *(Cysticercus cellulosae)*, the pork tapeworm *(Taenia solium)*, or rarely the beef tapeworm *(Taenia saginata)*. It occurs because of ingestion of eggs of the parasite, and autoinfection may occur in a human harboring the adult parasite in the intestine. The subcutaneous tissues, muscles, brain, eye, heart, and lung are invaded in that order of frequency. Tissue reaction is minimal until the larva dies, when there is a local inflammatory reaction and capsule formation. Increase in size of the cyst in the brain causes the signs and symptoms of an expanding tumor. In the eye the bladder worm is a translucent oval body 6 to 18 mm in length, without capsule, in which the head of the larva may be seen as a white spot. It may occur in the choroid, causing a retinal detachment, float free in the vitreous body or anterior chamber, or be found beneath the conjunctiva or in the orbit. Removal is the sole therapy, but rupture of the cyst is followed by a violent inflammation.

Ophthalmomyiasis. Invasion of the eye by the larval form (maggot) of flies in the order Diptera follows deposition of the eggs or larvae on the ocular surface by the adult fly, by a secondary vector such as a tick or mosquito, or by the patient's hands. The maggots bore their way into the eye, come to lie in the anterior chamber or vitreous cavity, and cause an endophthalmitis or iridocyclitis. Visual obstruction arises from the maggot in the visual line, from inflammation, from invasion of the optic nerve, from central retinal hemorrhage, or from retinal separation. A subretinal maggot may cause an ophthalmoscopically spectacular tracing of hypopigmented tracks beneath the sensory retina.

SARCOIDOSIS

Sarcoidosis is a chronic idiopathic disease characterized by the occurrence of epithelioid cell granulomas in nearly any organ system. The granuloma is similar to a tubercle but is without caseation and either resolves or is converted into an avascular, acellular hyaline tissue. Frequently it contains refractile or apparently calcified bodies in its giant cells. Mediastinal and peripheral lymph nodes, lungs, liver, spleen, skin, eyes, phalangeal bones, and parotic glands are most commonly affected. Most patients are black, and sarcoid is more prevalent in the southeastern states in both whites and blacks. It is more frequent in women than in men, and most patients are between 20 and 40 years of age.

Clinically, the disease is often first detected because of bilateral hilar adenopathy or the symptoms of cough, dyspnea, chest pain, or hemoptysis. Fever, weight loss, and arthralgia may be the initial signs. Uveitis, cutaneous plaques, papules, subcutaneous nodules, peripheral lymphadenopathy, or lassitude, fever, and malaise may usher in the disease. A leukopenia with a slight eosinophilia may be present. The erythrocyte sedimentation rate may be increased. Hyperglobulinemia is common among blacks. There may be increased serum and urinary muramidase (lysozyme) levels, a finding that also occurs with osteoarthritis and rheumatoid arthritis.

Reaction to the Kveim skin test (a granulomatous reaction occurring 4 weeks after injection of sarcoid spleen or lymph material) is positive in some 75% of the patients but is nonspecific and may be positive in other granulomatous diseases.

Ocular involvement is common but may be asymptomatic. In the lupus pernio type of skin sarcoidosis the skin of the eyelids may be involved. In all types of sarcoidosis the inferior conjunctival fornices may contain minute, translucent, slightly yellow, elevated lesions resembling follicles (Fig. 23-5). Serial section of

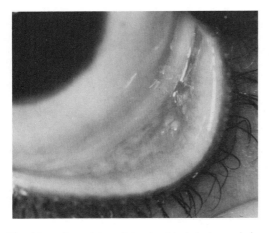

Fig. 23-5. Sarcoid nodules in the inferior cul-de-sac of a 23-year-old woman with advanced sarcoidosis.

such a lesion and skilled pathologic interpretation provide diagnostic material.

Keratoconjunctivitis sicca (p. 268) occurs frequently. Pseudotumor of the orbit may occur. The lacrimal gland may be enlarged, and the salivary glands may be affected.

Uveoparotid fever (Heerfordt disease), previously described in association with uveitis and parotid gland enlargement, is now recognized as being caused by sarcoidosis. A hypercalcemia may be associated with typical conjunctiva and corneal calcium infiltrates and band keratopathy.

The facial and optic nerves are the most common cranial nerves involved in meningeal sarcoidosis. There may be decreased or blurred vision, papilledema, optic atrophy, visual field defects, and pupillary abnormalities.

The chief ocular involvement is a chronic uveitis that may affect the anterior or posterior uvea. The anterior uveitis is associated with mutton-fat keratic precipitates, which may be deeply pigmented. Broad, flat posterior synechiae are common. Sarcoid nodules may appear on the surface of the iris or at the pupillary margin. Posterior uveitis is associated with "snowball" opacities in the vitreous. There may be a periphlebitis, with the adjacent exudates described as looking like candle-wax drippings. Sarcoid nodules may appear in the choroid, in the retina, or on the optic nerve head. Inflammation of the pars plana portion of the ciliary body occurs frequently, with cells in both the vitreous body and anterior chamber. There may be an associated edema of the central retinal region and the optic nerve with decreased central vision.

BIBLIOGRAPHY

Becker, Y.: The agent of trachoma. In Melnick, J. L., editor: Monographs in virology, vol. 7, Basel, Switzerland, 1974, S. Karger.

Bongiorno, F. J., Leavell, U. W., and Wirtschafer, J. D.: The black dot sign and North American cutaneous blastomycosis, Am. J. Ophthalmol. **78**:145, 1974.

Chumbley, L. C., and Kearns, T. P.: Retinopathy of sarcoidosis, Trans. Am. Ophthalmol. Soc. **69**:307, 1971.

Connor, D. H.: Current concepts in parasitology; onchocerciasis, N. Engl. J. Med. **298**:379, 1978.

Edwards, J. E., Jr., Foos, R. Y., Montgomerie, J. Z., and Guze, L. B.: Ocular manifestations of *Candida* septicemia; review of seventy six cases of hematogenous *Candida* endophthalmitis, Medicine **53**:47, 1974.

Fiala, M., Chatterjee, S. N., Carson, S., and others: Cytomegalovirus retinitis secondary to chronic viremia in phagocytic leukocytes, Am. J. Ophthalmol. **84**:567, 1977.

François, J., and Rysselaere, M.: Oculomycosis, Springfield, Ill., 1972, Charles C Thomas, Publisher.

Gass, J. D. M., and Lewis, R. A.: Subretinal tracks in ophthalmomyiasis, Arch. Ophthalmol. **94**:1500, 1976.

Gass, J. D. M., and Olson, C. L.: Sarcoidosis with optic nerve and retinal involvement, Arch. Ophthalmol. **94**:945, 1976.

Gitter, K. A., and Cohen, G.: Photocoagulation of active and inactive lesions of presumed ocular histoplasmosis, Am. J. Ophthalmol. **79**:428, 1975.

Harrison, H. R., English, M. G., Lee, C. K., and Alexander, E. R.: *Chlamydia trachomatis* infant pneumonitis, N. Engl. J. Med. **298**:702, 1978.

Hollenberg, M. J., Wilkie, J. S., Hudson, J. B., and Lewis, B. J.: Lesions produced by human herpesviruses 1 and 2, Arch. Ophthalmol. **94**:127, 1976.

Klein, M. L., Fine, S. L., Knox, D. L., and Patz, A.: Follow-up study in eyes with choroidal neovascularization caused by presumed ocular histoplasmosis, Am. J. Ophthalmol. **83**:830, 1977.

Krick, J. A., and Remington, J. S.: Toxoplasmosis in the adult; an overview, N. Engl. J. Med. **298**:550, 1978.

Locatcher-Khorazo, D., and Seegal, B. C.: Microbiology of the eye, St. Louis, 1972, The C. V. Mosby Co.

Marsh, R. J., Easty, D. L., and Jones, B. R.: Iritis and iris atrophy in herpes zoster ophthalmicus, Am. J. Ophthalmol. **78**:255, 1974.

Martin, R. G., Dawson, C. R., Jones, P., and others: Herpesvirus in sensory and autonomic ganglia after eye infection, Arch. Ophthalmol. **95**:2053, 1977.

Meredith, T. A., and Aaberg, T. M.: Hemorrhagic peripapillary lesions in presumed ocular histoplasmosis, Am. J. Ophthalmol. **84**:160, 1977.

Miller, B., and Ellis, P. P.: Conjunctival flora in patients receiving immunosuppressive drugs, Arch. Ophthalmol. **95**:2012, 1977.

Mizuno, K., and Watanabe, T.: Sarcoid granulomatous cyclitis, Am. J. Ophthalmol. **81**:82, 1976.

Mosier, M. A., Lusk, B., Pettit, T. H., and others: Fungal endophthalmitis following intraocular lens implantation, Am. J. Ophthalmol. **83**:1, 1977.

Murray, H. W., Knox, D. L., Green, W. R., and Susel, R. M.: Cytomegalovirus retinitis in adults; a manifestation of disseminated viral infection, Am. J. Med. **63**:574, 1977.

Rahi, A. H. S., and Garner, A.: Immunopathology of the eye, Philadelphia, 1976, J. B. Lippincott Co.

Rao, N. A., and Font, R. L.: Toxoplasmic retinochoroiditis, Am. J. Ophthalmol. **95**:273, 1977.

Raymond, L. A., Kerstine, R. S., and Shelburne, S. A., Jr: Preretinal vitreous membrane in subacute sclerosing panencephalitis, Arch. Ophthalmol. **94**:1412, 1976.

Rodrigues, M. M., Weiss, C. B., and Muncy, D. W.: Ophthalmomyiasis of the eyelid caused by *Cuterebra* larva, Am. J. Ophthal. **78**:1024, 1974.

Roth, A. M., and Purcell, T. W.: Ocular findings associated with encephalomyelitis caused by *Herpesvirus simiae*, Am. J. Ophthalmol. **84**:345, 1977.

Ryan, S. J., Jr: De novo subretinal neovascularization in histoplasmosis syndrome, Arch. Ophthalmol. **94**:321, 1976.

Ryan, S. J., Jr., and Smith, R. E., editors: Selected topics on the eye in systemic disease, New York, 1974, Grune & Stratton, Inc.

Sawelson, H., Goldberg, R. E., Annesley, W. H., Jr., and Tomer, T. L.: Presumed ocular histoplasmosis syndrome, Arch. Ophthalmol. **94**:221, 1976.

Schachter, J.: Chlamydial infections, N. Engl. J. Med. **298**:428, 540, 1978.

Schantz, P. M., and Glickman, L. T.: Current concepts in parasitology; toxocaral visceral larva migrans, N. Engl. J. Med. **298**:436, 1978.

Sher, N. A., Hill, C. W., and Elfrig, D. E.: Bilateral intraocular *Nocardia asteroides* infection, Arch. Ophthalmol. **95**:1415, 1977.

Shields, J. A., Lerner, H. A., and Felbert, N. T.: Aqueous cytology and enzymes in nematode endophthalmitis, Am. J. Ophthalmol. **84**:319, 1977.

Smith, T. W., and Burton, T. C.: The retinal manifestations of Rocky Mountain spotted fever, Am. J. Ophthalmol. **84**:259, 1977.

Tarazil, R. C.: Streptococcal immunology; protection versus injury, Ann. Intern. Med. **88**:422, 1978.

Chapter 24

HEREDITARY DISORDERS

Many ocular defects are transmitted by changes in genetic material. There may be associated systemic defects, but in many conditions, such as the corneal dystrophies, some cataracts, and some retinopathies, systemic abnormalities cannot be detected with present methods. McKusick lists 1,545 genetically determined variations in humans. Some 10% to 15% of these are confined to the eye, and an approximately equal number involve systemic abnormalities with ocular signs.

The genetic composition of each human being is determined by 22 pairs of autosomal chromosomes together with a pair of sex chromosomes, which are similar in the female (XX) and dissimilar in the male (XY). Each parent contributes an equal number of chromosomes to each individual. The male receives a Y chromosome from his father and an X chromosome from his mother. The female receives an X chromosome from each parent.

The chromosomes contain some 20,000 to 40,000 different pairs of genes, the unit of inheritance. The substance of a gene is deoxyribonucleic acid (DNA), which resides in the cell nucleus. The genetic information codified in DNA is transcribed to and passes into the cytoplasm on messenger ribonucleic acid (mRNA). Here the information on mRNA is translated within the ribosome. For a time it con-

trols the sequence of amino acids synthesized by means of transfer RNA (tRNA). The DNA responsible for designating the types and sequence of amino acids (structural gene) and transferring information to mRNA is controlled by two types of control gene: (1) an operator gene, which initiates the activity of mRNA synthesis, and (2) a regulator gene, which produces a repressor substance that stops the synthesis of mRNA.

Simply, replication of the gene depends on DNA synthesis. Growth, differentiation, and cell formation depend on RNA synthesis. The four bases in DNA (thymine, adenine, guanine, and cytosine) provide a code that governs the type and sequence of the 20 amino acids that form polypeptides and, in turn, enzymes and structural proteins. More than one gene may be involved in the synthesis of a particular protein.

Inherited disorders may involve one of several different mechanisms. A mutation that changes the sequence of bases in DNA may cause substitution of an amino acid (as occurs in hemoglobin sickle cell disease), an abnormality in protein synthesis, or premature termination of a polypeptide chain.

Each gene has a partner, or allele, located at the same position (locus) on the corresponding or homologous chromosome contributed by the other parent.

When these two allelic genes are similar and determine a similar characteristic, they are homozygous, and when they are different, they are heterozygous.

MENDELIAN INHERITANCE

The occurrence of a genetic defect is determined by the behavior of a pair of allelic genes. If the genetic abnormality requires a double dose of the abnormal gene (the homozygous state), the expression of the abnormality is considered to be recessive. If the condition may be fully expressed by a single dose of the affected gene, the condition is said to be dominant.

If the condition is carried on the sex chromosomes (X or Y), it is sex linked or X chromosome linked (Y chromosome abnormalities rarely manifest themselves because they can only occur in the homozygous male).

Autosomal defects are transmitted on the 22 nonsex autosomes. Both males and females are affected and can transmit the abnormality to both sons and daughters. An autosomal dominant condition is one that may be expressed in the heterozygous state, in which the individual has a normal partner gene (allele) located at the same position as the abnormal gene on the homologous chromosome contributed by the other parent. Autosomal dominant conditons involve mainly structural proteins rather than enzymes. Ocular conditions include aniridia (p. 290), granular corneal dystrophy (p. 269), and vitelliform central retinal degeneration (Best disease, p. 342). Often the presence of the abnormal gene cannot be recognized, and some generations are apparently skipped, because the carrier of the abnormal gene is clinically normal. When there is this lack of expression of the abnormality, the gene is called nonpenetrant. Heterozygous affected individuals mated to normal homozygotes will transmit the trait to half of the offspring; both sexes will be equally affected. The offspring of individuals heterozygous for a dominantly inherited trait will be one-fourth homozygous affected, one-half heterozygous affected, and one-fourth homozygous normal. The homozygous affected state may cause early death even though the heterozygous state may be clinically mild. Autosomal dominant traits may be recognized in human pedigrees by transmission from one generation to the next. Except when caused by mutation, every affected individual has at least one parent with the abnormal gene and may have affected offspring.

Autosomal recessive disorders are those conditions that require a double dose of the abnormal gene, as occurs in the homozygous state. In general, the autosomal homozygous affections are more severe than heterozygous affections and often cause inborn errors of metabolism. In the autosomal recessive trait, inheritance is from both parents who are heterozygous for the abnormal gene but, although clinically normal, often have subtle enzyme defects. When both parents are heterozygous for a recessive trait, the offspring will be one-fourth homozygous for the abnormal allele, one-fourth normal, and one-half heterozygous for the recessive trait. Since related individuals are more likely to be heterozygous for the same abnormal gene, consanguinity is more likely to produce offspring affected by a recessive disorder.

Most inborn errors of metabolism involve recessive inheritance. In general the conditions are clinically more severe than those involving dominant inheritance, which often involve structural proteins. A deficiency of a single enzyme has been demonstrated in many conditions.

Defects that are carried on the sex chromosomes may be heterozygous or homozygous in the female and heterozygous in the male. The female, having two X chromosomes and being either heterozygous or homozygous, can demonstrate either recessive or dominant behavior of a trait.

The male has one X chromosome and thus carries only one-half the complement of X chromosome–linked genes found in the female. There can be no father-to-son transmission, because the male transmits an X chromosome to his daughters and a Y chromosome to his sons.

On the average, half of the sons of heterozygous females will be normal and half will be affected. An affected male married to a normal female will have daughters who are all carriers and sons who are all normal. Carriers may be clinically abnormal. The carrier daughter will transmit the abnormality to one-half of her sons.

Dominant X chromosome–linked traits affect both males and females, who transmit the disorder to their offspring. The heterozygous female with one abnormal X chromosome received from her father may demonstrate subtle signs of the carrier state and transmits the trait to half of her sons and daughters. The heterozygous male transmits the trait to all of his daughters but not to any of his sons. X chromosome–linked dominance occurs in some instances of retinal pigmentary degeneration.

In recessive X chromosome–linked conditions the heterozygous female frequently shows evidence of the carrier state. Marked clinical manifestations of the abnormality are rare. In the heterozygous male, however, the deficiency is fully demonstrated. Ocular albinism, choroideremia (p. 292), central retinoschisis (p. 349), and color blindness are ocular examples of recessive X chromosome–linked disorders.

CHROMOSOMAL ABNORMALITIES

Chromosomal abnormalities arise from a basic alteration in morphogenesis in which there is an extra chromosome, a missing chromosome, small extra pieces of chromosomal material, pieces missing, or rearrangements within chromosomes. These alterations give rise to a genetic imbalance, which interferes with control mechanisms that manage the timeliness and sequential nature of morphogenesis. Often there is a growth deficiency, mental retardation, and hypoplasia of the middle facial structure. Because of disorders in the control system, epicanthal folds (p. 201) and a low nasal bridge occur. Generally, chromosomal abnormalities do not give rise to specific biochemical abnormalities but cause more generalized disorders that involve a number of systems. Redundant folds of skin in the posterior portion of the neck, up-slanting palpebral fissures, low-set and malformed auricles, and a simian palm crease all suggest chromosomal abnormalities.

Diagnosis of chromosomal aberrations requires staining by one of several methods that indicate specific bands in each of the chromosomes. Each chromosome is identified by its number, by its short or long arm, and by region or band number. Banding techniques provide identification of disorders arising from abnormalities involving almost every chromosome. Most chromosomal abnormalities rarely occur in otherwise normal individuals with a single malformation.

Deletion syndromes

Partial deletion of the short arm of chromosome 4 (Wolf syndrome) is associated with microcephaly, hemangioma of the brow, ocular hypertelorism (simulating exophthalmos), divergent strabismus, blepharoptosis, antimongoloid obliquity of the palpebral fissures, and coloboma of the iris.

Deletion of the short arm of chromosome 5 is characterized by a weak, shrill, mewing cry of the infant during the first few months of life because of hypoplasia of the larynx (cri du chat). There is severe mental retardation, failure to thrive, a birth weight usually less than 2,500 grams, microcephaly, and hypertelorism. In addition, there is an antimongoloid obliquity of the palpebral fissures, epicanthus, and an alternating esotropia. Further studies of denervation hypersensitivity of the iris are indicated.

Deletion of the long arm of chromosome 13 is sometimes associated with retinoblastoma (p. 353). Other signs of chromosome abnormality are usually present (95%), but the remaining infants may appear normal.

Deletion of the short arm of chromosome 18 is associated with microcephaly, hypertelorism, epicanthal folds, strabismus, and blepharoptosis. Deletion of the long arm is associated with midface hypoplasia and frequent eye defects, such as glaucoma, strabismus, nystagmus, tapetoretinal degeneration, and optic atrophy.

Numeral variation syndromes

Trisomy 13 syndrome. Trisomy 13 syndrome (Patau syndrome) is associated with multiple disorders. About 80% exhibit microphthalmia or iris coloboma with retinal dysplasia and ocular hypertelorism. There may be intraocular cartilage extending from the retrolental region to the sclera at the site of the iris coloboma. There are capillary hemangiomas in the glabellar region, cleft lip, and polydactyly. At least 80% of those affected have congenital heart defects.

Trisomy 18 syndrome. Trisomy 18 syndrome (Edward syndrome) is second only to Down syndrome in frequency. Affected infants are inactive, cry weakly, and develop poorly. Ocular changes, such as epicanthal folds, are common but relatively minor. Uveal colobomas, congenital glaucoma, corneal opacities, and microphthalmia have been described.

Trisomy 21 syndrome. Trisomy 21 syndrome (Down syndrome, mongolism) is the most common cause of mental retardation that can be recognized at birth. Most patients (95%) have 47 rather than 46 chromosomes with an extra chromosome 21 (trisomy 21; it is actually chromosome 22, but the earlier name remains). Some individuals with trisomy 21 (1:200) have an additional chromosome, so that they have 48 chromosomes. This disjunction is age dependent. If the mother is less than 20 years of age at the time of conception, the risk of producing a child with trisomy 21 is about 1 in 2,500 births. In a woman more than 45 years of age, the chance of having such a child is about 1 in 50. About 3.5% of patients with Down syndrome have the extra chromosome attached to another chromosome, often chromosome 14. This syndrome may be familial or sporadic. When familial, one of the parents has 45 chromosomes instead of the normal 46, with one of the small G-group chromosomes (21-22) translocated to another chromosome. If the mother has trisomy 21, about one half of the children have Down syndrome. Males with trisomy 21 are sterile. The remaining patients may have a mosaicism, or two different cell populations: one with trisomy 21 and the other normal. In such patients, the intelligence level is higher than expected and the phenotype is not fully expressed.

There are numerous typical physical findings: hypotonia; mental retardation; open mouth with thick protruding tongue; dental hypoplasia; hypoplasia of the nasal bones; angular overlapping helix, prominent antihelix, and small or absent earlobe; and excessive skin on the nape of the neck (noted in about 80% of the patients). Lips are broad, irregular, fissured, and dry. Hands are short and broad, and the fifth finger is usually abbreviated. The Moro reflex is absent in more than 80% of the cases. Intelligence quotients range from 25 to 70. There is a twentyfold increase in the association of the syndrome with acute leukemia.

The palpebral fissure is almond shaped, with the outer canthus higher than the medial canthus (mongoloid slant), and epicanthal folds are present. The iris is hypoplastic, and in early life whitish areas are present (Brushfield spots). Cataract (p. 389) occurs in about 60% of the patients. Esotropia, nystagmus, myopia, and blepharitis are common. In older groups keratoconus develops, often complicated by an acute corneal hydrops (p. 258) that heals with severe scarring.

Ophthalmoscopically, irrespective of the refractive error or the degree of skin or iris pigmentation, the fundus looks as it does in myopic or blonde individuals. Pigmentation of the retinal pigment epithelium and choroid is scanty, and the choroidal vasculature is easily visible. The optic disk appears more pink than normal because of a large number of retinal vessels crossing the disk margin.

Cat's-eye syndrome. Coloboma of the iris combined with anal atresia is a familial disorder that most likely involves chromosome 22 but is different from trisomy 22. There may be mosaicism or translocation of part of chromosome 22. Careful cytogenic studies are necessary in such patients. There is moderate developmental and mental deficiency, hypertelorism, antimongoloid slant of the eyes, microphthalmia, and sometimes optic atrophy. Preauricular skin tags are common, and renal abnormalities occur.

LYSOSOMAL STORAGE DISEASE

A lysosomal storage disease is an abnormality in which one of the acid hydrolase enzymes enclosed within the lysosome body is deficient and causes an excess of partially degraded metabolite. Presently some 35 inherited disorders can be classified as lysosomal storage diseases; in 20 of these the severe deficiency of a specific lysosomal hydrolase enzyme is known (Table 24-1). In many, electron microscopy of the conjunctiva will indicate abnormal lysosomes.

The lysosomes are intracellular vesicles containing many hydrolytic enzymes that split biologic compounds in a mild acid medium. In living cells, these enzymes are confined within the lysosome and can act only on material taken up by the cell. Four types of lysosomes are recognized: a primary lysosome and three types of secondary lysosome.

A primary lysosome is a small intracellular body that contains acid hydrolases synthesized by ribosomes. These enzymes accumulate in the granular endoplasmic reticulum and penetrate the Golgi apparatus, which forms an envelope containing the enzyme. A secondary lysosome arises when foreign matter enters the lysosome by either phagocytosis or pinocytosis. The engulfed material is progressively digested by hydrolytic enzymes that have been incorporated into the lysosome. If digestion is not complete, a lysosome called a residual body forms. In some cells these residual bodies are eliminated by reverse pinocytosis. In other cells they may be retained and accumulated. They are important in the aging process. The autophagic vacuole is a lysosome responsible for the economy of the cell itself.

The acid hydrolases of the lysosome are responsible for breaking ester bonds; glycosidases act at glycocytic linkages; phosphatases, sulfatases, and proteases act similarly. Thus far, it has not been demonstrated that the absence of lysosomal proteases causes disease. Additionally, different nonlysosomal particles called *peroxisomes* are rich in perioxidases and catylases. These particles are important in abnormalities such as neuronal ceroid lipofuscinosis (p. 488), in which lipid material accumulates.

The mitochondria, which participate in

Table 24-1. Summary of lysosomal disorders

Disorder	Enzyme deficiency	Metabolite primarily affected
Sphingolipidoses		
G$_{M1}$ gangliosidosis	β-Galactosidase	G$_{M1}$ ganglioside, fragments from glycoproteins
Krabbe disease	β-Galactosidase	Galactosyl ceramide
Tay-Sachs disease	Hexosaminidase A	G$_{M2}$ ganglioside
Sandhoff disease	Hexosaminidases A and B	G$_{M2}$ ganglioside, globoside
Gaucher disease	β-Glucosidase	Glucosyl ceramide
Fabry disease	α-Galactosidase	Trihexosyl ceramide
Metachromatic leukodystrophy	Arylsulfatase A	Sulfatide
Niemann-Pick disease	Sphingomyelinase	Sphingomyelin
Farber disease	Ceramidase	Ceramide
Mucopolysaccharidoses		
Type Eponym		
I Hurler	α-L-Iduronidase	Dermatan sulfate, heparan sulfate
II Hunter	Iduronate sulfatase	Dermatan sulfate, heparan sulfate
III Sanfillipo		
A subtype	Heparan N-sulfatase	Heparan sulfate
B subtype	N-Acetyl-α-glucosaminidase	Heparan sulfate
IV Morquio	Uncertain	Keratan sulfate
V Scheie	α-L-Iduronidase	Dermatan sulfate, heparan sulfate
VI Maroteaux-Lamy	N-Acetylgalactosamine sulfatase (arylsulfatase B)	Dermatan sulfate
β-Glucuronidase deficiency	β-Glucuronidase	Dermatan sulfate, heparan sulfate
Disorders of glycoprotein metabolism		
Fucosidosis	α-L-Fucosidase	Fragments from glycoproteins, glycolipids
Mannosidosis	α-Mannosidase	Mannose containing glycoproteins, glycopeptides, and oligosaccharides
Aspartylglycosaminuria	Amidase	Aspartyl-2-deoxy-2-acetamido glucosylamine
Other disorders with single enzyme defect		
Pompe disease	α-Glucosidase	Glycogen
Wolman disease	Acid lipase	Cholesterol esters, triglyceride
Acid phosphatase deficiency	Acid phosphastase	Phosphate esters
Multiple enzyme deficiencies (inherited as a single gene defect)		
Multiple sulfatase deficiency	Sulfatases (arylsulfatase A,B,C: steroid sulfatases; iduronate sulfatase; heparan N-sulfatase)	Sulfatide, steroid sulfate, mucopolysaccharide
I-cell disease and pseudo-Hurler polydystrophy	Almost all lysosomal enzymes deficient in cultured fibroblasts; present extracellularly	Mucopolysaccharide and glycolipids
Disorders of unknown cause		
Cystinosis	Accumulation of cystine in lysosomes	Cystine
Mucolipidoses I, IV	Ultrastructural evidence of lysosmal storage	Unknown

Modified from Neufeld, E. F., Lim, T. W., and Shapiro, L. J.: Annu. Rev. Biochem. **44:**357, 1975.

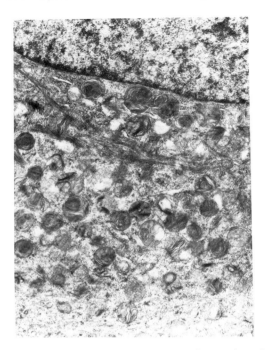

Fig. 24-1. Enlarged lysosomes within cultured fibroblasts in a lysosomal storage disease. All affected tissues show similar accumulation, and the deficient enzyme may be demonstrated in the culture media. (×19,000.)

the metabolism of carbohydrates and fats, are involved in a variety of myopathies with associated retinal degeneration. Closely related enzymes may have different substrates, and a deficiency may cause a variety of clinical manifestations.

The lysosomal disorders may affect skeletal growth, mental development, and central nervous system development. The severity varies greatly. They may be associated with characteristic facial changes. In some individuals there may be cloudy corneas; degeneration of the retinal ganglion cells with optic atrophy and a cherry-red spot at the fovea, where there are no inner layers of the retina; and retinal degeneration resembling that seen in retinal pigmentary degenerations.

The enzyme deficiency can be de-

tected in cultured fibroblasts of the affected individual or by amniocentesis before birth. The tissue-culture growth medium will indicate the enzyme deficiency, and electron microscopy will demonstrate the abnormal lysosomes (Fig. 24-1). Tears, urine, and hair follicles have been used for enzyme assay. In the mucopolysaccharidoses the abnormal storage substance may be detected in urine. The disorders are uncommon, and interest in them is high because of their indication of the nature of normal cell metabolism. Heterozygote screening for hexosaminidases A and B has been developed in many cities in the United States.

Sphingolipidoses

The sphingolipids are complex lipids that are important components of brain, nerve, and many membranes. Each contains one molecule of sphingosine, one molecule of an 18- to 26-carbon fatty acid, and a polar head group (Fig. 24-2). The combination of sphingosine and the fatty acid is called a ceramide. There are three major groups of sphingolipids: (1) sphingomyelins, the most abundant, which contain phosphorylcholine or phosphoroethanolamine as the polar head group; (2) neutral sphingolipids, which contain one or more sugars in the polar head group; and (3) acidic glycosphingolipids (gangliosides), which contain one or more molecules of sialic acid in the polar head group.

The sphingolipidoses are genetically determined metabolic defects characterized by the accumulation of excessive quantities of fatty substances in various tissues, giving rise to visceral, neural, and ocular manifestations. There are at least nine sphingolipid disorders and in each a different complex lipid accumulates. The abnormality occurs because of a deficiency of the catabolic enzyme necessary for the degradation of the excess lipid (Table 24-1). With the exception of Fabry dis-

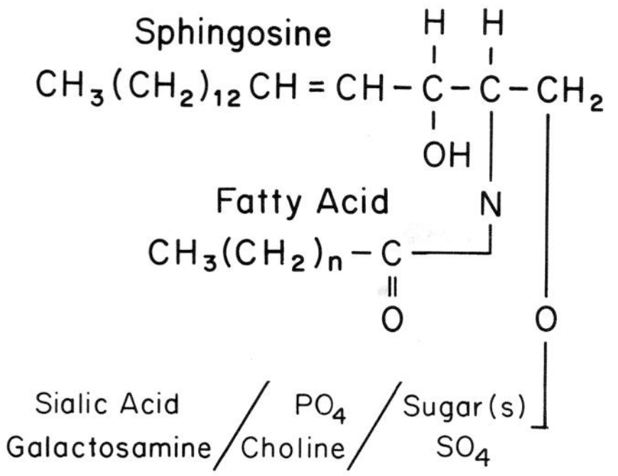

Sphingosine

$$CH_3(CH_2)_{12} CH = CH - \overset{\overset{\displaystyle H}{|}}{C} - \overset{\overset{\displaystyle H}{|}}{\underset{\underset{\displaystyle OH}{|}}{C}} - \overset{|}{\underset{|}{CH_2}}$$

Fatty Acid

$$CH_3(CH_2)_n - \underset{\underset{\displaystyle O}{\|}}{C} \overset{\displaystyle N}{\underline{\hspace{1cm}}}$$

O

Sialic Acid / PO₄ / Sugar(s)
Galactosamine / Choline / SO₄

Fig. 24-2. General chemical structure of the sphingolipids.

ease, which is an X chromosome–linked abnormality, each of the conditions is transmitted in an autosomal manner. Most result from the mating of heterozygotes in which each parent is a carrier. The enzyme deficiency may be demonstrated in cultured fibroblasts of parents or by assay of cultured fetal fibroblasts obtained by amniocentesis.

Niemann-Pick disease. Niemann-Pick disease (sphingomyelin lipidosis) is a collective term for a group of inherited abnormalities in which there is widespread accumulation of sphingomyelin and cholesterol in the reticuloendothelial and nervous systems and in the parenchymal cells of many organs. There is patchy destruction of ganglion cells and demyelination of many parts of the nervous system. Four types are described: A, acute, neuronopathic, sphingomyelinase deficient; B, chronic without central nervous system involvement, sphingomyelinase deficient; C, subacute, or juvenile, with neural involvement; D, Nova Scotia type. The sphingomyelinase assays are normal in types C and D. Rarely, an adult has visceral accumulation of sphingomyelin, but the cause is not known.

The conditions are transmitted as autosomal recessive traits and tend (46%) to involve children of Jewish parentage. Types A and C are the most common.

In type A, poor feeding may be the earliest sign, followed by retardation of physical and mental development. Nearly every organ may be infiltrated with lipid, and there is huge enlargement of the liver and spleen with abdominal distension, marked infiltration of lymph nodes and bone marrow, unexplained fever, and yellow-brown pigmentation of the skin. Involvement of the retina causes a cherry-red spot to develop in one or both eyes. Sometimes the central retinal region appears gray. Involvement of the nervous system causes a variety of sensory, motor, and psychic signs.

Type C has a later onset than type A and a more prolonged course, but eventually there is widespread neurologic involvement and death. Cherry-red spots are seen in the central retina late in childhood.

Accumulation of neutral sphingolipids. The main sphingolipidoses involving the accumulation of neutral sphingolipids are galactosylceramide lipidosis (Krabbe), diffuse angiokeratoma (Fabry), and glucosyl ceramide lipidosis (Gaucher).

Galactosyl ceramide lipidosis. Galactosyl ceramide lipidosis (globoid cell leukodystrophy, Krabbe disease) is an inherited abnormality of a sphingolipid that is normally concentrated in the myelin sheath. It has its onset in the first 6 months of life and results in death from emaciation at the age of 1 or 2 years. The disease begins with irritability and progresses to motor and mental deterioration. There is spasticity early, but patients become flaccid later. Blindness caused by optic atrophy occurs commonly. Deafness is common. There is no storage of sphingolipids in tissues, but there is an absence or deficiency of β-galactosidase, which normally degrades galactosyl ceramide resulting from myelin turnover. The globoid cell is characteristic. It resembles a large epithelial cell and occurs in demyelinated regions.

Diffuse angiokeratoma. Diffuse angio-keratoma (Fabry disease) is an X chromo-some–linked hereditary disorder charac-terized by a deficiency in the enzyme α-galactosidase, resulting in the accumu-lation of trihexosyl ceramide throughout the body tissues. Symptoms occur in early childhood, with episodes of excruciating pain in the extremities, fever, and angio-keratomatous skin lesions, particularly af-fecting the thighs and genitalia. There are fingerprint lines in the cornea caused by epithelial deposition of an abnormal substance. A star-shaped haze of the lens occurs. The veins of the conjunctiva and ocular fundus are abnormally tortuous. The fingerprint lines may occur in the corneas of female carriers. Death in the thirties and forties because of renal fail-ure can be prevented by renal transplan-tation. Galactose-free diets are used to reduce the chemical substrate, and kid-ney transplants appear to increase en-zyme activity.

Glucosyl ceramide lipidosis. Glucosyl ceramide lipidosis (Gaucher disease) in-cludes at least three rare familial dis-orders characterized by the accumulation of glucosyl ceramides in the reticuloen-dothelial system. The enzyme β-glucosi-dase, which catalyzes the cleavage of glu-cose from glucosyl ceramide, is deficient.

Type one may manifest itself at any age. Bleeding, thrombocytopenia, and intermittent infection occur, but there are no neurologic signs. Minor pingueculas occur.

Type two develops before the age of 6 months, and there is widespread neuro-logic involvement with mental retarda-tion, spasticity, hepatosplenomegaly, and eventually death from intercurrent infec-tion. Ocular signs are secondary to cranial nerve involvement.

Type three, or subacute Gaucher dis-ease, has its onset after the age of 6 months, and survival is from 2 to 20 years. The disease is dominated by the effects of an increasing mass of Gaucher cells in the liver, spleen, lymph nodes, and bone marrow. There is hepatosplenomegaly and lymphadenopathy, bone lesions causing spontaneous fractures, and in-volvement of the spleen and bone mar-row, with resultant pancytopenia often necessitating splenectomy. The skin is pigmented. Ultimately there is interfer-ence with blood cell formation and death from intercurrent infection.

A Gaucher cell is typically a large cell in which the cytoplasm has an irregular, streaked appearance resembling wrin-kled tissue paper. It stains strongly with periodic acid–Schiff reaction. There is a marked increase in acid phosphatase ac-tivity in plasma, tissues, and Gaucher cells themselves. Blood lipids are normal. The circulating vitamin B_{12}–binding pro-tein, transcobalamin II, and serum angio-tensin-converting enzyme are increased.

Large yellow-brown pingueculas may extend outward, with their bases at the cornea. These occur after childhood, are larger and darker than those occurring spontaneously in middle life, are asymp-tomatic, and require no treatment. Cen-tral retinal degeneration may occur, and corneal clouding has been described. Treatment is supportive.

Gangliosidoses. The acidic glycosphin-golipid (ganglioside) disorders include generalized G_{M1} gangliosidosis, which also has a juvenile variant; Tay-Sachs dis-ease; Sandhoff disease; and juvenile G_{M2} gangliosidosis. There is progressive mo-tor and mental deterioration with onset early in life and ultimately a fatal out-come. All are autosomal recessive condi-tions. In each there is storage of a specific ganglioside and absence or deficiency of a specific enzyme. The heterozygote may be detected by decreased enzyme activ-ity in the serum, and prenatal diagnosis is possible by amniocentesis.

Tay-Sachs disease, Sandhoff disease, and juvenile G_{M2} gangliosidosis involve storage of the same material, ganglioside G_{M2}. This compound is normally degraded by two enzymes, hexosaminidase A and B. In Tay-Sachs disease hexosaminidase A is absent and hexosaminidase B is deficient; in Sandhoff disease both hexosaminidase A and B are markedly deficient; and in juvenile G_{M2} gangliosidosis there is a moderate deficiency of hexosaminidase A.

Generalized gangliosidosis and juvenile G_{M1} gangliosidosis involve storage of ganglioside G_{M1}. In both conditions there is a marked deficiency of β-galactosidase, permitting the accumulation of the ganglioside.

Tay-Sachs disease. Tay-Sachs disease (infantile amaurotic familial idiocy) is an autosomal recessive abnormality that has its onset in the first year of life. The onset is insidious, with listlessness, retardation in development, or feeding difficulties. The most common initial symptom is a startled reaction to sound (hyperacusis). Vision is affected early, and there is inattentiveness, failure to move the eyes, or strabismus. Ophthalmoscopic examination may be normal initially, but soon the central retina shows a whitish area ophthalmoscopically that is approximately 2 disk diameters in size, with a small, reddish central area (cherry-red spot). Retinal and optic atrophy follows, with eventual blindness. As neurologic involvement progresses, convulsions or a state of decerebrate rigidity may occur. Death from bulbar involvement usually occurs at about the age of 30 months.

The white spot of the central retina is produced by swelling and degeneration of the numerous ganglion cells located there. The cherry-red spot results from the appearance of the choroidal circulation at the fovea centralis, where the inner layers of the retina are absent. Changes in the brain include enormously swollen and distorted ganglion cells. With a light microscope the neurons of the central, autonomic, and somatic nervous systems appear enormously swollen and distended. Electron microscopically, the neuronal deposits consist of concentric membranes called membranous cytoplasmic bodies. Nerve fibers arising from these cells are demyelinated, and this contributes to the optic atrophy.

The disorder has a carrier frequency of one in 30 for Ashkenazic (European) Jews and one in 300 for non-Jewish individuals.

Sandhoff disease. This condition is nearly identical to Tay-Sachs disease, but tubular epithelial cells contain lipids. It is distinguished from Tay-Sachs disease by the severe deficiency of hexosaminidase A and B.

Juvenile G_{M2} gangliosidosis. Onset is between ages 2 and 6 years, with ataxia, dysarthria, seizures, and eventual decerebrate rigidity. Cherry-red spots and blindness occur late, and patients die between 5 and 15 years of age.

Generalized gangliosidosis involves viscera as well as nervous tissue. Progressive cerebral degeneration develops early in life, and the infants die within 2 years. A cherry-red spot has been noted in about one-half the cases.

Ceramide lipidosis. Ceramide lipidosis (Farber disease) is a deficiency of ceramidase in which ceramides with a terminal alpha-galactosyl residue accumulate. Soon after birth infants develop tender and swollen joints and a hoarse weak cry because of deposition of ceramide in the joints and larynx. The tissue ceramide concentration is markedly increased, and G_{M3} ganglioside occurs in neuronal tissue. Cherry-red spots have been described in the central retina together with birefringent glycolipid in the retinal ganglion cell layer.

Metachromatic lipidosis. This is a group of autosomal recessive disorders in which sulfatides accumulate in myelin sheaths and viscera. The various types are distinguished by their time of onset: late infantile, the most common; multiple sulfatase deficiencies, with onset at age 1 to 3 years; and adult. Weakness, ataxia, dysarthria, ocular muscle palsies, and terminally severe mental retardation and spasticity occur. Optic atrophy and blindness eventually develop. Material that stains red with toluidine blue (metachromatic) is found in urinary sediment and collects in viscera and ganglion cells, including those of the retina. Leukocytes are deficient in arylsulfatase A activity.

Mucopolysaccharidoses

The mucopolysaccharides (proteoglycosaminoglycans) consist of compounds of long unbranched chains composed of disaccharide repeating units. One sugar is always a hexosamine and the other is hexuronic acid, with the exception of keratan sulfate, which contains galactose instead of hexuronic acid. All but hyaluronic acid and chondroitin contain sulfate groups. Hyaluronic acids provide viscosity to vitreous humor (p. 357), synovial fluid, and the umbilical cord but are apparently not involved in the genetic mucopolysaccharidoses. Chondroitin occurs in the cornea. The sulfated mucopolysaccharides are synthesized by connective tissue cells and are attached to proteins to form complex molecules.

Five main proteoglycosaminoglycans have been described: chondroitin-4-sulfate, chondroitin-6-sulfate, (formerly chondroitin A and C), dermatan sulfate (formerly chondroitin sulfate B), heparan sulfate (formerly heparitin sulfate), and keratin sulfate I (corneal) and II (skeletal). Chondroitin-4- and -6-sulfate are the most abundant mucopolysaccharides in the body but apparently are not directly involved in the mucopolysaccharidoses. Dermatan sulfate, which is present in the skin, tendons, heart valves, and aorta, is by far the major mucopolysaccharide in the majority of genetic mucopolysaccharidoses. Keratan sulfate in cartilage, nucleus pulposus, and cornea is found in abnormal amounts in Morquio disease.

Six distinct types (Table 24-2) of mucopolysaccharidoses have been identified on the basis of clinical and biochem-

Table 24-2. The mucopolysaccharidoses

Type	Eponym	Skeletal dysplasia	Mental retardation	Somatic changes	Corneal clouding
I	Hurler	Severe	Severe	Severe	Severe
II	Hunter				
	A. Severe	Severe	Severe	Severe	None
	B. Mild	Moderate	Slight to normal	Moderate	With aging
III	Sanfilippo				
	A. Sulfatase deficient	Slight	Severe		None
	B. Glucosoaminidase deficient	Slight	Severe		None
IV	Morquio	Severe	Slight to normal	Aortic regurgitation	Moderate
V	Scheie	Slight	Slight to normal	Aortic regurgitation	Severe
VI	Maroteaux-Lamy				
	A. Severe	Severe	None	None	Moderate
	B. Mild	Mild	None	None	Moderate

Hunter syndrome is inherited as an X chromosome–linked recessive trait; all others are autosomal recessive. Optic atrophy has been reported in all. Pigmentary degeneration of the retina has been described in all but IV and VI.

ical studies. There is tissue storage of acid mucopolysaccharide, which appears to be the product of the cells in which it appears.

Mucopolysaccharidosis I (Hurler syndrome) is a widespread systemic disorder usually evident within 6 months after birth. It is characterized clinically by skeletal deformities, limitations of joint movements, hernia, hepatosplenomegaly, cardiac abnormalities, deafness, mental retardation, and diffuse corneal clouding. Dermatan sulfate and heparan sulfate are found in urine and tissues, and dermatan sulfate is found in fibroblasts. There is increased ganglioside in the brain and absence of α-L-iduronidase in the tissues.

Typically the patient has a large and bulging head, the bridge of the nose is flattened and the nostrils are broad, and the posterior pharynx is occluded. The children are mouth breathers and have markedly carious teeth and a fetid breath.

The facies are apathetic, the tongue is enlarged and the facial features are coarse (Fig. 24-3). The neck is short, so that the head appears to rest directly upon the thorax. Kyphosis is common, as are deformities of the vertebrae. The broad hands have stubby fingers, and on roentgenologic study, the terminal phalangeal bones are found to be hypoplastic. Limitation of extension of the joints is striking. The abdomen is protuberant. Roentgenographic examination reveals a long and shallow sella turcica.

Clouding of the cornea is characteristic. The subepithelial area has the appearance of slightly glazed glass. The central cornea is more cloudy than the periphery, although histologically (Fig. 24-4) the deep epithelial layers of the periphery are more involved. The normal tension, absence of tearing, failure of the globe to enlarge, and associated physical changes exclude glaucoma as a cause of the cor-

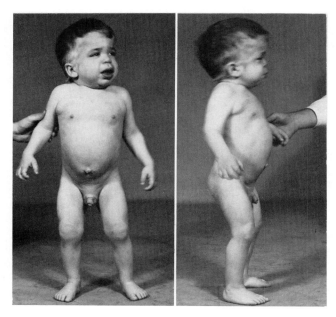

Fig. 24-3. Typical appearance of patient with mucopolysaccharidosis I (Hurler syndrome). (From Newell, F. W., and Koistenen, A.: Arch. Ophthalmol. **53:**45, 1955.)

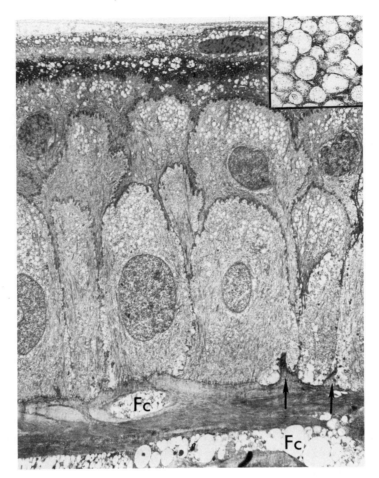

Fig. 24-4. Corneal epithelium in mucopolysaccharidosis I with numerous intracellular lysosomes (inset, ×17,000) filled with dermatan sulfate and keratan sulfate I. The Bowman membrane is destroyed, and the scarred anterior stroma sends projections *(arrows)* into the epithelium. Fibrocytic cells (Fc) have numerous lysosomes. (From Tripathi, R. C., and Ashton, N.: Application of electron microscopy to the study of ocular inborn errors of metabolism. In Bergsma, D., Bron, A. J., and Cotlier, E., editors: The eye and inborn errors of metabolism, New York, Alan R. Liss for The National Foundation—March of Dimes, BD:OAS **12**(3):69-104, 1976.) (Electron micrograph ×1,800.)

neal clouding. Rarely, increased intracranial pressure occurs, but the papilledema cannot be seen through the cloudy cornea. There is retinal infiltration with mucopolysaccharides and an extinguished electroretinogram.

Dermatan sulfate and heparan sulfate are found in the urine and tissues. Fibro-blast cultures synthesize dermatan sulfate, an abnormality that permits diagnosis by means of amniocentesis. There is increased ganglioside (p. 482) in the brain and decreased β-galactosidase in tissues, observations that raise questions regarding the relationship of this group of disorders to the sphingolipidoses. Treatment currently is directed toward replacement of "Hurler corrective factor" found in normal plasma and containing α-L-iduronidase.

Mucopolysaccharidosis II (Hunter syndrome) is inherited as an X chromosome–linked recessive trait. The patients clinically resemble those with Hurler disease, but clinical manifestations are less severe and grossly the corneas are clear, although there may be a slight corneal haze in occasional patients. Patients may survive into adulthood, and mental retardation may not occur. Laboratory findings resemble type I.

Other types of mucopolysaccharidoses occur less commonly.

Central macular corneal dystrophy, or Groenouw type II (hereditary corneal dystrophy), an autosomal recessive disorder involving only the cornea, is characterized by slowly progressive visual loss caused by the intracellular accumulation of a mucopolysaccharide within keratocytes. There is no abnormal excretion of mucopolysaccharides, and skin fibroblasts do not demonstrate an abnormal mucopolysaccharide metabolism. It is regarded as a local tissue abnormality.

Other lysosomal storage diseases

Fucosidosis. This is an autosomal lysosomal disease characterized by the absence or profound deficiency of α-L-fucosidase, resulting in a widespread accumulation of fucose-containing glycosphingolipids, oligosaccharides, and polysaccharides, together with an increased excretion of fucosides in the urine. Clinically, severe and mild phenotypes have been distinguished. The severe form causes a progressive psychomotor retardation and a moderate chondrodystrophy that somewhat resembles the mucopolysaccharidoses. Death occurs between 3 and 5 years of age. Survival to adolescence and beyond has been reported in the mild phenotype.

The skin changes of angiokeratoma corporis diffusum occur, and there are thin and tortuous veins in the conjunctiva and ocular fundus. Conjunctival biopsy shows cytoplasmic inclusions resulting from overloading of the lysosomal tissues. The endothelial cells of blood capillaries are filled with abnormal inclusions. Stored material is pathognomonic, and there may be clear vacuoles containing finely reticular material similar to that in mucopolusaccharidosis and less numerous dark inclusions.

Mannosidosis. This is a lysosomal storage disease that resembles muopolysaccharidosis clinically and is caused by tissue deficiency of α-mannosidase A and B, resulting in accumulation of mannose-rich glycoproteins, glycopeptides, and oligosaccharides in tissues and urine. There is a prominent metopic suture and coarse facies. Patients may demonstrate cardiac dysfunction, hepatosplenomegaly, and gibbus deformity. Connective tissue defects may include hernias, diastasis recti, and testicular hydrocele. Initial rapid growth is followed by slow growth and susceptibility to infection. Lens opacities develop in infancy in many patients. The usual type is located in the posterior cortex and appears ophthalmoscopically as radiating spokes of a wheel. A milder phenotype causes punctate lens opacities.

Mucolipidosis. This is a group of lysosomal storage diseases in which neither the storage substance nor the deficient enzyme has been recognized. All have inclusions in cultured fibroblasts. In mucolipidosis II (inclusion cell or I-cell disease), cloudy corneas were present in only one of ten instances. Except for this group, most patients have corneal clouding, skeletal dysplasia, mental retardation, and coarse features. Some have retinal degeneration. Death in adolescence is common.

Amaurotic familial idiocy. This obsolete

term characterizes two classes of disorders: the gangliosidoses (p. 482) and the neuronal ceroid lipofuscinoses. The diseases differ in the following ways: gangliosidosis is a lysosomal storage disease that involves the ganglion cell layer of the retina, causing a cherry-red spot, with the remainder of the sensory retina intact so that the electroretinogram is normal; neuronal ceroid lipofuscinosis is a peroxidase deficiency that involves mainly the photoreceptors, with the optic atrophy secondary to disturbance outside the ganglion cell layer so that the electroretinogram is extinguished.

Neuronal ceroid lipofuscinosis. Neuronal ceroid lipofuscinosis (Batten disease) is an autosomal recessive abnormality in which there is an excessive accumulation of ceroid lipofuscin in neurons. The disease may be divided into acute and chronic types plus an intermediate transitional and an atypical form. The chronic disease is associated with widespread deterioration of the rods and cones and the retinal pigment epithelium, with attenuation of blood vessels and optic nerve atrophy. The condition closely resembles that seen in the traditional primary pigmentary degeneration of the retina. The central retina has a granular appearance, and there may be peripheral pigment deposition. Motor and mental deterioration happens slowly, and visual loss may be the initial symptom.

The acute disease is ushered in by rapidly progressive, drug-resistant, mixed, often predominantly myoclonic seizures. Rapid mental and motor deterioration follows together with ocular changes similar to those in the chronic form. The transitional form combines the clinical and pathologic features of the acute and chronic disease forms with similar ocular changes. No visual impairment occurs in the atypical forms.

The disease arises from a peroxidase deficiency that may permit oxidation of unsaturated long chain fatty acids in the retinal pigment epithelium, so that photoreceptor synthesis is impaired.

In years past, neuronal ceroid lipofuscinosis has been given a variety of eponyms based on the age that eye symptoms appear: congenital (Norman-Wood), late infantile (Jansky-Bielschowsky), juvenile (Vogt-Spielmeyer or Batten-Mayou), and adult (Kufs-Hallervorden-Spatz).

HEPATOLENTICULAR DEGENERATION

Hepatolenticular degeneration (Wilson disease) is an uncommon autosomal recessive disorder characterized by widespread deposition of copper throughout the body, causing degenerative changes in the liver (cirrhosis), brain (particularly the basal ganglia), cornea (Kayser-Fleischer ring), kidneys, and joints. Clinical symptoms occur between 8 and 40 years of age. Cerebral or hepatic signs usually dominate the clinical picture. The pigmented corneal ring occurs in most patients and rarely may be the sole initial sign of the disease.

Cerebral signs involve (1) classical degeneration of the nucleus lentiformis (the part of the corpus striatum comprising the putamen and globus pallidus and lying just lateral to the internal capsule), with spasticity, rigidity, dysarthria, and dysphasia; or (2) pseudosclerosis (Westphal disease), with tremor as the major symptom. Personality disorders occur in the absence of motor involvement, and jacksonian epilepsy or hemiplegia may occur, as may a coma that persists for several weeks.

Cirrhosis of the liver, which may occur before neurologic involvement, varies from mild symptoms of hepatic dysfunction to portal hypertension with esophageal varices and hepatic coma.

Kidney involvement may cause aminoaciduria (predominantly of cystine but without calculi), albuminuria, impaired concentrating capacity, glycosuria, alkaline urine, increased uric acid excretion with a low serum uric acid level, hyperphosphaturia with a low serum phosphate level, and osteomalacia.

The Kayser-Fleischer ring is pathognomonic; it consists of a greenish yellow to golden yellow or tannish green ring at the corneoscleral limbus that involves the Descemet membrane. The posterior edge of the ring is always sharply demarcated at the point where the Descemet membrane terminates. Initially the ring occurs at the superior portion of the cornea. It then extends to form a complete circle at the periphery of the cornea. The ring consists of dense, nonuniform layers of unequal-sized copper granules in the Descemet membrane. Although the corneal stroma contains a markedly increased amount of copper, it is only visible in the Descemet membrane. Gonioscopic examination may be necessary to see the ring in early corneal involvement. Its early recognition is important because specific therapy is possible before hepatic and neurologic symptoms occur.

Less common is a sunflower cataract involving the anterior and posterior capsules. With biomicroscopy it appears as a powdery deposit of brilliantly colored material in browns, reds, blues, greens, and yellows that is located in the visual axis with deposits radiating peripherally, resembling the petals of a sunflower.

Brain involvement causes the expected ocular signs. Night blindness and degenerative changes in the peripheral retina seem to be unrelated to the primary disorder; however, retinal function has not been systematically studied.

Treatment consists of a low-copper diet, general management of hepatic cirrhosis, and administration of D-pencillamine, which chelates copper and increases its excretion. Successful treatment results in disappearance of the lens deposition followed by disappearance of the corneal ring and amelioration of hepatic and neurologic symptoms.

The diagnosis of asymptomatic Wilson disease in siblings of affected patients is important inasmuch as specific treatment dramatically improves what would otherwise be an inevitably fatal course.

MENKES KINKY-HAIR DISEASE

Menkes kinky-hair disease is an X chromosome–linked recessive hereditary disorder characterized by early psychomotor deterioration, seizures, spasticity, hypothermia, pili torti, late bone changes resembling scurvy, and fragmentation of internal elastic lamina causing vascular tortuosity. Levels of serum copper, copper oxidase, and ceruloplasmin are abnormally low, and a defect occurs in the intracellular transport of copper in the gut epithelium. Initially the eye develops normally, but later degeneration of ganglion cells takes place with loss of nerve fibers and optic atrophy. Mitochondria of surviving ganglion cells and photoreceptor inner segments are markedly swollen, with an electron-dense substance in the matrix of the mitochondria and pigment epithelium. Elastic tissue in the Bruch membrane is reduced.

AMYLOIDOSIS

Amyloidosis is a nonspecific disorder characterized by the local or generalized deposition of amyloid, a dichromatic, amorphous, fibrillar protein-polysaccharide with a distinctive ultrastructure. Clinically it may be classified as familial or nonfamilial, primary or secondary, systemic or localized. Eye involvement occurs most frequently with the primary type, whether systemic or localized.

In primary systemic amyloidosis, amyloid material is present in the conjunctiva, in the eyelids, in the uveal tract, and in the retina and vitreous body. The material is apparently secreted into the vitreous cavity without causing retinal abnormalities. Ophthalmoscopically, the vitreous opacities appear as veillike glasswool. Localized amyloidosis may include ocular proptosis. Rarely, patients with primary familial systemic amyloidosis have orbital amyloidosis, with deposition in the ciliary ganglion that may cause pupillary abnormalities. Additionally, external ophthalmoplegia, diplopia, and optic neuropathy have been reported in isolated cases of primary familial amyloidosis. Conjunctival biopsy material may indicate the accumulation of amyloid.

Lattice dystrophy of the cornea, an autosomal dominant abnormality, is the result of localized amyloidosis. A similar lattice dystrophy has also been seen in patients with familial systemic amyloidosis. In nonfamilial localized involvement of the skin, the lesions appear as centrally located, raised, gelatinous masses that resemble the hereditary lattice degeneration.

Early in the process, prominent perivascular sheathing may be observed in the retina. Amyloid in the vitreous body may originate from the walls of the retinal blood vessels.

Although medical treatment of amyloidosis is unsatisfactory, removal of the opacified vitreous body by means of a vitrectomy may improve vision.

CEREBROHEPATORENAL SYNDROME OF ZELLWEGER

The cerebrohepatorenal syndrome of Zellweger is an autosomal recessive abnormality that causes a generalized hypotonia, hepatomegaly, hypoprothrombinemia, cortical renal cysts, bilateral calcification of the patellae, and abnormalities of the central nervous system. There is apparent hypertelorism with hypoplasia of the supraorbital ridges, epicanthal folds, corneal opacification, glaucoma, cataract, Brushfield spots, nystagmus, rudimentary or irregular optic disks, narrow retinal blood vessels, and irregular pigmentation. Bilateral corneal edema is associated with paracentral iridocorneal adhesions and focal attenuation of the Descemet membrane. Selective degeneration of the outer nuclear layers and photoreceptors occurs mainly in the central retinal region.

INCONTINENTIA PIGMENTI

Incontinentia pigmenti is a rare skin disease in infant girls that is characterized by recurrent vesiculobullous dermatitis that resolves spontaneously and leaves irregularly pigmented atrophic scars on the trunk and lower extremities. The condition is an autosomal dominant abnormality that is lethal for male embryos; thus it is observed solely in girls. There may be a partial alopecia, delayed dentition, and malformed teeth. Mental retardation, seizures, and spastic paralysis may occur. Esotropia occurs in about one fifth of the patients. In about one sixth of the patients there may be total retinal detachment along with rosettes and fibrous tissue characteristic of retinal dysplasia. Optic atrophy, cataract, blue sclera, and nystagmus as well as conjunctival and retinal pigmentation have been reported. Some patients show a zone of abnormal arteriovenous connections and preretinal fibrotic tissue at the equator of the fundus. There is no retinal blood supply beyond this area, and progressive vascular changes require photocoagulation.

NORRIE DISEASE

Norrie disease is an X chromosome–linked recessive disorder in which boys are born with a gray vascularized mass behind the lens in each eye. Corneal degeneration begins at about the age of 1 year followed by cataracts at the age of 2 years. In early childhood the eyes begin to shrink. Hearing difficulties occur in about one third of the patients and mental retardation in about two thirds.

DISORDERS OF AMINO ACID METABOLISM

The major disorders of amino acid metabolism that affect the eye (Table 24-3) involve mainly the intermediate metabolism of either tyrosine or methionine. In albinism the biosynthesis of melanin from tyrosine is impaired because of a deficiency of tyrosinase or because of failure of tyrosine to enter cells containing tyrosinase. In alkaptonuria homogentisic acid produced in the metabolism of phenylalanine and tyrosine accumulates because the enzyme homogentisic acid oxidase is missing. In phenylketonuria (an abnormality associated with minimal ocular signs) plasma phenylalanine increases because L-phenylalanine is not oxidized to tyrosine. In homocysti-

nuria there is a defect in the metabolism of methionine to tyrosine. In tyrosinosis a metabolic abnormality results from excess tyrosine in the blood. All are autosomal recessive defects except ocular albinism, which is an X chromosome–linked disorder and, exceptionally, an autosomal disorder.

Many of these disorders as well as galactosemia (p. 390) and Wilson disease (p. 488) either induce or are associated with a renal transport defect (Table 24-5) that leads to a generalized aminoaciduria, glycosuria, and phosphaturia of the Lignac-Fanconi syndrome.

Gyrate atrophy (p. 292) is associated with an excess excretion of ornithine in the urine.

Albinism. Albinism is an inherited disorder of the pigment cell (melanocyte) system in the skin, hair, and eyes or in the eyes only. There is decreased or absent melanin, causing a fair complexion,

Table 24-3. Disorders of amino acid metabolism (other than albinism) that have ocular signs

Disease	Defect	Systemic involvement	Eye involvement	Laboratory findings
Alkaptonuria (homogentisic acid accumulates)	Absence of homogentisic acid oxidase	Arthritis (late), pigmentation (ochronosis) of cartilage and connective tissue, heart disease	Ochronosis of sclera and cornea	Homogentisic acid in urine (dark-colored urine if alkaline)
Homocystinuria (homocysteine not converted to cystathionine; homocystine accumulates)	Deficiency of cystathionine synthetase (in metabolism of methionine to cysteine)	Mental retardation, seizures, malar flush, fair skin, thromboembolism	Dislocated lenses, cataract, high myopia	Homocystine in urine
Phenylketonuria (phenylalanine excess)	Absence of phenylalanine hydroxylase (oxidation of L-phenylalanine to tyrosine)	Mental retardation, epilepsy, restlessness, hyperactive tendon reflexes, tremors	Light-colored iris, photophobia	Increased plasma phenylalanine, phenylpyruvic acid in urine
Tyrosinemia type II	Deficiency of p-hydroxyphenyl pyruvic acid oxidase	Painful hyperkeratosis of palms and soles, brain damage	Painful keratopathy	Excess tyrosine in plasma and urine
Sulfite oxidase deficiency	SO_3 to SO_4	Brain damage	Dislocated lenses	Excess sulfocysteine

blonde hair, and decreased vision. Melanocytes are derived from the neural crest and are normally located at the epidermal-dermal junction of the skin, hair bulb, pia-arachnoid, uveal tract, and retinal pigment epithelium. Melanocytes are present in albinism (unlike piebaldism, where they are absent).

Albinism may be divided into two main types: oculocutaneous and ocular (Table 24-4). The oculocutaneous type has at least four varieties, which are distinguished as tyrosinase-positive and tyrosinase-negative by the amount of pigment formed during incubation of hair follicles with L-tyrosine, by the degree of clinical severity, and by genetic data. Tyrosinase-negative albinism is characterized by a deficiency in tyrosinase, which catalyzes the conversion of tyrosine to dopa, which forms melanin after several additional metabolic steps. The tyrosine-positive type seems to arise from an abnormality in which tyrosine cannot penetrate the melanocyte cells containing tyrosinase. Tyrosinase-positive involvement is more common among blacks than whites, whereas tyrosinase-negative oculocutaneous albinism has about the same in-

cidence in both races. Hair and skin in tyrosinase-negative oculocutaneous albinism are usually white and do not darken with age. In tyrosinase-positive albinism, pigmentation of the hair and skin tends to darken with age. The exposed skin in both types becomes erythematous and does not tan when exposed to ultraviolet light.

Ocular albinism is limited to the uveal tract and retinal pigment epithelium. It occurs in three forms: (1) X chromosome–linked with normal color vision, (2) X chromosome–linked with an atypical protanomaly, and (3) mild autosomal (possibly dominant) punctate type. The first type is more common and is closely associated with the Xg blood group. In general, this type of albinism, as well as the Chediak-Higashi type, is the result of disturbance in the melanosome structure characterized by giant pigment granules. Macromelanosomes may be found in both the skin and the eyes, and future studies should include electron microscopy of skin samples.

The severity of depigmentation is variable, and the fundus may resemble a blonde fundus with the choroidal vasculature visible. The foveal reflex is absent, and some pigment and irregular areas of hyperpigmentation may be in clumps or stripes at the periphery; this may be caused by lyonization of the X chromosome. The iris transmits light to a variable degree. Some, but not all, female carriers have a partial iris transillumination and may have coarse pigment in the midperiphery of the fundus. The pigmentation of the fundus of the female carrier may be caused by inactivation of the X chromosome in mosaicism. The often present pendular nystagmus may be diagnosed as a congenital nystagmus rather than being recognized as the result of the ocular albinism.

The iris in infants is light gray in color and translucent so that red light is re-

Table 24-4. Types of albinism

Disease	Defect
Oculocutaneous albinism	
Tyrosinase-positive	Transport defect of tyrosine into cell
Tyrosinase-negative	Deficiency of tyrosinase
Yellow-mutant form with hemorrhagic diathesis	
Ocular albinism	Giant pigment granules in melanosome
X chromosome–linked Normal color vision Atypical protanomaly Autosomal (dominant?)	
Chediak-Higashi syndrome (partial cutaneous and partial ocular albinism)	Neutropenia, giant lysosomal granules

flected from the fundus. The iris of carriers of the tyrosinase-negative defect is translucent to light directed into the eye through the sclera. Failure of the retinal pigment epithelium (which is present but does not contain melanin) to absorb light results in failure of the fovea centralis to develop. Visual acuity is reduced. An ocular nystagmus is present. Visual acuity is disproportionately poorer for distance than for near, and often normal schooling is possible although the distance visual acuity is 6/60 (20/200). The decreased vision is associated with a high incidence of strabismus. The outstanding symptom is photophobia with extreme intolerance to light. Ophthalmoscopic examination indicates a bright orange-red reflex with prominent choroidal vessels that are normally obscured by the retinal pigment epithelium. The retinal vessels are normal.

A number of ocular defects occur in association with albinism, such as hypoplastic iris, heterochromia iridis (p. 293), mixed astigmatism (p. 435), and severe myopia (p. 434). Rarely there may be deaf-mutism or mental retardation.

In the tyrosinase-positive type, the increasing pigmentation of the eye with age may be associated with improved visual acuity and decreased nystagmus.

Albino animals, including humans, have misrouted retinal ganglion cell axions so that some temporal fibers decussate rather than remain on the same side. The visual-evoked potential to monocular stimulation is abnormally small. The lateral geniculate body is abnormal, with fusion of adjacent layers that received the abnormal crossed fibers. In humans, the normal lateral geniculate body has six layers. In human albinism, instead of six layers there are three, the result of fusion between adjacent layers.

Treatment of albinism is directed toward accurate correction of the refractive error and the strabismus if present.

The use of a strong reading addition for near work may be helpful. Colored lenses are used to reduce the amount of light entering the eye. Contact lenses with a central clear area surrounded by a pigmented area to simulate the normal pupil and iris have not been found to improve vision but are helpful in reducing photophobia.

The Chediak-Higashi syndrome is a rare autosomal recessive disorder characterized by oculocutaneous albinism, severe pyogenic infections, neutropenia, neurologic defects, lymphomatous infiltration, and death before the age of 7 years from infection or hemorrhage. The disease is associated with giant lysosomal granules in neutrophils, monocytes, and hepatocytes. The ocular signs and symptoms are those of albinism.

Alkaptonuria and ochronosis. Alkaptonuria is a rare hereditary disorder in which homogentisic acid, produced in the metabolism of phenylalanine and tyrosine, is not metabolized because of the absence of the enzyme homogentisic acid oxidase. Homogentisic acid is a normal intermediate in the metabolism of throsine, and the enzyme for its oxidation is normally present in the liver, kidney, and possibly other tissues.

In affected individuals, homogentisic acid is actively excreted by the kidney and appears in the urine (alkaptonuria) in large amounts. It causes the urine to have a dark color or to become dark after standing, provided the urine is alkaline and large amounts of ascorbic acid are not simultaneously excreted. The substance reduces Benedict reagent and may give false-positive tests for reducing substance in the urine.

Clinically alkaptonuria is characterized by homogentisic acid in the urine and generalized pigmentation of cartilage and other connective tissue (ochronosis), which in turn causes arthritis. The pigmentation is most prominent in the eyes,

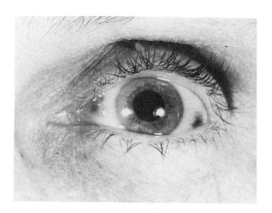

Fig. 24-5. Ochronosis involving the sclera in the palpebral fissure area. (From Hatch, J. L.: Arch. Ophthalmol. **62**:575, copyright 1959, American Medical Association.)

ears, and nose, and it becomes evident between the ages of 20 and 30 years. The ocular pigmentation arises from deposits of homogentisic acid metabolites in the collagen bundles of the cornea, sclera, and elastic tissue of the conjunctiva, which degenerate. The deposits appear on both globes in the palpebral fissure just in front of the insertions of the horizontal rectus muscle; they are oval in shape and have a slate-gray pigmentation (Fig. 24-5). Biomicroscopy of the cornea reveals tiny, round, golden brown deposits at the level of the Bowman membrane within the palpebral fissure. The concha and the antihelix of the ears have a drab blue-gray color. There is a tendency toward valvular heart disease, calcification of the heart valves, and atherosclerosis; myocardial infarction is a common cause of death.

Phenylketonuria. Phenylketonuria is an abnormality in which there is an absence of phenylalanine hydroxylase in the liver, causing an accumulation of phenylalanine in the plasma and phenylpyruvic acid in the urine. Those afflicted are born with normal neurologic and intellectual capacity but deteriorate progressively during the first 5 or 6 years of life. Phen-

ylpyruvic acid in the urine is demonstrated by an olive green color when 5% ferric chloride is impregnated on filter paper or tested on a wet diaper.

The accumulation of phenylalanine and its metabolites in pigmented cells causes a competitive inhibition of tyrosinase. A defect similar to that in albinism may occur, so that the patient has lightly pigmented hair and skin and blue eyes. Other ocular changes are not specific and are related to the brain damage. Treatment is directed to a low-phenylalanine diet.

Homocystinuria. Homocystinuria is an autosomal recessive disorder of the metabolism of methionine to cysteine. Normally, homocysteine transulfurates serine to form cystathionine in a reaction catalyzed by the enzyme cystothionine synthetase, which is deficient in homocystinuria.

The main ocular finding is dislocation of both lenses (p. 375), which may cause a secondary glaucoma. A cataract may be present. Peripheral retinal degeneration may be associated with retinal separation (p. 348).

There may be personality disorders suggesting schizophrenia and mental deficiency in about two thirds of the cases. There is progressive endothelial denudation leading to progressive arterial and venous thrombosis. Osteoporosis and scoliosis are common.

The cyanide nitroprusside urine color test is used for screening. A positive reaction indicates the need for urine chromatography to quantitate the abnormality. In over one half of the patients, administration of pyridoxine (vitamin B_6) in a dosage 100 to 1,000 times the usual daily requirement clears the urine of homocystine and may prevent vascular accidents. Folate may be required additionally.

Tyrosinemia type II. Tyrosinemia type II (Richner-Hanhart syndrome) is an auto-

Table 24-5. Renal tubule transport defects

Disease	Defect	Inheritance	Systemic involvement	Eye involvement	Laboratory findings
Nephropathic cystine storage disease (Lignac-Fanconi syndrome)	Abnormal compartmentalization of cystine	Autosomal recessive	Vitamin D–resistant rickets, acidosis, polyuria, dehydration, infection	Cystine crystals in conjunctiva and cornea, retinal pigmentation	Aminoaciduria, glycosuria, hypophosphatemia, elevated alkaline phosphatase
Benign cystinosis	Same as nephropathic	Autosomal recessive	None	Corneal and conjunctival crystals	Normal
Oculocerebrorenal syndrome (Lowe)	Not known	X chromosome–linked recessive	Rickets, mental retardation, hypotonia	Congenital cataract, glaucoma, corneal opacities	Aminoaciduria, proteinuria

somal recessive disorder with painful corneal lesions that occur shortly after birth, painful hyperkeratosis of the palms and soles, and brain damage. There is a deficiency of *p*-hydroxyphenyl pyruvic acid oxidase, leading to an excess of tyrosine in the plasma and urine. Within weeks of birth there is photophobia, lacrimation, corneal opacification and neovascularization (pseudoherpetic keratitis), poor conjunctival translucence, conjunctival plaques, and papillary hypertrophy. During the first year of life painful hyperkeratosis of the palms and soles develops without involvement of other parts of the skin. Severe neurologic and mental defects follow. Treatment with a diet low in tyrosine and phenylalanine (Mead Johnson 3200 AB diet) corrects the disorder.

There are no eye or skin abnormalities in tyrosinemia type I (splenomegaly, hepatomegaly, cirrhosis, fever, edema, aminoaciduria, phosphaturia, and renal rickets) or in the transient disorder of premature infants, neonatal tyrosinemia.

Sulfite oxidase deficiency. Sulfite (SO_3) is oxidized to sulfate (SO_4) by the enzyme sulfite oxidase, a deficiency of which results in dislocated lenses, severe brain damage, and an accumulation of sulfocysteine.

Renal tubule transport defects. Cystine storage disease (Lignac-Fanconi syndrome) and the oculocerebrorenal syndrome (Lowe) arise from a disturbance in renal function with impaired tubular reabsorption (Table 24-5). This causes an excessive amino acid excretion and gives rise to complex metabolic disturbances often associated with rickets and ocular changes.

Nephropathic cystine storage disease (Lignac-Fanconi syndrome). Childhood, or nephropathic, cystine storage disease ocurring early in life is characterized by widespread deposition of L-cystine crystals in the kidneys, liver, spleen, bone marrow, lymph nodes, conjunctiva, cornea, and uveal tissues. Cystine accumulates within lysosomes until crystals form and the cell dies.

The disease becomes evident between the fourth and sixth months of life with symptoms related to faulty resorption of water from the renal tubule and subsequent dehydration. There is failure to grow, emesis, recurrent fever, a severe form of rickets resistant to vitamin D in the usual doses, chronic acidosis, polyuria, and dehydration. An aminoaciduria involves a number of amino acids. There is progressive kidney damage, and chronic glomerulonephritis develops. There may be a terminal vascular hypertension and ophthalmoscopic signs of severe vascular hypertension and papilledema. Death usually ensues from uremia or intercurrent infection.

Crystalline deposits in the conjunctiva and the cornea are pathognomonic of cystine storage disease. Good illumination and magnification are required for their demonstration because of their small size. They appear as tinsellike, fine refractile crystals or fine white dots uniformly scattered over the entire cornea, predominantly in the anterior stroma (although the corneal bodies appear the same clinically as the conjunctival crystals, they do not have the same x-ray diffraction pattern and may not be cystine). In the conjunctiva the crystals are superficial and tend to aggregate in the walls of blood vessels. Photophobia is marked, but visual acuity seems normal. Ophthalmoscopically there is peripheral patchy depigmentation with pigment clumps that often form small rings. The retinal pigmentary changes precede corneal and conjunctival involvement. The posterior pole, disk, and blood vessels are normal.

Treatment is directed toward correction of the acidosis and dietary supplementation of phosphate and potassium. Vitamin D should be used only as re-quired to correct the rickets. Supplementary calcium may be necessary until the skeleton is normal, but hypercalcemia must be prevented. A cystine-free diet may be helpful. In the terminal stages, renal transplant is indicated.

The renal changes of the disorder also occur in galactosemia (p. 390), Wilson disease (p. 488), fructose intolerance, tyrosinemia (p. 494), and the oculocerebrorenal syndrome (p. 389).

Benign cystinosis. Benign cystinosis is an autosomal recessive disorder in which cystine crystals are found in the eye and bone marrow. There are no kidney signs or retinal pigmentation. The cystine level is much lower than in the nephropathic type. Attention is usually directed to the disorder only when the crystals are seen in the cornea and conjunctiva.

Oculocerebrorenal syndrome. Oculocerebrorenal syndrome (Lowe syndrome) is an X chromosome–linked recessive abnormality in which the affected male demonstrates hypotonia, osteoporosis, and failure to thrive. There is a renal tubular acidosis and aminoaciduria. Congenital cataract may be the first sign and may involve the entire lens or be confined to the fetal nucleus. The female carrier has punctate lens opacities. Congenital glaucoma occurs in slightly more than one

Table 24-6. Disorders of carbohydrate metabolism

Disease	Defect	Inheritance
Galactosemia	1. Deficiency of hexose-1-phosphate uridyl transferase	Autosomal recessive
	2. Galactokinase deficiency	Autosomal recessive
Hepatorenal glycogenosis (Gierke)	Deficiency of glucose-6-phosphatase	Autosomal recessive
Generalized glycogenosis (Pompe)	Deficiency of alpha-glucosidase (?), deficiency of acid maltase (?)	Autosomal recessive (?
Glucose-6-phosphate dehydrogenase deficiency		X chromosome linked

half of the males. The poor vision causes nystagmus and strabismus. The pupil may be miotic and may not dilate with any mydriatics (p. 389).

Miscellaneous disorders. An abnormal aminoaciduria is often seen in patients with congenital cataract or in those with congenital glaucoma. In one large family, central retinal degeneration was seen in 25 of 70 members with aminoaciduria. In another group composed of individuals having mental retardation and congenital cataract, there was an excessive urinary excretion of glycine and alanine. The metabolic basis of these disorders has not been investigated.

Spherophakia and dislocated lenses have been seen in hyperlysinemia associated with growth and mental retardation, seizures, and muscular asthenia. Imidazole aminoaciduria was associated with pigmentary retinopathy and mental retardation in one family. Increased urinary oxalic acid with pigmentary retinopathy has been described.

DISORDERS OF CARBOHYDRATE METABOLISM

Diabetes mellitus (p. 511) is clinically the most important abnormality of carbohydrate metabolism. Galactosemia (Table 24-6) is an abnormality in which there is failure to convert galactose to glucose and lactose. The glycogen storage diseases do not have prominent ocular changes; but in Gierke disease, peripheral corneal clouding has been noted, and in Pompe disease, glycogen is found in retinal ganglion cells, corneal endothelium, pericytes of the retinal capillaries, extraocular muscles, and ciliary muscle.

Galactosemia. Galactose is a hexose that differs from glucose in the configuration of the hydroxyl group of the fourth carbon. It is a component of many complex polysaccharides, but normally nearly all dietary galactose is converted to glucose. Lacoste, the main carbohydrate of milk, is split in the intestine into its two component hexoses, glucose and galactose.

The enzyme galactokinase catalyzes the reaction of galactose and adenosine triphosphate to galactose-1-phosphate and adenosine diphosphate. In infants the enzyme hexose-1-phosphate uridyl transferase catalyzes the reaction of galactose-1-phosphate and uridine diphosphate glucose to uridine diphosphate galactose and glucose-1-phosphate. The enzyme uridine diphosphate galactose-4-epimerase then catalyzes the reaction of uridine diphosphate galactose to uridine diphosphate glucose (p. 390).

Systemic involvement	Eye involvement	Laboratory findings
Mental retardation, hepatospleno-megaly, vomiting, dehydration	Cataracts	Reducing substance in urine (galactose), albuminuria, aminoaciduria, erythrocyte deficiency of hexose-1-phosphate uridyl transferase
None	Cataracts	Reducing substance in urine, erythrocyte deficiency of galactokinase
Retarded growth, adiposity, hepato-megaly, eruptive xanthomas	Peripheral corneal glycogen deposition	Hypoglycemia, hyperglyceridemia, hypercholesterolemia, acidosis, hyperuricemia
Lethal, anorexia, muscle weakness, tongue enlargement, cardiac and CNS involvement	Clinically negative, but glycogen deposition in eye	Requires muscle biopsy
Hemolytic anemia	Color blindness, optic nerve atrophy, cataract	Decreased enzyme activity, anemia

There are two types of galactosemia: (1) galactokinase deficiency, which is uncommon, and (2) hexose-1-phosphate uridyl transferase deficiency, the more common type.

Galactokinase deficiency galactosemia is an autosomal recessive disorder in which galactose is not metabolized and is excreted either unchanged or as galactose alcohol (galactitol) through the action of aldose reductase. Bilateral cataract appears to be the sole physical abnormality. The diagnosis is based on an absence of galactokinase in erythrocytes. The high blood galactose level and galactosuria will not be diagnosed if tests for reducing substance are done with glucose-specific agents (as in test tapes) or in the absence of milk ingestion.

The uridyl transferase deficiency is transmitted as an autosomal recessive disorder. The afflicted children are usually normal at birth, but cataracts have been found in the fetus at the fifth month of gestation. Usually, shortly after birth as the infant begins to ingest milk, he develops feeding problems along with vomiting, diarrhea, and failure to thrive. Progressive cataracts occur, initially with an increase in nuclear refractive power (as in senile nuclear sclerosis) and with the appearance of a drop of oil in the center of the lens. In other cases a zonular type of opacity develops. If galactose is removed from the diet, cataracts either will not develop or, if present, will not progress. The cataracts appear to arise from the conversion by aldose reductase of excess galactose in the lens to its alcohol, which diffuses poorly through the lens capsule and causes imbibition of water (p. 90).

Systemically, there is hepatomegaly along with abdominal distension and sometimes jaundice and ascites. Cirrhosis may develop. Mental retardation is evident early. Albuminuria, aminoaciduria, and impaired liver function may be present.

Treatment involves exclusion of milk and other galactose-containing foods from the diet. Soybean milk or casein hydrolysate is usually substituted. If treatment is instituted early, mental retardation, cataract formation, and impairment of hepatic function may be avoided.

Glucose-6-phosphate dehydrogenase deficiency. This is a variable disorder involving primarily the erythrocytes and manifesting itself mainly by a hemolytic anemia after ingestion of antimalarial drugs containing 8-aminoquinaline. Its ophthalmic interest arises because of the similarity of the anaerobic metabolism of the lens and the erythrocyte. It is transmitted mainly as an X chromosome–linked deficiency. Its most common variants are the Western type, occurring predominantly in blacks, and the Mediterranean type found in that area.

Protanomaly and deuteranomaly (p. 101) occur commonly in the disorder. The genes for protos and deuteros perception appear to lie relatively far apart on the X chromosome with the gene for glucose-6-phosphate dehydrogenase between them. Optic atrophy of an X chromosome–linked type has been described. The level of glucose-6-phosphate dehydrogenase in the lens parallels that of the erythrocyte, but although cataract has been described, its incidence is only slightly higher than in the normal black population.

DISORDERS OF LIPID METABOLISM

The plasma lipoproteins function as vehicles to transport lipids in the blood and to maintain them in a stable colloidal form. They consist of four groups: (1) chylomicrons, (2) very low-density or pre-beta-lipoproteins, (3) low-density or beta-lipoproteins, and (4) high-density or alpha-lipoproteins.

Dietary (exogenous) glycerides are carried on lipid-protein complexes—chylomicrons—large enough to be seen with the light microscope. These enter the bloodstream from the intestinal lymphatics through the thoracic duct and are hydrolyzed by the enzyme lipoprotein lipase in adipose tissue, liver, heart, and other organs, and the constituent fatty acids are resynthesized into triglyceride. The deposition or mobilization of fat is regulated by the presence or absence of food, particularly carbohydrates, and the presence or absence of activities requiring fat for sudden energy.

Glycerides arise either from endogenous synthesis, mainly in the liver, or from dietary fat. Plasma glycerides of endogenous origin are transported predominantly on a very low-density pre-beta-lipoprotein. This is composed predominantly of glycerides (50% to 70%), with a small amount of cholesterol (10% to 25%) and phospholipid (15% to 25%) and a minute amount of protein (2% to 15%).

Plasma fatty acids are derived from adipose tissue triglycerides and are bound to protein. The complex releases the fatty acids at sites of utilization. When the amount of fatty acids in the plasma exceeds the capacity of the tissues to utilize them, they are converted by the liver to triglycerides and may give rise to an endogenous hyperlipemia.

Plasma cholesterol is mainly in the esterified form, whereas free cholesterol is the major fraction in tissues. Cholesterol is esterified by lecithin cholesterol acyl transferase, which is activated by high-density (alpha) lipoproteins. Cholesterol is derived from the diet and from intestinal biliary sterols synthesized into cholesterol in the liver.

The phospholipids are relatively constant and are present mainly as "biologic detergents" to promote stability at the oil-water interface formed by lipoproteins and plasma. Beta-carotene is converted in the intestine to vitamin A alcohol (retinol) and ester and is transported together with other carotenes to the bloodstream in association with chylomicrons. Retinol is transported with a high-density protein in the blood, but the carotenes together with vitamins D, E, and K are found mainly in beta-lipoproteins.

The alpha-lipoproteins (high-density proteins) are composed of about 50% protein, 30% phospholipids, 18% cholesterol, and 2% triglycerides. The beta-lipoproteins (low-density proteins) are composed of about 25% protein, 22% phospholipids, 43% cholesterol, and 10% triglycerides. Some 90% of the cholesterol and phospholipid in the plasma is contained in the lipoprotein.

A deficiency or excess of lipoproteins may be associated with ocular signs. In general, the basic disorders are detected by measurement of serum cholesterol and plasma in a postabsorptive state and by examination of refrigerated serum for chylomicrons.

A-beta-lipoproteinemia. A-beta-lipoproteinemia (acanthocytosis, Bassen-Kornzweig syndrome) is an autosomal recessive disorder in which the gene responsible for synthesis of beta-lipoprotein is absent. Serum lipoprotein is not detectable, the erythrocytes are abnormally shaped (acanthocytosis), and pigmentary degeneration of the retina leads to blindness. Progressively severe atactic neuropathy and cardiac conduction defects lead to death in early adult life.

The disease is evidenced in infancy by retarded growth, abdominal distension, and steatorrhea. Cholesterol and phospholipid levels are extremely low and chylomicrons absent. In childhood, malabsorption becomes less severe, but muscle weakness, nystagmus, and degeneration of the posterior lateral columns and cerebellar tracts occur. Pigmentary degeneration of the retina (p. 340) is evident at age 8 to 10 years. There is pigment clumping in the central retinal region and bright dots in the periphery. Night blindness parallels the retinal degeneration. Cataract may occur. Progressive palsy of the medial recti muscles along with exotropia, dissociated nystagmus on lateral gaze, mild blepharoptosis, and ophthalmoplegia have been described in about one third of the patients.

Retinal changes are improved by parenteral administration or large oral doses of vitamin A. Treatment is directed toward adequate nutrition, despite severe fat intolerance, combined with large amounts of vitamins A and E.

Familial alpha-lipoprotein deficiency (Tangier disease). Familial absence of normal alpha- (high-density) lipoproteins in plasma is an autosomal recessive disorder characterized by the deposition of cholesteryl esters in histiocytes in the tonsils (pathognomonic) and bowel mucosa, combined with peripheral sensory neuropathy. The high-density lipoproteins in the plasma are reduced 50% to 90%, the triglyceride levels are increased, and the cholesterol and phospholipid concentrations are low.

Most individuals are heterozygous for the disorder, and the defect is not symptomatic. The tonsils may be markedly enlarged and of orange color or have stripes of orange alternating with the usual red color. The cornea may be diffusely infiltrated with fine dots visible only with the biomicroscope. Visual acuity is apparently not affected. In individuals with the homozygous defect, psychomotor retardation, polyneuropathy, and pigmentary degeneration of the retina occur.

Lecithin cholesterol acyl transferase deficiency. Lecithin cholesterol acyl transferase normally esterifies cholesterol and, when absent, cellular production of cholesterol is not inhibited. Liproprotein lipase (clearing enzyme) activity decreases so that only very low-density lipoproteins and chylomicrons are cleared. Cholesterol, triglyceride, and phospholipid levels increase. Clinically there is proteinemia, normochromic anemia with a hemolytic component, and

turgid plasma. The corneal stroma is infiltrated with grayish particles that are pronounced at the corneoscleral limbus, where they simulate the appearance of a corneal arcus. Premature arteriosclerosis occurs from the hyperlipoproteinemia.

Hyperlipoproteinemia. For the most part, the ocular involvement in hyperlipoproteinemia, although sometimes of diagnostic significance, is only incidental to the abnormal metabolism. The major ocular manifestations of hyperlipoproteinemia include lipemia retinalis, corneal arcus, xanthelasma, and ophthalmoscopic signs of atherosclerosis involving the central retinal artery before it bifurcates into arterioles.

Lipemia retinalis (p. 520) occurs because of an excessive number of chylomicrons in the plasma. It occurs in a familial form in fat-induced hyperchylomicronemia type II, in which an absence of low-density lipoprotein receptors prolongs their turnover. It is far more common in carbohydrate-induced (particularly in diabetic ketosis and in pancreatitis and alcoholism) low-density hyperlipoproteinemia (types IV and V). In types IV and V, lipemia retinalis is exceptional in the primary type and much more common

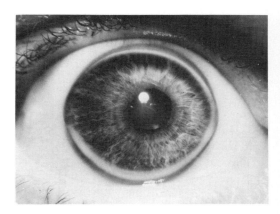

Fig. 24-6. Corneal arcus begins at the corneal periphery above and below and progresses to involve the entire corneal circumference.

in secondary types. Usually a triglyceride concentration in excess of 2,000 mg/100 ml is associated with chylomicrons, giving the appearance of lipemia retinalis.

Corneal arcus (gerontoxon, arcus senilis, embryotoxon, p. 255) is a deposition of phospholipid and cholesterol in the corneal stroma and anterior sclera. Generally, it appears as a deep, sharply defined, yellowish white ring, frequently incomplete, in the cornea concentric to the corneoscleral limbus (Fig. 24-6). It involves the entire thickness of the cornea but is usually most marked in the Descemet membrane and least marked in the midstroma. The area nearest blood vessels is clear, but when corneal neovascularization is present, the opacity affects that area preferentially.

Corneal arcus is not related to diabetes, vitamin deficiencies, obesity, hypertension, exercise, or alcohol intake. It is correlated with xanthamatosis, but its association with serum lipids is disputed. However, white subjects who are less than 50 years old, who smoke, and who have corneal arcus have higher serum lipid levels and a twofold higher risk of heart attack than others.

Xanthelasma (p. 212) is a cutaneous deposition of lipid occurring most commonly in the skin of the eyelids near the medial canthus. Xanthelasma does not occur with hyperchylomicronemia but is common in other hyperlipoproteinemias, which are often associated with xanthomas of tendons, particularly the Achilles tendon, and tuberous xanthomas over extensor surfaces.

Atherosclerosis (p. 543) is a vascular abnormality characterized by focal necrosis and thickening of the intima, lipid deposition in the intima and subintima, and hyperplastic and degenerative changes in the muscular coat of the artery, particularly in the internal elastic lamina. Atherosclerosis does not cause symptoms or functional changes unless there is obstruction or a focal decrease in the blood supply to a region, but it is distinctly localized in distribution. Therefore, the presence of atherosclerosis in one vessel does not indicate a similar involvement in another vessel.

Heredopathia atactica polyneuritiformis (Refsum disease, phytanic acid storage disease). Patients with this autosomal recessive disorder accumulate phytanic acid (a 20-carbon branched chain fatty acid) from dairy fat and cattle fat because of an enzymatic block in its degradation. The chief signs are retinal pigmentary degeneration (p. 340), cerebellar ataxia, peripheral neuropathy, and increased cerebrospinal fluid protein without pleocytosis. The initial signs relate to defective dark adaptation and constricted visual fields of pigmentary degeneration of the retina. Onset is in childhood, but diagnosis may be delayed until middle years. The retinal changes and deafness are followed by lower eyelid weakness, drop foot, and loss of deep tendon reflexes. Ataxia, intention tremor, and nystagmus suggest cerebellar involvement. There may be a mild ichthyosis, miotic pupils, anosmia, and nonspecific changes in the electrocardiogram. A thin layer of lipid may occur in urine and serum; the phytanic acid level is markedly increased.

Cultured fibroblasts of homozygotes indicate the absence of phytanic acid α-hydrolase, an enzyme that is responsible for the first step in phytanic acid degradation. There is a reduced amount in heterozygotes. Long remissions occur and exacerbations are triggered by fever, surgery, and pregnancy. Improvement may follow long-term exclusion of dietary dairy fat and cattle fat, the dietary source of phytanic acid, but the slow course and tendency to spontaneous remission make evaluation difficult.

Cerebrotendinous xanthomatosis. Cerebrotendinous xanthomatosis is an abnormality of cholesterol metabolism in which there are juvenile cataracts, xanthomas of the Achilles tendons, dull-normal intelligence, and cerebellar ataxia. Ataxia occurs after puberty and is followed by spinal cord involvement and pseudobulbar paralysis, which results in death. The blood cholesterol level is normal or minimally increased, but dihydrocholesterol (cholestanol), which is cholesterol without its 5,6 double bond, is deposited in the tendons. The condition appears to be an autosomal recessive disorder.

BIBLIOGRAPHY

Ahmad, A., and Pruett, R. C.: Fundus in mongolism, Arch. Ophthalmol. **94:**772, 1976.

Arbisser, A. I., Murphree, A. L., Garcia, C. A., and Howell, R. R.: Ocular findings in mannosidosis, Am. J. Ophthalmol. **82:**465, 1976.

Beckerman, B. L., and Rapin, I.: Ceroid lipofuscinosis, Am. J. Ophthalmol. **80:**73, 1975.

Bergsma, D., Bron, A. J., and Cotlier, E., editors: The eye and inborn errors of metabolism, New York, 1976, Alan R. Liss, Inc.

Bienfang, D. C., Kuwabara, T., and Pueschel, S. M.: Richner-Hanhart syndrome, Arch. Ophthalmol. **94:**1133, 1976.

Brook, J. G., Lees, R. S., Yules, J. H., and Cusack, B.: Tangier disease (α-lipoprotein deficiency), J.A.M.A. **238:**332, 1977.

Cartwright, G. E.: Diagnosis of treatable Wilson's disease, N. Engl. J. Med. **298:**1347, 1978.

Cotlier, E., Reinglass, H., and Rosenthal, I.: The eye in the partial trisomy 2q syndrome, Am. J. Ophthalmol. **84:**251, 1977.

Cross, H. E., Hansen, R. C., Morrow, G. III, and Davis, J. R.: Retinoblastoma in a patient with a 13QXP translocation, Am. J. Ophthalmol. **84:**548, 1977.

Ferry, A. P., and Lieberman, T. W.: Bilateral amyloidosis of vitreous body, Arch. Ophthalmol. **94:**982, 1976.

Franceschetti, A., François, J., and Babel, J.: Chorioretinal heredodegenerations, Springfield, Ill., 1974, Charles C Thomas, Publisher.

François, J.: Ocular manifestations of inborn errors of carbohydrate and lipid metabolism, Basel, Switzerland, 1975, S. Karger.

Fulton, A. B., Howard, R. O., Albert, D. M., and others: Ocular findings in triploidy, Am. J. Ophthalmol. **84:**859, 1977.

Garcia-Castro, J. M., and DeTorres, L. C. R.: Nic-

titating membrane in trisomy 18 syndrome, Am. J. Ophthalmol. **80:**550, 1975.

Ginsberg, J., Bofinger, M. K., and Roush, J. R.: Pathologic features of the eye in Down's syndrome with relationship to other chromosomal anomalies, Am. J. Ophthalmol. **83:**874, 1977.

Goebel, H. H., Zeman, W., and Damaske, E.: An ultrastructural study of the retina in the Jansky-Bielschowsky type of neuronal ceroid-lipofuscinosis, Am. J. Ophthalmol. **83:**70, 1977.

Goldberg, M. F., editor: Genetic and metabolic eye disease, Boston, 1974, Little, Brown & Co.

Goldsmith, L. A., and Reed, J.: Tyrosine-induced eye and skin lesions, J.A.M.A. **236:**382, 1976.

Goodman, R. M., and Gorlin, R. J.: Atlas of the face in genetic disorders, ed. 2, St. Louis, 1977, The C. V. Mosby Co.

Guillery, R. W., Okoro, A. N., and Witkop, C. J., Jr.: Abnormal visual pathways in the brain of a human albino, Brain Res. **96:**373, 1975.

Guillery, R. W., and Updyke, B. V.: Retinofugal pathways in normal and albino axolotls, Brain Res. **109:**235, 1976.

Haddad, R., Font, R. L., and Friendly, D. S.: Cerebro-hepato-renal syndrome of Zellweger, Arch. Ophthalmol. **94:**1927, 1976.

Hahnenberger, R. W.: Differences in optokinetic nystagmus between albino and pigmented rabbits, Exp. Eye Res. **25:**9, 1977.

Harley, R. D., editor: Pediatric ophthalmology, Philadelphia, 1975, W. B. Saunders Co.

Havel, R. J.: Classification of the hyperlipidemias, Annu. Rev. Med. **28:**195, 1977.

Jay, M.: Ophthalmology series. Vol. 2: The eye in chromosome duplications and deficiencies, New York, 1977, Marcel Dekker, Inc.

Kearns, W. P., and Wood, W. S.: Cerebrotendinous xanthomatosis, Arch. Ophthalmol. **94:**148, 1976.

Kenyon, K. R., and Kidwell, E. J.: Corneal hydrops and keratoconus associated with mongolism, Arch. Ophthalmol. **94:**494, 1976.

Kenyon, K. R., and Sensenbrenner, J. A.: Electron microscopy of cornea and conjunctiva in childhood cystinosis, Am. J. Ophthalmol. **78:**68, 1974.

Kurz, G. H., Shakib, M., Sohmer, K. K., and Friedman, A. H.: The retina in type 5 hyperlipoproteinemia, Am. J. Ophthalmol. **82:**32, 1976.

Letson, R. D., and Desnick, R. J.: Punctate lenticular opacities in type II mannosidosis, Am. J. Ophthalmol. **85:**218, 1978.

Levy, N. S., Dawson, W. W., Rhodes, B. J., and Garnica, A.: Ocular abnormalities in Menkes' kinky-hair syndrome, Am. J. Ophthalmol. **77:**319, 1974.

Libert, J., Toussaint, D., and Guiselings, R.: Ocular findings in Niemann-Pick disease, Am. J. Ophthalmol. **80:**975, 1975.

Libert, J., Van Hoof, F., Farriaux, J.-P., and Toussaint, D.: Ocular findings in I-cell disease (mucolipidosis type II), Am. J. Ophthalmol. **83**:617, 1977.

Margolis, S., Siegel, I. M., Choy, A., and Breinin, G. M.: Oculocutaneous albinism associated with Apert's syndrome, Am. J. Ophthalmol. **84**:830, 1977.

Mullaney, J.: Ocular pathology in trisomy 18 (Edwards' syndrome), Am. J. Ophthalmol. **76**:246, 1973.

Neufeld, E. F., Lim, T. W., and Shapiro, L. J.: Inherited disorders of lysosomal metabolism, Annu. Rev. Biochem. **44**:357, 1975.

Newell, F. W., Matalon, R., and Meyer, S.: A new mucolipidosis with psychomotor retardation, corneal clouding, and retinal degeneration, Am. J. Ophthalmol. **80**:440, 1975.

O'Donnell, F. E., Jr., Hambrick, G. W., Jr., Green, W. R., and others: X-linked ocular albinism; an oculocutaneous macromelanosomal disorder, Arch. Ophthalmol. **94**:1883, 1977.

O'Donnell, J. J., Sandman, R. P., and Martin, S. R.: Gyrate atrophy of the retina; inborn error of L-ornithine: 2-oxoacid aminotransferase, Science **200**:200, 1978.

O'Grady, R. B., Rothstein, T. B., and Romano, P. E.: D-group deletion syndromes and retinoblastoma, Am. J. Ophthalmol. **77**:40, 1974.

Pearce, W. G., and Sanger, R.: X mapping in man; evidence against direct measurable linkage between ocular albinism and deutan colour blindness, J. Med. Genet. **13**:319, 1976.

Rosenman, R. H., Brand, R. J., Sholtz, R. I., and

Jenkins, C. D.: Relation of corneal arcus to cardiovascular risk factors and the incidence of coronary disease, N. Engl. J. Med. **291**:1322, 1974.

Sears, M. L.: Browning of the lens in generalized albinism, Am. J. Ophthalmol. **77**:819, 1974.

Segal, S.: Disorders of renal amino acid transport, N. Engl. J. Med. **294**:1044, 1976.

Stanbury, J. B., Wyngaarden, J. B., and Fredrickson, D. S., editors: The metabolic basis of inherited disease, New York, 1978, McGraw-Hill Book Co.

Tripp, J. H., Lake, B. D., Young, E., and others: Juvenile Gaucher's disease with horizontal gaze palsy in three siblings, J. Neurol. Neurosurg. Psychiatry **40**:470, 1977.

Vannas, A., Hogan, M. J., Golbus, M. S., and Wood, I.: Lens changes in a galactosemic fetus, Am. J. Ophthalmol. **80**:726, 1975.

Walton, D. S., Robb, R. M., and Crocker, A. C.: Ocular manifestations of group A Niemann-Pick disease, Am. J. Ophthalmol. **85**:174, 1978.

Weleber, R. G., Walknowska, J., and Peakman, D.: Cytogenetic investigation of cat-eye syndrome, Am. J. Ophthalmol. **84**:477, 1977.

Wiebers, D. O., Hollenhorst, R. W., and Goldstein, N. P.: The ophthalmologic manifestation of Wilson's disease, Mayo Clin. Proc. **52**:409, 1977.

Yee, R. D., Herbert, P. N., Bergsma, D. R., and Biemer, J. J.: Atypical retinitis pigmentosa in familial hypobetalipoproteinema, Am. J. Ophthalmol. **82**:64, 1976.

Yunis, J. J., editor: New chromosomal syndromes, New York, 1977, Academic Press, Inc.

Chapter 25

ENDOCRINE DISEASE AND THE EYE

The endocrine system and the nervous system provide the major pathways for transfer of information between cells in different parts of the body. The endocrine system is effective through the delivery of hormones, which regulate the rate at which enzymes and other proteins are manufactured, affect the enzymes of metabolic pathways, or alter the permeability of cell membranes. There are two ways in which hormones gain entry into target cells: (1) the steroid hormones, such as the glucocorticoids, the mineralocorticoids, estradiol, and testosterone, are lipid soluble and pass directly through the membranes of the target cells; and (2) other hormones, such as insulin, thyroxin, and triiodothyronine, are transported in the blood attached to specific carrier proteins. Because of their size, shape, or electrical charge, they are unable to pass through cell membranes. Instead, they attach themselves to highly specific hormone receptors on the target cell's surface. The binding is weak, and unless the hormone is acted upon, it is soon released, leaving the receptor open to accept similar molecules.

Once the hormone is bound to the cell receptor, it is effective by stimulating the cell to produce adenyl cyclase, which converts adenosine triphosphate into cyclic adenosine monophosphate (cyclic AMP). The cyclic AMP is then released into the cell cytoplasm, where it signals the cell's biochemical machinery to produce the characteristic secretion of the cell. The hormone is considered the first messenger, and the cyclic AMP the second messenger. The cyclic AMP is degraded by the enzyme phosphodiesterase into a physiologically inactive form of adenosine monophosphate.

The adenyl cyclase thus must be located in the cell membrane and face inward to release the cyclic AMP within the cell. Adenyl cyclase has a similar function in the transmission of nervous impulses, and the cyclic nucleotides are involved in changes in ion permeability, activation of enzymes, synthesis and release of neural transmitters, intracellular movements, carbohydrate metabolism, and other functions.

THYROID GLAND

The hypothalamus secretes a thyrotropin-releasing hormone (TRH), which causes release of the thyrotropin-secreting hormone (TSH) of the pituitary gland. Pituitary TSH carrier protein binds to receptor sites on thyroid gland membranes and controls (1) the rate of trapping circulating iodide; (2) the enzymes that synthesize thyroxin (T_4) from two molecules of diiodotyrosine and that synthesize triiodothyronine (T_3) from one molecule of monoiodotyrosine and one molecule of diiodotyrosine; and (3) the activation of adenyl cyclase, which catalyzes the formation of cyclic AMP. This in turn provides an intracellular mechanism for proteolysis of thyroglobulin and release of T_3 and T_4 into the circulation. Both the hypothalamus and the pituitary gland have a feedback control so that the level of secretion of TRH and TSH vary inversely with the serum concentration of T_3 and T_4. Circulating T_4 is mainly (85%) bound to serum thyrotoxin–binding globulin (TBG), to a T_4-binding prealbumin, and to albumin. Only the minute amount circulating in the free form is metabolically active. Circulating T_3 is less strongly bound to TBG, and the amount circulating in the free form is eight to ten times greater than T_4.

The serum of some individuals contains at least two IgG immunoglobulins that are distinct from TSH and that stimulate the thyroid gland: long-acting thyroid stimulator (LATS), or thyroid-stimulating antibody (TSA); and (2) LATS protector (LATS-P), or human-specific thyroid stimulator (HTS). Both bind to thyroid gland membranes at a site similar or identical to TSH receptor sites. LATS is associated with a neutralizing factor in thyroid microsomes and cell sap. LATS-P is the neutralizing factor present in the serum of possibly all patients with Graves disease (including those in whom LATS is not detected). LATS-P immunoglobulin is human specific, stimulates human thyroid tissue in vivo and in vitro, and binds human TSH thyroid membrane receptor sites. LATS is regarded as less specific than LATS-P. Increased LATS is seen particularly in patients with pretibial edema and to a lesser extent in patients with thyroid ophthalmopathy.

The occurrence of these immunoglobulins in the serum of patients who have hyperthyroidism with ocular signs (Graves disease) suggests that the disease is caused by an immunologic abnormality in which immune globulins develop that have thyroid cell receptors as the antigen. The most popular theories relate to (1) primary abnormalities of the TSH receptor site; (2) a disturbance in cell-mediated immunity; (3) interaction between thymic lymphocytes, thyroid antigen stimulatory B-lymphocytes, and LATS-P production; or (4) a reduction in controlling T-lymphocyte production, leading to increased autoantibody formation by the B-cells. The exophthalmos-producing factor (in the Atlantic minnow) of the pituitary gland (EPF) does not appear to be a factor in human disease.

Hyperthyroidism

Hyperthyroidism is a systemic abnormality arising from an excessive concentration of thyroid hormones in the blood, usually endogenous in origin. This causes widespread neuromuscular changes and increased tissue metabolism. In some patients ocular signs occur, but hyperthyroidism appears to be the same with or without eye changes. Hyperthyroidism with eye signs is known as endocrine exophthalmos, endocrine ophthalmopathy, thyrotoxic or thyrotropic exophthalmos, and Graves disease (Basedow disease). Clinically there are three main manifestations: hyperthyroidism, ophthalmopathy, and pretibial myxedema. Ophthalmopathy may be present with, without, before, or after hyperthyroidism.

The onset of the systemic disease is usually insidious, with fatigue, tachycardia, and weight loss despite an increased appetite. There may be a fine tremor of the fingers and tongue, heat intolerance, and excessive sweating. The systolic blood pressure increases, atrial arrhythmias occur, and the pulse pressure widens; in individuals over 40 years of age there may be cardiac failure. Muscle weakness may be marked, and true myasthenia gravis occurs.

The serum T_4 is measured by competitive protein binding, by radioimmunoassay, or by column chromatography. T_3 is usually measured by radioimmunoassay. The thyroid radioactive test is performed by administering radioactive iodine or pertechnetate either orally or intravenously and measuring the uptake of these isotopes by the thyroid gland. The thyroid suppression test assesses whether thyroid function is controlled by normal homeostatic mechanisms. It is of particular value when ocular signs of hyperthyroidism occur in the absence of other clinical signs. The uptake of radioactive iodine or radioactive pertechnetate is measured; then $100\mu g$ of T_3 is given daily for a week, and the uptake is measured a second time. The administration of T_3 daily for 1 week does not suppress the uptake of radioactive isotope by the abnormal thyroid gland. If the gland is normal, the uptake is suppressed.

Ocular signs. In somewhat more than half of the patients with hyperthyroidism, eye signs (ophthalmopathy) appear some-

Table 25-1. Ocular signs of thyroid dysfunction

I. Eyelids
  A. Eyelid retraction (Dalrymple)*
    1. Increased by attentive gaze (Kocher) or by conjunctival instillation of epinephrine; decreased by adrenergic blockage (guanethidine locally or block of superior cervical ganglion); forehead does not wrinkle on upward gaze (Joffroy)
  B. Eyelid lag (von Graefe)
    1. Delay of upper eyelid in following globe in downward gaze (common in thyrotoxicosis)
  C. Infrequent blinking (Stellwag)
  D. Miscellaneous signs
    1. Globe lags behind upper eyelid on upward gaze (Means)
    2. Lower eyelid lags behind globe on upward gaze (Griffith)
    3. Increased pigmentation of skin (Jellinek)
II. Orbital congestion*
  A. May be associated with fullness of eyelids (Enroth)
  B. May prevent eversion of upper eyelid (Gifford)
III. Exophthalmos
  A. Bilateral* or unilateral*
    1. Eyelid retraction exaggerates or simulates appearance
  B. Compressible
    1. Common type in thyrotoxicosis
  C. Solid (noncompressible)
    1. Common type following medical or surgical treatment of thyrotoxicosis
IV. Extraocular muscles
  A. Contracture of ocular muscle usual
    1. Inferior rectus preventing upward gaze
    2. Most common following thyroid ablation
  B. Weakness of convergence (Möbius)
V. Corneal involvement
  A. Irritation from rapid drying of precorneal tear film
  B. Keratitis from failure of eyelids to cover cornea adequately in sleep
  C. Severe keratitis from rapidly developing exophthalmos
VI. Optic nerve disease
  A. Most common following thyroid ablation
  B. Papillitis or retrobulbar neuritis
  C. Papilledema
    1. Neuroretinal edema

*May occur at any stage of thyroid dysfunction.

time in the course of the disease. These may be unilateral or bilateral and mild or severe. They may precede frank hyperthyroidism or may occur long after the thyroid abnormality has been ameliorated. The severity of ocular signs (Table 25-1) does not parallel any currently recognized clinical or laboratory manifestation of the disease or any abnormality of the thyroid, pituitary, or other endocrine glands. The ocular changes involve retraction of the eyelids and an increase in the volume of the orbital contents, causing an exophthalmos (Fig. 25-1). In some patients, contracture of extraocular muscles occurs, often associated with signs of congestion of the orbital contents. Rarely, optic neuropathy occurs.

The initial eyelid change of hyperthyroidism is usually retraction of the upper eyelid. The sclera in the 12 o'clock meridian is exposed, and there is widening of the palpebral fissure, giving a wide-eyed, staring appearance. Rarely, the sclera is exposed in the 6 o'clock meridian without exophthalmos. There is often failure of the upper eyelid to follow the globe in downward gaze (eyelid lag).

The ocular signs of thyroid disease arise from two sources: (1) sympathetic overactivity, which causes many of the eyelid signs, and (2) increased volume of the orbital contents. Sympathetic over-

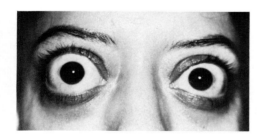

Fig. 25-1. Extreme exophthalmos in a 29-year-old woman who developed the condition gradually without signs of orbital congestion or ocular muscle weakness.

activity and contraction of the smooth muscles of the orbit have been considered an important cause inasmuch as stimulation of the cervical sympathetic nerve in dogs causes marked exophthalmos and eyelid retraction. The smooth muscle in the orbit of humans is too scanty to produce an exophthalmos when stimulated. Eyelid retraction in hyperthyroidism does not parallel the increase in T_4 that potentiates the action of epinephrine. However, the adrenergic nervous system may contribute to upper eyelid retraction and the eyelid lag in downward gaze, but does not have a role in the pathogenesis of exophthalmos. Eyelid signs may be unilateral or bilateral and differ in severity. They occur in the absence of exophthalmos and often precede it. They are much more sensitive to amelioration of the thyroid abnormality than is the exophthalmos.

When severe exophthalmos develops rapidly, the globe is not protected by the eyelids, and an exposure keratitis occurs (keratitis e lagophthalmos, p. 267), which can lead to corneal necrosis. The disease may be caused by an autoimmune reaction involving thyroid antigens and lymphocytes to retro-orbital tissues.

A number of changes increase the volume of the orbital contents. Because few orbits have been studied pathologically, there is inadequate evidence to conclude that the process is the same in all patients. The ocular muscles are inflamed, may increase three to six times in mass, and have a pale, swollen, pink appearance. Eventually, fibrous tissue replacement occurs. Lymphocytes and plasma cells infiltrate the tissues, and an acid mucopolysaccharide appears. Possibly, the acid mucopolysaccharide is responsible for marked water binding within the orbit and resultant exophthalmos. The cause is not known, but antigen-antibody reactions within the orbit are blamed. A fundamental defect in

T-cell function may impair tolerance to thyroid antigens. Immune complexes may accumulate within the orbit and release vasoactive amines. Inasmuch as the orbit has no lymphatics posterior to the conjunctiva, it may be uniquely vulnerable to autoimmune disease.

Exophthalmos. As a rule, the term *exophthalmos* relates to any abnormal prominence of the eyes, whereas the term *ocular proptosis* is reserved to describe a unilateral prominence. Both eyes are usually involved in thyroid disease, although one orbit may be more markedly involved than the other.

The exophthalmos develops gradually or suddenly after eyelid retraction, with increased prominence of the eyes, sensitivity to light, conjunctival irritation, and sometimes conjunctival hyperemia. If the exophthalmos increases slowly, extreme degrees may develop, whereas signs of orbital congestion develop if the increase is rapid.

Exophthalmos has not been produced in experimental animals by the administration of the thyroid or pituitary hormones (corticotropin, ACTH, gonadotropin, growth hormone, and prolactin). No hormone or antibody has been demonstrated to cause exophthalmos or to be consistently associated with exophthalmos. An exophthalmos-producing substance (EPS) from serum, or one composed of polypeptide fragments of the pituitary thyroid-stimulating hormone, irregularly causes exophthalmos in goldfish or the Atlantic minnow or increases the uptake of radioactive sulfur in the harderian gland of the guinea pig or mouse.

Orbital congestion. Signs of marked orbital congestion may develop quickly (Fig. 25-2). The eyelids become puffy and full. The conjunctiva becomes chemotic and injected. The conjunctival vessels may be so congested as to lead to a diagnosis of conjunctivitis or the suspicion of a carotid artery–cavernous sinus fistula. Chemosis of the palpebral conjunctiva may be marked, and the closed eyelids may not entirely cover the globe. Edema of the conjunctiva may be so marked as to evert the lower eyelid, and tearing be-

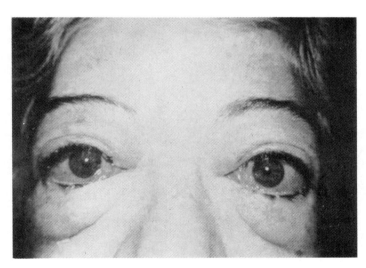

Fig. 25-2. Orbital congestion with eyelid edema, chemosis, and rapidly developing exophthalmos in a 57-year-old woman.

comes a prominent symptom. Orbital congestion may occur without increased prominence of the globes, but more often there is a rapid increase in exophthalmos during this period. If the cornea is not protected by the eyelids, a keratitis e lagophthalmos may develop, causing rapid loss of vision and loss of the eye from corneal necrosis if not effectively treated.

Extraocular muscle contracture. An extraocular muscle contracture may develop at any time in the course of thyroid disease. Severe congestion of the orbit may limit ocular movement mechanically. If there is interference with the Bell phenomenon, in which the cornea is usually rotated upward and outward with eyelid closure, the cornea may be exposed. A weakness of convergence arises from mechanical inefficiency of the medial recti muscles in rotating the exophthalmic globes inward.

Muscular contracture may develop in hyperthyroidism in the absence of exophthalmos, but more commonly it arises after adequate and appropriate treatment of moderately severe exophthalmos. The inferior rectus muscle is often fibrosed, causing an inability to rotate one or both

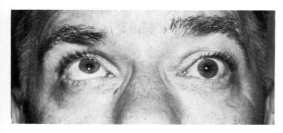

Fig. 25-3. Inability to turn the left eye upward after therapy for hyperthyroidism. The condition arises from a contracture of the inferior rectus muscle that prevents the normal elevators from rotating the eye upward. The contracture may develop without exophthalmos. Myasthenia gravis associated with thyroid disease may cause an isolated muscle paresis but does not cause contracture.

eyes upward, which creates a vertical diplopia (Fig. 25-3). If contracture develops in the eye commonly used for fixing, there may be marked secondary deviation of the fellow eye (p. 416). Contracture of the muscle is demonstrated by the forced duction test (p. 417).

Optic nerve involvement. In occasional individuals, papilledema, papillitis, or retrobulbar neuritis may develop. There are associated visual field changes characteristic of the involvement: enlargement of the blind spot, central scotomas, and sometimes peripheral field constriction. Vision is markedly reduced in patients with papillitis and in those with retrobulbar neuritis.

Patients who develop such optic nerve complications often have restriction of ocular movements and varying degrees of exophthalmos. Optic neuropathy, like other ocular involvements of hyperthyroidism, may develop long after the original disease has been corrected. Extremely large amounts of systemic and retrobulbar corticosteroids are used in therapy. Treatment must be continued for long periods; usually the corticosteroid dosage may be titrated against the response of the visual acuity. Orbital decompression or radiation therapy of the orbits is used if corticosteroids fail or are contraindicated.

Euthyroid Graves disease. Some patients develop ophthalmopathy of Graves disease with no signs of thyroid disorder. They do not have goiter or thyroid antibodies, and there is no evidence of LATS-P or normal thyroid suppressibility. This condition possibly arises from an autoimmune reaction of the orbit or from an effect of circulating exophthalmogenic factors of immunologic or hypophyseal origin rather than dependence on transfer of antigens and sensitized lymphocytes from the thyroid gland to the retro-orbital tissues.

Medical treatment. Treatment of thyroid

disease is unsatisfactory insofar as the eyes are concerned. Correction of hyperthyroidism usually eliminates eyelid retraction, and the exophthalmos appears to regress, although it may well increase 1 or 2 mm. Despite the increase, the eyes appear less prominent without the eyelid retraction. If ocular signs are marked, it is generally agreed that antithyroid drugs or radioactive iodine should be used in small, fractionated doses and that euthyroid and hypothyroid conditions should be avoided. Even though ocular signs of hyperthyroidism are present, antithyroid drugs should not be administered if there are no laboratory signs of hyperthyroidism.

Medical treatment of established exophthalmos is difficult. Prevention of orbital congestion by sleeping with the head on pillows may be helpful. Methyl cellulose eye drops may give comfort. Prevention of corneal desiccation by shielding or by use of ophthalmic ointments may help if the eyelids do not cover the eyes in sleep. Hypothyroidism should be corrected. Corticosteroids given systemically in large doses may be helpful.

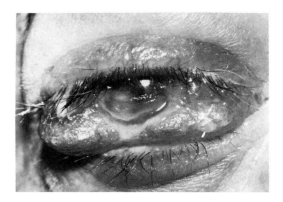

Fig. 25-4. Keratitis e lagophthalmos that developed after amelioration of hyperthyroidism in a 25-year-old woman. Loss of the eye was prevented by lateral (Berke) decompression of the orbit combined with a temporary tarsorrhaphy.

Surgical treatment. Loss of vision in thyroid disease occurs because of either keratitis e lagophthalmos (Fig. 25-4), other corneal involvement, or optic neuritis. Inflammation of the cornea usually requires orbital decompression or tarsorrhaphy, whereas the optic neuritis often responds to systemic corticosteroids. In severe orbital congestion with exposure of the cornea, orbital decompression is the treatment of choice. The decompression through the maxilla (Ogura procedure) is currently favored.

Cosmetic improvement of exophthalmos persisting after correction of the hyperthyroidism is not fully satisfactory. If the exophthalmos developed gradually and congestion is not present, a lateral blepharoplasty narrows the palpebral fissure and improves the cosmetic appearance. Retraction of the upper eyelid persisting after correction of the hyperthyroidism has been adequately treated by recessing the Müller smooth muscle of the eyelid. In severe cases, implantation of preserved sclera into the eyelid provides additional correction.

Correction of the fibrous replacement of an extraocular muscle with contracture is often disappointing. The procedure must be delayed until spontaneous improvement is unlikely, usually a year or more after the onset of the muscle weakness. The contracted muscle can then be recessed.

PARATHYROID GLANDS

The level of ionic calcium in body fluids is regulated by two hormones: specific hormone from the parathyroid glands and calcitonin from the ultimobranchial body. The parathyroid glands are two pairs of minute structures closely related to the dorsal surface of the thyroid gland on either side of the midline. The cells of the ultimobranchial body are embedded in the parafollicular area of the thyroid gland (C-cells) and in the parathyroid.

The parathyroid hormone causes a rise in serum calcium concentration in response to a fall of the ionized plasma calcium level. The active metabolite of vitamin D, 1,25 dihydrocholecalciferol, which is activated by parathormone, is essential to its action. Calcitonin is secreted by C-cells in response to hypercalcemia.

Hypercalcemia and hyperphosphatemia. In hypercalcemia and hyperphosphatemia, calcium crystals are deposited in the cornea and conjunctiva. In the cornea, the deposits are subepithelial, usually most marked near the corneoscleral limbus in the palpebral fissure (band keratopathy, p. 256). The conjunctiva is injected, particularly in the palpebral fissure, and glasslike, glistening crystals may be seen with the biomicroscope. The deposits disappear when the blood calcium becomes normal.

Calcification in otherwise normal eyes is seen in juvenile rheumatoid arthritis (Still disease), hyperparathyroidism, milk-alkali syndrome, sarcoidosis, hypervitaminosis D, thyrotoxicosis, post–uremic phosphate depletion, widespread malignant disease, and myeloma. Calcium deposition occurs locally in pathologic conditions of the eye such as uveitis, corneal scarring, and degenerating eyes.

Hypocalcemia. Decreased secretion of the parathyroid hormone results in a lowered serum calcium level, an increased serum phosphorus level, and decreased urinary excretion of both calcium and phosphorus. A decreased serum calcium level gives rise to a clinical picture dominated by manifestations of tetany and neuromuscular hyperexcitability. In milder cases there is numbness and tingling of the extremities or in the area around the lips. Hoarseness may occur. In more severe cases carpopedal spasm and laryngeal stridor are seen. Generalized convulsions are common. Latent tetany is elicited by the Chvostek sign, in which tapping the finger over the facial nerve causes twitching of the muscles of the mouth and, in severe cases, of the nose and eyelids. The Trousseau sign consists of carpal spasm, with evocation of the so-called obstetric hand that follows nerve ischemia when the arm is constricted by a sphygmomanometer cuff.

Cataracts develop when the blood calcium falls to a level at which neuromuscular hyperexcitability is observed. Lens changes are bilateral and involve formation of lens fibers predominantly in the subcapsular region. As lens damage progresses, small, discrete, punctate opacities and crystals of different shapes and colors develop. Similar opacities may be found in myotonic dystrophy, cretinism, and Down syndrome.

Calcification of basal ganglia, increased intracranial pressure, and papilledema may occur in hypoparathyroidism. Care must be taken to distinguish brain tumor from hypoparathyroidism with convulsive seizures and papilledema.

Children with idiopathic hypoparathyroidism (girls 2:1) develop chronic recurrent keratoconjunctivitis with corneal neovascularization. Superficial moniliasis involving the face and nails occurs simultaneously; later an adrenal insufficiency that may be fatal (78%) develops.

DIABETES MELLITUS

Diabetes mellitus (Gr. *diabetes,* a siphon; *mellitus,* honey) is a complex and widespread disorder of metabolism in which insulin is absent (juvenile-onset diabetes and after pancreatectomy) or decreased (maturity-onset diabetes). This leads to hepatic overproduction of glucose with underutilization by peripheral cells, resulting in hyperglycemia, glycosuria, and water loss.

Diabetes is the major systemic disease causing blindness and is the leading cause of blindness in individuals aged 40 to 60 years. Diabetics have 20 times the blindness found in all the population.

Table 25-2. Ocular signs of diabetes mellitus

I. Ocular fundi
  A. Background retinopathy
    1. Microaneurysms
    2. Deep and superficial hemorrhages
    3. Chronic edema residues (hard exudates)
    4. Cotton-wool patches (soft exudates; histologically, cytoid bodies)
    5. Venous dilation and venous beading
    6. Dilated, tortuous, kinked intraretinal vessels; intraretinal "shunt" vessels (intraretinal microangiopathy)
    7. Cystoid central retinal edema
      a. Peripheral retinal edema
    8. Areas of capillary nonperfusion
    9. Abnormally permeable blood vessels
  B. Proliferative retinopathy
    1. New blood vessels (with and without fibrous proliferation)
      a. Peripheral only
      b. Disk only
      c. Both peripheral and disk
  C. Vitreous hemorrhage
    1. Fundus can be seen
    2. Fundus completely obscured
  D. Lipemia retinalis
  E. Preretinal membrane
  F. Optic disk
    1. Neovascularization
    2. Atrophy
II. Oculomotor nerves
  A. Neuropathy with muscle paralysis (pupil frequently spared in N III involvement)
III. Visual acuity
  A. Transient variations in refraction
  B. Photopsia and diplopia in cerebral hypoglycemia
  C. Decreased accommodation
  D. Depressed in cataract, vitreous hemorrhage, central retinal edema, and central retinal detachment
  E. Blindness from proliferative retinopathy
  F. Diplopia in ophthalmoplegia caused by neuropathy
IV. Intraocular pressure
  A. Decreased in acidosis
  B. Increased in rubeosis of iris (sometimes)
V. Conjunctiva
  A. Sludging of blood; tortuous, constricted blood vessels
VI. Cornea
  A. Wrinkling of Descemet membrane
  B. Decreased corneal sensation (trigeminal nerve neuropathy)
VII. Iris
  A. Hydrops of pigment epithelium (transient glycogen storage, disappears with normal blood glucose)
  B. Rubeosis
  C. Minute "holes" in pigment epithelium
VIII. Lens
  A. Variation in refractive power (hyperglycemia)
  B. Snowflake ("sugar") cataract (growth-onset diabetes)
  C. Earlier onset of senile cataract

The rate of blindness peaks at ages 65 to 74; the rates are reduced thereafter. Among diabetics there is an increased risk of blindness among white women, white men, and nonwhite men and a high risk of blindness among nonwhite women. Retinopathy, neuropathy, and nephropathy increase in frequency with the duration of the diabetes and are often seen in the same patient. Many of the ocular, neural, and renal complications of diabetes may be caused by the direct conversion of glucose to its alcohol (glucitol or L-sorbitol) by the enzyme aldose reductase (p. 90). Almost every portion of the eye may be affected in diabetes (Table 25-2).

Retinopathy

Retinopathy is the most important ocular manifestation of diabetes. The introduction of insulin in 1921 followed by the sulfonamides in 1937 and the antibiotics thereafter prevented premature death of the diabetic from coma or infection. Since then the ocular, renal, and cardiovascular complications have emerged as the chief complications of the disease. Only unoperated senile cataract in patients unwilling to have surgery and glaucoma cause more adult blindness in the United States than diabetic retinopathy. Nearly 2% of all diabetics are blind from the retinopathy solely.

Diabetic retinopathy does not occur

because of concurrent atherosclerosis or vascular hypertension.

The severity of the retinopathy generally parallels the duration of the disease and the adequacy of control, particularly in the first 5 years after its onset, but not the severity of the diabetes. Diabetic control has little effect once the retinopathy begins. The severity and rapidity of involvement of the two eyes may be unequal, and even in the same eye one area may progress while another recedes.

The retinopathy involves retinal capillaries, particularly at the posterior pole of the eye between the superior and inferior temporal blood vessels. The choriocapillaris is involved solely in the generalized thickening of basement membranes and never in retinopathy. The visual acuity is a poor index of the severity of the retinopathy. If the fovea centralis is not affected, there may be excellent vision with advanced retinopathy, whereas a single lesion involving the fovea may markedly reduce vision.

Retinopathy may be divided into (1) background retinopathy and (2) proliferative (neovascular) retinopathy. Background retinopathy includes microaneurysms, hemorrhages (retinal and preretinal), hard exudates, soft exudates (cotton-wool patches), intraretinal microvascular abnormalities, nonperfusion of capillary beds, abnormal vascular permeability, retinal edema, and venous dilation and tortuosity. Proliferative retinopathy has, in addition to the changes of background retinopathy, new blood vessel formation, which may be with or without fibrous proliferation. It is subdivided into that occurring within 1 disk diameter of the optic disk or on the disk and that occurring peripherally. Retinal detachment from vitreous traction may occur and is divided into that which is 4 disk diameters or less in extent and that which is more.

Grading the severity of changes in diabetic retinopathy is difficult; clinical studies usually compare photographs of the patient's fundus with standard photographs. Classification as background or proliferative retinopathy is often descriptive enough, but fluorescein angiography indicates that in some areas the capillaries may no longer perfuse the retina. Blood vessels become permeable, and it is evident that serum proteins and electrolytes must be leaking into the eye. In controlled studies the retina is often "mapped" with a collage of fundus photographs and changes specifically described. In advanced diabetic retinopathy, even though the fundus can be seen adequately with the ophthalmoscope, the quality of fundus photographs is poor because of opacities in the ocular media.

The prognosis for vision is good if only background retinopathy is present. The prognosis improves if only microaneurysms are present and there are no hemorrhages or deposits. If proliferative retinopathy is present, the visual prognosis is considerably worse and loss of vision may be abrupt. Fibrovascular proliferative disease is more serious than neovascularization without fibrous tissue. Proliferative changes near the optic disk have a worse prognosis that changes more than 1 disk diameter away. With aging, the severity of retinopathy lessens.

Background retinopathy. Retinal microaneurysms are the most characteristic ocular lesion of diabetes, but they also occur in retinal vein closure, Coats disease, glaucoma, and many systemic diseases (hypertension, pernicious anemia, pulseless disease). However, in no other disease do as many microaneurysms occur as in diabetes. Those associated with diseases other than diabetes are located on the arterial side (thus in the nerve fiber layer of the retina, p. 33) rather than on the venous side of the capillary circulation and in the periphery rather than at the posterior pole. The microaneurysms occur only in the retina and do not occur in tissues other than the retina.

Microscopically, microaneurysms consist of minute spherical or ovoid distentions ranging from 20μ to 200μ in size, located on the venous side of the capillary network at the level of the inner nuclear layer. The resolving power of the direct ophthalmoscope is approximately 70μ to 80μ. Thus the majority of retinal microaneurysms are not seen with the ophthalmoscope. This is partially appreciated when the retina is viewed after intravenous injection of fluorescein (Fig. 25-5) or is seen histologically after trypsin diges-

tion of the retina. Microaneurysms become hyalinized, packed with stagnated erythrocytes, bleed into their walls, and are not visualized except histologically.

Ophthalmoscopically, microaneurysms appear as minute, deep, round, red bodies similar to hemorrhages. They may be distinguished from deep small hemorrhages by their unchanging appearance and their location far from blood vessels. Microaneurysms develop at the sites of degenerated capillary pericytes (mural cells).

Possible causes of capillary closure are loss of capillary tone, edema of the sur-

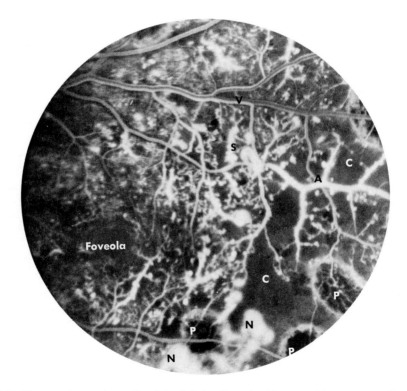

Fig. 25-5. Fluorescein angiograph of the left fundus of a 27-year-old woman with juvenile-onset diabetes mellitus (early venous phase). There are numerous microaneurysms and dilated, kinked, tortuous retinal vessels (intraretinal microangiography). There are areas of capillary nonperfusion. Two xenon photocoagulation scars *(P)* are outlined with fluorescein. Areas of neovascularization *(N)* leak fluorescein. The wall of a branch of the superior temporal artery stains with fluorescein *(A)*, indicating a breakdown of endothelial integrity. A shunt vessel *(S)* connects the artery and vein.

rounding retina, reduced capillary perfusion pressure, or endothelial proliferation. This results in the channeling of blood into a few distended capillaries, which become shunt vessels, or in arteriovenous anastomosis. With capillary closure there is retinal damage, which, if acute enough, causes cotton-wool patches. Fluorescein angiography makes evident additional capillary abnormalities appearing as fusiform aneurysms, capillary leakage, dilation of capillaries, and shunt vessels. Clinically, they are associated with severe progressive retinopathy. Fluorescein angiography may demonstrate large areas of capillary nonperfusion. The patients often have only a mild background retinopathy.

The retinal hemorrhages of diabetes do not differ from hemorrhages seen in other conditions. Small round hemorrhages are located in the inner nuclear layer of the retina, the cells of which are arranged so compactly that the hemorrhage cannot spread. Most hemorrhages are larger than microaneurysms and tend to disappear.

Flame-shaped hemorrhages located in the nerve fiber layers of the retina commonly reflect the distribution of the nerve fibers. Similar hemorrhages are seen in hypertension, blood dyscrasias, papilledema, and central vein obstruction.

Preretinal hemorrhages spread between the internal limiting membrane and the nerve fiber layer of the retina and have a "blot" appearance. Some may show a fluid level with bed rest. Acute trauma and subarachnoid and subdural hemorrhage may produce a similar hemorrhage. Preretinal hemorrhages tend to burst into the vitreous body, causing immediate obscuration of vision.

The deposits of diabetes are divided into hard exudates (waxy exudates, chronic edema residues) and soft exudates (cotton-wool patches, p. 325). Hard exudates (Fig. 25-6) consist of multiple small, glistening, yellow-white areas that gradually coalesce and become larger and confluent. They have a hard, waxy appearance and are often more yellowish than those seen in aging sclerosis. They are fatty infiltrates that occur in areas of retinal edema and are composed of free fatty material within the retina and of microglia that phagocytize the fat.

Soft exudates, or cotton-wool patches, are microinfarcts in the nerve fiber layer of the retina secondary to acute vascular insufficiency and occlusion of terminal arterioles. The lesions are less conspicuous than those of vascular hypertension and may be overlooked. They do not occur after retinal neovascularization.

Dilation of retinal veins occurs sometime before or during the course of nearly every instance of retinopathy. All of the veins or only a branch becomes engorged and dilated, and there may be a granular blood flow. There may be dilated segments of veins ("beading"). Although

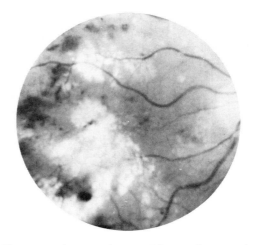

Fig. 25-6. Chronic edema residues at the posterior pole of the right eye in a 50-year-old patient. Although the other signs of background retinopathy are minimal, the deposits in the fovea reduce vision to 20/200.

the picture resembles an impending central vein closure, the veins pulsate normally with pressure on the globe, and there are no adjacent retinal hemorrhages.

Rarely, the central retinal region has a yellowish tinge in diabetics (xanthosis fundi diabetica), but the change is not significant.

Central retinal edema is a common cause of visual loss in nonproliferative retinopathy and can be diagnosed only by means of careful ophthalmoscopic study and fluorescein angiography. Detachment of the central retina occurs late in proliferative retinopathy and causes irremediable loss of central vision.

Proliferative retinopathy (Fig. 25-7). The development of new blood vessels in and anterior to the retina heralds a serious change in the visual prognosis of diabetic retinopathy. The vessels arise most commonly from a retinal vein near an arteriovenous crossing at the posterior pole and next most commonly from the surface of the optic disk. The superior

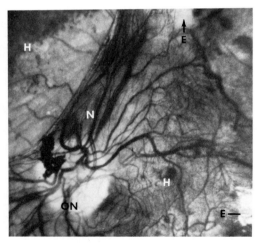

Fig. 25-7. Diabetic proliferative retinopathy with a sheath of new blood vessels *(N)* arising from the optic nerve *(ON)*. There are scattered retinal hemorrhages *(H)* and hard exudates *(E)*.

temporal vein is the most common retinal location; the inferior temporal, superior nasal, and inferior nasal veins are involved in that order.

Initially there is a collection of delicate lacelike naked vessels that are extremely permeable. The vessels then become more fibrous in appearance, with connective tissue proliferation surrounding them, and there may be loss of transparency of the adjacent retina. During this period, there may be severe retinal hemorrhages and vitreous hemorrhages. As the vessels become fibrosed, they may appear to decrease in size and number. As long as the vitreous remains in contact with the retina, the blood vessels seem to extend only as a flat sheet along the inner retinal surface.

If the vitreous body contracts, blood vessels adherent to its posterior face may rupture and cause hemorrhage or drag the retina inward and cause retinal detachment. This process proceeds for years with fibrous blood vessels growing into the vitreous gel. However, the vessels gradually regress and contract, and the eye is likely to be blind, with the full extent of the damage obscured by the blood-filled vitreous.

Vitreous hemorrhage may cause sudden loss of vision, or when less severe, a mist of red may obscure vision. In young individuals it may be quickly absorbed, but often after repeated episodes or in elderly persons the blood may persist indefinitely. The hemorrhage may produce a black ophthalmoscopic reflex or cause all fundus details to be blurred. As the blood absorbs, large vitreous floaters are visible. Vitreous hemorrhage always has a serious visual prognosis, because it often reflects vitreous contraction and the onset of the final stages of proliferative retinopathy.

Vitrectomy (p. 361) removes vitreous blood and fibrous proliferation that cause traction detachment of the retina. The instrumentation is complex, and the procedure may be complicated by the need to remove the lens and by inadvertent damage to the retina. However, many patients previously considered hopelessly blind can benefit from vitrectomy, and every physician must be certain that his patients who are blind because of vitreous hemorrhage have been recently examined for possible vitrectomy.

Treatment. Medical treatment of diabetic retinopathy is not satisfactory. Although careful control of diabetes during the first 5 years of the disease apparently minimizes the severity or delays the onset of retinopathy, it seemingly has little or no effect on the established condition. Currently, major attention is directed toward photocoagulation of the retina with the argon laser or xenon arc lamp in proliferative retinopathy on the surface of the optic disk or on new blood vessel formation elsewhere in the retina and in severe background retinopathy in which there is central retinal edema.

In some patients photocoagulation is

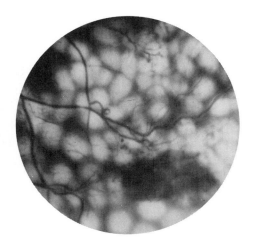

Fig. 25-8. Appearance of the retina immediately after photocoagulation at areas of origin of new blood vessels.

followed by nearly complete disappearance of all signs of diabetic retinopathy, although one may see the remnants of previous areas of neovascularization still present (Fig. 25-8). The results of argon laser and xenon arc photocoagulation in diabetic retinopathy have been evaluated by a National Eye Institute collaborative group. These investigators limited treatment to one eye of individuals having visual acuity of 6/30 (20/100) or better in both eyes and having either proliferative changes in at least one eye or severe nonproliferative changes in both eyes. They used extensive "scatter" photocoagulation (panretinal photocoagulation, retinal ablation) and focal treatment of new vessels on the surface of the retina, or argon laser treatment of new vessels on the retina. Photocoagulation improved visual prognosis and is indicated in both eyes with proliferative retinopathy. The prognosis is better in eyes with proliferative retinopathy when it does not involve the disk than when the disk is involved.

In proliferative retinopathy not involving vessels on the disk, the University of Chicago group uses focal photocoagulation to surround the area of new blood vessel formation. Mainly, no attempt is made to direct photocoagulation on the new-formed blood vessels, because this can cause bleeding into the vitreous.

In patients with blood vessels near or on the disk, the retina is ablated by treatment divided into four or five sessions with a maximum of 500 bursts per session. Excessive treatment at one session may cause extensive damage to the eye. Generally, some 1,500 to 2,500 photocoagulation burns are directed to peripheral areas of the retina not involving the region encompassed by the superior and inferior temporal vascular arcades. In extensive photocoagulation the treatment may be carried out more rapidly with the xenon arc photocoagulator. With this photocoagulator one can have a larger burn diameter, but it is more difficult to reach the periphery of the fundus.

In central retinal edema in nonproliferative retinopathy, we photocoagulate areas of nonperfusion of the retina as indicated by fluorescein angiography. We tend to limit the photocoagulation to the temporal side of the eye above and below the central retina. Generally, we photocoagulate superiorly first; if there is improvement in vision, we do not photocoagulate the inferior retina.

We judge the severity of the retinopathy in terms of areas of nonperfusion of the retina and in terms of leakage from major retinal blood vessels. All new blood vessels tend to leak, but leakage in established blood vessels in diabetes carries a serious prognosis.

It is not known whether photocoagulation is of value in background retinopathy. Background retinopathy tends to wax and wane, and whether therapy is effective is difficult to judge. However, I believe that such eyes should not be treated unless new blood vessels develop or severe retinal edema occurs or if background retinopathy is particularly severe at the posterior pole. Any sign of vitreous hemorrhage is an indication that blood vessels should be photocoagulated in that area. Damage by photocoagulation may be minimized by repeated treatments with relatively few burns each session.

Other ocular manifestations

Rubeosis of the iris. Rubeosis of the iris (p. 295) is a vascular proliferation of the iris vessels that becomes evident at the pupillary margin and in the anterior chamber angle. It also occurs spontaneously and following central vein closure. The glaucoma that occurs is resistant to both medical and surgical treatment.

Hydrops of the iris. Glycogen may accumulate in the pigment epithelium of the iris. Alcohol-fixed sections of eyes that have been enucleated during a period of high blood glucose concentration indicate the glycogen in dilated and vacuolated cells (Fig. 25-9). Clinically, the condition may be suspected by observing the release of pigment into the anterior chamber after dilation of the pupil or after iridectomy in diabetics.

Diabetic cataract. The lens may be involved in diabetes by transient changes in refractive power, early and more frequent senile cataract, and juvenile diabetic cataract ("sugar" cataract, p. 390).

Juvenile cataracts secondary to diabetes occur 10 to 20 years after the onset of growth-onset diabetes. Diabetic cataract develops rapidly and decreases vision soon after its onset. Both eyes are involved, often simultaneously. Typi-

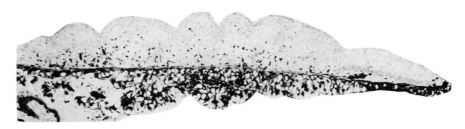

Fig. 25-9. Hydrops of the iris with the accumulation of glycogen in cystlike spaces in the pigment epithelium of the iris. (Courtesy Bertha A. Klien.)

cally, the opacity consists of small flaky opacities (snowflakes) and water clefts located in the anterior or posterior cortex immediately beneath the lens capsule. Control of the diabetes with restoration of normal blood glucose levels stops progression of the opacity. In persistent hyperglycemia a complete (mature) lens opacity may form within 48 hours, but progress is usually more gradual. Diabetic retinopathy may prevent good vision after cataract extraction.

Neuropathy. Paralysis of ocular muscles innervated by the third or the sixth cranial nerve (Fig. 25-10) occurs relatively rarely in diabetes. Characteristically, a middle-aged to elderly individual with mild overt diabetes or chemical diabetes has a sudden onset of diplopia and muscle paralysis associated with a homolateral headache of an intensity severe enough to lead one to suspect intracranial aneurysm. There may be a history of previous Bell palsy or similar neurologic disease. Neuropathy involving other areas may or may not be present. Signs of meningeal irritation do not occur. If the third cranial nerve is involved, the pupil will most likely be spared (in 17 of 24 cases), in contrast to pupillary paralysis, which occurs commonly in cerebral tumors and aneurysms. The paralysis disappears spontaneously within several weeks if the diabetes is of

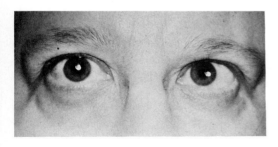

Fig. 25-10. Paralysis of the left lateral rectus muscle in a 62-year-old woman with adult-onset diabetes mellitus.

short duration, or it persists up to 6 months if the diabetes has been present for a long time, particularly if poorly controlled.

Unilateral frontal headache and oculomotor paralysis are characteristic of aneurysms of the intracranial portion of the carotid artery (p. 529). The sparing of the pupil, the laboratory signs of diabetes, normal spinal fluid, and absence of meningeal irritation suggest that the disease is caused by diabetes.

Other causes of ophthalmoplegia besides intracranial aneurysms include tumors (roentgenographic changes), leukemia (blood count), ophthalmoplegic migraine (history), head trauma, demyelinating disease (painless onset), myasthenia gravis (painless onset), and cerebrovascular disease.

Variations in refractive error. Hyperglycemia may be associated with or followed by increased refractive power of the lens, resulting in a change in the refractive error in the direction of myopia. After the blood glucose level has been normal for several days, the refractive power of the lens decreases, and the change is in the direction of hyperopia. The exact mechanism of the change is not known, but it is assumed that during hyperglycemia there is an increased glucose content of the lens cortex with imbibition of water, causing the lens to become thicker and thus increasing its refractive power.

The visual acuity parallels the change in refraction. Refraction during hyperglycemia varies, often markedly, from that during an interval of normal blood glucose concentration. Paralysis of accommodation by means of a cycloplegic drug does not affect the induced refractive error. Correcting lenses, often quite different from those usually worn, improve vision to normal. Diagnosis is not difficult in a known diabetic, but the variation in refraction and visual acuity may be the first indication of diabetes mellitus, particularly in the growth-onset type.

A similar change in refractive power may be produced in nondiabetic individuals by drugs, particularly sulfonamides. An actual change in the total refractive power of the eye, as occurs in diabetes, should be differentiated from that occurring with sustained accommodation ("spasm of accommodation"), which is neutralized with drugs that paralyze accommodation.

Subjective visual symptoms. Patients with diabetes mellitus without organic changes in the eyes may complain of photopsia (p. 151), not unlike that observed in migraine, or of double vision during periods of hypoglycemia. These symptoms are presumably of cerebral origin and are abolished by increasing the blood glucose level.

Intraocular pressure. Ciliary body secretion is sensitive to the plasma bicarbonate level. A low intraocular pressure is associated with diabetic acidosis, and the hypotension may be augmented by the concurrent dehydration.

Glaucoma in diabetes is a complication of neovascularization of the iris (rubeosis of the iris, p. 295). Diabetes mellitus occurs more commonly in patients with primary open-angle glaucoma, but proliferative retinopathy occurs less commonly in diabetic patients with glaucoma.

Lipemia retinalis. Lipemia retinalis is an uncommon abnormality of the ocular fundus that arises when the triglyceride concentration of the blood exceeds 2,000 mg/100 ml and is combined with low-density lipoproteins. Ophthalmoscopically, the normal color and size contrast between the arteries and the veins of the fundus are lost, and the vessels become engorged until they stand out like neoprene casts in bold relief. If the triglyceride concentration exceeds 3%

or 4%, the color of the blood column changes from salmon pink to a yellow-white-cream color. The choroid appears pinkish rather than red. Vision is not affected, and there are no ocular symptoms.

The condition occurs most commonly in diabetic acidosis, usually in growth-onset diabetes. It may occur also in familial and secondary hyperlipidemia.

Recognition of the ophthalmoscopic picture may establish a presumptive diagnosis of diabetic coma. More often a milky, opalescent serum is noted in blood removed for laboratory testing, and the fundi are then studied.

Associated renal changes

Growth-onset diabetes commonly causes death in the fifth decade of life from renal failure. The fundi of many of these patients show an unusual combination of diabetic retinopathy with superimposed changes of severe vascular hypertension (p. 549). There may be papilledema, diabetic deposits, cotton-wool spots of hypertension, angiospasm, hemorrhages, and microaneurysms.

Renal biopsy with study by means of light and electron microscopy indicates that in every case of diabetic retinopathy there are typical diabetic changes in the kidney. Electron microscopy shows specific marked infolding and thickening of the glomerular basement membranes. Intercapillary glomerulosclerosis is a less specific lesion, but it is likely to occur in every instance of diabetic retinopathy—in all probability it precedes the ocular lesion. However, it is of patchy distribution. Not all renal biopsy specimens are taken from an area of involvement, and unless serial sections are made of kidneys removed after death, the lesion may be missed.

BIBLIOGRAPHY

Allison, A. C.: Self-tolerance and autoimmunity in the thyroid, N. Engl. J. Med. **295:**821, 1976.

Bajandas, F. J., and Smith, J. L.: Optic neuritis in hypoparathyroidism, Neurology (Minneap.) **26:** 451, 1976.

Bresnick, G. H., Davis, M. D., Myers, F. L., and de Venecia, G.: Clinicopathologic correlations in diabetic retinopathy, Arch. Ophthalmol. **95:**1215, 1977.

Cavalieri, R. R., and Rapoport, B.: Impaired peripheral conversion of thyroxine to triiodothyronine, Annu. Rev. Med. **28:**57, 1977.

Ditzel, J., and Poulsen, J. E., editors: Diabetic microangiopathy, Aalborg, Denmark, 1975, Microcirculation Laboratory.

Dyer, J. A.: The oculorotary muscles in Graves' disease, Trans. Am. Ophthalmol. Soc. **74:**425, 1976.

James, W. A., and L'Esperance, F. A., Jr.: Treatment of diabetic optic nerve neovascularization by extensive retinal photocoagulation, Am. J. Ophthalmol. **78:**939, 1974.

L'Esperance, F. A., Jr.: Ocular photocoagulation; a stereoscopic atlas, St. Louis, 1975, The C. V. Mosby Co.

Mandelcorn, M. S., Blankenship, G., and Machemer, R.: Pars plana vitrectomy for the management of severe diabetic retinopathy, Am. J. Ophthalmol. **81:**561, 1976.

Ravin, J. G., Sisson, J. C., and Knapp, W. T.: Orbital radiation for the ocular changes of Graves' disease, Am. J. Ophthalmol. **79:**285, 1975.

Solomon, D. C., Chopra, I. J., Chopra, U., and Smith, F. J.: Identification of subgroups of euthyroid Graves's ophthalmopathy, N. Engl. J. Med. **296:**181, 1977.

Stieglitz, L. N., Kind, H. P., Kazdan, J. J., and others: Keratitis with hypoparathyroidism, Am. J. Ophthalmol. **84:**467, 1977.

Unger, R. H., and Orci, L.: The role of glucagon in the endogenous hyperglycemia of diabetes mellitus, Annu. Rev. Med. **28:**119, 1977.

Urrets-Zavalia, A.: Diabetic retinopathy, Paris, 1977, Masson & Cie Editeurs.

Vagenakis, A. G., and Braverman, L. E.: Thyroid function tests—which one? Editorial, Ann. Intern. Med. **84:**607, 1976.

Werner, S. C.: Modification of the classification of the eye changes of Graves' disease, Am. J. Ophthalmol. **83:**725, 1977.

Chapter 26

THE CENTRAL NERVOUS SYSTEM AND THE EYE

A wide variety of diseases of the central nervous system may be associated with involvement of the eye or its adnexa or may give rise to ocular symptoms. Some require elaborate instrumentation and study to diagnose, whereas others are immediately evident. Even the most cursory physical examination should indicate that the optic disks are flat, the eyes move normally, and the pupils are round and equal, and constrict with light.

OPTIC NERVE

Optic nerve atrophy (p. 371) may be complete or partial, and it may arise from disease within the eye (such as glaucoma or retinal ganglion cell degeneration) or from disease of the optic nerve or tract. If optic nerve atrophy is preceded by papilledema or inflammation, it is called secondary; if not, it is called primary.

Inflammation of the optic nerve (termed retrobulbar neuritis when involving the optic nerve posterior to the eye or papillitis when involving the intraocular portion of the optic nerve) is nearly always monocular and reduces visual acuity. In the retrobulbar variety there are no ophthalmoscopic signs of the disorder, but the pupil is invariably defective in its constriction to light (p. 286).

Papilledema is generally bilateral, is associated with good vision early in its course, is never present when the lamina cribrosa is clearly visible, and is usually associated with disappearance of spontaneous or induced retinal vein pulsation.

VISUAL PATHWAY

Lesions in the retina and in the optic nerve anterior to the decussation of nasal retinal fibers in the optic chiasm cause a visual field defect in one eye only (p. 162). A lesion of the chiasm involves decussating nasal fibers and causes blindness in the temporal half of each visual field, a bitemporal hemianopia. Lesions posterior to the chiasm involve nerve fibers that originate from both eyes. The visual field defect is bilateral and involves the right or the left portion of the entire visual field. A left homonymous hemianopia indicates that the nasal fibers of the left eye and the temporal fibers of the right eye are involved posterior to the chiasm. After synapse in the lateral geniculate body, visual fibers from each eye are superimposed. A visual field defect arising from disease in these fibers is the same in each eye (congruous defect).

PUPILS

The pupils (Chapter 14) are normally round and approximately equal, and both constrict when the retina of one eye is stimulated with light. Adhesion of the iris to the cornea or the lens, atrophy, or surgical excision of a portion of the pupillary margin gives rise to a pupil that is not round.

Lesions in the afferent pathway for the pupillary reflex, as in optic atrophy or optic neuritis, impair pupillary constriction to light (p. 286). Horner syndrome arises from interruption of the sympathetic nerve fibers to the dilatator pupillae muscle. The pupil is miotic and does not dilate when cocaine is instilled into the eye; there is an associated blepharoptosis and failure of sweating on the involved side. Adie syndrome involves parasympathetic postganglionic nerves of the ciliary ganglion in which pupillary constriction is absent or delayed. Argyll Robertson pupils (miotic and irregular pupils that fail to constrict to light but constrict to convergence) occur in tabes dorsalis.

Unilateral mydriasis after a head injury suggests a skull fracture on the side of pupillary dilation. Generally, pupillary fibers are interrupted with resultant mydriasis in oculomotor nerve interruption caused by tumors, aneurysms, and injuries and are not affected in disorders such as diabetic neuropathy. With midbrain hypoxia the pupils dilate, but otherwise the pupils constrict in coma. Unilateral mydriasis caused by topical instillation of drugs such as atropine, by ocular injury, or by acute angle-closure glaucoma does not constrict after instillation of 1% pilocarpine, but that caused by oculomotor nerve disease or injury constricts readily after pilocarpine instillation.

MOTOR NERVES

The motor nerves to the eye may be involved in a variety of abnormalities resulting from trauma, hemorrhage, cerebral edema, inflammation, neoplasm, aneurysms, or demyelination.

Oculomotor nerve. Complete paralysis of the oculomotor nerve (N III) causes blepharoptosis of the upper eyelid and paralysis of the superior rectus, medial rectus, inferior rectus, and inferior oblique muscles. The pupil is dilated and does not contrict to light or convergence, and there is loss of accommodation (internal ophthalmoplegia). When the unimpaired fellow eye fixes, the paralyzed eye is turned outward by the action of the lateral rectus muscle (N VI).

Lesions in the oculomotor nerve nucleus tend not to involve the pupil or the ciliary muscle. Tumors in the midbrain or the pineal body produce Parinaud syndrome, in which there is supranuclear conjugate palsy of vertical gaze (inability to elevate or to depress the eyes on command). Often the pupils are dilated and do not react to light.

Involvement of the fibers of the oculomotor nerve passing through the red nucleus causes Benedikt syndrome, in which there is homolateral oculomotor paralysis, contralateral dyskinesia, and contralateral intention tremor of the arm only. There may be an associated contralateral hemianesthesia.

Involvement of fibers near the ventral surface of the brain in the cerebral peduncle interrupts pyramidal fibers and causes Weber syndrome, which results in homolateral oculomotor paralysis, contralateral hemiplegia, and paralysis of the tongue and lower part of the face.

Interruption of the oculomotor nerve in the cavernous sinus is likely to be associated with involvement of the fourth and sixth cranial nerves. Involvement in the superior orbital fissure may affect sympathetic nerve fibers, so that pupillary dilation is not marked.

The third cranial nerve is particularly likely to be involved in tuberculosis or syphilitic meningitis and in herpes zoster. The nerve is often spared in purulent meningitis, which is more likely to involve the sixth cranial nerve. All of the ocular motor nerves are involved in cavernous sinus thrombosis, and the motor involvement is likely to precede pupillary involvement. The syndrome of the superior orbital fissure involves all of the motor and sensory nerves of the eye, including the sympathetic nerves. It may be produced by suppuration in the sphenoidal sinus, skull fracture, hemorrhage, or tumor.

After paralysis of the third cranial nerve, aberrant regeneration of the nerve fibers may give rise to a pseudo–von Graefe phenomenon in which the fibers originally distributed to the inferior rectus muscle innervate the levator palpebrae superioris muscle. Thus, when an attempt is made to look downward, the inferior rectus muscle is ineffective, but the eyelid rises. Aberrant regeneration of the branch intended for the medial rectus muscle into the sphincter pupillae muscle causes constriction of the pupil when an attempt is made to rotate the eye nasalward. If nerve fibers destined for the superior rectus muscle abnormally regenerate into the levator palpebrae superioris muscle, attempts to elevate the eye are associated with abnormal elevation of the eyelid. With closure of the eyelids, as in sleep, an abnormal Bell phenomenon occurs in which the upper eyelid elevates rather than closes.

Trochlear nerve. Disorders of the trochlear nerve (N IV) affect the superior oblique muscle, which rotates the eye downward when it is adducted. Diplopia is particularly marked when one is reading. The involved eye is higher than the fellow eye, the head is tilted to the sound side, the face is rotated to the sound side, and the chin is depressed. When the head is tilted to the involved side, the involved eye moves higher.

Secondary contracture of the inferior oblique muscle may occur rapidly after superior oblique muscle paralysis, and the resulting hypertropia in upward gaze may be larger than that in downward gaze.

Abducent nerve. Disorders of the abducent nerve (N VI) affect the lateral rectus muscle, causing inability to turn the eye laterally beyond the midline. The unopposed action of the medial rectus muscle causes esotropia. When attempts are made to abduct the eye, the palpebral fissure may widen. The long intracranial course of the nerve, its angulation over the sphenoidal bone, and its free position in the cavernous sinus make it vulnerable in skull fractures, increased intracranial pressure, and purulent meningitis.

Gradenigo syndrome is caused by an osteitis of the petrous tip of the pyramidal bone and follows mastoid and middle ear infections on the homolateral side. It is associated with sixth cranial nerve paralysis, pain on the same side of the face from fifth cranial nerve involvement, and deafness. Acoustic neuromas are associated with deafness, sixth cranial nerve involvement, facial paralysis caused by seventh cranial nerve involvement, and papilledema.

Internuclear ophthalmoplegia. When the pontine center for horizontal gaze sends a message to turn the eyes to the right or left, the impulse passes through the medial longitudinal fasciculus (p. 62) to the motor nerve nuclei involved in the action. A lesion in the medial longitudinal fasciculus impairs the signal reaching the third nerve nuclei, so that the adducting eye does not cross the midline on lateral gaze and the abducting eye shows a coarse nystagmus. There is a vertical nystagmus on upward gaze. Convergence, which is not mediated by impulses through the medial longitudinal fasciculus, may or may not be affected. In early internuclear ophthalmoplegia adduction may be slowed, but there is an exodeviation in lateral gaze and orthophoria in primary gaze.

Bilateral internuclear ophthalmoplegia is most commonly caused by multiple sclerosis. It also occurs with brain stem tumors, syphilis, encephalitis, and trauma and may be simulated by myasthenia gravis. Unilateral involvement is the result of an infarct of a small branch of the basilar artery.

SPACE-OCCUPYING INTRACRANIAL LESIONS

An intracranial tumor, abscess, aneurysm, or hemorrhage may produce characteristic ocular signs and symptoms (pituitary adenoma, craniopharyngioma, chiasmal gliomas) combined with general signs and symptoms arising from increased intracranial pressure and local signs arising from irritation or damage to a specific part of the brain.

Focal symptoms. Focal symptoms may be divided into (1) those arising from a supratentorial location and (2) those arising from an infratentorial location. The supratentorial group includes the cerebral hemispheres with their frontal, temporal, parietal, and occipital lobes; the pituitary gland, chiasm, and surrounding area; the anterior and middle fossa; and the diencephalon, including the third ventricle. The infratentorial group includes the cerebellopontine angle, the cerebellar hemispheres and vermis, the pons, and the medulla oblongata. Tumors in the mesencephalon may expand in a supratentorial or an infratentorial direction.

Supratentorial tumors. The ocular symptoms of supratentorial tumors differ widely. Visual field defects occur commonly, as do optic atrophy and papilledema. Involvement of ocular movements is less common than with infratentorial tumors.

Chiasmal syndrome. Interference with the decussating axons arising from the nasal half of each retina gives rise to a bitemporal hemianopia combined with optic atrophy. The hemianopia is often more advanced in one eye than the other. When caused by a pituitary lesion impinging on the chiasm from below, the field defect begins in the superior temporal fields and progresses inferiorly (Fig. 26-1).

A large variety of lesions may give rise

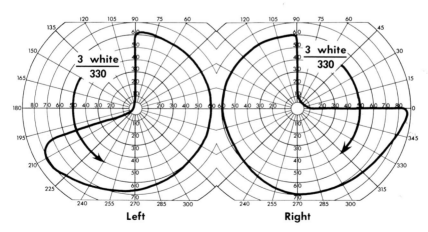

Fig. 26-1. Early field defect in the chiasmal syndrome that begins in the superior temporal field and progresses inferiorly. (Modified from Harrington, D. O.: The visual fields; a textbook and atlas of clinical perimetry, ed. 4, St. Louis, 1976, The C. V. Mosby Co.)

to the chiasmal syndrome: tumors and inflammation of the chiasm, pituitary gland tumors, aneurysms, basal meningitis, injuries, and abnormalities of the structures surrounding the dorsum sellae.

PITUITARY ADENOMAS. Classically, pituitary adenomas are classified by their hematoxylin-eosin staining characteristics: eosinophilic (acromegaly), basophilic (Cushing syndrome), and chromophobe (space-occupying lesion with hypopituitarism and chiasmal compression). New immunochemical and staining methods provide a functional classification into adenomas with and without clinically manifest endocrine activity (Table 26-1). The latter group is most likely to cause ocular signs; but in many patients, long before the chiasm is involved there is amenorrhea in women or loss of libido and potency in men. Measurement of the prolactin level when such symptoms occur can lead to early effective treatment.

Table 26-1. Functional classification of pituitary adenoma

With clinically manifest endocrine activity
  Growth hormone–producing (acromegaly)
  Prolactin-producing (amenorrhea, galactorrhea
    [Forbes-Albright syndrome])
  Adrenocorticotropic hormone–producing (Cushing
    syndrome, pituitary adenoma expansion after
    adrenalectomy in Cushing syndrome [Nelson
    syndrome])
  Thyroid stimulation–producing (hyperthyroidism or
    hypothyroidism)
  Multiple homone–producing (acromegaly [growth
    homone and prolactin, adrenocorticotropic
    hormone and prolactin])
Without clinically manifest endocrine activity
  Adenomas with increased prolactin production
    (amenorrhea or impotency, no galactorrhea)
  Adenomas with decrease of normal hormones
  Adenomas without hormone production
    (oncocytoma—a mitochondrial disorder)

Modified from Landolt, A. M.: Changing concepts of structure and function in pituitary adenomas. In Glaser, J. S., editor: Neuro-ophthalmology, vol. 9, St. Louis, 1977, The C. V. Mosby Co.

The ocular signs of adenoma follow typical ballooning and uniform enlargement of the sella, thinning of the floor, and erosion of the clinoid processes. Suprasellar tumors that cause chiasmal signs give rise to ocular changes before roentgenographic changes.

Involvement of the optic chiasm causes a "cloudy" or "foggy" decrease in vision. Complaint of bilateral hemianopia occurs late. The field defect initially involves the superior temporal quadrant and then spreads to the inferior quadrant (Fig. 26-1).

Development of optic atrophy lags behind the field defect. Often the degree of atrophy in the two eyes differs markedly.

CRANIOPHARYNGIOMAS. Craniopharyngiomas originate from epithelial remnants of the Rathke pouch and may be primarily intrasellar (rare) or suprasellar. About one third occur in children and adolescents and the remainder in individuals more than 20 years of age.

In children, the tumor invades the third ventricle early and causes internal hydrocephalus with papilledema. In adolescents, decreased anterior pituitary secretion may cause dystrophia adiposogenitalis (Fröhlich syndrome), cachexia (Simmonds disease), or dwarfism (Lorain disease). Hypothalamic involvement may cause diabetes insipidus, lethargy, and hyperthermia. In adults, a fluctuating chiasmal syndrome that involves the two eyes unequally occurs. An associated hypopituitarism causes impotence or amenorrhea with loss of libido; obesity; fine, silky skin with loss of body hair; and decreased beard growth in men. Involvement of the hypothalamus causes diabetes insipidus, lethargy, and hyperthermia.

Visual field involvement is typically asymmetric with a tendency to initial involvement of the temporal fields, but defects tend to be far advanced in one eye before involvement of the fellow eye. Because of the cystic nature of the tumor, there may be fluctuation in the visual field even without treatment. Suprasellar calcification demonstrated roentgenographically is helpful in diagnosis. Typically the roentgenographic changes occur after the visual changes.

Frontal lobe tumors. Frontal lobe tumors may reach a huge size or may cause increased intracranial pressure without localizing signs. Mental symptoms frequently dominate the clinical picture with the development of a striking change in character—apathy, euphoria, and a peculiar, silly jocularity (moria). Involvement of the Broca area causes a motor aphasia, whereas involvement of the anterior angular gyrus may cause focal epilepsy. An atrophic optic disk does not develop papilledema, but the Foster Kennedy syndrome of ipsilateral optic atrophy and contralateral papilledema is rare.

Temporal lobe tumors. Temporal lobe tumors cause uncinate seizures with unpleasant olfactory or gustatory hallucinations. There may be psychomotor epilepsy or paroxysmal visual hallucinations. The visual hallucinations are typically of the formed type in which the subject sees scenes such as landscapes. Involvement of the optic tract causes a homonymous hemianopia that is incongruous (that is, of a different extent or intensity in the two eyes). A homonymous superior quadrantanopia, indicating involvement of the Flechsig-Archambault-Meyer loop, occurs in only about one third of the cases but is pathognomonic of temporal lobe involvement.

Parietal lobe tumors. Parietal lobe tumors involve the posterior central gyrus, with disturbance of position sense, two-point discrimination, and stereognosis on the contralateral side. Disturbances in reading (dyslexia, alexia) and writing (agraphia) may occur. Late in the course a homonymous hemianopia may develop.

Inferior homonymous quandrantanopia is uncommon but pathognomonic of parietal lobe involvement.

Occipital lobe tumors. Occipital lobe tumors manifest themselves almost solely by ocular signs. Tumors elsewhere in the brain may easily injure the posterior cerebral artery and cause occipital lobe ocular signs. A homonymous hemianopia exactly similar (congruous) in the two eyes is the characteristic sign of occipital lobe involvement. The margin of the seeing-blind area often leaves a 2° or 3° opening surrounding the fixation point (central retinal sparing). Visual hallucinations are typically of the unformed type and consist of bursting balloons of light like those of migraine. They occur rarely. Increased intracranial pressure occurs early in the course of the disease and progresses rapidly, and severe papilledema is common.

Midbrain tumors. Pineal tumors and tumors of the midbrain cause Parinaud syndrome, in which there is a conjugate paralysis of the vertical gaze. The pupils may not react to light but will react to convergence, and there may be paralysis of the oculomotor and trochlear nerves. (Parinaud oculoglandular syndrome is a conjunctival granuloma with preauricular adenopathy [p. 223].)

Infratentorial tumors. Infratentorial tumors cannot involve the visual pathways, and disturbance in ocular motility is their chief ocular manifestation. They tend to produce embarrassed intracranial circulation earlier than do supratentorial tumors.

Cerebellar tumors. Cerebellar tumors cause ataxia, asynergy, dysmetria, and weakness. Ataxia and asynergy are demonstrated by the knee-to-heel test and in testing for diadochokinesis. Dysmetria is demonstrated in the finger-to-finger test. Weakness occurs on the same side. There is a distinct tendency to fall toward the side of the lesion. Acute cerebellar lesions disturb posture, and the patient may be unable to stand or sit up. There is a loss of skeletal muscle tone and coordination.

The earliest ocular sign is jerk nystagmus (p. 538), which is usually horizontal and accentuated on lateral gaze. Lesions in the vermis cause vertical nystagmus that is accentuated on upward gaze. Papilledema occurs early and may be the initial sign of disease. Other ocular signs are secondary to increased intracranial pressure.

Cerebellopontine angle tumors. Cerebellopontine angle tumors are mainly acoustic neuromas causing cerebellar signs, with lesions of the fifth, sixth, seventh, and eighth cranial nerves. Impairment of hearing occurs initially, followed by cerebellar signs with nystagmus and then cranial nerve involvement. The facial nerve is frequently impaired, initially with a tic and later with blepharospasm. Involvement of the fifth cranial nerve causes corneal anesthesia. Increased intracranial pressure occurs late.

Tumors of the pons and medulla. Tumors of the pons and the medulla are prone to cause disturbance of the abducent nucleus or distrubance of horizontal conjugate gaze. Horizontal jerk nystagmus occurs occasionally, combined with vertical nystagmus. It is usually absent when the eyes are in the primary position and becomes more marked as the eyes are turned toward the side of the lesion. Palsies of the third cranial nerve are uncommon. Corneal anesthesia from trigeminal nerve involvement is common. Increased intracranial pressure does not occur.

Increased intracranial pressure. The general signs and symptoms of increased intracranial pressure are severe bioccipital and bifrontal headaches that awaken the patient from sleep or are present on awakening, vomiting that may or may not be expected (projectile),

sphincter incontinence, mental torpor, and unsteady gait. The headache is aggravated by coughing, sneezing, or defecating, all of which increase intracranial pressure. Typically the headache is relieved by vomiting that occurs without nausea. Later in the course of the condition the vagus nerve effect causes slowed pulse, lowered pulse pressure, and increased respiratory rate. There is a clouding of consciousness that varies from somnolence to deep coma to a delirium to an organic psychosis.

The main ocular sign of increased intracranial pressure is bilateral papilledema (p. 370). In the absence of ocular or orbital disease, papilledema suggests brain tumor (or a tumor equivalent) to be the most likely cause. However, many brain tumors do not cause papilledema or are diagnosed before it develops; thus the absence of papilledema does not exclude increased intracranial pressure. Other ocular signs of increased intracranial pressure occur relatively late. Extraocular muscle paresis, particularly unilateral lateral rectus muscle paralysis, occurs but is not of localizing value. The oculomotor nerve may be compressed at the tentorial notch in the transtentorial herniation syndrome, with unilateral mydriasis and loss of the direct light pupillary reflex. Later the ocular muscles weaken, causing blepharoptosis. Initially the pupillary response to light and convergence is normal, but later it is lost. Exophthalmos is bilateral when caused by increased intraocular pressure. Unilateral proptosis suggests orbital invasion by a tumor rather than increased intracranial pressure.

Benign intracranial hypertension. In this chronic condition, fat young women develop papilledema, headache, and increased intracranial pressure with no other neurologic signs. The cerebrospinal fluid is normal, and computed tomography indicates small or normal-sized ventricles. Repeated lumbar punctures, sometimes as frequent as daily, relieve the headache, and recovery is gradual. Corticosteroids and acetazolamide are used in the treatment.

Papilledema also develops with vascular hypertension (p. 546), chronic emphysema, chronic fibrosing meningeal disease, Addison disease, corticosteroid withdrawal, vitamin A overdosage, and hypothyroidism.

CEREBROVASCULAR DISEASE

It is possible to include only a few of the abnormalities of the brain that result from pathologic processes of the blood vessels or blood (Table 26-2). Stroke caused by hemorrhage in hypertensive vascular disease or vascular occlusive disease with cerebral ischemia both with and without infarction ranks only after

Table 26-2. Cerebrovascular disorders with ocular signs

I. Occlusive vascular disorders
  A. Thrombotic
    1. Intracranial (sudden onset)
    2. Carotid (transient ischemic attacks)
  B. Embolic
    1. Retinal arteries (cholesterol: glistening yellow; fibrin-platelet: white)
II. Cerebral aneurysms
  A. Infraclinoid
    1. Carotid artery within cavernous sinus
    2. Carotid-cavernous sinus fistula
  B. Supraclinoid
    1. Carotid artery
    2. Middle cerebral artery
    3. Anterior cerebral artery
    4. Basilar artery
III. Subarachnoid hemorrhage
  A. Vascular hypertension
  B. Ruptured supraclinoid aneurysm
  C. Angiomas and arteriovenous malformations
IV. Arteritis
  A. Infectious disease (syphilis, tuberculosis, and so on)
  B. Connective tissue disorders (giant cell arteritis of aorta or cerebral vessels, Wegener arteritis, and so on)

heart disease and cancer as a major cause of death in the United States.

Carotid-vertebral-basilar artery occlusive disease. About 40% of all cerebrovascular accidents are caused by atherosclerosis within the extracranial portions of the carotid and the vertebral-basilar system. Occasional instances are caused by severe angulation, with kinking of arteries or occlusive disease from atheromatous ulceration in the ascending arch of the aorta or the subclavian artery.

Incomplete occlusion of the carotid and the vertebral-basilar system is characterized by episodes of transient ischemic attacks (TIAs) that appear suddenly, last 5 minutes to 24 hours, and disappear without residue. TIAs have the same clinical pattern and occur with increasing frequency; about 50% of the patients will have a serious stroke in an average of 3 years. Of the remainder, one half will continue to have attacks, and the others will recover without further trouble.

Sudden complete occlusion causes loss of consciousness with contralateral motor and sensory defects known as a "stroke." Most often, sudden attacks occur from emboli and are not preceded by a TIA. Gradual development of complete occlusion may be compensated for by collateral circulation, and the symptoms resemble those of the preceding TIA.

The symptoms of TIA are caused by a temporary hypoxia in terminal portions of the cerebrovascular tree. Transient decrease in vision varying from slight blurring to complete loss of light perception occurs in 80% to 90% of patients with carotid or vertebral-basilar insufficiency.

Carotid artery. The internal carotid arterial system or its branches (ophthalmic, anterior choroidal, anterior cerebral, and middle cerebral arteries) supply the frontal and parietal lobes, part of the temporal lobe, the corpus striatum, and the internal capsule. Occlusive disease is associated with contralateral impairment of motor or sensory function of the hand, arm, leg, or lower portion of the face. Ischemia involving the left middle cerebral artery causes aphasia in right-handed persons. Unconsciousness simulating syncope occurs when an anterior cerebral artery is compromised.

The chief ocular symptom of carotid artery ischemia is transient loss of vision in one eye, called amaurosis fugax. It consists of sudden contraction of the visual field of one eye, varying from hemianopia to loss of light perception. The pupillary light reflex is absent. The retinal arteries are markely attenuated during an attack. Vision gradually returns within a few minutes. Permanent visual loss does not occur. Amaurosis fugax may also occur in migraine (p. 541), impending central artery closure (p. 333), and giant cell arteritis (p. 565).

Repeated attacks of amaurosis fugax may give rise to an ophthalmoscopic picture of cotton-wool patches in one eye, probably caused by small infarcts secondary to vascular insufficiency. In patients with hypertension, the occluded carotid artery may protect the retinal vasculature from the signs of arteriolar sclerosis or even hemorrhages and papilledema.

In both carotid and vertebral-basilar system insufficiency there may be showers of emboli. Cholesterol emboli are observed near or at the bifurcation of retinal arterioles and appear as bright, yellowish orange plaques. With massage on the globe, they tumble to the periphery. Platelet emboli appear as small, white bodies in the arteries (p. 541).

Rarely, venous stasis retinopathy develops on the same side as the diseased artery in carotid insufficiency. There are dilated retinal veins, sludging of venous blood, microaneurysms, and small retinal hemorrhages. Neovascularization may develop on the surface of the optic disk. If only the diseased eye is examined without reference to the nearly normal fellow eye, the abnormality might be mistaken for the retinopathy of diabetes, impending central vein occlusion, or pulseless disease.

Pulsation in the affected internal carotid artery may be diminished or absent. Palpation through the oropharynx is more reliable than through the neck. Even with complete occlusion of the internal carotid artery, there may be normal pulsation of the common or external carotid artery.

Auscultation of the neck and the mediastinum may reveal a bruit best heard over the bifurcation of the internal and external carotid arteries. The bruit of occlusive disease of the vertebral arteries is best heard over the supraclavicular area and is sometimes accentuated by turning the patient's head to the opposite side.

Measurement of the pressure in the ophthalmic arteries with the ophthalmodynamometer has its greatest application in carotid artery insufficiency. The measurement is made by increasing the intraocular pressure until the central retinal artery is seen to pulsate on the optic disk. Most patients with carotid artery occlusive disease that reduces the lumen 90% or more have a 15% to 25% reduction in the systolic pressure of the ophthalmic artery on the side of the occlusive disease. In about one fourth of the patients with proved disease the pressure is the same or higher on the involved side.

Compression of the carotid artery may produce syncope suggestive of an insufficiency of the vascular supply of the contralateral anterior cerebral artery. In vertebral-basilar artery insufficiency there may be syncope or convulsive movements. Compression is not recommended and can produce permanent complete occlusion.

Angiography demonstrates the site and extent of the occlusion but carries the risk of permanent complications. It is reserved preferably for distinguishing between carotid occlusive disease, cerebral infarction, and tumor in patients who have symptoms of recent onset, do not have brain infarcts, and are good candidates for surgery if necessary.

Vertebral-basilar system. The vertebral-basilar arterial system supplies the brain stem, cerebellum, occipital lobe, and a portion of the temporal lobe. The vertebral system arises from the two vertebral arteries, which are the first branches of the subclavian arteries. The vertebral arteries traverse the neck in the vertebral canals of the cervical vertebrae and unite within the cranium to form the basilar artery. The basilar artery supplies branches to the brain stem and the cerebellum, and the posterior cerebral artery supplies branches to the occipital lobe. The posterior communicating arteries connect the vertebral-basilar system with the carotid circulation.

Intermittent insufficiency of the vertebral-basilar arteries causes TIA with complicated and widespread neurologic signs. Involvement tends to be bilateral when the basilar artery is occluded and unilateral when one vertebral artery is the site of the occlusion.

Involvement of the cochlear-vestibular system causes vertigo, nausea, and a staggering gait. Auditory system symptoms include partial deafness and unilateral tinnitus. There may be parethesia, hemiplegia, or hemiparesis. Headache, dysarthria, dysphagia, and hiccupping occur.

Many patients note ocular symptoms for many months before complete occlusion. There may be blurred vision, diplopia, transient homonymous hemianopia, and scintillating scotomas. Blurring is usually bilateral, and the individual is occasionally momentarily blind. There are no ocular signs, and the condition is not discovered unless examination is made at the time of an attack.

Complete thrombosis causes a congruous homonymous hemianopia and motor involvement of the eyes. There may be paresis of conjugate gaze, with a conjugate deviation to one side. Internuclear ophthalmoplegia (p. 524) may be identical with that seen in multiple sclerosis. Horizontal or rotatory nystagmus is frequent. Horner syndrome is occasionally present (p. 285).

Recognition of the TIA is important in preventing the development of permanent cerebrovascular disease. Differential diagnosis includes migraine, epilepsy, carotid sinus syncope, and Ménière syndrome. Diagnostic steps should include ausculation of the neck for bruit, ophthalmoscopy for emboli, comparison of the radial pulses and brachial blood pressure in the two arms, computed tomography, and ophthalmodynamometry.

Possible causes, such as giant cell arteritis, vascular hypertension, and neurosyphilis, should be excluded in the elderly. Infection of the tonsillar bed is a cause in children. Systemic lupus erythematosus, polyarteritis nodosa, pulseless disease, and thrombocytopenia from leukemia must be excluded in older persons. A sudden decrease in blood pressure or alteration in the heart rhythm or rate may be the cause.

Surgery to correct ischemic attacks is limited to the extracranial portion of the carotid artery system. It may be indicated for patients who have symptoms of recent onset but who do not have brain infarction or widespread atherosclerotic disease. In other patients, anticoagulation may be used. Aspirin, which decreases platelet adhesiveness, is currently popular. Control of vascular hypertension and investigation of its cause are desirable.

Aortic arch syndrome. The aortic arch syndrome is a chronic disorder arising from obstruction of the subclavian and the carotid arteries. It includes pulseless disease, reversed coarctation of the aorta, and the subclavian steal syndrome. Symptoms arise from insufficiency of the cerebral blood supply and are similar to those described in carotid and vertebral-basilar insufficiency.

Pulseless disease is a giant cell arteritis of the aorta of unknown etiology that occurs mainly in young Japanese women. It is associated with retinal neovascularization, venous engorgement, microaneurysms, and arterial and venous occlusions. The radial pulse is absent. There may be widespread ischemic changes involving the head and the upper extremities.

Reversed coarctation of the aorta occurs in aortic arch occlusion and is a disorder of collateral circulation in which blood reaches the head, neck, and upper extremities through the intercostal, scapular, axillary, posterior and inferior thyroid, inferior epigastric, and internal mammary arteries.

The subclavian steal syndrome arises in stenosis or occlusion of the first portion of the subclavian artery. Blood flows up the contralateral vertebral artery and down the opposite vertebral artery to supply the subclavian artery distal to the area of occlusion. Symptoms arise from cerebral ischemia in the area of distribution of the vertebral-basilar system. A bruit in the subclavicular area and reduction of pulse and blood pressure in the ipsilateral arm suggest the diagnosis.

Brachial-basilar insufficiency arises in patients with occlusive disease of the proximal segment of the subclavian artery who develop transient ischemic vertebral-basilar symptoms when the arm is exercised. The symptoms arise, as in the subclavian steal syndrome, from retrograde blood flow through the ipsilateral vertebral artery.

Infraclinoid aneurysms. Dilation of the internal carotid artery within the cavernous sinus occurs most commonly in women during or after the fifth decade of life. The artery gives off no major branches in this location, and atheroma-tous plaque formation is common. The cavernous sinus contains the motor nerves to the eye and the ophthalmic and maxillary divisions of the trigeminal nerve. An expanding aneurysm thus gives rise to an ophthalmoplegia of all motor nerves and pain and paresthesia in the face. In infraclinoid aneurysms, unlike supraclinoid aneurysms, corneal and facial sensitivity is reduced.

The most conspicuous sign is an insidious, slowly progressive ophthalmoplegia, with all muscles of the eye involved. The pupil does not constrict to light but may not be dilated because of interruption of sympathetic nerve fibers on the surface of the artery. Pain is a relatively minor symptom. There is pain or paresthesia of the face, the side of the head, about the eye, or along the nose on the same side. Corneal anesthesia usually occurs and is usually associated with anesthesia of the face.

The gradual onset is suggestive of tumor, and arteriography is often necessary for exact diagnosis. Large infraclinoid aneurysms are probably reinforced by the walls of the cavernous sinus and do not rupture. Although it is likely that most spontaneous arteriovenous fistulas represent rupture of an aneurysm, usually they are so small before rupture that they do not cause signs of an aneurysm.

If untreated, infraclinoid aneurysms follow one of two patterns. Complete thrombosis of the aneurysm may occur, with resultant spontaneous cure, leaving a residual loss of ocular motility. The artery may expand anteriorly within the cavernous sinus, causing erosion of the optic foramen and the superior orbital fissure, with compression and atrophy of the optic nerve and a proptosis. The development of proptosis is frequently concealed by blepharoptosis. Venous drainage of the orbit is not involved, and there is no chemosis or congestion of bulbar vessels. Posterior expansion may involve the petrous portion of the temporal bone and the acoustic nerve, causing ipsilateral deafness.

The treatment of choice is gradual occlusion of the internal carotid artery, provided arteriography indicates adequate filling of the middle and anterior cerebral arteries on the side of the aneurysm from the contralateral carotid artery and provided there is no untoward effect from digital compression of the common carotid artery for 15 minutes. Patients should be less than 60 years old and should require the operation because of severe pain, failing vision, or exophthalmos.

Carotid artery–cavernous sinus fistula. The rupture of an infraclinoid aneurysm shunts blood from the carotid artery into the cavernous sinus, creating an arteriovenous fistula. The arterial blood passes into channels draining the cavernous sinus, and congestion of the superior ophthalmic vein draining the orbit causes visual loss, diplopia, headache, and pain.

Carotid-cavernous fistulas are traumatic (75%) or spontaneous. The traumatic fistula follows skull fracture, particularly basilotemporal fracture. A latent period may occur before the onset of symptoms. Spontaneous fistulas occur most commonly in middle-aged women, presumably

from rupture of aneurysms so small that they did not cause symptoms before rupture. Many may be caused by dural shunts occurring between meningeal branches of the carotid system and dural veins in the region of the cavernous sinus.

The outstanding sign is unilateral or bilateral proptosis (Fig. 26-2), which may pulsate. A bruit synchronous with the pulse is present and can be heard by the patient as a rushing, roaring sound. The increased venous pressure with stasis causes chemosis (Fig. 26-3), eyelid swelling, congested conjunctival and retinal veins, and hemorrhages. The abducent nerve may be involved or, less commonly, the third, fourth, or seventh. Visual failure is common from impairment of arterial and venous retinal circulations. Secondary glaucoma may not be diagnosed but may be the chief cause of visual loss. Tonography indicates increased arterial pulsation.

The ideal treatment is early ligation of the internal carotid artery in the neck combined with simultaneous intracranial clipping of the internal carotid artery and the ophthalmic artery. The anastomoses between the external carotid artery and the ophthalmic artery will maintain vision in about 75% of patients in whom the ophthalmic artery is clipped. The rec-

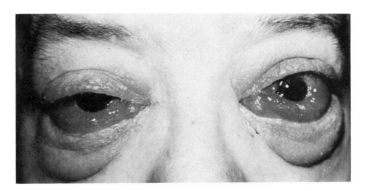

Fig. 26-2. Severe orbital congestion and bilateral proptosis in a spontaneous carotid artery–cavernous sinus fistula in a 57-year-old woman.

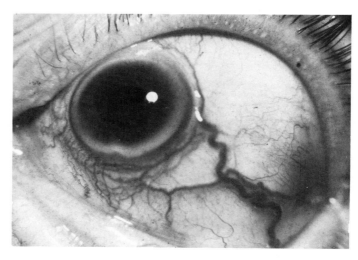

Fig. 26-3. Congested conjunctival vessels in a long-standing carotid artery–cavernous sinus fistula. The dilated blood vessels that surround the corneoscleral limbus are sometimes called "caput medusa."

ommendations described for infraclinoid aneurysms must be followed. Failure to treat promptly patients who would benefit leads to irreversible changes.

Supraclinoid aneurysms. Supraclinoid aneurysms usually arise at the bifurcation of the internal carotid artery into the middle and anterior cerebral arteries or at the junction of the internal carotid artery with the posterior communicating artery. Congenital berry aneurysms are common in this region, but the majority of patients are middle-aged or older. Women are involved more frequently, and hypertension is present in many patients.

Symptoms occur suddenly, with severe unilateral headache and pain about the face and eye. Pain in the medial canthal region is particularly characteristic. The pain arises from meningeal irritation and not from direct involvement of the trigeminal nerve as occurs in infraclinoid aneurysms. Simultaneously with the headache, or within 72 hours, an oculomotor paralysis develops, with blepharoptosis, exotropia, pupillary dilation, and failure of accommodation.

The prognosis for life is poorer with supraclinoid aneurysms than with infraclinoid aneurysms. Death occurs from subarachnoid hemorrhage or from bleeding into the brain. Untreated patients may experience no further episodes, presumably because of intravascular clotting, or may have recurrent attacks. Recovery with regeneration of the oculomotor nerve is seldom complete. A pseudo–von Graefe phenomenon is frequently present (p. 524), and pupillary abnormalities are observed. There may be loss of pupillary constriction, causing dilation of the pupil with light and constriction with convergence. The pupil may be widely dilated with no reaction to light or convergence.

Aneurysms of the middle and anterior cerebral arteries. Aneurysms if the middle and anterior cerebral arteries are particularly prone to cause defects in the visual fields. Optic atrophy is usually present. The visual field changes are bilateral and tend to be variable. An anterior cerebral artery aneurysm may cause a bitemporal hemianopia that begins in the inferior temporal quadrant rather than in the superior temporal quadrant, as in early pituitary gland adenoma. With aneurysm of the middle cerebral artery there may be loss of vision in one eye and a hemianopia in the fellow eye. Subarachnoid hemorrhage is common.

Basilar aneurysms. Congenital berry aneurysms may arise rarely at the anterior end of the basilar artery where it divides into the posterior cerebral arteries or at the posterior end where the vertebral arteries join to form the basilar arteries. The basilar artery is also the most common artery in the body to be affected with atherosclerosis.

The symptoms of basilar-vertebral aneurysms are variable and not characteristic. Dizziness, diplopia, and blurring of vision are the most common symptoms. There may be involvement of motor nerves on the brain stem, occipital headache, deafness, memory impairment, and coma. Diagnosis is often not made until autopsy.

Subarachnoid hemorrhage. The chief causes of spontaneous bleeding into the space between the arachnoid and the pia mater are (1) vascular hypertension, (2) ruptured supraclinoid aneurysms, and (3) angiomas or arteriovenous malformations. Less common causes include blood dyscrasias, necrosis of metastatic or glial brain tumors, and spinal varices.

Subarachnoid hemorrhage is characterized by a sudden, violent head pain of shocking severity followed by photophobia and stiffness of the legs. Unconsciousness persisting for a few hours to days may follow. Later there may be rigidity of the neck and spine. Lumbar puncture, in which only a few drops of fluid should be removed, indicates fresh blood. Bilateral carotid arteriography is indicated to determine whether the circle of Willis is normal and to determine the adequacy of the blood supply from the contralateral side.

The ocular signs are mainly those described for unruptured supraclinoid aneurysms. In addition, there may be sudden loss of vision, papilledema, and exophthalmos. An uncommon but pathognomonic ocular sign is bilateral subhyaloid hemorrhage, which develops at the posterior pole adjacent to the optic disk and develops a fluid level after rest or breaks into the vitreous.

Treatment must be individualized, but modern microsurgical techniques have decreased mortality, although the morbidity is still high. Surgical treatment should be carried out immediately in patients who are conscious or semiconscious, provided the collateral circulation is adequate. Gradual occlusion of the common carotid artery in the neck is moderately effective in subarachnoid hemorrhage arising from ruptured aneurysms of the internal carotid or posterior communicating artery. The treatment of choice is exposure of the aneurysm and either clipping it, coating it with plastic, or inducing intravascular thrombosis by means of an electric current, animal hair, or wire placed in the arterial wall.

DIABETES MELLITUS NEUROPATHY

Diabetes mellitus (p. 511) in rare instances is complicated by a neuropathy involving the cranial motor nerves. There is a severe unilateral headache usually followed by an abducent weakness. More rarely there is an oculomotor nerve palsy that does not involve the pupil in 75% of the instances. Diabetes mellitus neuropathy is usually distinguished from supraclinoid aneurysms by paralysis of the abducent nerve, which is rarely involved separately in an aneurysm. The sparing of the sphincter pupillae muscle aids in the diagnosis of diabetes. Generally, if the pupil is not involved, the cause is medical, whereas if it is involved, the cause is an aneurysm or tumor.

tated. The slow component of the nystagmus is in the direction of the displacement of endolymph in the semicircular canals, which causes deviation of the eyes to the opposite side. Thus, if the body is rapidly rotated to the right, the nystagmus during rotation has its slow component to the left. When rotation stops, the slow component is to the right.

Vestibular nystagmus can be conveniently studied by rotation of the body or by caloric irrigation of the external auditory canal, which sets up convection currents in the semicircular canals. Most attention is directed to study of the horizontal canals that involve mainly the medial and lateral recti muscles. Stimulation of the vertical canals causes vertical and torsional nystagmus, making complicated analysis necessary.

Vestibular nystagmus occurs in diseases of the end organ, its nuclei, or its central nervous system connections. Peripheral disease may be associated with vertigo, tinnitus, and deafness. The onset is abrupt. The nystagmus is horizontal and rotary and tends to decrease in the course of the disease. The common diseases causing peripheral involvement are labyrinthitis and Ménière disease.

Involvement of the vestibular nuclei and the central nervous system connections causes a static or increasing nystagmus. Spontaneous vertical nystagmus is virtually always of central origin; spontaneous rotary nystagmus suggests involvement of vestibular nuclei. Both types may be triggered by administration of barbiturates. Nystagmus may occur in multiple sclerosis, encephalitis, vascular disease (particularly occlusion of the posteroinferior cerebellar artery), and cerebellar and cerebellopontine lesions. The latter are likely to produce nystagmus that varies with the position of the head. The fast component is toward the side of the lesion.

DEMYELINATIVE DISEASE

Destruction of the myelin sheath of nerve fibers occurs in a variety of disorders: multiple sclerosis, neuromyelitis optica (Devic disease), subcortical encephalopathy (Schilder disease), and postinfectious disseminated encephalitis. These conditions may all affect vision through involvement of the optic nerve or optic radiation. In addition, they may cause ocular muscle weakness.

Multiple sclerosis. Multiple sclerosis (MS) is a chronic, remittent disease of the spinal cord and brain. It typically involves the white matter of the brain and is characterized by disseminated areas of demyelination of glial scar formation. It rarely affects individuals before 15 years of age. The rate rises rapidly to peak at age 30 and then rapidly decline, with only an occasional case with onset after age 55. Women are affected more often than men (1.7:1). The incidence and death rate are relatively high in the northern regions of the United States and Canada and low in the South. The initial factor may be a slow virus infection and the second mechanism an autoimmune reaction that destroys myelin. The average duration of the disease is 27 years, and in most patients there are remissions without permanent neurologic residue.

Retrobulbar neuritis is the initial episode of the disease in 15% of the patients, whereas in another 25%, paresis of an ocular muscle occurs. Of patients hospitalized because of MS, 70% have or have had retrobulbar neuritis. The fully developed disease is characterized by the Charcot triad of nystagmus, scanning speech, and optic atrophy. Visual-evoked potential (p. 104) often shows a delay in the signal's latency. Sheathing of peripheral retinal veins occurs in about 5% of the patients. Diplopia occurs because of an internuclear ophthalmoplegia or because of palsies of individual muscles.

Neuromyelitis optica. Neuromyelitis optica appears to be an acute MS. It is characterized by a bilateral acute optic neuritis with a transverse inflammation of the spinal cord. The disease may occur at any age. There are prodromal signs of headache, sore throat, fever, and malaise. The visual loss occurs rapidly, with blindness or near blindness developing within a few days. Ascending paralysis and sensory disturbances occur within a few weeks before or after blindness. Patients may die within a month, or there may be complete remission with recurrences. There is no treatment.

Subcortical encephalopathy. Subcortical encephalopathy (Schilder disease) affects children and adolescents and is characterized by progressive involvement of the brain with loss of vision, spastic paralysis, deafness, mental deterioration, and death in a few months to a year. Papilledema occurs in the majority of patients.

Postinfectious encephalitis. Encephalitis may develop after viral infections such as measles, mumps, varicella, and vaccinia. It most commonly follows measles, and the mortality of patients with measles encephalitis is 10%. There may be papilledema, papillitis, or retrobulbar neuritis. Recovery of vision is usual.

DYSAUTONOMIA

Familial dysautonomia. Familial dysautonomia or familial autonomic dysfunction (Riley-Day syndrome) is an autosomal recessive neurologic disorder largely confined to Ashkenazic Jews. A unique combination of ocular findings occurs: absence of overflow tears (alacrima), corneal hypesthesia, exotropia, and pupillary constriction after instillation of 0.1% pilocarpine. The cause of the disorder is unknown but appears to arise from impaired elaboration or release of a neurohumoral transmitter agent, possibly acetylcholine.

Many systemic defects occur: vasomotor instability with excessive sweating, skin blotching from eating or excitement, orthostatic hypotension, cyclic vomiting, fixed heart rate with episodes of tachycardia, and episodic fever. There is a striking indifference to pain, but proprioception and vibration sense are normal. There may be self-mutilation or mutilation from trauma. The patients are unsteady and uncoordinated and are unable to perform fine repetitive movements or to ride a bicycle. Response to touch stimuli is excessive (dysethesia). Deep tendon reflexes are absent or hypoactive. Emotions are labile, and patients are often sullen and uncommunicative; breath-holding is common in infancy. Few patients survive to adulthood, and most succumb to pneumonia, cardiovascular collapse, and intercurrent illness after a progressively downhill course during childhood.

The fungiform papillae of the tongue, the site of most of the taste buds, are absent. Disturbed swallowing causes drooling, feeding problems, and sometimes aspiration pneumonia. Intradermal injection of 1:1,000 histamine causes a wheal but not the usual flare.

The initial finding may be the absence of tears in a crying infant who has a feeding problem. By the age of 2 years, the child drools constantly, is undernourished, and walks on his toes with a stumbling gait. High fever of unexplained origin is common and sometimes is accompanied by convulsions.

In about one half of the patients, deficient lacrimation is associated with chronic, indolent, corneal ulcers that cause little or no pain because of the reduced corneal sensation. Intermarginal eyelid adhesions may be required. The Schirmer test (p. 232) indicates reduced tear formation. Myopia occurs in about 80% of the patients, and about one third of these have more than 1.5 diopters difference in the refractive error in the two eyes (anisometropia). Exotropia occurs in about two thirds of the patients, but it is not clear whether this is secondary to decreased vision arising from keratitis or myopia or is caused by a central defect.

Constriction of the pupil after instillation of 0.1% pilocarpine (also seen in Adie syndrome [p. 285]) reflects a parasympathetic denervation hypersensitivity. The pupillary sympathetics respond normally.

Ocular differential diagnosis includes congenital absence of the lacrimal gland and anhidrotic hereditary ectodermal dysplasia, in each of which the corneal sensitivity is normal. Keratoconjunctivitis sicca occurs in later years and, in addition to punctate or filamentary keratitis, has a stringy, mucoid discharge not present in autonomic dysfunction. Vitamin A deficiency with keratomalacia presents feeding problems, decreased tearing, and corneal ulcers, but the conjunctiva is affected initially and loses its luster, with dry spots appearing in it in contrast to the glistening, normal-appearing conjunctiva in autonomic dysfunction. Neuroparalytic keratitis is usually unilateral, follows trigeminal nerve injury, and has no associated systemic findings.

Acute pandysautonomia. Acute pandysautonomia occurs with no sex predilection in previously healthy individuals. Instances have been reported in individuals as young as 6 years and as old as 49 years. Interference with accommodation causes a blurring of vision for near work and may precede or accompany other signs of generalized autonomic dysfunction. Systemic signs of impaired sympathetic and parasympatheic function are usually initially severe and include orthostatic hypotension with a fixed heart rate, decreased salivation, anhidrosis, atony of the bladder, diarrhea, constipation, im-

potence, and abnormal flushing of the skin.

The pupils are dilated and react poorly to light stimulation. There may be atrophy of the iris sphincter later in the disease. The pupils are hypersensitive to dilute concentrations of pilocarpine but fail to dilate after topical instillation of 4% cocaine or 1% hydroxyamphetamine. The pupils dilate when 0.1% epinephrine is administered, suggesting a sympathetic postganglionic block with denervation hypersensitivity.

The cause is not known, but current attention is directed to an autoimmune disorder. The disease tends to be self-limited, with recovery occurring 2 to 3 years after its onset. In some patients a keratoconjunctivitis sicca may develop.

Subacute sclerosing panencephalitis. This is a slow measles-virus infection in which there is a long asymptomatic period between the introduction of the infectious agent and the appearance of the clinical illness. It usually develops before 11 years of age (80%) in previously well children who have had measles at an unusually early age. Mental deterioration is followed by severe motor involvement. Focal retinitis of the central retina is followed by pigment proliferation and gliosis. Cortical blindness, papilledema, and optic atrophy may occur with associated cranial nerve lesions. Death occurs within 1 year of onset.

HEADACHE

Iridocyclitis (p. 295), high intraocular pressure (p. 404), impending zoster ophthalmicus (p. 461), and temporal arteritis (p. 565) cause orbital pain. Retrobulbar neuritis (p. 367) is associated with pain behind the eye aggravated by ocular movements. The ocular muscle palsy of diabetic neuropathy begins with severe retrobulbar pain. Increased intracranial pressure (p. 528), subarachnoid hemorrhage (p. 538), and intracranial aneurysms cause severe headaches, sometimes localized to one orbit. Refractive errors (p. 432) are commonly thought to cause discomfort and pain in the head, but usually the cause is vascular, neurologic, or psychogenic.

Migraine. This is a specific, periodic, throbbing, hemicranial head pain that begins before the age of 20 years and recurs less frequently with advancing years. There is often a family history of similar head pain. Classic migraine is preceded by an aura consisting of bright spots or zigzag lines (scintillating scotoma) that may be followed by a homonymous hemianopia. A severe hemicrania follows with nausea, vomiting, photophobia, exhaustion, and sleep. Ergot preparations give relief if administered early in the attack. The headache persists for several hours or days and then clears without residue.

Transient oculomotor nerve paralysis with exotropia, blepharoptosis, and pupillary dilation occurs in rare cases as the headache is receding. In some individuals the oculomotor paresis becomes permanent. It is debatable whether such a paresis constitutes a specific entity of ophthalmoplegic migraine or whether it reflects bleeding of a supraclinoid aneurysm. Carotid arteriography is usually negative. On the basis of age of onset, aura, history of migraine, response to medication, and ophthalmoplegia developing as the headache recedes, it seems likely that ophthalmoplegic migraine is a definite disease.

Methysergide, a serotonin antagonist, wholly prevents attacks. It may cause a retroperitoneal fibrosis with ureteral obstruction, hydronephrosis, and vascular hypertension together with mediastinal fibrosis and sclerosing cholangitis. Associated with these signs may be bilateral pseudotumor of the orbit. This group of signs may also be unrelated to ingestion of the drug.

Recurrent nocturnal orbital (cluster) headaches. These are characterized by constant, unilateral orbital localization; occurrence in men between 20 and 50 years of age; and onset within 2 to 3 hours of falling asleep. There is lacrimation, sometimes flush and edema of the cheek, and sometimes Horner syndrome (p. 285). The nostril is blocked, and this is followed by rhinorrhea. The attack disappears within several hours. The attacks recur nightly for days or weeks (hence, cluster) and then may disappear for years.

Some pains behind the eye, nose, or upper jaw associated with a blocked nostril are described as neuralgia affecting specific nerves; sphenopalatine (Sluder), petrosal, vidian, and ciliary (Charlin). They probably are instances of cluster headache or variants thereof.

Paratrigeminal syndrome (of Raeder). This consists of severe daily unilateral headaches with Horner syndrome minus anhydrosis and often with lacrimation and conjunctival injection. Men are commonly affected (7:1). The average age of onset is 46 years. The attacks last 1 or 2 months and rarely recur.

BIBLIOGRAPHY

Harrington, D. O.: The visual fields, ed. 4, St. Louis, 1976, The C. V. Mosby Co.

Kimball, R. W., and Hedges, T. R.: Amaurosis fugax caused by a prolapsed mitral valve leaflet in the midsystolic click, late systolic murmur syndrome, Am. J. Ophthalmol. **83**:469, 1977.

Lindenberg, R., Walsh, F. B., and Sacks, J. G.: Neuropathology of vision; an atlas, Philadelphia, 1973, Lea & Febiger.

Neupert, J. R., Brubaker, R. F., Kearns, T. P., and Sundt, T. M.: Rapid resolution of venous stasis retinopathy after carotid endarterectomy, Am. J. Ophthalmol. **81**:600, 1976.

Yee, R. D., Trese, M., Zee, D. S., and others: Ocular manifestations of acute pandysautonomia, Am. J. Ophthalmol. **81**:740, 1976.

Chapter 27

CARDIOVASCULAR DISORDERS

The ocular fundus is the sole location where small arteries, arterioles, and their accompanying veins may be readily examined during life. These blood vessels are subject to the same diseases as similar-sized vessels elsewhere but, additionally, are responsive to conditions, such as glaucoma or retinitis pigmentosa, that have no systemic counterpart. Since the venous pressure must exceed the intraocular pressure or the eye will collapse, this is a highly specialized vascular bed, and changes in retinal vessels must be extrapolated to similar changes in the cardiac, cerebral, or renal blood vessels with considerable caution.

Careful observers are increasingly reluctant to deduce the general vascular state from the appearance of the retinal blood vessels. There is little problem in accelerated hypertension when papilledema, cotton-wool patches, and hemorrhages are present, but this occurs rarely. The main difficulty arises in subtle changes in caliber and arteriovenous crossings that seem to occur as part of the aging process but may be seen in younger patients with vascular hypertension.

A number of cardiovascular disorders of the eye have been discussed: corneal arcus and the increased incidence of myocardial infarction before the age of 50 in men who smoke (p. 255), amaurosis fugax in occlusive disease of the carotid artery

(p. 530), occlusive disease of the central retinal artery and vein and their branches (p. 330), giant-cell vasculitis (p. 565), and cerebrovascular disease (p. 529).

This chapter is mainly directed to discussion of age-related retinal vascular changes, arteriosclerosis of the central retinal artery, and the arteriolar sclerosis of vascular hypertension that affects branches of the central retinal artery. Particulars concerning the ophthalmoscopic examination are discussed elsewhere (pp. 174 and 321).

AGING (INVOLUTIONARY SCLEROSIS)

Abnormalities of the retinal blood vessels are common in elderly persons and occasionally occur in younger individuals who do not have and have not had vascular hypertension. The outstanding ophthalmoscopic characteristic of involutionary sclerosis is localized involvement of medium-sized retinal arterioles, with much of the vasculature appearing to be normal. There is loss of brilliant light reflexes, from the retinal surface, and the retina reflects a coarser texture. The light reflex from the convex surface of arterioles is of diminished intensity and more diffuse than is normal. There may be generalized widening of the arteriovenous crossing that is less marked than the crossing changes in arteriolar sclerosis. A slight reduction in the caliber of arterioles may occur. Associated with the vascular changes are degenerative changes such as drusen (p. 343) and atrophic changes in the choroid about the optic disk and the central and peripheral retina.

The changes of involutionary sclerosis occur with aging and do not necessarily parallel any aging processes elsewhere in the body. Their cause is not known, but in all probability they are the consequence of loss of elasticity and arteriolar fibrosis.

ARTERIOSCLEROSIS

Arteriosclerosis is a nonspecific, broadly inclusive term that describes all processes in which hardening and thickening of the arterial coat have occurred. The three conditions generally included in the term are Mönckeberg medial sclerosis, atherosclerosis, and diffuse arteriolar sclerosis. Mönckeberg medial sclerosis affects medium-sized arteries, particularly in the extremities; there is never ocular involvement. Atherosclerosis affects large and medium-sized arteries; the central retinal artery and its branches immediately adjacent to the optic disk may be involved. Diffuse arteriolar sclerosis involves all arterioles in the body in a similar manner. It occurs solely as a result of vascular hypertension.

Retinal vein obstruction (p. 330) from any causes gives rise to changes in adjacent arterioles identical with those occurring in aging and arteriolar sclerosis. It is postulated that the venous stasis gives rise to a local toxin affecting the arterial wall. The adjacent vein disease and the focal localization of the arterial changes indicate the cause.

Atherosclerosis

Atherosclerosis is a vascular abnormality characterized by focal necrosis and thickening of the intima, with intimal and subintimal lipid deposition associated with hyperplastic and degenerative changes in the wall of the artery, particularly of the internal elastic lamina. The disease may affect arteries of all diameters, but it has a predilection for the aorta and tends to involve arteries to the heart, brain, and extremities. The condition is absent in puberty, but thereafter its extent and severity increase with advancing years. Atheromas are symptomless unless there is frank obstruction or localized decrease in blood supply to a region. The lesions may be multiple, but atheromas in one vessel do not indicate atheromas in another. Their cause is unknown, but they are associated with vascular hypertension, turbulence eddies within blood vessels, hyperlipoproteinemia (p. 500), and heredity.

Atherosclerosis of retinal vessels. Ocular atherosclerosis involves the central retinal artery either within the optic nerve or in its branches immediately adjacent to the optic disk.

Atheroma formation in the central retinal artery within the optic nerve may cause constriction of the artery and displace the retinal arterioles toward the disk. As the bifurcations of arterioles are drawn onto the disk, more blood vessels cross the disk margins, the retinal vessels become straighter, and the bifurcations occur at more acute angles. Reduction in the lumen of the central retinal artery by an atheroma decreases blood flow and narrows the arterial caliber.

Atheromas in branches of the central artery near the optic disk cause subtle changes. Localized indentations in the wall of the artery result in reduction in caliber of the lumen as the result of projection of an atheromatous plaque into the lumen. Fibrosis causes a whitish or opaque area in the wall of the involved blood vessel.

Occlusion. Ocular atherosclerosis may obstruct the central retinal artery or vein. Occlusion of the central retinal artery (p. 333) causes a pale coagulation necrosis of the inner layers of the retina. The fovea centralis, which lacks inner layers, is not involved and thus appears red (normal) relative to the surrounding edematous and pale retina. The entire arterial tree becomes markedly attenuated. Branch arterial occlusion (p. 334) causes a pale coagulation necrosis of the inner layers of the retina in the region of distribution of the involved vessel, the caliber of which is markedly attenuated. A scotoma with very sharp margins corresponding to the involved area can be demonstrated in the visual field.

A cholesterol embolus dislodged from an atheromatous plaque in the carotid artery appears as a glistening, crystalline body within a retinal artery, often at a vessel bifurcation (Fig. 27-1, A). The embolus may cause an amaurosis fugax (p. 530) or retinal ischemia (p. 335). Patients with cholesterol emboli have many signs: atherosclerosis of large blood vessels, transient cerebral ischemic attacks (p.

529), and abnormal electrocardiograms. Observation of such an embolus should lead to a full study of the patient's vascular status.

A fibrin embolus arises from a damaged heart valve or other cardiac lesion. It is dull white to yellowish with soft margins and is less likely to be lodged at a vessel bifurcation (Fig. 27-1, B).

Arteries and veins are bound together in a common adventitial sheath at the lamina cribrosa and at arteriovenous crossings within the eye. Atheromatous plaque formation in the artery may impinge on the lumen of the vein, giving rise to venous closure at the lamina cribrosa (central retinal vein occlusion) or closure at one of the crossings (branch vein occlusion). Glaucoma enhances the likelihood of venous closure, since the increased intraocular pressure favors stagnation of blood and thrombus formation. Atheromatous disease is inferred when involvement within the optic nerve causes sud-

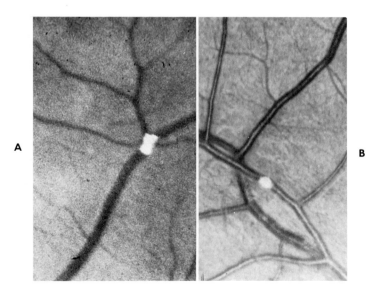

Fig. 27-1. A, Cholesterol embolus at bifurcation of a branch of a retinal artery in a 57-year-old woman with an atheroma of the common carotid artery. **B,** Fibrin embolus in the inferior temporal artery of the left eye of a 23-year-old man with mitral regurgitation after rheumatic heart disease. Four months later, the embolus was no longer present. There were no symptoms.

den loss of vision. The lesion cannot be seen with the ophthalmoscope.

Arteriolar sclerosis

Arteriolar sclerosis indicates a prolonged, significant increase in blood pressure that causes thickening of the walls and narrowing of the lumen of arterioles. The vascular involvement is generalized, and thus all arterioles throughout the body are affected to a similar degree, in contrast to the spotty, plaquelike involvement of atherosclerosis.

One of two of changes occurs in arteriolar sclerosis.

1. Replacement fibrosis develops in slowly increasing, moderately severe hypertension, associated chiefly with a rise of the systolic blood pressure in the range of 170 to 200 mm Hg, with the diastolic pressure usually less than 100 mm Hg. There is increased collagen and elastic tissue in all layers of the blood vessel and eventual complete loss of cellular detail.

2. Hyperplastic thickening and fibrinoid necrosis occur as acute, severe reactions to a sudden marked increase in the blood pressure in which the systolic blood pressure exceeds 200 mm Hg and the diastolic blood pressure exceeds 120 mm Hg. The diffuse thickening of arteriolar walls, if severe, may lead to necrosis. Hyperplastic thickening and fibrinoid necrosis occur only in vessels containing muscle fibers. Vessels that have been the site of involutionary sclerosis or prior replacement fibrosis are not involved. These changes appear to protect the arterioles from the effects of severe hypertension, and they may explain the infrequency of hyperplastic thickening and fibrinoid necrosis in the age group in which involutionary sclerosis is seen.

Replacement fibrosis and fibrinoid necrosis cause two main groups of ophthalmoscopic changes (Table 27-1). If ophthalmoscopy in a patient with known vascular hypertension indicates no arteriolar sclerosis, then the hypertension either is not severe or is of recent onset. If the changes of replacement fibrosis are present, the disease is of long duration and has affected arterioles throughout the body similarly. If the ophthalmoscopic changes are those of hyperplastic thickening and fibrinoid necrosis, the hypertension is severe, is likely of recent onset,

Table 27-1. Ophthalmoscopic signs of arteriolar sclerosis

Replacement fibrosis: long-duration, moderately severe hypertension	Fibrinoid necrosis: recent-onset, severe hypertension
Attenuation of arterioles	Severe attenuation of arterioles
Arteriovenous crossing changes	Edema of retina
Concealment	Cotton-wool patches
Depression or elevation	Hemorrhage
Deviation	Papilledema
Stenosis	Ophthalmoscopic changes of replacement fibrosis may
Changes in vascular light reflex	precede above signs or remain after condition is
Irregularities of caliber	corrected
Widening	
Copper-wire arteries	
Silver-wire arteries	
Sheathing	
Tortuosity	
Hard, shiny exudates	
Hemorrhage	

and may be associated with renal insufficiency, encephalopathy, and impairment of cardiac function.

Retinal vascular changes. The retinal blood vessels in health are transparent tubes with blood visible inside. The oxygenated blood within arteries is brighter red than that in veins. With ophthalmoscopy, a light streak is reflected from the convex wall of arteries, presumably from the medial coat. With replacement fibrosis, the blood vessel wall becomes less transparent, and the thickening of the medial coat is reflected in variation in the light reflex. Attention is directed mainly to blood vessels after they have traversed a little distance on the surface of the retinal to avoid confusion arising from congenital anomalies associated with the optic disk. The difficulty of interpretation is emphasized in the critical study by Salus of the accuracy of his own ophthalmoscopy, a field in which he was preeminent. In a careful experiment, he found his diagnosis correct in only 70% of hypertensive patients and in only 50% of arteriosclerotic patients. In young adults who did not have arteriosclerosis and whose features and figures were covered except for their eyes, he diagnosed arteriosclerosis in more than 50%.

Attenuation of arterioles. Attenuation of the arterioles is the most consis-tent sign of hypertension but is the most difficult finding to interpret. Both generalized and local constriction may be observed, but only the generalized attenuation appears to result from vascular spasm. Attenuation is best appreciated by observation of arterioles beyond their second bifurcation, where they seem to become thin red threads that disappear from view at the equator. The ophthalmoscopic change is observed in severe vascular hypertension occurring in young individuals who have not developed replacement fibrosis.

Errors arise because of concealment of arteries by retinal edema and dilation of veins, making arteries appear narrower. Many believe that the arteriovenous ratio is not significant and that attention should be directed to the diameter of the arteries.

Arteriovenous crossing changes. Replacement fibrosis of a retinal arteriole produces a variety of changes at locations at which it crosses over or under a vein. The earliest and most subtle change is loss of translucency of the arteriole so that the vein can no longer be seen beneath the vessel. The generalized variations in arteriovenous crossing changes are observed solely in arteriolar sclerosis and serve to differentiate it from the occasional crossing change seen in in-

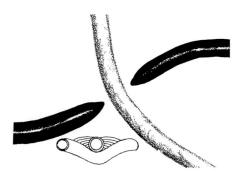

Fig. 27-2. Tapering concealment of the vein appearing as "nicking."

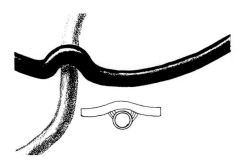

Fig. 27-3. Elevation of the vein over the artery.

volutionary sclerosis. The arteriovenous crossing changes in arteriolar sclerosis are as follows.

1. *Concealment.* The underlying vein is concealed because of loss of transparency of the wall of the retinal arteriole, which is caused by thickening of its wall. The venous blood column appears to terminate abruptly on either side of the crossing. Alternatively, there may be a tapering type of concealment, with the vein fading on either side of the crossing. The concealment appears to cause a narrowing of the vein, commonly described as "nicking" (Fig. 27-2). The venous lumen is not narrowed.

2. *Depression or elevation.* A vein may be deflected deep into the retina or may hump abruptly over the artery (Fig. 27-3). The thickening of the wall of the arterioles causes displacement of the vein.

3. *Deviation.* Displacement of a vein at the point of crossing is characterized by an abrupt turn in the course of the vein just as it reaches the artery (Fig. 27-4). At a similar distance beyond the artery it again assumes the same direction as before the crossing. This gives the vein an S-shape bend. Compared with arterial pressure, the lower pressure in the vein permits it to be deflected from its course or compressed with greater ease.

4. *Stenosis.* Because of compression or constriction at the arteriovenous crossing, the vein distal to the crossing becomes dilated and swollen (Fig. 27-5). The crossing is concealed, and thereafter the vein has a normal diameter.

Changes in light reflex. In the early days of ophthalmoscopy, much attention was directed to light reflected from the surface of blood vessels. Modern study now focuses little attention on correlating systemic disease with the light reflex.

The major changes in light reflex are as follows.

1. *Irregularities in caliber.* Widening of the light reflex does not occur uniformly. Initially there are areas of normal width combined with areas of decreased width. This has been interpreted as a sign of focal vasospasm; but unlike generalized vasospasm, it does not disappear with correction of the hypertension. It is the easiest of the light reflex abnormalities to observe.

2. *Widening of the light reflex.* The earliest sign of arteriolar sclerosis is widening of the central light reflex from arterioles. Instead of a bright central line, it becomes broader and softer with less distinct borders.

3. *Copper-wire arteries.* As the reflex broadens, it eventually occupies most of the width of the blood vessel. Early ophthalmoscopists used reflected light hav-

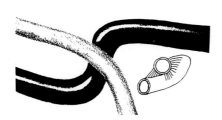

Fig. 27-4. Deviation of the vein out of its path.

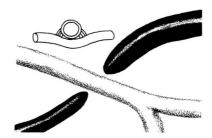

Fig. 27-5. Compression of the vein at the arteriovenous crossing, causing stenosis of the distal vein.

ing less intensity than the modern direct ophthalmoscope provides and described the burnished, metallic reflections as copper-wire arteries.

4. *Silver-wire arteries.* As replacement fibrosis continues, the vessel wall obscures the blood column, and the arteriole appears as a whitish tube containing a red fluid. This is not the white, threadlike appearance of the artery that follows occlusion of the central retinal artery.

5. *Sheathing.* Sheathing may occur as a result either of arteriolar sclerosis or of an atheromatous plaque involving an artery adjacent to the optic disk. Normally arterioles near the disk are sheathed with glial tissue. In arteriolar sclerosis, white parallel lines appear at arteriovenous crossings and encase the arteriole, giving rise to the appearance of a white, fibrous-looking cord. Sheathing also occurs in vessels after a vasculitis subsides, and the arteries appear as white cords long after an arterial occlusion.

6. *Tortuosity.* In fibrous replacement the arterioles increase in length and diameter, with resultant increased tortuosity. This may also be a congenital condition (Fig. 27-6), and its occurrence in hypertension can be evaluated solely by repeated observation.

Cotton-wool patches. Cotton-wool patches (p. 325) occur in fibrinoid necrosis when the diastolic blood pressure exceeds 120 mm Hg. They are located in the nerve fiber layer of the retina at the posterior pole, number usually less than 10, and are about one third of the disk diameter in size (Fig. 27-7). They result from an ischemic infarct of the retina caused by occlusion of an arteriole. The occlusion is thought to be caused by fibrinoid arteriolar necrosis or severe spasm giving rise to abnormal endothelial permeability. Similar cotton-wool patches may also be seen in collagen diseases and in a number of other diseases not necessarily associated with vascular

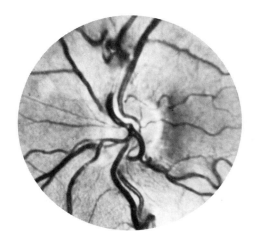

Fig. 27-6. Congenital tortuosity of retinal veins in a 27-year-old man with normal vision.

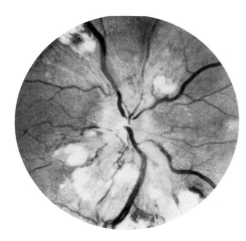

Fig. 27-7. A 39-year-old woman with fibrinoid necrosis. Her blood pressure is 250/160. Vision is 6/7.5 (20/25) in each eye. The disk margins are slightly blurred superiorly. The arterioles are extremely attenuated. There are numerous cotton-wool patches.

hypertension but in which there is generalized endothelial damage. Cotton-wool patches are described histologically as microinfarcts containing cellular organelles. They may reflect impaired axoplasmic transport (p. 95).

Hard deposits. Hard deposits develop in areas of chronic retinal edema and are composed of free fat and fat-laden microglia. These exudates are observed mainly at the posterior pole, vary in number from a few to 50 or more, and are scattered throughout the outer plexiform layer of the retina. In severe hypertension they may be concentrated around the fovea centralis, creating a star-shaped figure.

Hemorrhages. Hemorrhages in arteriolar sclerosis are located in the nerve fiber layer and are splinter or flame shaped and minute (p. 323).

Papilledema. The development of hypertensive encephalopathy is associated with the development of papilledema. As in papilledema from brain tumor or other intracranial masses, there is initial congestion of the optic disk with obliteration of the physiologic optic cup. Blurring of the upper and lower nasal margins follows, accompanied by venous dilation. The veins do not pulsate. Early in the course there is edema and swelling of the retina, which has a wet, watery appearance with many highlights. With increasing venous dilation, superficial flame-shaped hemorrhages occur. Visual acuity remains good, but the blind spots are enlarged, as demonstrated by testing on the tangent screen (p. 162). If the primary hypertension is corrected, the ophthalmoscopic changes may disappear without residue.

Choroidal changes. The vasculature of the choroid cannot be seen distinctly with the ophthalmoscope, but vascular changes of the choroid parallel those elsewhere in the body and the eye. Atherosclerosis of choroidal vessels is common, but the rich anastomoses minimize ischemia. Severe hypertension may result in fibrinoid necrosis of the choroidal arterioles. The retinal pigment epithelium becomes necrotic, and there may be atrophy of the sensory retina along with the formation of bright yellow Elschnig spots three to four times the diameter of a retinal artery. The older lesions have central pigment clumps, and there may be focal retinal detachment. Choroidal vessels show an early involutionary sclerosis, which precedes that of the retinal arterioles.

GRADING OF HYPERTENSION

The grading of the ocular changes secondary to vascular hypertension has caused much confusion. Every grading system is a form of medical shorthand used to group patients with similar changes. Unless everyone caring for a patient uses the same grading system, the grading of disease findings confuses, rather than clarifies, the diagnosis. It is far more instructive to describe and to interpret the changes seen ophthalmoscopically than to use a grading method.

Keith-Wagener-Barker grouping. This classification relates solely to the grouping of the retinal changes associated with vascular hypertension and arteriolar sclerosis. It is not intended to be applied to involutionary sclerosis of aging or atherosclerosis. Inasmuch as hypertension causes generalized, diffuse changes, one should not use the classification for focal changes or for changes secondary to retinal inflammation with venous stasis. Both eyes should have similar changes; involvement of only one eye suggests impaired internal carotid circulation on the side of the normal eye (p. 529). Glaucoma tends to minimize the ophthalmoscopic changes of vascular hypertension.

Group I. The light reflex from arterioles is brightened, and there is an increased luster with a burnished copper-wire or polished silver-wire appearance. There is moderate arteriolar attenuation often combined with focal constriction. No marked changes are seen in arteriovenous crossings, although there may be widening with increased translucency of the arteriole, making the underlying vein nearly invisible. Patients in this group have an essential benign hypertension with adequate cardiac and renal function; the heart size and the electrocardiogram are usually normal. The majority of cases of hypertension fall into this group. The vascular changes of the fundi are virtually identical with those occurring in aging sclerosis without hypertension. With adequate treatment of the hypertensive disease, the ophthalmoscopic changes will probably not progress.

Group II. The light reflex has a definite burnished copper-wire or polished silver-wire luster. Arteriovenous crossing changes may be marked and include all the various abnormalities. The arterioles are about half the size of normal, and there are areas of localized constriction. Hard, shiny deposits as well as minute linear hemorrhages may develop late in the course of the disease. These patients have a more sustained hypertension with higher diastolic pressure than those in Group I. Their cardiac and renal functions tend to be normal, but cardiomegaly may develop, along with corresponding changes in the electrocardiogram. Angina pectoris and proteinuria may also be present.

Group III. Marked attenuation of the arterioles occurs. The retina appears wet and edematous. One or more cotton-wool patches and hemorrhages are present. The significant change is the cotton-wool patch. These patients have a diastolic blood pressure of more than 120 mm Hg. Depending on the cause of hypertension, there may be cardiac symptoms, changes in the electrocardiogram, and renal changes of proteinuria and insufficiency.

Group IV. The patients in Group IV have all of the ophthalmoscopic signs of those in Group III, in addition to papilledema. The degree of papilledema may vary from blurring of the disk margins to complete obliteration of the disk structure. Cardiac and renal functions may be seriously impaired. Papilledema and cotton-wool patches may disappear shortly before death.

• • •

A number of systemic abnormalities cause the angiospastic retinopathy of Groups III and IV, and with their correction the ophthalmoscopic appearance of the fundus may be restored to normal. However, if the condition has persisted for some time and if considerable fibrinoid necrosis has occurred, after the blood pressure has been restored to normal, the fundus will resemble that seen in Group II. The originators of this classification did not describe hard, shiny deposits as occurring in Group II. A serious error is introduced if such deposits are the basis for classifying the fundus disease as Group III.

ECLAMPSIA, PHEOCHROMOCYTOMA, AND GLOMERULONEPHRITIS

The retinal manifestation of these diseases is entirely related to the vascular hypertension they produce. In years past, ophthalmologists used the term "renal retinopathy" to describe the hypertensive fundus changes that occurred with chronic renal disease. Many internists disliked the term because of the implication that the fundus changes reflected a specific renal abnormality rather than the hypertension. The fundi show advanced arteriolar sclerosis. Superimposed on these changes is the gradual development of cotton-wool patches and hemorrhages. The combination suggests a severe hypertensive vascular disease that has been present for a long period.

In true eclampsia the hypertensive vascular changes occur in a fundus that has not previously been the site of vascular change. The rapid onset of a severe hypertension gives rise to a generalized arteriolar spasm. Cotton-wool patches occur along with much retinal edema, giving the retina a wet, edematous, "shot silk" appearance. The hemodynamic disturbances may be so severe that a bilateral retinal detachment occurs without holes in the retina. Once the hypertension is corrected, the fundi rapidly return to normal.

Pheochromocytoma and unilateral renal disease cause hypertension with the fundus changes of severe hypertension without antecedent vascular disease. Usually the hypertension develops more slowly than that seen in eclampsia, and the retina is less edematous. If the condition is corrected early in the course of the hypertension, the fundus returns to normal. If the condition has persisted for some time before correction of the hypertension, the hemorrhages and deposits disappear, but the arteriolar constriction and variation in caliber tend to persist. The ophthalmoscopic picture is not unlike that seen in elderly individuals with treated hypertension.

RENAL TRANSPLANTATION

About one third of patients receiving a kidney transplant develop some type of ocular complication. Many have had severe hypertension for many years before the transplant, and their retinal blood vessels have severe changes of arteriolar sclerosis. Except when the donor kidney is obtained from an identical twin, nearly all patients develop signs of rejection and require prolonged therapy with immunosuppressive drugs. Following successful transplantation, there is a period of severe hypertension, and in many patients the preexisting arteriolar sclerosis limits the capacity of the vasculature of the eyes to respond to another episode of hypertension. Posterior subcapsular cataracts (p. 379), seldom reducing vision below 6/12 (20/40), develop in about one fourth of the patients. The incidence parallels the high corticosteroid dosage. Corticosteroid-induced glaucoma (p. 399) may occur but less frequently than when the corticosteroid is instilled topically. Acute retinitis caused by cytomegalic inclusion disease or fungi occurs in 5% to 10% of the patients. Many blood transfusions combined with a need for large doses of immunosuppressive agents predispose to the retinitis.

BIBLIOGRAPHY

Ballantyne, A. J., and Michaelson, I. C.: Textbook of the fundus of the eye, ed. 2, Baltimore, 1970, The Williams & Wilkins Co.

Blodi, F. C., Allen, L., and Frazier, O.: Stereoscopic manual of the ocular fundus in local and systemic disease, vol. 2, St. Louis, 1970, The C. V. Mosby Co.

Cogan, D. G.: Major problems in internal medicine. Vol. 3: Ophthalmic manifestations of systemic vascular disease, Philadelphia, 1974, W. B. Saunders Co.

Fine, S. L., Patz, A., and Orth, D. H.: Sights and sounds in ophthalmology. Vol. 2: Retinal vascular disorders; diagnosis and management, St. Louis, 1976, The C. V. Mosby Co.

Keith, N. M., Wagener, H. P., and Barker, N. W.: Some different types of essential hypertension; their course and prognosis, Am. J. Med. Sci. **197:** 332, 1939.

Nover, A.: The ocular fundus, ed. 3, translated by F. Blodi, Philadelphia, 1974, Lea & Febiger.

Patz, A.: Retinal vascular diseases, N. Engl. J. Med. **298:**1451, 1978.

Pavlin, C. R., Deveber, G. A., Cook, G. T., and Chisholm, L. D.: Ocular complications in renal transplant recipients, Can. Med. Assoc. J. **117:** 360, 1977.

Pfaffenbach, D. D., and Hollenhorst, R. W.: Morbidity and survivorship of patients with embolic cholesterol crystals in the ocular fundus, Am. J. Ophthalmol. **75:**66, 1973.

Chapter 28

DISORDERS OF THE HEMATOPOIETIC SYSTEM

Abnormalities in the number of cells, their shape, their membranes, their metabolism, their survival time, or their immunologic functions may cause marked ocular alterations. Sometimes changes in the eye lead to the appropriate tests, as in some hemoglobinopathies and macroglobulinemias. In other instances the ocular changes are only incidental to the blood disease. This topic is so encompassing that reference will be made here mainly to those diseases in which there are more or less specific ocular changes.

HEMOGLOBINOPATHIES

Hemoglobin consists of a protein molecule, globin, bound to four molecules of heme, an iron and protoporphyrin compound. The globin is composed of two pairs of amino acid chains that differ in the sequence and composition of their constituent amino acids. Four normal amino acid chains occur in humans: alpha, beta, gamma, and delta. Separate pairs of allelic genes control their structure.

Normal adult hemoglobin (Hb A) comprises mainly (97%) a pair of alpha amino acid chains and a pair of beta amino acid chains. Normal adults also have a minor amount of hemoglobin (3%) composed of a pair of alpha chains and a pair of delta chains (Hb A_2). Fetal hemoglobin (Hb F), which is normally formed in trace amounts after birth, contains a pair of alpha chains and a pair of gamma chains.

An alteration in the sequence of amino acids in the amino acid chains may cause changes in the shape, oxygen affinity, electrophoretic mobility, pliability, solubility, and life span of the hemoglobin molecule. Most variations of clinical significance (Table 28-1) involve the beta chain. The variants are tabulated according to the position in the amino acid chain in which the substitution has occurred. Thus, sickle hemoglobin (Hb S) is designated $\alpha_2\beta_2^{6\ glu \rightarrow val}$ indicating that valine has been substitued for glutamic acid in the sixth position of the beta chain. Hb C has a structure of $\alpha_2\beta_2^{6\ glu \rightarrow lysine}$

Sickle cell anemia or homozygous Hb S disease arises when each parent provides one gene for the abnormal hemoglobin. There is from 70% to 98% Hb S and the remainder is Hb F, normal fetal hemoglobin. In sickle cell trait, or heterozygous Hb SA disease, one parent provides the gene for sickle cell hemoglobin, and the other provides the gene for normal hemoglobin. Homozygous Hb C

Table 28-1. Hemoglobinopathies of major ophthalmic interest

Sickle cell anemia: SS disease ($\alpha_2\beta_2^{6\ glu\rightarrow val}$ and $\alpha_2\beta_2^{6\ glu\rightarrow val}$)
  Each parent provides Hb S
Sickle cell trait: SA disease ($\alpha_2\beta_2^{6\ glu\rightarrow val}$ and $\alpha_2\beta_2$)
  One parent provides Hb S and one parent provides normal Hb A
Sickle cell hemoglobin C disease: SC disease ($\alpha_2\beta_2^{6\ glu\rightarrow val}$ and $\alpha_2\beta_2^{6\ glu\rightarrow lysine}$)
  One parent provides Hb S and one parent provides Hb C
Hemoglobin C trait: AC disease ($\alpha_2\beta_2$ and $\alpha_2\beta_2^{6\ glu\rightarrow lysine}$)
  One parent provides normal Hb A and one parent provides Hb C
Sickle cell β-thalassemia: S-β-thalassemia ($\alpha_2\beta_2^{6\ glu\rightarrow val}$ and $\alpha_2\delta_2$)
  One parent provides Hb S and one parent provides β-thalassemia

causes a mild hemolytic anemia and no sickle cell disease. However, if one parent provides a gene for Hb C and the other for Hb S, the resultant Hb SC combination leads to a particularly severe retinopathy. The abnormal hemoglobin causes abnormal oxygen binding, which results in thrombi, anemia, susceptibility to infection, and impaired growth and development. Blunt trauma to the eye is more likely to cause severe hyphema and vitreous hemorrhage in those with Hb S.

Heterozygous SA involves about 9% of blacks in the United States. These individuals are frequently asymptomatic; the major sign is painless hematuria arising from thrombosis and infarction of the kidney papillae.

In patients with homozygous Hb S disease, low oxygen tension may lead to infarction of the spleen, brain, and lungs. Symptoms and signs arise from sickling. Sickled erythrocytes trapped in capillaries cause stasis, anoxia, and decreased pH, resulting in further sickling, thrombosis, and infarction. The disease becomes manifest as Hb F replaced by Hb S. There are episodic attacks of abdominal or joint pain or aplastic anemia. Patients have increased susceptibility to many infectious agents. Cerebrovascular accidents, aseptic necrosis of bones, ulcers, and hepatic and hematologic disorders occur.

The ocular lesions arise from the intravascular changes either in the conjunctiva or in the retinal vessels. The conjunctival changes are asymptomatic and consist of multiple, short, comma-shaped or distorted capillary segments that appear separated from the vascular network. Unlike the retinal changes, they are most severe in SS disease, mild in SC disease, and rare in SA disease.

The most marked changes are retinal. Typically, lesions are in the temporal periphery with arteriolar occlusions followed by arteriolar-venular anastomoses (shunts) and aneurysmal dilations, arborizing vascular networks, focal constriction, dilation, and sheathing (Fig. 28-1, *A* and *B*). Neovascularization and fibrous proliferation are followed by vitreous hemorrhage and finally by retinal separation. In addition to the sickle cell retinopathy, angioid streaks (also associated with pseudoxanthoma elasticum and Paget disease) have been observed (see Fig. 16-17).

Whites of Mediterranean ancestry or blacks who develop hemolytic anemia, angioid streaks, recurrent vitreous hemorrhages (Eales disease), or a hemorrhagic retinopathy should have hemoglobin electrophoresis. In patients with Hb S, the ocular fundi, particularly the peripheral portions, should be studied through a maximally dilated pupil. Correction of retinal separation in patients with hemoglobinopathies is difficult, since encircling bands (p. 351) may cause necrosis of the anterior segment.

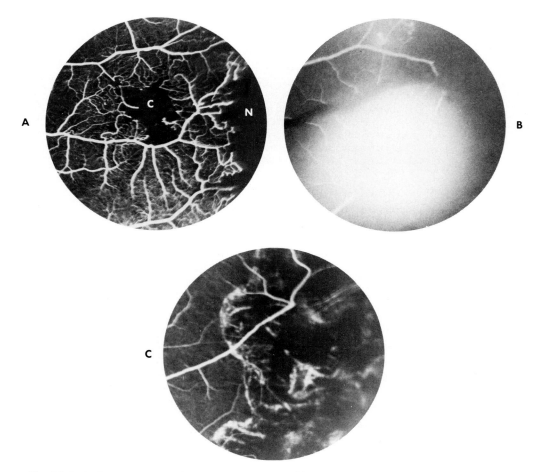

Fig. 28-1. A, Late venous angiogram in a 23-year-old woman with sickle cell hemoglobin C disease. Because of arteriolar occlusion there is a central area *(C)* of failure of capillary filling with fluorescein. There is distal occlusion in the periphery and early neovascularization adjacent to this area *(N)*. **B,** In the extreme periphery new blood vessels leak fluorescein. **C,** The new blood vessels have been destroyed by xenon photocoagulation of the retina.

Photocoagulation of newly formed blood vessels by means of a xenon arc photocoagulator (Fig. 28-1, *C*) or laser may minimize bleeding into the vitreous.

THALASSEMIA SYNDROMES

The thalassemia ("the sea") syndromes are hereditary abnormalities in which the rate of normal hemoglobin synthesis is impaired and in which the number of alpha or beta chains may be insufficient.

The major group arises because of a deficiency in the rate of synthesis of beta chains (beta-thalassemia) and substitution of delta chains. A deficiency of alpha chains (alpha-thalassemia) is more difficult to recognize and less clinically severe.

Hemolytic anemia and excessive deposition of iron in spleen, liver, and kidneys dominate the systemic aspects of the condition. The onset is in infancy, and the children have mongoloid facies with prominent epicanthal folds. There may be neovascularization of the peripheral retina as in sickle cell disease. The thalassemia syndromes may be combined with sickle cell hemoglobinopathies.

POLYCYTHEMIA

Polcythemia is an uncommon hematologic disorder in which there is an absolute increase in red blood cells. In primary polycythemia there is hyperactivity of all hematopoiesis, causing a panmyelosis. Secondary polycythemia arises because of conditions causing excessive release of erythropoietin, which is absent or reduced in the primary type. Secondary polycythemia occurs in response to persistent low oxygen tension in mountain dwellers and in patients with chronic lung disease, hypernephromas and cysts of the kidney, cerebellar hemangiomas, uterine myomas, and congenital heart disease.

Ocular symptoms are related to blood hyperviscosity and include dilation of conjunctival vessels and retinal vein dilation (cyanosis retinae), which appears as an impending vein closure. There may be retinal vein occlusion (p. 330) with visual loss. Ocular abnormalities may disappear with venesection. Papilledema has been reported as a complication of polycythemia without brain tumor. Transient loss of vision may occur. Retinal artery spasm has been reported.

LEUKOCYTE ABNORMALITIES

Stem cells from bone marrow may mature to B-lymphocytes or T-lymphocytes. B-lymphocytes mature under control of "bursal equivalent" cells (gut-associated lymphoid tissue: Peyer patches, appendix, and others), whereas T-lymphocytes mature under control of the thymus gland.

Thymus-dependent lymphocytes have a variety of functions. Although they do not secrete immunoglobulins, sensitized T-cells release lymphokines when in contact with an antigen. Lymphokines attract, activate, and prevent macrophages from leaving the site of antigen–T-cell interactions. The macrophages modify the antigen to stimulate B-cells to form immunoglobulins. The lymphokines increase vascular permeability. Some T-cells have a direct injurious effect on cells. K-cells, or killer cells, may reject cancer cells, although it is not entirely clear that they are T-cells.

B-lymphocytes form five soluble immunoglobulins (antibodies) that combine specifically with the provocative antigen. Immunoglobulin G (IgG) is the smallest but most common antibody molecule and contains the most anti-infectious antibodies. The concentration of immunoglobulin A (IgA) in plasma is second only to that of tears; IgA is formed locally in submucosal surfaces and participates in infections of mucous membranes of the mouth, gut, and conjunctiva. It is the major immunoglobulin of the tears. Immunoglobulin M (IgM) is the largest of the immunoglobulins (macroglobulins) and is confined to the vascular compartment in order to combat bacteremias. Its synthesis is inversely proportional to the concentration of IgG. The rheumatoid factor is an autoantibody of the IgM type. Immunoglobulin D (IgD) has an unknown function. Immunoglobulin E (IgE) has an affinity for basophils and mast cells and, on contact with an antigen, degranulates mast cells, releasing histamine and other vasoactive amines. It is responsible for immediate hypersensitivity reactions, such as atopic dermatitis, allergy, vernal conjunctivitis, and giant papillary conjunctivitis in contact lens wearers.

Immunoglobulin-producing B-lymphocytes further mature to immunoglobulin-producing and -secreting lymphocytes (plasma cells). Malignant or abnormal deviation can occur at any one of the steps in maturation. Thus chronic lymphatic leukemia is postulated to be a B-cell deviation, which in most cases is a malignant clonal deviation in a cell capable of producing but not secreting IgM. Multiple myeloma and Waldenström macroglobulinemia are considered to be a clonal deviation in a plasma cell capable of both producing and secreting an immunoglobulin (plasma cell).

Multiple myeloma. This is a neoplasm of plasma cells that elaborates an excess of a single immunoglobulin. The other immunoglobulins are present in decreased amounts. There are multiple osteolytic lesions ("punched out" type), anemia, proteinuria, myeloma (M-) proteins in the serum, and Bence Jones protein (subunits of the involved immunoblobulin) in the urine. If IgG is involved, there may be a fraction causing hyperviscosity of the blood (p. 555) or another fraction that precipitates at temperatures below 37° C and redissolves on warming (cryoglobulins).

The ocular signs may be divided into two main groups: (1) those arising from the neoplasm itself, such as orbital tumor, compression of cranial nerves within the orbit or head, and papilledema, and (2) those arising from blood viscosity changes, such as retinal hemorrhage and vascular occlusion. Cysts of the pars plana that are filled with protein, possibly a myeloma globulin, are found in about one third of the eyes removed at autopsy from patients with multiple myeloma.

Diffuse uveal accumulation of leukocytes may occur. Sludging and dilation of conjunctival blood vessels occur in cryoglobulinemia, and the signs may be accentuated by irritating the conjunctiva with cold water. Treatment consists of cytotoxic agents, ambulation, and adequate hydration.

Waldenström macroglobulinemia. This is a plasma cell abnormality involving plasma cells that produce and secrete

IgM. Onset of the disease is in the fifth or sixth decade and is characterized by severe anemia, lymphadenopathy, splenomegaly, and hepatomegaly suggestive of chronic lymphatic leukemia. The IgM globulins give rise to cryoglobulins and increased viscosity of the blood, which may give rise to vascular occlusions involving almost any system.

The main ocular signs relate to the blood hyperviscosity, which produces a spectacular fundus appearance of dilated veins, hemorrhages, cotton-wool patches, and exudative retinal detachment (p. 349). Treatment is by means of cytotoxic agents. When increased blood viscosity causes severe ocular or systemic symptoms, plasmaphoresis may cause prompt improvement.

Corneal dystrophy may occur in both multiple myeloma and Waldenström macroglobulinemia. The deposits are clinically suggestive of cholesterol. The dystrophy has appeared as early as 5 years before the onset of overt disease.

Leukemia. Leukemia is a disease of unknown cause of the blood-forming tissue characterized by abnormal proliferation of a precursor of one of the types of leukocytes. It may be classified as acute or chronic according to the maturity of cells in the peripheral blood or bone marrow and according to the cell type involved: myelocytic, monocytic, or lymphocytic. Its greatest incidence is before the fifth and after the fiftieth year of life.

The clinical features arise from infiltration of tissues, hemorrhage, and infection. Infiltration commonly involves the liver, spleen, and lymph nodes. Subperiosteal infiltration causes bone pain, and pathologic fractures may occur.

Infiltration and direct extension into the central nervous system may involve cranial nerves with ophthalmoplegia, deafness, or Ménière syndrome. Leukemic meningitis is common in treated cases, presumably because the chemical antileukemic agents do not cross the blood-brain barrier, so that leukemic cells proliferate in the meninges. Internal hydrocephalus may occur, with headache, nausea, increased cerebrospinal fluid pressure, and papilledema. Hydrocephalus may occur in an infant.

Infections are common, particularly infections of the oral cavity, skin, and rectum. Fungi and usually nonvirulent organisms may be involved, possibly because of predisposition secondary to antibiotic and corticosteroid therapy.

The diagnosis is made by hematologic examination. Types of treatment include corticosteroids, antimetabolites, irradiation (with radioactive phosphorus in chronic leukemias), and supportive treatment.

The ocular changes in leukemia arise from infiltration and hemorrhage involving the conjunctiva, sclera, retina, and choroid. Acute forms of leukemia are far more likely to cause ocular signs than chronic forms, but in both types, changes are likely to be reversible with remission. There is no clinical difference in ocular changes in lymphocytic leukemia and in myelogenous leukemia.

The conjunctiva is subtly and frequently involved in acute leukemias, with a slight thickening near the corneoscleral limbus arising from leukemic infiltrates. Infiltrates in the sclera are found on histologic study but do not cause clinical signs. The main ophthalmoscopic signs are as follows: (1) change in color of blood column caused by anemia or high leukocyte concentration; (2) dilated, tortuous veins of irregular caliber; (3) gray-white lines on either side of a vessel; (4) hard, yellow-white exudates and occasionally cotton-wool patches; (5) superficial and deep hemorrhages, commonly with a white spot (Fig. 28-2), leading on occasion to (6) vitreous hemorrhage. The choroid is often packed with leukemic cells, but visual symptoms are absent.

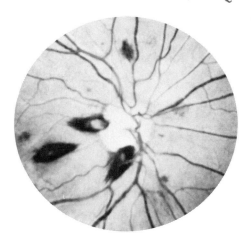

Fig. 28-2. Retinal hemorrhages in a 19-year-old man with acute myelogenous leukemia. The white spots at the center of the hemorrhage are leukocytes.

Hemorrhage usually occurs when the platelet count is less than 20,000/mm³. It may involve the mucous membranes, skin, kidney, conjunctiva, orbit, and retina. The retinal hemorrhage may be a large preretinal collection of blood with a meniscus. Subarachnoid hemorrhage may cause death.

Leukemic infiltration may give rise to obstruction of lacrimal drainage with the occurrence of a typical dacryocystitis. Intracranial infiltration may cause papilledema and cranial nerve abnormalities. Orbital infiltration may cause a severe proptosis.

Neoplasms. Lymphomas, lymphosarcomas, reticulum cell sarcoma, and Hodgkin disease are closely related neoplasms that affect lymphoid tissue and cause symptoms because of infiltration, compression, or obstruction of vital tissues or organs. The onset is insidious, the course is long, and diagnosis is based on the histologic study of involved tissue.

The ocular changes include the following: (1) eyelid involvement, with painless, progressive infiltration; (2) a characteristic subconjunctival tumor, frequently with smooth surfaces in the lower cul-de-sac; and (3) orbital or lacrimal gland enlargement, with proptosis causing diplopia, ocular compression, and the like.

Treatment is individualized as to site of involvement and symptoms and includes surgery, irradiation, chemotherapy, and corticosteroids. Commonly the ocular manifestations can be resolved with a dosage of radiation too low to cause cataract.

HEMORRHAGE (SYSTEMIC)

Optic atrophy is a rare complication of severe hemorrhage. The hemorrhage is often spontaneous from bowel lesions rather than traumatic. Loss of vision occurs either immediately or several days later. The arteries and the veins are small, the retina is pale, and the optic disk may be swollen. Cotton-wool patches may occur. There may be permanent, complete blindness, or vision may improve to normal. More often the vision remains at the 6/60 (20/200) level, and optic atrophy is evident. The arteries remain constricted. Acute blood loss may also cause visual defects from cortical interference, with no ocular fundus changes.

Chronic anemia or an acute anemia may cause a transient loss of vision in one or both eyes. The symptoms are most suggestive of occlusive disease involving the carotid-basilar system. Hypoxia secondary to hemorrhage may aggravate the visual defects of open-angle glaucoma.

RETICULOENDOTHELIAL SYSTEM DISORDERS

Unlike the abnormalities of lipid metabolism described in Chapter 24, there is no demonstrable metabolic defect in unifocal eosinophilic granuloma, multifocal eosinophilic granuloma (Hand-Schüller-Christian disease), Letterer-Siwe disease, or juvenile ocular xanthogranuloma (nevoxanthoendothelioma). Lipid, when present, is liberated as part of a locally destructive, inflammatory, and probably infectious process.

Eosinophilic granuloma, both focal and multifocal, represents a nonneoplastic response of well-differentiated histiocytes to an unknown stimulus. Letterer-Siwe disease is a lymphomatous proliferation of poorly differentiated histiocytes. Juvenile ocular xanthogranuloma may represent a transitional form between the solely cutaneous involvement of nevoxanthoendothelioma and the systemic involvement of the other conditions.

Different histopathologic pictures may develop simultaneously in the same patient. The characteristic four stages are as follows: (1) a histiocytic proliferative stage with accumulation of eosinophils, (2) vascular granulomatous stage, (3) diffuse xanthomatous stage with abundance of "foam" cells, and (4) fibrous dysplasia stage.

Unifocal eosinophilic granuloma. Unifocal eosinophilic granuloma is an abnormality localized to bone that may have one, several, or many areas of histiocytic proliferation, with eosinophils. There is no intracellular lipid accumulation. An orbital bone may be involved with a circumscribed osteolytic granuloma demonstrable on roentgenographic examination.

Multifocal eosinophilic granuloma (Hand-Schüller-Christian disease). This is an idiopathic, nonspecific type of histiocytic proliferation occurring usually before the age of 10 years. It is characterized by the development of multiple lipid granulomas. The classic triad is polyuria, exophthalmos, and skull defects. The polyuria arises from a diabetes insipidus caused by a deficiency of antidiuretic hormone secondary to involvement of the tubercinereum and the hypothalamus. Histiocytic lesions commonly involve the skull, particularly the temporoparietal region, and give rise to otitis media. The skeletal involvement is painless and in the skull gives rise to large, confluent areas with a maplike roentgenographic appearance. Growth abnormalities are commonly present. Exophthalmos is often present and arises from orbital accumulation of granulomatous tissue that may be combined with granulomas of orbital bones. Ophthalmoplegia, papilledema, and loss of vision may follow either mechanical displacement or actual infiltration of the skull or orbit.

The skeletal lesions, but not the visceral manifestations, respond to localized roentgen-ray therapy. The polyuria tends to resist treatment, and the occurrence of spontaneous improvement suggests involvement of the adrenal glands, the anterior pituitary gland, or the hypothalamus. Corticosteroids and ACTH have been helpful, as has chemotherapy, sometimes in combination with corticosteroids.

Letterer-Siwe disease. This is a rapidly fatal disease of infancy characterized by fever, osseous lesions, hemorrhage, progressive anemia, and hepatosplenomegaly. Ocular signs may be secondary to skull involvement.

Juvenile ocular xanthogranuloma (nevoxanthoendothelioma). This is an ocular complication of what is usually considered to be a disease solely of the skin. Inconspicuous, small, yellow-orange plaques on the head and trunk develop during the first 5 years of life. They disappear without treatment. If removed for histologic study, the scar may be infiltrated with a similar plaque.

When there is ocular involvement, there may be frank bleeding into the anterior chamber, which may cause secondary glaucoma. Glaucoma with enlargement of the globe may occur without a hyphema. The iris and the ciliary body are infiltrated with histiocytes, which become fused to form giant (Teuton) cells. The ocular disease is sensitive to small doses of radiation.

Other causes of hyphema, such as retinoblastoma, leukemia, injury, and persistent primary vitreous, should be excluded. The occurrence of typical skin lesions should distinguish secondary glaucoma from congenital glaucoma caused by either a malformation of the chamber angle or neurofibromatosis of von Recklinghausen.

BIBLIOGRAPHY

Galinos, S., Rabb, M. F., Goldberg, M. F., and Frenkel, M.: Hemoglobin SC disease and iris atrophy, Am. J. Ophthalmol. **75**:421, 1973.

Jampol, L. M., Goldberg, M. F., and Busse, B.: Peripheral retinal microaneurysms in chronic leukemia, Am. J. Ophthalmol. **80**:242, 1975.

Madigan, J. C., Jr., Gragoudas, E. S., Schwartz, P. L., and Lapus, J. V.: Peripheral retinal neovascularization in sarcoidosis and sickle cell anemia, Am. J. Ophthalmol. **83**:387, 1977.

Moschandreou, M., Galinos, S., Valenzuela, R., and others: Retinopathy in hemoglobin C trait (AC hemoglobinopathy), Am. J. Ophthalmol. **77**:465, 1974.

Raichand, M., Goldberg, M. F., Nagpal, K. D., and others: Evaluation of neovascularization in sickle cell retinopathy, Arch. Ophthalmol. **95**:1543, 1977.

Sorr, E. M., and Goldberg, R. E.: Traumatic central retinal occlusion with sickle cell trait, Am. J. Ophthalmol. **80**:648, 1975.

Chapter 29

DISORDERS OF CONNECTIVE TISSUE, JOINTS AND STRIATED MUSCLE, AND SKIN

DISORDERS OF CONNECTIVE TISSUE

The specialized cells of the eye as well as other parts of the body are supported by connective tissue fibers embedded in a nonstructural matrix. The connective tissue consists of (1) cellular elements, (2) collagenous and elastic fibers, and (3) ground substance.

The cellular elements are derived from mesenchyme and include (1) fibroblasts, which are responsible for the elaboration of the endogenous elements of connective tissue; (2) macrophages, which are histiocytes that function as phagocytes; (3) mast cells, which are implicated in the formation of heparin and possibly of hyaluronic acid, and which are rich in histamine and serotonin; (4) lymphocytes that produce antibodies; and (5) lymphocytes, which carry the genocopy of antigenic determinants that are transmitted to immunologically competent cells.

The main fibrous elements of connective tissue are collagen and elastic fibers. Collagen is a fibrous protein of high tensile strength that has characteristic striations with regular bands at intervals of 64 nm. It contains two unique amino acids, hydroxyproline and hydroxylysine, as well as large amounts of proline and glycine. The hydroxyl group on the hydroxylysine is conjugated to galactose or glucosyl galactose.

Elastic fibers are extensible structures stained by orcein and digested by elastase. They are found in tissues characterized by extensibility, such as arteries, skin, and some ligaments.

The ground substance (from the German words *grund substanz,* meaning fundamental) is the extracellular, extrafibrillar, amorphous matrix of connective tissue. Some components are derived from the fibroblast, such as acid mucoprotein, acid mucopolysaccharide, and soluble collagen (procollagen). Additionally, the ground substance contains water molecules such as glucose, cell metabolites, plasma proteins, and similar substances reflecting the passage of metabolites between cells.

The connective tissue (collagen) disorders (Table 29-1) are a heterogeneous group of maladies in which fibrinoid material is deposited in the ground substance of connective tissue and inflammation of connective tissue is widespread. Some patients respond favorably

Table 29-1. Connective tissue disorders

I. Hereditary disorders
  A. Marfan syndrome
  B. Pseudoxanthoma elasticum
  C. Ehlers-Danlos syndrome
    1. Gravis
    2. Mitis
    3. Benign hypermobile
    4. Ecchymotic (vascular)
    5. X chromosome–linked
    6. Ocular
  D. Osteogenesis imperfecta
II. Acquired disorders
  A. Seropositive conditions
    1. Sjögren syndrome
    2. Rheumatoid arthritis
      a. Juvenile rheumatoid arthritis (including Still disease)
    3. Systemic lupus erythematosus
  B. Seronegative conditions
    1. Polyarteritis of unknown etiology
      a. Ankylosing spondylitis
      b. Psoriatic arthritis
      c. Reiter syndrome
    2. Necrotizing arteritis and other forms of vasculitis
      a. Polyarteritis nodosa
      b. Hypersensitivity angiitis
      c. Wegener granulomatosis
      d. Giant cell arteritis
      e. Takayasu disease (pulseless disease) (p. 532)
      f. Cogan syndrome (p. 265)
    3. Other conditions
      a. Ulcerative colitis
      b. Crohn disease
      c. Behçet syndrome
      d. Erythema nodosum
      e. Relapsing polychondritis
      f. Sarcoidosis (p. 471)
      g. Amyloidosis (p. 489)
      h. Polymyositis and dermomyositis
      i. Progressive systemic sclerosis (scleroderma)

to corticosteroid therapy, and this has led to use of the term "collagen disease" for any disorder of obscure etiology that improves with corticosteroid therapy.

Marfan syndrome. This is a widespread autosomal dominant systemic abnormality of connective tissue. The major manifestations include ectopia lentis, aortic dilatation, dissecting aneurysm of the aorta, and multiple skeletal defects, particularly excessive length of long bones. The pubis-to-sole measurement is characteristically in excess of the pubis-to-vertex measurement, and the arm span is in excess of the height. The more distal bones tend to demonstrate excessive length (arachnodactyly: spider fingers). There is a weakness of the joint capsule, causing flatfoot, hyperextensibility of the joints, recurrent dislocation of the hip, and kyphoscoliosis. Pigeon breast (pectus excavatum) may occur. Frequently the patient has a long, narrow face and a highly arched palate, and prognathism is present.

Subluxation of the lens is the outstanding ocular change. Characteristic deformities of the chamber angle are present (Fig. 29-1). The lens is usually dislocated upward and inward, and the zonular fibers are drawn taut in the inferior temporal quadrant. Ectopia lentis may be suspected only because of the abnormal mobility of the iris (iridodonesis), which lacks the support of the lens. The lens may be smaller than normal and may be spherical. In some patients, ectopia lentis may be the only stigma of the Marfan syndrome.

Patients with this abnormality tend to be myopic and to develop retinal degeneration, and subsequent retinal detachment is more common than in normal individuals. The retinal degeneration is apparently related to an elastic fiber defect and not to the myopia. Heterochromia iridis, translucence of the iris diaphragm, keratoconus, megalocornea, and blue scleras may be present. In general, surgical removal of the subluxated lens is not indicated (p. 376). Complications are common, and surgery should be deferred unless necessitated by glaucoma that has not responded to medical therapy.

The major differential diagnosis in-

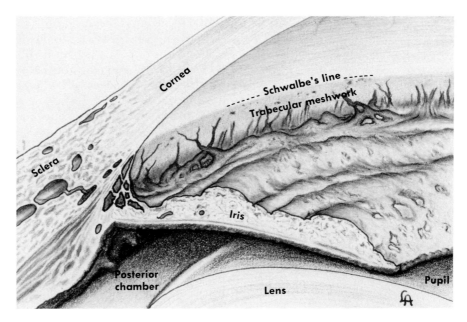

Fig. 29-1. Chamber angle anomalies in a patient with Marfan syndrome. There are coarse, pigmented, densely packed pectinate ligament fibers bridging the anterior chamber angle and inserting into the trabecular zone. The lens is dislocated. (From Burian, H. M., von Noorden, G. K., and Ponseti, I. V.: Arch. Ophthalmol. **64**:671, 1961.)

volves other causes of ectopia lentis, particularly homocystinuria (pp. 376 and 494) or Weill-Marchesani syndrome (p. 375).

Pseudoxanthoma elasticum. This is a generally autosomal recessive abnormality characterized by changes in the skin, cardiovascular system, and eyes. The basic defect is presumably in the elastic fibers, and widespread systemic changes occur because of involvement of the muscular arteries. The skin of the face, neck, axillary folds, inguinal folds, cubital areas, and periumbilical areas becomes lax and grooved, redundant and relatively inelastic, and resembles coarse-grain Moroccan leather. Involvement of the small muscular arteries may cause hemorrhages in the gastrointestinal tract, which must be distinguished from those that occur with peptic ulcer. Similarly, hemorrhages may occur in the brain, kidney, uterus, bladder, and nose. A severe hyper-

tension that aggravates the hemorrhagic tendency commonly occurs.

The characteristic ocular change is angioid streaks (see Fig. 18-1) (Grönblad-Strandberg, p. 345), a bizarre network of pigmented lines involving particularly the posterior pole and often associated with preretinal neovascularization and focal chorioretinal atrophy. Ultimately there is involvement of the central retina with disciform degeneration.

Ehlers-Danlos syndrome. This generalized systemic disorder is clinically characterized by hyperextensibility of the joints, kyphoscoliosis, and hyperelastic skin (India rubber-men). The skin is fragile and easily bruised ("cigarette paper"), and pseudotumor may occur at pressure points. Multiple internal abnormalities occur with arterial aneurysms, diaphragmatic hernia, and congenital defects of the heart, the respiratory and gastrointestinal tracts, and the genitalia.

The skin of the eyelids is often involved. Epicanthal folds may be present. The eyelids are easily everted. Esotropia is common, as are blue scleras, and glaucoma has been recorded. Additionally, there may be ectopia lentis, proliferative retinopathy, hemorrhages into the retina, and detachment of the retina.

There are a variety of types. In the hydrolysine-deficient type there is a deficiency of lysyl hydrolase, which catalyzes the hydroxylation of lysine to hydroxylysine, and weakening of collagen cross-linking. Ocular abnormalities predominate in this type. Microcornea or megalocornea, extreme thinning of the cornea, corneal rupture caused by slight trauma, ectopia lentis, cataract, and retinal separation occur. All patients with blue scleras should be warned against contact sports, because the thinning of their corneas (fragilitas oculi) predisposes to rupture.

Osteogenesis imperfecta. This is mainly an autosomal dominant disorder in which there are bright blue scleras, otosclerosis, loose-jointedness, hernia, and multiple long-bone fractures with minimal trauma. There is dwarfism with short legs and a large head.

The scleras in patients with osteogenesis imperfecta are vividly blue. The color, described as robin's egg blue, slate blue, and Wedgewood blue, is apparently caused by thinning of the sclera so that the choroid is seen beneath. Often the corneoscleral limbus is white, resulting in a Saturn ring. Corneal arcus is common. The eyes are frequently hyperopic, and there may be keratoconus, megalocornea, and maculas of the cornea. The fundamental defect suggests that there is failure of maturation of collagen, which remains in the reticulum fiber stage.

Treatment is symptomatic.

Sjögren syndrome. This is a chronic connective tissue disease that occurs predominantly in women (90% of the cases). It is manifested by keratoconjunctivitis sicca (dry eyes), xerostomia (dry mouth), and chronic arthritis. There is dryness of the eyes, nose, mouth, pharynx, tracheobronchial tree, vagina, stomach, and skin together with lymphocytic and plasma cell infiltration of the salivary glands and, occasionally, of the lacrimal glands, which causes enlargement. Histologic and immunologic abnormalities suggest involvement of both T-cell and B-cell mechanisms.

The disorder predominantly affects middle-aged women but may have its onset at extremes of 5 and 72 years. The syndrome may include dry skin, pancreatitis, interstitial nephritis, hepatobiliary disease, thyroid abnormalities, and lymphoma. Excessive proliferation and abnormal distribution of lymphoid and plasma cells may impair function of major organs,

Keratoconjunctivitis sicca (p. 268) (L. *siccus*, dry) causes burning or smarting of the eyes, sometimes associated with severe photophobia. The symptoms are aggravated by a dry, hot environment. Occasionally, a filamentary keratitis occurs in which minute horns of epithelium extend from the corneal surface. A yellowish white, thick, tenacious secretion may gather on the inner corner of the eyelids. Large areas of the conjunctival and corneal epithelium may be absent, and the tissues stain with rose bengal or fluorescein. The Schirmer test (p. 232) indicates less than a 5-mm wetting of the filter paper strip. The enzyme lysozyme (muramidase) (p. 85) is decreased. Dryness of the mouth (xerostomia) causes burning pain and paresthesia of the mouth and tongue with atrophy of the lip and oral mucous membrane. Patients are unable to swallow a tablet of medication without drinking water.

The laboratory signs indicate a widespread abnormality of immunologic mechanisms. B-cell lymphocytes synthesize large amounts of IgG and IgM, including rheumatoid factor. There are often autoantibodies directed against the salivary, lacrimal, and thyroid glands, as well as against the smooth muscle, salivary ducts, and mitochondria. The sedimentation rate is increased. A chronic viral infection may be present.

Treatment is often unsatisfactory, and death may occur from infection. The dry eye (p. 268) is treated with artificial tears and by avoiding conditions that favor the rapid evaporation of tears, such as hot, dry rooms. Artificial tears may be instilled as often as every 30 or 60 minutes. Closure of the lacrimal puncta to conserve the remaining tears is not often effective and is used only in severe cases.

In some patients malignant lymphomas develop. In severe progressive disease, treatment by means of immune suppression seems useful.

Rheumatoid arthritis. This is a chronic systemic disease of unknown cause that has a familial tendency and onset between the ages of 25 and 50 years. Women are affected more commonly (75%). The onset is insidious, with pain and swelling in one or more joints that may become chronic and involve all joints with contraction and deformity. There may be constitutional disturbances such as lymphadenopathy, splenomegaly, fever, tachycardia, leukocytosis, and increased sedimentation rate. Subcutaneous nodules occur at sites of pressure over bones. They vary in size from 2 or 3 mm to 3 cm in diameter. They are composed of a central necrotic area surrounded by a zone of fibroblasts enveloped in a zone of granulation tissue.

The ocular manifestations are caused by an inflammatory-exudative alteration in connective tissue elements. Ocular changes are fairly common, so that the possibility of associated rheumatoid arthritis, especially ankylosing spondylitis, must be considered in every case of nongranulomatous iritis and scleral inflammation.

Iritis may precede or follow the acute

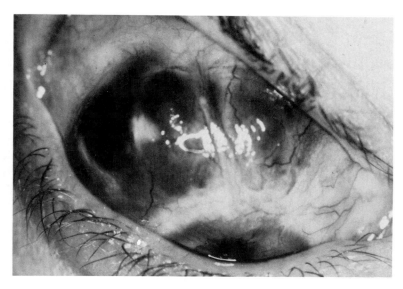

Fig. 29-2. Scleromalacia perforans in a 39-year-old woman with rheumatoid arthritis. The condition has remained unchanged for the past 10 years.

disease but usually accompanies it. Most attacks are mild, may involve either eye, and may be recurrent. The severity of the attack varies. It responds quickly to systemic and local corticosteroids. In some patients the inflammation is extremely severe and is unresponsive to therapy, with progression to secondary glaucoma and cataract formation. About 4% of the patients with rheumatoid arthritis develop iritis.

Development of rheumatoid nodules in the sclera causes scleromalacia perforans (Fig. 29-2) in which the sclera appears to melt away. Additionally, rheumatoid nodules in the sclera may cause a massive granuloma (brawny scleritis or annular scleritis), in which there is massive scar formation, or necroscleritis nodosa, limited to small areas of the anterior sclera.

Juvenile rheumatoid arthritis (Still disease). This uncommon disease is identical to adult rheumatoid arthritis. It occurs insidiously at about the time of second dentition. Systemic signs of fever, leukocytosis, splenomegaly, lymphadenopathy, and hepatomegaly are common. Iridocyclitis (15%) tends to be bilateral and resistant to treatment. Secondary cataract may develop. A band-shaped keratopathy (90%) develops, with a deposition of calcium in the superficial layers of the cornea. It usually accompanies the iridocyclitis. Posterior inflammation is uncommon, but bilateral retinal separation may occur. A similar keratopathy occurs in degenerated eyes, with excessive vitamin D intake, and in hypercalcemia.

Ankylosing spondylitis (Marie-Strümpell disease). This is an inflammatory disease of the hip and shoulder joints that causes back pain, has a variable course, and involves white young men predominantly (90%). Acute anterior uveitis occurs in 20% to 30% of the patients. The diagnosis is often suggested when a young man with uveitis has difficulty in adjusting himself to the chin-rest of a biomicroscope. Histocompatability typing indicates that 90% to 95% of spondylitic patients have HLA-B27 antigen, as contrasted with 7% in the normal white population. Individuals with Reiter syndrome (p. 304) and acute anterior uveitis also have HLA-B27 antigens but less often than those with ankylosing spondylitis.

Giant cell arteritis. Giant cell arteritis (temporal arteritis, cranial arteritis) is a chronic inflammatory disease of segments of large and medium-sized arteries in persons more than 60 years of age. It may be identical to polymyalgia rheumatica, in which there is fever, headache, and pain in the muscles and joints. The erythrocyte sedimentation rate is increased. In temporal arteritis the arteries are painful, tender, and prominent, with nodularity and frequently erythema of the overlying skin. Pain on chewing is a common complaint.

Some 1 to 4 weeks after the onset of the disease, sudden loss of vision may arise caused by occlusion of the central retinal artery or of the short posterior ciliary arteries that supply the optic nerve. There may be branch occlusion of retinal arteries, hemorrhage, exudates, and occasionally ocular pain. Often both eyes are affected, the second eye from 1 to 21 days after the first.

Palsies of external ocular muscles, especially of the lateral recti muscles, may occur. Loss of vision may occur in some patients without obvious evidence of temporal artery involvement, but biopsy of the temporal artery may indicate the typical histiocytes, epithelioid cells, and multinucleated giant cells in intima and media adjacent to a highly fragmented or absent elastic lamina. Some patients appear curiously unconcerned about the devastating loss of vision.

The diagnosis of giant cell arteritis should be considered in all cases of sudden loss of vision, ocular vascular occlusion, and unexplained ophthalmoplegia in individuals more than 60 years of age. If ocular symptoms are associated with an increase in the sedimentation rate, temporal artery biopsy should be performed, since the rate is increased during the actual disease. Serum alkaline phosphatase is also increased.

Once vision is lost it seldom improves, but remarkable recovery has been reported. Corticosteroids should be administered before permanent visual loss has occurred.

Systemic lupus erythematosus. This is a generalized systemic disorder that may involve nearly any system and may be associated with severe constitutional signs. Young women are affected predominantly. The disease appears to arise from a hyperreactive immunologic system, which causes the synthesis of anticell, anticytoplasmic, and antinuclear antibodies. Fever, a rash on the face with a "butterfly" distribution, and an arthralgia may occur. Glomerulonephritis, pericarditis, myocardial and endocardial lesions, or pleurisy may develop. Mental changes, convulsions, and cranial nerves may be involved, with diplopia, nystagmus, and decreased vision. Leukopenia caused by a decrease in mononuclear cells is common. Excessive IgG is present, and there is an increased fibrinogen and erythrocyte sedimentation rate, false-positive tests for syphilis, and positive flocculation tests. Lupus erythematosus may simulate almost any clinical disease, and the diagnosis may be neglected because of failure to associate successive involvement of different systems with the same disease.

External involvement of the eye is mainly erythema and puffiness of the eyelids when involved in the "butterfly" rash. Keratoconjunctivitis sicca has been known to occur. The most common ocular sign is cotton-wool patches (p. 325) at the posterior pole. The lesions appear during a toxic phase of the disease and disappear with remission. They appear first as soft, white spots that become sharply delineated and gradually disappear over a 1-month to 3-month period. They are not associated with hypertensive vascular disease. Changes other than cotton-wool patches have been described rarely: secondary optic atrophy, superficial and deep retinal hemorrhages, and arterial and venous occlusion. Chloroquine is widely used in therapy and may itself cause retinal damage (p. 141).

Systemic sclerosis (scleroderma). This is a systemic disease with symptoms that may involve any system. The cutaneous signs are widespread leathery skin, which becomes atrophic and pigmented and fixed to underlying structures. The eyelids lose their elasticity and then become thin, smooth, and shiny. Cutaneous signs may not occur. Major systemic involvement includes Raynaud phenomenon, dysphagia, pulmonary insufficiency, pulmonary hypertension, cardiac signs, polymyositis, and rheumatoid arthritis. Abnormal gamma globulins resemble those of systemic lupus erythematosus.

Sjögren syndrome (p. 563) may occur. An atypical uveitis, with graying of the eyelashes (poliosis), vitiligo, and dysacousia (Vogt-Koyanagi syndrome, p. 308), has been described. Cotton-wool patches may occur on the retina without vascular hypertension.

Dermatomyositis. This is an acute or chronic disease of middle life characterized by edema, dermatitis, and multiple muscle inflammation. It often follows an infection, and in patients more than 40 years of age may be associated with a neoplasm (20%). A peculiar periorbital edema associated with a reddish brown erythema of the eyelids (heliotrope) may occur. Ophthalmoplegia, nystagmus, and episcleritis have been described. A retinopathy with cotton-wool patches may be present.

Polyarteritis (periarteritis nodosa). This is a necrotizing angiitis that causes a variety of symptoms depending on the blood vessels involved. Men are involved more frequently (75%), usually between the ages of 20 and 50 years. Constitutional symptoms of fever, weight loss, and arthralgia occur. Symptoms include abdominal pain, renal disease often causing a vascular hypertension when healed, peripheral neuritis, myocardial infarction, pulmonary infiltration, and asthma. Leukocytosis is present, often with marked eosinophilia, and the sedimentation rate is increased. The disease is often fatal, but remissions and recovery occur. Symptomatic relief follows administration of corticosteroids.

Involvement of cerebral vessels may cause subarachnoid hemorrhage, headache, vertigo, and convulsions. There may be involvement of motor nerves of the eye or decreased vision with involvement of the optic tracts or radiation.

Local involvement of ocular vessels causes conjunctival chemosis and scleral necrosis. Involvement of the pericorneal arcade may be followed by corneal necrosis beginning at the corneoscleral limbus. Periarteritis of the choroidal vessels has been found histologically with no history or signs of disturbed function. Ophthalmologic findings are common, although often the eyes are not examined. Hypertensive retinopathy with papilledema, cotton-wool patches, and vasospasm may follow renal disease and be in no way different from any other vascular hypertension. Cotton-wool patches may develop as a toxic sign unrelated to hypertension, as in the other collagen diseases.

Miscellaneous connective tissue disorders. A variety of conditions with prominent ocular signs may be classified in the group of connective tissue disorders. Rei-

ter syndrome (urethritis, conjunctivitis, uveitis, p. 304) and Behçet syndrome (aphthous ulcers, uveitis, p. 304) are discussed in the section on uveitis. Cogan syndrome (p. 265), in which there is interstitial keratitis, deafness, and vestibular signs, is described in the diseases of the cornea. Polyarteritis nodosa (25%) and vasculitis have also been described. A reported relationship with histocompatibility antigen HLA-B17 was not found in ten instances. The several aortic arch inflammations that may be variants of polyarteritis are described in Chapter 26. A variety of localized ocular disorders arise because of connective tissue abnormalities but are seldom classed as such, including pterygia, pingueculas, corneal dystrophies, and keratoconus.

MUSCLE DISORDERS

Myotonic dystrophy. This is an autosomal dominant disorder that affects not only muscular tissue but causes widespread ocular involvement, testicular and ovarian atrophy, endocrine changes, and mental deterioration. There is muscle wasting, often of the extremities, and inability of muscles to relax after voluntary contraction. Cardiac muscle is often involved. Frontal baldness, atrophy of the muscles of mastication, enophthalmos, and blepharoptosis of the upper eyelid combine to produce a long, expressionless, hawklike face. The onset is often in the third or fourth decade of life, although the myotonia may cause persistent closure of the eyelids after crying in infancy.

Cataract is the most common ocular finding and may precede muscular weakness. The lens opacities may be minute, brilliantly colored specks (iridescent dust) or snowball shaped. They seldom progress enough to cause visual disturbance. Blepharoptosis of the upper eyelid and weakness and rigidity of the extraocular muscle are almost constant in later years. Myofibrils, which are originally irregular, eventually disappear. The pupils are miotic and react sluggishly to light. Granular pigmentation in the central retina occurs together with impaired dark adaptation and reduced scoptic electroretinogram.

Myasthenia gravis. This is a chronic disease of skeletal muscle characterized by easy fatigability of muscle groups. Adults with myasthenia gravis have several different antibodies directed against the receptors of acetylcholine that contribute to the adult form of the disease.

In approximately 15% of the cases, unilateral or bilateral blepharoptosis and ophthalmoplegia constitute the only evidence of the disease. In an additional 40% of cases, ocular signs are combined with skeletal or oropharyngeal weakness. There are no ocular signs in the remainder. In patients with otherwise profound ophthalmoplegia, there may be twitchlike or quiver movements that are highly characteristic of myasthenia gravis. They are elicited by asking the patient to change his gaze from downward to straight ahead. There may be a rapid movement of the eyes of 3° to 4° described as quiver, lightning, twitchlike, or jellylike oscillations. An eyelid twitch may also occur.

Women are affected in 75% of the cases when the age of onset is less than 35 years; thereafter there is no sex predilection. Weakness is often exacerbated in the premenstrual period in young women.

The diagnosis is based on the history of fluctuations in strength and confirmed by the administration of edrophonium (Tensilon). (Atropine sulfate, 0.4 mg, should be available to counteract cholinergic toxicity.) Edrophonium is administered intravenously in a dosage of 2 to 10 mg; if myasthenia gravis is present, relief of blepharoptosis, improvement of speech, and generalized muscle strengthening will occur within 30 to 60 seconds and persist 2 to 3 minutes, although the effect

of the drug may be unusually short. The extraocular muscles are resistant to cholinergic effects, and ophthalmoplegia may not be grossly responsive, although diplopia may decrease slightly, intraocular pressure may increase, and electromyography of an affected ocular muscle may show increased activity.

Hyperthyroidism occurs in some 3% to 8% of patients with myasthenia gravis and must be excluded. A myasthenialike syndrome occurs in association with oat cell carcinoma of the lung, presumably on a toxic basis.

The classic treatment for systemic myasthenia gravis is anticholinesterase medication. Blepharoptosis of the upper eyelid responds well, but the extraocular muscle paresis may be resistant. The instillation of 0.25% eserine solution into the conjunctival cul-de-sac may be helpful.

Erythema multiforme (Stevens-Johnson syndrome). This is an acute perivascular inflammatory systemic disease that varies in severity from mild skin and mucous membrane lesions to a severe, sometimes fatal systemic disorder. Ophthalmologists describe the disease with ocular involvement as Stevens-Johnson syndrome. The disease affects all ages. The cause is unknown, but the condition is associated with infectious agents and drugs. Topical sulfacetamide sodium, topical anesthetics, systemic sulfonamides, acetazolamide, phenytoin (Dilantin), and antibiotics have all been implicated as sensitizing agents.

The onset is variable, with mild to severe constitutional symptoms of fever, malaise, myalgia, and arthralgia and the symptoms of an upper respiratory tract infection. Skin and mucous membrane lesions develop 1 to 14 days later, often with systemic reaction. The skin lesions develop symmetrically and in crops and vary considerably in appearance. Vesicles and bullae may develop on preex-

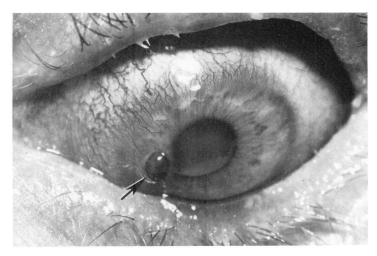

Fig. 29-3. Spontaneous corneal perforation in a 17-year-old man who had erythema multiforme at the age of 4 years. The iris has prolapsed into the corneal opening *(arrow),* and there is ciliary injection and corneal neovascularization.

isting central retinal papules or wheals. A pale white center may be surrounded by shades of erythema, called iris, target, or bull's-eye lesions. Ulcerations and scaling take place with healing, leaving pigmented and depigmented areas. The mouth, pharynx, vagina, and rectum may have erosions and ulcerations. These heal, leaving scarred areas that suggest the diagnosis long after the disease has cleared.

The skin of the eyelids may be involved. A conjunctivitis develops, varying in severity from catarrhal to pseudomembranous. There may be marked swelling of the eyelids. An acute iritis may occur. In severe cases the cornea may perforate (Fig. 29-3), resulting in loss of the eye. The active inflammation may persist for weeks. Treatment during the acute phase is mainly supportive. Secondary bacterial infection may be combated with antibiotics; corticosteroids may be used.

With healing there are often adhesions between the tarsal and the bulbar conjunctivae (symblepharon). Trichiasis is common. The most marked symptoms arise from keratoconjunctivitis sicca caused by scarring of the orifices of the lacrimal glands. The eyes are dry, uncomfortable, and injected. Corneal vascularization occurs easily. Infection may occur. Treatment is by means of soft contact lenses and artificial tear substitutes and by transplantation of the Stensen duct of the parotid gland to provide saliva as a substitute for tears.

BIBLIOGRAPHY

Albert, D. M., Ruchman, M. C., and Keltner, J. L.: Skip areas in temporal arteritis, Arch. Ophthalmol. **94:**2072, 1976.

Brenkman, R. F., Oosterhuis, J. A., and Manschot, W. A.: Recurrent hemorrhage in the anterior chamber caused by a (juvenile) xanthogranuloma of the iris in an adult, Doc. Ophthalmol. **42:**329, 1977.

Drachman, D. B.: Myasthenia gravis, N. Engl. J. Med. **298:**136, 186, 1978.

Drachman, D. B., Angus, C. W., Adams, R. N., and others: Myasthenic antibodies cross-link acetylcholine receptors to accelerate degradation, N. Engl. J. Med. **298:**1116, 1978.

Eberl, R., and Rosenthal, M., editors: Organic manifestations and complications in rheumatoid arthritis, Stuttgart, 1976, Schattauer.

Fulton, A. B., Lee, R. V., Jampol, L. M., and others: Active giant cell arteritis with cerebral involvement, Arch. Ophthalmol. **94:**2068, 1976.

Huston, K. A., Hunder, G. G., Lie, J. T., and others: Temporal arteritis, Ann. Intern. Med. **88:**162, 1978.

Judisch, G. F., Waziri, M., and Krachmer, J. H.: Ocular Ehler-Danlos syndrome with normal lysyl hydroxylase activity, Arch. Ophthalmol. **94:**1489, 1976.

Kanski, J. J.: Anterior uveitis in juvenile rheumatoid arthritis, Arch. Ophthalmol. **95:**1794, 1977.

Key, S. N. III, and Kimura, S. J.: Iridocyclitis associated with juvenile rheumatoid arthritis, Am. J. Ophthalmol. **80:**425, 1975.

Kuwabara, T., and Lessell, S.: Electron microscopic study of extraocular muscles in myotonic dystrophy, Am. J. Ophthalmol. **82:**303, 1976.

Maumenee, I. H.: Hereditary connective tissue diseases involving the eye, Trans. Ophthalmol. Soc. U.K. **94:**753, 1974.

Moutsopoulos, H. M., and Chused, T. M.: B lymphocyte antigens in sicca syndrome, Science **199:**1441, 1978.

Ruben, Z.: Ophthalmic sulfonamid-induced Stevens-Johnson syndrome, Arch. Dermatol. **113:**235, 1977.

Spalter, H. F.: The visual prognosis in juvenile rheumatoid arthritis, Trans. Am. Ophthalmol. Soc. **73:**554, 1976.

Vassilopoulos, D., Alevizos, B., and Spengos, M.: Cataract and gamma-glutamyl cycle in myotonic dystrophy, Ophthalmologica **174:**167, 1977.

Appendices

Appendix A

GLOSSARY

ablepharon absence of the eyelids.

abnormal (anomalous) retinal correspondence condition in which corresponding points on the two retinas do not have the same relative direction in space.

> *disharmonious* angle of abnormality is less than the angle of strabismus.
>
> *harmonious* angle of abnormality is the same as the angle of strabismus.

accommodation process by which the refractive power of the lens is increased through contraction of the ciliary muscle (N III), causing an increased thickness and curvature of the lens.

accommodative esotropia inward deviation of the eyes characteristically more marked for near than far and increased by ciliary muscle contraction in accommodation.

achromatopia color blindness; often applied to complete color blindness.

after-cataract opacity of posterior capsule after extracapsular lens extraction.

after-image visual sensation occurring after the stimulus causing it has ceased.

agnosia inability to recognize objects by sight with ability to recognize by touch; a sign of lesions of the angular gyrus of the parieto-occipital fissure.

agraphia (visual) loss of ability to write.

albinism inherited absence or deficiency of tyrosinase characterized by an absence or decrease of melanin in the skin, hair, and eyes.

alternating cross-eyes deviation of the eyes in which either eye may be used for fixation while the other deviates.

amaurosis nearly obsolete term indicating loss of vision.

amblyopia subnormal visual acuity.

> *ex anopsia* functional, refractive, sensory, or strabismic amblyopia now preferred.
>
> *functional* cortical inhibition as in refractive or strabismic amblyopia.
>
> *refractive* arises from a refractive error, particu-

larly a marked difference in refraction of the two eyes (anisometropia).

> *relative* associated with sensory amblyopia on which is superimposed an inhibition as in strabismic amblyopia.
>
> *sensory* caused by organic disease such as optic atrophy, central retinal degeneration, or cataract.
>
> *strabismic* associated with crossing of the eyes that occurs before the establishment of normal visual acuity in each eye; there appears to be active inhibition of perception of the retinal image transmitted by one eye.

ametropia optical condition in which parallel rays of light do not focus on the retina; a refractive error.

angioid streaks abnormality of the elastic layer of lamina basalis (Bruch membrane) giving rise to pigmented striations of the ocular fundus; associated with a variety of systemic diseases such as pseudozanthoma elasticum, sickle cell disease, and osteitis deformans (Paget disease) and a variety of generalized diseases affecting the elastic lamina of blood vessels.

angle of anomaly (abnormality) in strabismus, the degree an eye deviates from parallelism.

angle-closure glaucoma ocular abnormality in which the intraocular pressure increases, often quickly, because the anterior aqueous humor is mechanically prevented from reaching the trabecular meshwork.

angstrom (Å) unit of wavelength equal to 10^{-10} meter (nanometer now preferred [10^{-9} meter]).

aniridia almost total absence of iris.

aniseikonia optical condition in which the retinal images in the two eyes are of different sizes.

anisocoria condition in which the pupils of the two eyes are of unequal size.

anisometropia condition in which the refractive errors in the two eyes are different.

ankyloblepharon condition in which the margins of the eyelids are fused together.

anomalous (abnormal) retinal correspondence con-

573

dition in which corresponding points on the two retinas do not have the same relative direction in space.

anomalous trichromatism defect of color vision in which there appears to be a deficiency of one of the cone pigments (*see also* deuteranomaly, protoanomaly, tritanomaly).

anophthalmia absence of the eye.

aphakia absence of the crystalline lens of the eye.

aqueous flare Tyndall beam observed with a biomicroscope when excessive protein is present in the anterior aqueous humor.

aqueous humor fluid that fills the posterior and anterior chambers.

arcuate scotoma area of blindness in the field of vision of characteristic arc shape; caused by interruption of a nerve fiber bundle in the retina; most often seen in glaucoma.

arcus cornealis deposition of lipid in the peripheral cornea mainly in the aged (arcus senilis; gerontoxon) and rarely in youth (arcus juvenilis; embryotoxon).

argyria discoloration of the skin or mucous membranes produced by prolonged administration of silver salts with deposition of metallic silver in tissue.

asteroid hyalosis fixed opacities composed of a calcium lipid complex that occur in an otherwise normal vitreous body; there are no symptoms.

asthenopia ill-defined ocular discomfort arising from use of the eyes.

astigmatism optical condition in which the refractive power is not uniform in all meridians; when regular, there are two main meridians of refractive power; when irregular, there are a number of meridians of different power.

avulsion of caruncle term usually applied to a laceration involving inner one sixth (lacrimal portion) of lower eyelid with rupture of the inferior canaliculus.

axis, visual the straight line connecting an object seen with the foveola.

band keratopathy deposition of calcium in the cornea most marked in the horizontal meridian; occurs in degenerating eyes, hypercalcemia, hypophosphatemia, and juvenile arthritis (of Still).

bedewing of cornea subepithelial corneal edema, often associated with sudden prolonged increase in intraocular pressure or wearing of contact lenses for an excessively long period (Sattler veil).

Bell palsy peripheral paralysis of the facial nerve (N VII).

Bell phenomenon upward and outward deviation of the eyes occurring in sleep or with forcible closure of the eyelids.

Bergmeister papilla small mass of glial cells that surrounds the hyaloid artery in the center of the optic disk; occasionally it persists and obliterates the physiologic cup of the optic disk.

biomicroscope microscope for examining the eye; consists essentially of a dissecting microscope combined with a light source that projects a rectangular light beam that can be changed in size and focus.

Bitot spot highly refractile mass with silver-gray hue and a foamy surface that appears on the bulbar conjunctiva in vitamin A deficiency.

blennorrhea conjunctivitis.

blepharitis inflammation of the margin of the eyelids; occurs in squamous (seborrheic) and ulcerative forms.

blepharochalasis relaxation of the skin of the eyelid caused by atrophy of the elastic tissue; the upper eyelid is commonly involved, and a fold of tissue hangs over the eyelid margin.

blepharoclonus exaggerated reflex blinking.

blepharophimosis narrowing of the palpebral fissure, often associated with excessive distance between the inner canthi and drooping of the upper eyelid (blepharoptosis).

blepharoplasty plastic surgery of the eyelids.

blepharoptosis drooping of the upper eyelid caused by paralysis of the oculomotor nerve (N III) or the sympathetic nerves or by excessive weight of the upper eyelids.

blepharospasm tonic spasm of the orbicularis oculi muscle.

blind spot (of Mariotte) area of blindness in the visual field marking the site of the optic nerve in the eye where there are no photoreceptors.

blindness inability to see; defined by Internal Revenue Service as reduction of best corrected visual acuity to 6/60 (20/200) or less in better eye or restriction of the visual field to 20° or less; defined by Social Security Agency as reduction of vision in best corrected eye to 1.5/60 (5/200) or less; in industry, reduction of the best corrected visual acuity to less than 6/60 (20/200).

color see deuteranopia, protanopia, tritanopia, deuteranomly, protanomaly, tritanomaly.

cortical caused by a lesion in the cortical visual center.

night inefficient dark adaptation so that vision is markedly reduced in reduced illumination.

snow inability to open the eyes to see; secondary to ultraviolet keratitis.

blowout fracture of orbit fracture of the roof of the maxillary sinus with prolapse of the intraorbital contents into the antrum; there is enophthalmos, blepharoptosis, inability to turn the eye upward, and usually infraorbital anesthesia.

blue sclera abnormality in which the sclera is thin and has a blue appearance arising from the underlying pigmented choroid.

bobbing disordered ocular movements in comatose

patients with lower pontine lesions; intermittent rapid downward movement of eyes with slow return to primary position.

Brushfield spots transient whitish areas in the iris at birth that occur in Down syndrome and in many normal children.

buckling operation for retinal separation with resection of a portion of the sclera and implantation of foreign material to indent the eye.

buphthalmos enlargement of the eye usually occurring as a result of congenital glaucoma.

campimeter alternative term for perimeter.

canaliculitis inflammation of the lacrimal canaliculi, often caused by fungus infection.

candela unit of luminous intensity; one candela is defined as the luminous intensity of $1/60$ of a square centimeter of projected area of a blackbody radiator operating at the temperature of solidification of platinum.

candle power luminous intensity as expressed in candelas.

carotid-cavernous fistula rupture of a carotic aneurysm into the cavernous sinus (infraseller) that causes an increased venous pressure in the sinus; also occurs with dural shunt.

cataract an opacity of the crystalline lens.

central serous choroidopathy condition characterized by separation of the sensory retina from the pigment epithelium in the central retinal area by a serous fluid.

centrocecal scotoma area of blindness in the field of vision involving both the fixation point and the blind spot (cecum); characterizes toxic amblyopias.

cerclage operation for retinal separation placing encircling band around the sclera at the equator.

chalazion chronic lipogranuloma of a meibomian gland.

chalcosis deposition of copper in tissues.

Charcot triad nystagmus, intention tremor, and scanning speech, all of which occur as a late sign in demyelinating disease, particularly multiple sclerosis.

chemosis edema of the conjunctiva.

cherry-red spot ophthalmoscopic appearance of the fovea centralis (which contains only the outer layers of the retina adjacent to the choroid) when surrounded by either edematous or lipid-filled inner layers of the retina, as occurs in occlusion of the central retinal artery, in amaurotic familial idiocy, and in Neimann-Pick disease.

choristoma tumor of a tissue not normally belonging in an area.

choroideremia X chromosome–linked abnormality characterized by atrophy of the choriocapillaris and degeneration of the retinal pigment epithelium.

choroiditis inflammation of the choroid.

chromatic aberration imperfection of an image produced by variations in the refractivity of the various wavelengths of white light.

chrysiasis deposition of gold in connective tissue of skin.

C.I.E. observer hypothetical observer having color-vision sensitivity recommended in 1931 by Commission Internationale de l'Eclairage (C.I.E.).

circinate retinopathy rare monocular disorder, mainly in elderly women, characterized by an oval zone of small, discrete, coalescing white spots engirdling the central retinal area.

closed-angle glaucoma angle-closure glaucoma.

collarette junction of ciliary and pupillary zones of iris.

collyrium eyewash.

coloboma fissure of a part of the eye.

commotio retinae traumatic lesion of the posterior pole with edema and hemorrhage following contusion of the anterior ocular segment.

complementary after-image after-image in which the hue is approximately complementary to the hue of the sensation produced by the original stimulus.

complementary chromaticities pairs of different samples of light that produce an achromatic (colorless) stimulus when combined in suitable proportions.

complementary colors pairs of samples of light that have complementary chromaticities; also the proper relative amounts of luminous flux to produce an achromatic (colorless) mixture.

congruous field defects visual field defects that are exactly the same in extent and intensity in both eyes; characterizes lesions in the optic radiation and occipital cortex.

conical cornea keratoconus.

conjugate ocular movements similar ocular movements of both eyes, such as eyes right, eyes left, eyes up, eyes down (version).

conjunctivitis inflammation of the conjunctiva.

consensual light reflex constriction of the pupil in the fellow eye when the retina is stimulated by light.

conus of optic disk condition in which the choroid and retinal pigment epithelium do not extend to the optic disk, allowing the sclera to be observed ophthalmoscopically at its margin.

convergence simultaneous movement of both eyes forward to fix a nearby object (vergence).

corectopia displacement of pupil from its normal position.

corresponding points areas on the two retinas that have the same directional value in space.

cotton-wool patches a microinfarct causing acute edema of the nerve fiber layer of the retina (cytoid body).

couching an ancient surgical procedure of displacing the lens from the optical axis.

cover-uncover test alternate covering and uncovering of one eye to distinguish between a phoria and a tropia.

craniosynostosis premature fusion of cranial bone sutures.

Credé prophylaxis instillation of 1% silver nitrate in the eyes of a newborn infant to prevent gonococcal conjunctivitis.

crescent, myopic term applied to a conus of the optic disk in myopia.

cryopexy retinal separation procedure with a freezing probe.

cryotherapy procedure carried out with a freezing probe.

cryptophthalmos congenital absence of eyelids.

cup/disk ratio ratio of horizontal diameter of physiologic cup of optic disk to diameter of disk.

cyanosis retinae old term for vascular dilation in hyperviscosity of blood syndromes.

cyclectomy excision of a portion of the ciliary body.

cyclitis inflammation of the ciliary body.

cyclocryotherapy destruction of a portion of ciliary body by freezing to reduce the quantity of aqueous humor produced in glaucoma.

cyclodialysis surgical procedure for glaucoma to establish a communication between the anterior chamber and the suprachoroidal space.

cyclodiathermy destruction of a portion of the ciliary body by diathermy to reduce the quantity of aqueous humor produced in glaucoma.

cycloplegia paralysis of the ciliary muscle giving rise to paralysis of accommodation.

cylinder in optics, a lens with no refracting power in one meridian and maximal refracting power in the meridian at right angles to this.

dacryoadenitis inflammation of the lacrimal gland, often chronic and caused by a granulomatous disease; acute dacryoadenitis occurs with mumps and infectious mononucleosis.

dacryocystitis inflammation of the lacrimal sac that usually results from interference with lacrimal drainage.

dacryocystorhinostomy surgical procedure in which the mucous membrane of the lacrimal sac is anastomosed with the mucous membrane that lines the middle meatus of the nose in order to establish lacrimal drainage.

dacryostenosis atresia of the lacrimal duct.

dark adaptation biochemical and neurologic process by which the eye becomes more sensitive to light.

dendritic keratitis inflammation of the corneal epithelium by *Herpesvirus hominis.*

denervation supersensitivity sensitivity to neural effector substance that follows postganglionic interruption of the nerve supply of organs innervated by the autonomic nervous system.

descemetocele herniation of the basement membrane of the corneal endothelium.

detachment, retinal separation of the sensory retina from the retinal pigment epithelium.

deuteranomaly form of anomalous trichromatism for which there appears to be a deficiency of green-sensitive cones so that there is poor green-purple and red-purple discrimination, green insensitivity, and normal luminosity function.

deuteranopia form of dichromatism in which there are only two cone pigments present and there is complete insensitivity to green.

deviation

   primary ocular deviation seen in paralysis of an ocular muscle when the nonparalyzed eye is used for fixation.

   secondary ocular deviation seen in paralysis of an ocular muscle when the paralyzed eye is used for fixation.

   supranuclear binocular paralysis of the volitional ocular movements arising because of abnormalities in the frontal or occipital cortex.

dialysis of retina separation at the ora serrata of the sensory retina from the retinal pigment epithelium.

diaphanoscopy transillumination of a body cavity; used in ophthalmology to demonstrate the diminution of pigment in the iris (pigmentary dispersion syndrome) in the female carriers of albinism or to diagnose intraocular tumors.

dichromatism abnormality of color vision in which only two of the three cone pigments are present; mixtures of two, rather than the normal three, components are necessary and sufficient to match all colors (protanopes, red absent; deuteranopes, green absent; tritanopes, blue absent).

diopter unit of measurement of the refractive power of lenses equal to the reciprocal focal length of the lens expressed in meters.

diplopia double vision; simultaneous perception of two grossly dissimilar images.

   crossed double vision in which the image arising from the right is observed to the left of the image arising from the left eye; associated with conditions in which the eyes turn outward.

   uncrossed condition in which the image of the right eye is to the right of the image arising from the left eye; observed in conditions in which the visual axes of the eye are directed toward each other, as in esotropia.

disciform degeneration of central retina secondary type of central retinal degeneration arising from subretinal neovascularization.

disciform keratitis stromal type of corneal inflammation, roughly circular in shape, often seen as secondary stromal involvement to herpes simplex keratitis.

disinsertion of retina retinal dialysis at the ora serrata in which the sensory retina is separated from the retinal pigment epithelium.

dislocation of lens condition in which the crystalline lens is completely unsupported by the zonular fibers so that the lens is free, either in the vitreous body or in the anterior chamber.

distichiasis supernumerary row of eyelashes.

drusen hyaline excrescences of the retinal pigment epithelium or acellular laminated bodies of the optic nerve.

dry eye keratoconjunctivitis sicca.

ductions ocular movements of one eye only.

dyslexia psychologic abnormality in which, despite adequate intelligence, motivation, and instruction, and in the absence of a physical handicap, emotional disturbance, or cultural deprivation, an individual fails to master printed and written language.

dysmetria abnormality of ocular movements in which there is an overshoot of the eyes when an attempt is made to fixate an object.

dystrophy noninflammatory developmental, nutritional, or metabolic abnormality.

eccentric fixation visual abnormality in which a retinal area other than the fovea centralis is used for visual fixation.

ecchymosis extravasation of blood beneath the skin.

ectasia of sclera localized bulging of the sclera lined with uveal tissue; a staphyloma.

ectopia displacement or malposition, especially congenital.

ectropion turning outward of the margin of the eyelid occurring in spastic, cicatricial, and paralytic forms.

electromagnetic spectrum range of radiant energy that has a variable frequency and a constant velocity (energy = Planck's constant × frequency).

electro-oculogram (EOG) ratio of standing potential between retina and cornea in light and dark adaptation.

electroretinogram (ERG) action potential that follows stimulation of the retina.

embryotoxon arcus cornealis (arcus juvenilis).

emmetropia refractive condition in which no refractive error is present with accommodation at rest.

emphysema, orbital air in the orbit; generally follows traumatic rupture of a nasal sinus, particularly the lamina papyracea of the ethmoid bone.

endogenous uveitis inflammation of the uveal tract arising from causes within the body in contrast to that introduced from outside the body, as in injuries (exogenous).

endophthalmitis purulent inflammation of the intraocular contents.

enophthalmos recession of the eye within the orbit.

entropion inward turning of the eyelid, observed in cicatricial, spastic, and paralytic forms.

enucleation removal of the eye.

epicanthus vertical fold of skin on either side of the nose (epicanthal fold).

epidemic keratoconjunctivitis inflammation of the cornea and conjunctiva by adenovirus type 8 or 19.

epiphora tearing in which faulty drainage of tears permits their overflow.

episcleritis localized inflammation of the superficial tissues of the sclera.

epithelial downgrowth epithelization of the interior of the eye that may follow faulty wound healing of the anterior ocular segment.

erosion, corneal a recurrent loss of corneal epithelium that may follow minor injury.

erysiphake instrument that uses a vacuum to grasp the lens in cataract extraction.

esodeviation inward deviation of the eye.

esophoria latent inward deviation of the eye in which, with binocular vision suspended, the eyes deviate inward.

esotropia manifest inward deviation that occurs with both eyes open.

essential atrophy of iris rare, progressive, unilateral disease of the iris in which there is a patchy loss of all layers of the iris, causing a distorted and migrating pupil and often a secondary glaucoma.

evisceration in ophthalmology, the surgical procedure in which the intraocular contents are removed, retaining the cornea (sometimes) and the sclera.

exenteration, orbital removal of all of the orbital tissues, including the eye and its nervous, vascular, and muscular connections.

exfoliation of lens capsule condition in which the anterior lens capsule degenerates and appears to be wiped from the lens by the movement of the iris; true exfoliation follows infrared injury to the lens; pseudoexfoliation is more common; the cause is unknown.

exodeviation turning outward of the eyes.

exophoria latent outward deviation of the eyes in which, with binocular vision suspended, the eyes deviate outward.

exophthalmos abnormal protrusion of the eyes.
  endocrine associated with abnormalities of the thyroid gland.
  ophthalmoplegic inability to move the eye because of exophthalmos.
  pulsating associated with a carotid-cavernous fistula.

exotropia outward deviation of the eyes.

extorsion temporal rotation of 12 o'clock corneal meridian.

eye

   cat's yellow reflex in retinoblastoma.

   dominant preferred eye for monocular fixation.

   exciting initially injured eye that gives rise to sympathetic ophthalmia in fellow eye, the sympathizing eye.

   fixating in strabismus, the eye directed to the object of regard.

   reduced, schematic simplified eye used in optics.

   squinting deviating eye in strabismus.

Farnsworth-Munsell color test contains 84 colors arranged in order of increasing hue.

field of vision area simultaneously visible to an eye without movement.

fixation the coordinated accommodation and ocular movements that maintain the image of objects on the retina.

flare, aqueous *see* aqueous flare.

floater object seen in the field of vision that originates in the vitreous body; the most common floaters are muscae volitantes, minute residues of the hyaloid vasculature seen in bright, uniform illumination.

fluorescein angiography serial photography of ocular fundus after intravenous administration of fluorescein solution.

fluorescence reradiation of energy with increase of wavelength by an absorbing substance.

flutter, ocular involuntary intermittent to-and-fro movements of eye occurring in cerebellar disease.

flux short form for radiant flux, or luminous flux, according to context.

focus point of convergence of light rays; starting point of disease.

follicles, conjunctival lymphatic hypertrophy in response to conjunctival inflammation.

foot-candle unit of illuminance equal to one lumen incident per square foot.

foot-lambert unit of luminance.

fornix in ophthalmology the reflection of the conjunctiva from the eyelid to the eye.

Fuchs black spot area of proliferation of the retinal pigment layer in the central retina; occurs in degenerative myopia.

Fuchs dystrophy corneal abnormality in which there is initially a degeneration of the endothelium followed sometimes by epithelial changes.

funduscope inasmuch as many organs have a fundus, a more precise term for the instrument used in ophthalmoscopy is *ophthalmoscope*.

fusion reflex; the stimulus to unify images falling upon retinal areas that have the same directional value in space.

   fusion with amplitude blending of the similar images from the two foveas into a single perception (Grade 2).

   simultaneous central retinal perception (normal correspondence) ability of the brain to receive and appreciate images from the fovea of each eye simultaneously.

   stereopsis blending of slightly dissimilar images from the two eyes with the perception of depth.

fusion-free position of the eyes when binocular vision is suspended.

gerontoxon a corneal arcus of lipid (arcus senilis).

glare sensation produced by brightnesses within the visual field that are sufficiently greater than the luminance to which the eyes are adapted to cause annoyance, discomfort, or loss in visual performance and visibility.

glaucoma ocular disease with increased intraocular pressure.

gonioscope optical instrument for studying the angle of the anterior chamber of the eye.

goniosynechiae adhesions between the iris and cornea at the anterior chamber angle.

goniotomy operation for congenital glaucoma in which the trabecular meshwork in the region of the canal of Schlemm is incised.

hallucinations perception without external stimulus that may occur in every field of sensation; formed visual hallucinations are composed of scenes, and unformed are composed of sparks, lights, and the like; formed hallucinations characterize temporal lobe disturbances, and unformed visual hallucinations characterize occipital lobe disorders.

hamartoma a localized tumor composed of an abnormal proportion of a single tissue element of tissues normally present in the areas.

Hassall-Henle bodies hyaline deposits of the Descemet membrane that occur with aging.

Henle layer outer plexiform layer of the retina in radiation from the foveola.

Hering's law of equal innervation impulse to each muscle involved in turning the eyes in the same direction.

heterochromia of iris condition in which the irises of the two eyes are different colors.

heterophoria condition in which there is a latent tendency of the eyes to deviate that is prevented by fusion.

heterotropia condition in which the eyes deviate; a strabismus.

hippus spasmodic dilation and contraction of the pupil independent of stimulation with light.

hole, retinal break in the continuity of the sensory

retina so that there is a communication between the vitreous cavity and the potential space between the sensory retina and the retinal pigment epithelium.

homonymous in ophthalmology, having the same side of the field of vision; thus a right homonymous hemianopia is right half-blindness and arises from a defect involving the nasal fibers of the right eye that decussate and the noncrossing fibers of the left eye; the lesion is on the left side, posterior to the optic chiasm.

hordeolum acute inflammation caused by infection of one of the sebaceous glands of Zeis; a sty; the term "internal hordeolum" is sometimes applied to a chalazion.

horopter plane in space that localizes the visual direction of corresponding retinal points.

Hudson-Stähli line pigmented iron line of the cornea.

hydrops of iris vacuolization of the iris pigment layer when these cells are filled with glycogen in diabetes mellitus.

hyperopia refractive state of the eye in which the parallel rays of light would come to focus behind the retina if not intercepted by it.

   absolute cannot be neutralized completely by accommodation so that there is indistinct vision both for near and for distance.

   axial caused by abnormal shortness of the anteroposterior diameter of the eye.

   latent portion of total hypermetropia that cannot be overcome, or the difference between the manifest and total hypermetropia.

   manifest amount of hypermetropia indicated by the strongest convex lens a patient will accept while retaining normal visual acuity.

   total entire hypermetropia, both latent and manifest.

hyperphoria tendency for the eyes to deviate vertically that is prevented by binocular vision

hypertelorism excessive width between two organs; in ocular hypertelorism there is increased distance between the eyes that is often associated with mental deficiency and exotropia.

hypertropia deviation of the eyes in which one eye is higher than the other.

hyphema blood in the anterior chamber.

hypopyon pus in the anterior chamber.

hypotony, ocular diminished ocular pressure.

illuminance luminous flux incident per unit area of a surface.

image visual impression of an object formed by a lens or mirror.

   false in diplopia, the image arising in the deviating eye.

   Purkinje images reflected from the surface of the cornea, the anterior surface of the lens, and the posterior surface of the lens.

   real in optics, the inverted image in which refracted rays pass through the image point.

   true in diplopia, the image received by the nondeviating eye.

   virtual in optics, the erect image in which the refracted rays do not pass through the image point but appear to come from it.

incongruous field defects visual field defects that are dissimilar in the two eyes; occur in lesions involving that portion of the visual pathways anterior to the lateral geniculate body.

infrared radiation portion of the electromagnetic spectrum that has a wavelength of more than 700 nm and less than 10,000 nm.

interstitial keratitis inflammation of the corneal stroma with neovascularization, often complicating congenital syphilis.

intorsion nasal rotation of 12 o'clock corneal meridian.

intrascleral nerve loop condition in which a long ciliary nerve loops in the anterior sclera; gives rise to a minute dark spot of uveal tissue on the sclera.

iridectomy cutting out of a part of the iris.

   peripheral removal of a portion of the peripheral iris.

   sector removal of an entire sector, extending usually from the pupillary margin to the root of the iris.

iridencleisis surgical procedure to correct glaucoma in which an incision is made at the corneoscleral limbus and the iris is incarcerated in the wound to create a filtering wick between the anterior chamber and subconjunctival space.

iridescent vision halos around lights, particularly in corneal edema.

iridocyclitis inflammation of the iris and ciliary body.

iridodialysis separation of the base of the iris from the ciliary body; the main cause is blunt trauma to the eye.

iridodonesis tremulousness of the iris; occurs following loss of support after lens removal.

iridoplegia paralysis of the sphincter pupillae muscle of the iris.

iridoschisis separation of the mesodermal layer of the iris from the ectodermal layer.

iris bombé condition in which the pupil is adherent to the lens so that aqueous humor accumulates in the posterior chamber.

iris coloboma defect of the iris that occurs either as a congenital abnormality or after iridectomy.

iritis inflammation of the iris.

irradiance density of radiant flux incident on a surface.

Ishihara color plates device for screening for color discrimination using forms composed of different colored dots.

isopter curve of equal sensitivity in the visual field.

joule ten million ergs.

K reading corneal curvature as measured with keratometer.

Kayser-Fleischer ring golden deposit of copper in the periphery of the Descemet membrane observed in hepatolenticular degeneration (Wilson disease).

keratectomy excision of the cornea.

keratic precipitates clumps of leukocytes adhering to the corneal endothelium in uveal tract inflammation; customarily divided into mutton-fat (macrophages and epithelioid cells) and punctate (lymphocytes and plasma cells).

keratitis inflammation of the cornea.

keratocele hernia of the Descemet membrane through the cornea; a descemetocele.

keratoconjunctivitis simultaneous inflammation of the cornea and conjunctiva.

keratoconus conical protrusion of the cornea.

keratomalacia softening of the cornea, often occurring in severe vitamin A deficiency.

keratome knife with a triangular blade used for corneal incision.

keratometer instrument for measuring the radius of curvature of the cornea.

keratomycosis keratitis caused by fungus infection.

keratoplasty transplantation of a portion of the cornea.
  lamellar replacement of superficial layers.
  partial replacement of a portion of the cornea.
  penetrating replacement of entire thickness of the cornea; may be partial or total.
  total replacement of entire cornea.

keratotomy incision of the cornea carried out in years past to limit the spread of an ulcer.

Koeppe nodule accumulation of epithelioid cells at the pupillary margin in granulomatous uveitis.

Krukenberg spindle accumulation of pigment on the corneal endothelium in the shape of a vertical spindle that occurs in pigmentary glaucoma.

lacrimation secretion of tears.

lagophthalmos condition in which the globe is not entirely covered with the eyelids closed.

lambert unit of luminance.

laser acronym for *l*ight *a*mplification by *s*timulated *e*mission of *r*adiation; the laser produces a nearly monochromatic and coherent beam of radiation.

lens glass or other transparent material used optically to modify the path of light.
  bifocal spectacles that contain two foci, usually arranged with the focus for distance above and a smaller segment for near below; such lenses are used in the correction of presbyopia and to relieve excessive accommodation in accommodative strabismus of children.
  colored selectively absorb or reflect certain wavelengths of light.
  contact worn beneath the eyelids.
  crystalline transparent biconvex tissue located behind the pupil and in front of the vitreous.
  omnifocal spectacles that contain both near and distance portions with gradual increase in reading power.
  prism transparent solid with triangular ends and two converging sides; separates white light into its spectral components and bends rays of light toward its base; used to measure or to correct ocular muscle imbalance.
  safety lens resistant to shattering made either of plastic or by means of case-hardening, coating, or lamination.

lensometer instrument for determining the refractive power of a lens.

lenticonus rare abnormality of the lens characterized by a conical prominence on the anterior or posterior lens surface.

leukocoria whitish reflex caused by intraocular mass.

leukoma opacity of the cornea; a less marked opacity is a macula, and the least type of opacity is a nebula.
  adherent corneal opacity to which the iris is adherent.

light that portion of the electromagnetic spectrum that gives rise to a sensation through stimulation of the retina.

lumen unit of luminous flux equal to the flux in a unit of solid angle (one steradian) from a uniform point source of one candela.

luminance luminous flux per unit of solid angle emitted per unit of projected area.

luminosity ratio of lumens per watt of any kind of radiant energy.

luminous emittance density of luminous flux emitted from a surface.

luminous flux rate of flow of luminous energy.

lux unit of illuminance equal to one lumen per square meter.

lysozyme (muramidase) antibacterial enzyme found in tears, leukocytes, egg albumin, and plants; mainly destructive of nonpathogenic bacteria.

macula minute corneal opacity.

macula lutea yellow spot; the ill-defined retinal area surrounding the fovea centralis.

mandibulofacial dysostosis hereditary hypoplasia of zygoma and mandible.

megalocornea cornea with a diameter of 12 mm or more.

melanocytoma nevus with giant melanosomes on the surface of the optic disk.

metamorphopsia condition in which objects appear distorted.

microaneurysms capillary outpouching in the retina in diabetes mellitus, pulseless disease, hypertension.

microcornea cornea with a diameter of less than 9 mm.

microphakia anomaly in which the crystalline lens is abnormally small.

microphthalmia condition in which the eyeball is abnormally small.

micropsia disturbance of visual perception in which objects appear smaller than their true size.

microtropia strabismus of less than 5°.

millimicron unit of wavelength equal to 10^{-9} meter; nanometer now preferred.

miosis condition in which the pupil is constricted.

miotic pertaining to or characterized by constriction of the pupil.

Mittendorf dot opacity of the posterior lens capsule marking the site of hyaloid artery attachment.

Mooren ulcer chronic keratitis in the aged.

morgagnian cataract hypermature cataract in which the cortex is liquefied, permitting the lens nucleus to float within the capsule.

mural cells pericytes in retinal capillary walls.

muscae volitantes remnants of the fetal hyaloid system that appear as opacities in the vitreous humor (floaters).

mydriasis dilation of the pupil.

myopia optical condition in which parallel rays of light come to focus in front of the retina.

　axial caused by abnormal length of anteroposterior diameter of the eye.

　degenerative associated with conus of optic disk and retinal abnormalities.

　refractive caused by increased index of refraction of the lens, as in nuclear sclerosis.

Nagel anomaloscope device for mixing two colors to match a third; used for analysis of color perception.

nanometer (nm) unit of wavelength equal to 10^{-9} (one one-billionth) meter; formerly called millimicron ($m\mu$).

nebula of cornea minor opacity of the cornea.

neurotrophic keratitis keratitis arising because of anesthesia of the cornea.

nodal points locations in an optical system toward and from which are directed corresponding incident and transmitted rays that make equal angles with the optic axis.

nystagmus oscillatory movement of the eye.

　end-position involuntary rhythmic movement of the eyes observed when in extreme positions of gaze.

jerk occurs with a fast and a slow phase.

labyrinthine occurs when the labyrinths are irritated or diseased (synonym, vestibular nystagmus).

miner's nystagmus caused by darkness.

optokinetic occurs in normal individuals when a succession of moving objects traverse the field of vision such as occurs when gazing out of the window of a moving vehicle at a succession of stationary objects (synonym, railroad nystagmus).

pendular approximately equal in each direction.

rotatory eye partially rotates around the visual axis.

open-angle glaucoma condition of increased intraocular pressure in which the aqueous humor has access to the trabecular meshwork.

ophthalmia conjunctivitis.

ophthalmodynamometer instrument for measuring blood pressure in the ophthalmic artery through observation of collapse of the central retinal artery.

ophthalmoplegia paralysis of the ocular muscles.

　externa paralysis of the external ocular muscles.

　interna paralysis of the muscles of the iris and the ciliary body.

　total combination of both intrinsic and extrinsic paralysis

ophthalmoscope instrument for examining the interior of the eye.

　direct provides an upright image of about 15 diameters magnification.

　indirect convex lens is held in front of the eye and an inverted image is observed; provides a magnification of about four times, but allows examination of a more peripheral portion of the fundus than direct ophthalmoscopy.

opsoclonus irregular jerks of the eyes in all directions in cerebellar disease.

optic atrophy atrophy of the optic nerve.

orbitonometer instrument for measuring resistance to compression of orbital contents.

orthophoria tendency for the eyes to be parallel; normal ocular muscle balance.

orthoptics technique of providing correct and efficient visual responses, usually by the form of visual training; these measures include the treatment of functional amblyopia, management of convergence insufficiency, and diagnosis of muscle imbalance and strabismus.

pannus subepithelial fibrovascular tissue in the cornea.

Panum area spatial area surrounding the horopter in which objects are viewed with stereopsis; outside this area, diplopia occurs.

papilla small nipplelike eminence.

Bergmeister small mass of glial tissue on the surface of the disk.

lacrimal small conical eminence on the upper and lower eyelid at the inner canthus pierced by the lacrimal punctum; particularly evident in the elderly.

optic a misnomer in that the optic disk does not project into the eye.

papilledema passive edema of the optic disk.

papillitis inflammation of the optic nerve at the level of the disk.

perimeter instrument used to measure the visual field.

persistent hyperplastic vitreous abnormality arising from failure of the hyaloid system to regress.

phacoemulsification fragmentation of the lens with ultrasound combined with aspiration.

phakomatoses group of hereditary diseases characterized by the presence of spots, tumors, and cysts in various parts of the body; types recognized as associated with ocular findings are tuberous sclerosis, Lindau–von Hippel disease, Recklinghausen disease, Bourneville disease, and Louis-Bar syndrome (*see also* syndrome).

phlyctenule localized lymphocytic infiltration of the conjunctiva.

phosphene sensation of light produced by electrical or mechanical stimulation of the visual system.

photocoagulation use of laser or xenon arc energy to coagulate portions of the retina under direct observation.

photophobia ocular discomfort induced by bright lights.

photopsia subjective sensation of sparks or flashes of light that occur in some pathologic conditions of the optic nerve, the retina, or the brain.

phthisis bulbi degenerative shrinkage of the eye.

pinguecula small yellowish white subconjunctival elevation composed of elastic tissue located between the corneoscleral limbus and the canthus.

pits incomplete coloboma of the optic disk, sometimes associated with central serous choroidopathy.

Placido disk device composed of concentric black and white lines that is reflected onto the anterior surface of the cornea to detect astigmatism.

pleoptics a method of reestablishing foveal fixation.

poliosis condition characterized by the absence of pigment in the hair; poliosis of the eyelashes occurs in sympathetic ophthalmia, syphilis, and Vogt-Koyanagi bilateral uveitis.

polycoria condition of multiple pupils; true polycoria if surrounded with sphincter muscle.

presbyopia refractive condition in which there is a diminished power of accommodation arising from impaired elasticity of the crystalline lens, as occurs with aging.

proptosis forward displacement of any organ.

protanomaly form of anomalous trichromatism for which, in a red-green mixture, more than the normal amount of red is required than for a normal observer.

protanopia form of dichromatism in which red and bluish green are confused, and relative luminosity of red is much lower than for a normal observer.

pseudoisochromatic plate see Ishihara color plates.

pseudopapillitis blurring of optic disk margins in hyperopia.

pseudostrabismus appearance of crossed eyes caused by epicanthal folds or a visual axis not centered in the pupil.

pterygium abnormality arising basically in the cornea in which a triangular patch of conjunctiva extends into the cornea; apex of the patch points toward the pupil.

pupil aperture in the iris of the eye for the passage of light.

Adie abnormality in the reaction of the pupil to light and associated with hypotonic deep reflexes.

Argyll Robertson pupil that does not constrict to light but constricts to convergence; pupils are small, unequal in size, and irregular; seen mainly in tabes dorsalis.

cat's-eye pupil with a white reflex when light is directed into it; most commonly associated with retinoblastoma.

pupillary membrane anomaly of the iris, usually minor, in which there is failure of the fetal pupillary membrane to atrophy; often a persistent strand extends between the iris collarette and the anterior lens capsule.

Purkinje shift luminosity curve of dark-adapted individual peaks at 500 nm, whereas the luminosity curve of light-adapted individual peaks at 550 nm; indicates two types of retinal photoreceptors.

quadrantanopia loss of one quadrant of the visual field; homonymous inferior considered pathognomonic of parietal lobe involvement; homonymous superior vascular lesion of temporal loop of the visual radiation.

radiance radiant intensity per unit of projected area.

radiant absorptance ratio of absorbed radiant flux to incident flux.

radiant emittance radiant flux emitted per unit area of a source.

radiant energy energy being transferred, unaccompanied by transfer of matter.

radiant flux rate of transfer of radiant energy.

radiant intensity flux radiated per unit of solid angle.

radiant power alternative term for radiant flux.

radiant reflectance ratio of reflected radiant flux to incident flux.

red eye lay term applied to any condition with dilation of conjunctival or ciliary blood vessels.

reflex involuntary, invariable, adaptive response to a stimulus.

accommodation constriction of the pupils when the eyes converge for near vision; an associated reaction and not a reflex.

auditory brief closure of the eyelids resulting from a sudden sound.

conjunctival (eyelid) closure of the eyelids induced by touching the conjunctiva (also called corneal reflex).

consensual light (crossed) constriction of the pupil when the opposite retina is stimulated with light.

cutaneous pupillary (ciliospinal) dilation of the ipsilateral pupil on pinching of the skin on one side of the neck.

direct light contraction of the sphincter pupillae muscle induced by stimulation of the retina with light (also called pupillary reflex).

eye compression (oculocardiac) decrease of heartbeat caused by pressure on the eye.

fixation direction of the eye so that an image remains on the fovea centralis of each eye.

foveolar bright dot of light arising from the foveola when an ophthalmoscope light is directed on the region of the fovea centralis.

lacrimal secretion of tears induced by irritation of the cornea and conjunctiva.

red red glow of light seen to emerge from the pupil when the interior of the eye is illuminated.

refraction deviation of rays of light when passing from one transparent medium into another of a different density.

retinal correspondence (*see* abnormal retinal correspondence).

retinitis inflammation of the retina.

retinoblastoma malignant retina tumor of infancy.

retinopathy noninflammatory degenerations of the retina.

retinopexy surgical procedure to correct retinal detachment by means of diathermy.

retinoschisis retinal abnormality in which the sensory retina splits at the level of the inner plexiform layer.

retinoscopy objective method of determining the refraction of the eye by observing the movements of the reflection of light from the eye (skiascopy).

retrobulbar neuritis inflammation of the optic nerve occurring without involvement of the optic disk.

retrolental fibroplasia retinopathy of prematurity; a condition of cicatricial neovascularization of the retina that occurs predominantly in infants who weigh less than 1,500 grams at birth.

rubeosis iridis neovascularization of the iris.

saccadic movements following movements in ductions and versions.

salmon patch central area of intense vascularization that occurs in interstitial keratitis with the confluence of all blood vessels at the center of the cornea.

Sattler veil subepithelial corneal edema that occurs after prolonged wearing of a contact lens.

scintillating scotoma an unformed visual hallucination with flashing, bursting lights occurring in occipital lobe disorders, particularly migraine.

scleritis inflammation of the sclera.

scleromalacia perforans degenerative condition of the sclera in which localized rheumatoid nodules cause necrosis.

sclerosing keratitis inflammation in which the cornea becomes white and opaque, resembling the sclera.

scotoma area of blindness in the field of vision.

scotopic adaptation adaptation to low levels of luminance at which only rod vision is operative.

serous chorioretinopathy term applied to limited separation of the sensory layer of the retina from the pigment epithelium layer by fluid.

siderosis chronic inflammation of the eye caused by a retained iron foreign body within the eye.

slit lamp see biomicroscope.

Snellen letter letter so constructed that at a given distance from the eye it subtends an angle of 5 minutes, with each portion of the letter subtending an angle of 1 minute.

squamous blepharitis seborrheic inflammation of the eyelid margins.

squint cross-eyes (strabismus).

staphyloma ectasia of the wall of the eye lined with the uveal tract.

Stiles-Crawford effect light passing through the center of the pupil of the eye is more effective in evoking the sensation of brightness than the same amount of light passing through an equal area near the edge of the pupil.

strabismus condition in which the eyes are not simultaneously directed to the same object.

comitant deviation of the eye in which there is no ocular muscle paralysis and the degree of crossing is the same in all directions of gaze.

noncomitant deviation of the eyes from parallelism in which a muscle is paretic or paralytic.

sty purulent inflammation of a gland of Zeis; hordeolum.

subconjunctival hemorrhage bleeding beneath the conjunctiva, often occurring spontaneously.

subhyaloid hemorrhage hemorrhage between the sensory retina and the vitreous body; a meniscus level is often present.

subluxation of lens condition of the lens when a

portion of the supporting zonule is absent and the lens lacks support in one or more quadrants.

suppression physiologic mental process whereby the retinal image transmitted by one eye is ignored.

sursumversion upward rotation of the eyes.

symblepharon adhesion between the palpebral and bulbar conjunctivae.

sympathetic ophthalmia granulomatous uveitis that follows in the opposite eye when there are penetrating injuries of one eye; the eye secondarily affected is called the sympathizing eye, and the injured eye is called the exciting or activating eye.

syndrome group of symptoms and signs that occur together; disease or definite morbid process having a characteristic sequence of symptoms; may affect the whole body or any of its parts.

A and V cross-eyes in which the eyes are closer together in looking up than down (A) or closer looking down than up (V).

Adie see pupil.

Alport familial hemorrhagic nephritis, nephropathy, deafness, and anterior lenticonus (sometimes spherophakia or anterior polar or posterior cortical cataract).

Anton form of anosognosia in which the patient denies his blindness; usually accompanied by confabulation, with the patient claiming to see objects in the blind field.

Axenfeld anomaly posterior corneal arcus, glaucoma (and hypertelorism).

Bassen-Kornzweig progressive ataxic neuropathy associated with retinal pigmentary degeneration and a crenated appearance of erythrocytes (A-beta-lipoproteinemia).

Batten-Mayou neuronal ceroid lipofuscinosis.

Behçet aphthous ulcers (canker sores) of mouth and genitalia combined with uveitis, iritis, and hypopyon.

Benedikt hemianesthesia and involuntary movements of a choreiform nature in the extremities on the side opposite to the lesion in the medial lemniscus and region of the red nucleus.

Berlin disease perimacular retinal edema following trauma (commotio retinae).

Best disease autosomal dominant vitelliruptive central retinal degeneration characterized by a central retinal lesion with an ophthalmoscopic appearance of an egg fried "sunny side up" and associated in this stage with good vision; when egg is "scrambled," vision deteriorates.

Bielschowsky-Lutz-Cogan internuclear ophthalmoplegia with medial rectus muscle paralysis for versions, intact convergence, and nystagmus of abducted eye.

Bourneville disease mental deficiency, tuberous sclerosis, and adenoma sebaceum; glaucoma and conjunctival and retinal tumors may occur.

Bowen disease intraepithelial epithelioma; when the eye is affected, it commonly involves the conjunctiva at the corneoscleral junction in chronically irritated eyes.

cavernous sinus thrombosis of the cavernous sinus with third, fourth, and sixth cranial nerve palsy, edema of the face and eyelids, and infection.

cerebellopontine angle tumor ataxia, tinnitus, deafness, ipsilateral paralysis of the sixth and seventh cranial nerves, involvement of the fifth cranial nerve, vertigo, and nystagmus.

Chediak-Higashi disease recessive albinism with leukocytic inclusions.

chiasmal optic atrophy and bitemporal hemianopia.

Coats disease chronic progressive retinal abnormality characterized by retinal deposits and malformation of retinal blood vessels.

Cogan 1. nonsyphilitic interstitial keratitis with associated nerve deafness. 2. oculomotor apraxia with absence of voluntary ocular movements with full random movements. Fixation by jerky head movements with overshooting.

Collins (Franceschetti) mandibulofacial dysostosis.

crocodile tears spontaneous lacrimation that occurs with the normal salivation of eating; follows facial nerve paralysis and is caused by aberrant regenerating nerve fibers so that some destined for the salivary glands go to the lacrimal gland.

Crouzon disease craniofacial dysostosis with eyes widely separated.

Devic disease subacute encephalomyopathy with severe demyelination of optic nerves.

Down mongolism.

Doyne autosomal dominant drusen of retinal pigment epithelium.

Duane retraction narrowing of the papebral fissure on the side on which the lateral rectus muscle is paralyzed when the patient looks toward the opposite side.

Eales disease vasculitis of the retinal vessels characterized by inflammation, occlusion, neovascularization, and recurrent retinal hemorrhages, occurring particularly in young men.

Ehlers-Danlos widespread systemic disorder with overextensibility of joints, hyperelasticity of the skin, fragility of the skin, and pseudotumors following trauma; there may may be epicanthal folds, esotropia, blue sclera, glaucoma, ectopic lenses, proliferating retinopathy, and acanthocytosis.

Fabry X chromosome–linked sphingolipidosis with deficiency of α-galactosidase.

syndrome—cont'd

Foster Kennedy *see* syndrome, Kennedy.

Foville paralysis of the limbs on one side of the body and of the face on the opposite side together with loss of power to rotate the eyes to that side.

Franceschetti (Collins) mandibulofacial dysostosis.

François dyscephaly, microphthalmia, and cataract.

Fuchs unilateral heterochromia, inflammation of the iris and ciliary body, and secondary cataract.

Gaucher disease familial disorder characterized by splenomegaly, skin pigmentation, and pigmented pingueculas.

Goldenhar mandibulofacial dysostosis with epibulbar dermoids and vertebral anomalies.

Gradenigo palsy of the lateral rectus muscle (N VI) and severe unilateral headache in suppurative disease of the middle ear.

Graves disease hyperthyroidism, goiter, and exophthalmos (Basedow, Parry).

Grönblad-Strandberg angioid streaks of the fundus and pseudoxanthoma elasticum of the skin.

Gunn (Robert Marcus Gunn) unilateral blepharoptosis with marked opening of the eye during chewing.

Hallerman-Streiff mandibulofacial dysostosis with microphthalmia and congenital cataract (François).

Hand-Schüller-Christian disease insidious and progressive abnormality in children characterized by exophthalmos, diabetes insipidus, and softened areas in the bones, particularly in femurs and in bones of the skull, shoulder, and pelvic girdle.

Harada Vogt-Koyanagi syndrome combined with retinal detachment.

Heerfordt disease uveitis, fever, and parotid gland swelling; now recognized as a manifestation of sarcoidosis.

hepatolenticular degeneration (Wilson) abnormality of copper metabolism associated with progressive degeneration of the liver and lentate nucleus, mental retardation, and a brownish ring (Kayser-Fleischer) composed of copper at the periphery of the cornea.

Horner sympathetic nerve paralysis with miosis, blepharoptosis, and anhydrosis of the face.

Hunter X chromosome–linked form of mucopolysaccharidosis (type I) in which the corneas remain clear until the third decade.

Hurler (gargoylism) autosomal recessive mucopolysaccharidosis (type II) characterized by dwarfism with short, kyphotic spinal column; short fingers; depression of bridge of the nose; heavy, ugly facies; stiffness of joints; cloudiness of the cornea; retinal degeneration; hepatosplenomegaly; and mental retardation.

Hutchinson interstitial keratitis, deafness, and notched, narrow-edged permanent incisors in congenital syphilis.

Hutchison neuroblastoma with orbital metastasis.

Irvine-Gass cystoid central retinal edema with corneal-vitreous adhesions after cataract extraction.

Jensen disease chorioretinitis adjacent to the optic disk (juxtapapillary).

Kennedy (Foster Kennedy) ipsilateral optic atrophy and contralateral papilledema in frontal lobe tumors, aneurysms, or abscesses.

Kimmelstiel-Wilson hypertension, retinopathy, and intercapillary glomerulosclerosis in diabetes mellitus.

Kufs disease late juvenile form of cerebromacular degeneration.

Laurence-Moon-Biedl inherited disturbance of the pituitary gland characterized by girdle-type obesity, hypogenitalism, mental retardation, polydactyly, and pigmentary retinal degeneration.

Leber autosomal recessive retinal aplasia.

Leber disease sex-linked form of retrobulbar neuritis occurring at about the age of 20 years.

Letterer-Siwe disease nonfamilial reticuloendotheliosis of early childhood.

Lignac-Fanconi cystinosis with renal rickets (Abderhalden–de Toni–Debré).

Lindau disease angioma of the central nervous system, particularly in the cerebellum, and associated Lindau–von Hippel disease with angioma of the cerebellum, retina, pancreas, and kidney.

Louis-Bar cerebellar ataxia with oculocutaneous telangiectasia.

Lowe oculocerebrorenal X chromosome–linked glaucoma, cataract, growth and mental retardation, and aminoaciduria.

Marcus Gunn *see* syndrome, Gunn.

Marfan spider fingers and toes (arachnodactyly), ectopia lentis, cardiovascular defects, and widespread defects of elastic tissue.

Marinesco-Sjögren autosomal stationary cerebellar ataxia, mental retardation, cataract, and oligophrenia.

Maroteaux-Lamy mucopolysaccharidosis type III.

Mikulicz chronic lymphocytic infiltration and enlargement of the lacrimal and salivary glands (Sjögren).

milk-alkali hypercalcemia induced by peptic ulcer management with milk and calcium carbonate.

Millard-Gubler paralysis of sixth and seventh

syndrome—cont'd
    cranial nerves and contralateral hemiplegia of extremities.

    Möbius 1. migraine headache with recurrent oculomotor paralysis (ophthalmoplegic migraine). 2. bilateral lateral rectus and facial nerve paralysis.

    Morquio-Brailsford mucopolysaccharidosis type IV.

    Neimann-Pick disease heredofamilial lipid disorder mainly caused by sphingomyelinase deficiency.

    Oguchi disease autosomal recessive night blindness found almost exclusively in Japanese.

    orbital apex oculomotor paresis and neuralgia resulting from involvement of structures at the apex of the orbit by a tumor, often a neoplasm of the nasopharynx.

    osteogenesis imperfecta (van der Hoeve) bone fragility, blue sclera, and deafness.

    Ota nevus pigmented nevus of the eyelids, nose, and zygomatic and frontal regions.

    Paget disease bone thickening and thinning, sometimes with angioid streaks.

    paratrigeminal (Raeder) rare abnormality caused by a lesion of the semilunar ganglion and related sympathetic fibers from the carotid plexus; characterized by trigeminal neuralgia; often followed by sensory loss on the affected side of the face, weakness and atrophy of the muscles of mastication, miosis, and blepharoptosis.

    Parinaud 1. conjunctivitis associated with palpable preauricular lymph nodes. 2. paralysis of convergence in upward gaze, usually associated with lesions of the tectum.

    Peter anomaly adherent corneal leukoma with absence of the Descemet membrane and endothelium.

    Posner-Schlossman glaucomacyclitic crisis; recurrent cyclitis with glaucoma.

    Purtscher disease traumatic angiopathy of the retina.

    Raeder see syndrome, paratrigeminal.

    Recklinghausen disease autosomal dominant neurofibromatosis.

    Refsum disease (heredopathia atactica polyneuritiformis) autosomal recessive pigmentary degeneration of the retina with polyneuritis, deafness, and cerebellar signs with excretion of phytanic acid.

    Reiter disease disease of males marked by initial diarrhea and followed by urethritis, conjunctivitis, and migratory polyarthritis.

    Rieger autosomal dominant mesodermal dysgenesis of the cornea and iris; corneal opacities, hypoplastic iris, iridotrabecular adhesions, and posterior corneal arcus occur.

    Riley-Day (familial autonomic dysfunction) reduced or absent tears, postural hypotension, excessive sweating, corneal anesthesia, exotropia, and absence of taste buds.

    Rollet orbital apex syndrome with involvement of the second, third, fourth, fifth, sixth, and sympathetic nerves.

    Roth spot retinal hemorrhage with white center in subacute bacterial endocarditis.

    Rothmund (-Thomson; Bloch-Stauffer) autosomal recessive congenital cataract with skin telangiectasis and pigmentation.

    Sanfilippo mucopolysaccharidosis type III.

    Scheie mucopolysaccharidosis type V.

    Sjögren keratoconjunctivitis sicca, xerostomia, enlargement of the parotic gland, and polyarthritis.

    Stargardt disease fundus flavimaculatus with atrophic central retinal degeneration.

    Stevens-Johnson form of erythema multiforme characterized by constitutional symptoms and marked inflammation and later by scarring of the conjunctiva and oral mucosa.

    Stilling-Duane-Türk an abnormality of ocular musculature innervation with absence of abduction combined with retraction of the globe and blepharoptosis on adduction.

    Sturge-Weber-Dimitri disease nevus flammeus (port wine), often associated with glaucoma.

    Tay-Sachs disease infantile amaurotic familial idiocy; a sphingolipidosis.

    Usher autosomal recessive pigmentary degeneration of the retina with congenital nerve deafness.

    Vogt-Koyanagi bilateral uveitis, poliosis, vitiligo, alopecia, and dysacousia.

    Waardenburg-Klein autosomal dominant hypertrophy of the root of the nose, heterochromia iridis, white forelock, and deafness.

    Weber paralysis of the oculomotor nerve (N III) on the same side as the lesion and spastic hemiplegia on the side opposite the lesion with increased reflexes and loss of superficial reflexes.

    Weill-Marchesani short fingers and toes, compact body, glaucoma, and spherophakia.

    Wilson autosomal recessive deficiency of ceruloplasmin with cirrhosis of the liver, lenticular degeneration, and deposition of copper in the periphery of the Descemet membrane (Kayser-Fleischer ring).

synechiae adhesion between the iris and adjacent structures.

    anterior adhesion between the iris and the cornea.

    peripheral anterior occurs with unrelieved attacks of angle-closure glaucoma; may occur following injury or surgery when the anterior chamber does not form.

posterior adhesion between the iris and the lens as occurs commonly in uveitis.

talbot unit of light equal to one lumen-second.

tangent screen instrument used for the study of the field of vision within 30° of the fixation point; testing is carried out 1 or 2 meters from the eye; called tangent because it would be tangent to the arc of a perimeter.

tapetoretinopathy hereditary degeneration of the retinal pigment epithelium and sensory retina.

tarsorrhaphy operation in which the eyelids are sutured together, as in lagophthalmos.

temporal arteritis giant cell arteritis.

tonography test by means of which the amount of fluid forced from the eye by a constant pressure during a constant period is determined.

tonometer instrument for measuring ocular tension.
 applanation instrument used to measure intraocular pressure that does not indent the globe.
 Schiøtz indentation type of instrument.

torsion rotation of eye about its anteroposterior axis.

trachoma cicatrizing conjunctivitis caused by *Chlamydia trachomatis.*

TRIC agents acronym derived from *tr*achoma and *i*nclusion *c*onjunctivitis, members of the psittacosis–lymphogranuloma venereum–trachoma *(Chlamydia)* group of microorganisms.

trichiasis condition in which there are supernumerary lashes.

tritanopia form of dichromatism in which there are only two cone pigments present and there is a complete insensitivity to blue.

uveitis inflammation of the uveal tract.

vergence binocular disjugate rotations of the eyes as in convergence and divergence.

vernal conjunctivitis inflammation of the conjunctiva presumably caused by allergy and characterized by giant papillary hypertrophy of the conjunctiva.

version binocular conjugate movements of the eyes.

VISC acronym for *v*itreous *i*nfusion *s*uction *c*utter used in vitreous surgery.

vision
 binocular faculty of using both eyes synchronously, with diplopia.
 color ability to distinguish subjectively a large variety of wavelengths of light in the visible spectrum.
 photopic vision in bright illumination.
 scotopic vision in dim illumination or vision following the biochemical or neurologic changes occurring in dark adaptation.

visual angle angle that an object or detail subtends at the point of observation; usually measured in minutes of arc.

visual field locus of objects or points in space that can be perceived when the head and eyes are kept fixed; the field may be monocular or binocular.

visual line that line which connects a point in space with the fovea centralis.

visuscope a modified ophthalmoscope that projects a fixation pattern onto the fundus.

xanthelasma flat, sharply circumscribed deposits of lipid in the eyelids, sometimes associated with hypercholesterolemia.

yellow spot term applied to macula lutea.

BIBLIOGRAPHY

Bergsma, D., editor: The second conference on the clinical delineation of birth defects, Part VIII. Eye, Baltimore, 1971, The Williams & Wilkins Co.

Geeraets, W. J.: Ocular syndromes, ed. 3, Philadelphia, 1976, Lea & Febiger.

Gellis, S. S., and Feingold, M.: Atlas of mental retardation syndromes, Washington, D.C., 1970, U.S. Government Printing Office.

Goodman, R. M., and Gorlin, R. J.: The face in genetic disorders, St. Louis, 1970, The C. V. Mosby Co.

Gorlin, R. J., and Pindborg, J. J.: Syndromes of the head and neck, New York, 1969, McGraw-Hill Book Co.

Jablonski, S.: Illustrated dictionary of eponymic syndromes and diseases and their syonyms, Philadelphia, 1969, W. B. Saunders Co.

Lebensohn, J. E.: An anthology of ophthalmic classics, Baltimore, 1969, The Williams & Wilkins Co.

Nema, H. V.: Ophthalmic syndromes, Scarborough, Ontario, 1973, Butterworth & Co. (Canada) Ltd.

Roy, F. H.: Ocular differential diagnoses, Philadelphia, 1972, Lea & Febiger.

Appendix B

A NOTE ON GENERAL REFERENCES

The normal eye and the abnormal eye are richly described in many monographs, atlases, and systems. The *System of Ophthalmology,* edited by Sir Stewart Duke-Elder, provides a comprehensive review of clinical and basic ophthalmology. The three-volume *Clinical Neuro-ophthalmology* by Frank B. Walsh and William F. Hoyt surveys anatomy, toxicology, and other topics not suggested by the title. The *Handbooks of Sensory Physiology* and Davson's six-volume *Physiology of the Eye* are unusually comprehensive. The Mosby atlases by Donaldson, by Gass, and by Patz and his coworkers provide a wide coverage of anterior segment and fundus disorders. Duane's new loose-leaf *Clinical Ophthalmology* is most helpful.

Reviews are published in the *Survey of Ophthalmology* and in *International Ophthalmology Clinics.* The annual publications of the meetings of the New Orleans Academy of Ophthalmology and the Bascom Palmer Eye Institute provide surveys of general ophthalmology topics and reports of neuro-ophthalmology topics.

Abstracts of ophthalmic reports are available in the *American Journal of Ophthalmology, Excerpta Medica,* and *Ophthalmic Literature.* A 5-year index of the *American Journal of Ophthalmology* including abstracts appeared in May 1978. The *Year Book of Ophthalmology* abstracts recent literature and provides comments. The Medline system, of course, provides an unexcelled key to recent medical publications.

Previous editions of this textbook provide many references to classical studies.

Appendix C

CENTRAL VISUAL ACUITY: DISTANCE, SNELLEN

Feet	Meters	Reduced	Percent loss of central vision
20/16	6/5	1.2	0
20/20	6/6	1.0	0
20/25	6/7.5	0.8	5
20/30	6/9	0.66	9
20/40	6/12	0.5	15
20/50	6/15	0.4	25
20/60	6/18	0.33	35
20/80	6/24	0.25	40
20/100	6/30	0.2	50
20/200	6/60	0.1	80
20/300	6/90	0.066	85
20/400	6/120	0.05	90
20/800	6/240	0.025	95

Appendix D

COMMON ABBREVIATIONS

+	Convex lens
−	Concave lens
Δ	Prism diopters
A	Ocular tension by Goldmann applanation tonometer; initial negative deflection of electroretinogram; accommodation
AC/A	Accommodation convergence/accommodation ratio
Acc	Accommodation
ARC	Abnormal retinal correspondence; anomalous retinal correspondence
Ax	Axis of cylindrical lens
B	Large positive defection of electroretinogram; base of prism
C	Coefficient of outflow in tonography; cylinder
cc	Cum correction (with lenses)
CF	Counting fingers
cyl	Cylindrical lens
D	Diopter; dextro: right
dd	Disk diameters (1.5 mm)
E	Esophoria for distance
E′	Esophoria for near
EOM	Extraocular muscles; extraocular movements
ET	Esotropia for distance
ET′	Esotropia for near
FC	Finger counting

HM	Hand movements
HT	Hypertropia
IOL	Intraocular lens
IOP	Intraocular pressure
J-1	Jaeger test type number 1
K	Refractive power of cornea
KP	Keratic precipitates
LPerc	Light perception
LProj	Light projection
NLP	No light perception
NPA	Near point accommodation
NPC	Near point convergence
OD	Oculus dexter: right eye
OS	Oculus sinister: left eye
OU	Oculi uterque: both eyes
PD	Interpupillary distance; prism diopters
P_o	Intraocular pressure
S	Spherical lens; sinister: left
SC	Sine correction (without lenses)
TT	Tactile tension of eye
VA	Visual acuity (without correction)
VA_{cc}	Visual acuity with correction
VA_{ph}	Visual acuity with pinhole
VA_{sc}	Visual acuity without correction
X	Exophoria distance
X′	Exophoria near
XT	Exotropia distance
XT′	Exotropia near

INDEX